Lens Disorders

Lens Disorders
A Clinical Manual of Cataract Diagnosis

Nicholas Phelps Brown MD FRCS FRCOphth
Director, Clinical Cataract Research Unit, Nuffield Laboratory of Ophthalmology, Oxford University, Oxford, UK

Anthony J. Bron BSc FRCS FRCOphth
Professor of Ophthalmology, Clinical Cataract Research Unit, Nuffield Laboratory of Ophthalmology, Oxford University, Oxford, UK

BUTTERWORTH
HEINEMANN

Butterworth-Heinemann Ltd
Linacre House, Jordan Hill, Oxford OX2 8DP

A member of the Reed Elsevier plc group

OXFORD LONDON BOSTON
MUNICH NEW DELHI SINGAPORE SYDNEY
TOKYO TORONTO WELLINGTON

First published 1996

British Library Cataloguing in Publication Data
Brown, Nicholas Phelps
Lens Disorders: Clinical Manual of Cataract Diagnosis
I. Title II. Bron, Anthony J.
617.7

ISBN 0 7506 1482 X

Library of Congress Cataloguing in Publication Data
Brown, N. A. Phelps (Nicholas Anthony Phelps)
Lens Disorders: a clinical manual of cataract diagnosis / N.A.P. Brown, A. J. Bron.
p. cm.
Includes bibliographical references and index.
ISBN 0 7506 1482 X
1. Cataract—Diagnosis. I. Bron, Anthony J. II. Title.
[DNLM: 1. Cataract—diagnosis. 2. Cataract—physiopathology.
3. Lens, Crystalline—physiology. WW 260 B879L 1995]
RE451.B765 1995 94-32580
617.7'42075—dc20 CIP

Composition by Genesis Typesetting, Rochester, Kent
Printed in Scotland by Cambus Litho Ltd, Glasgow

Contents

Preface

The authors have been passionately devoted to the study of the lens of the eye in a working association beginning 25 years ago and resulting in the establishment of the Clinical Cataract Research Unit at the Department of Ophthalmology and Nuffield Laboratory of Ophthalmology, Oxford. During these years our knowledge and understanding of the lens, including much learned from others, has gradually accumulated. This is a process that can never be complete, but we feel that the time is ripe to share our experience with others.

The book is intended to give a broad introduction to the lens of the eye and to cataract. It is designed to be readable by the novice optometrist, ophthalmologist and researcher, as well as to be of value to the experienced worker.

Before being presented with the features of lens disorders and cataract the reader is led gently through the basic science of the lens: its growth, structure and transparency, and the methods of its examination.

The section on cataract is set out in such a way that it may be used as a clinical reference manual. Particular attention has been given to the description of cataract in a morphological order, which should allow the ready identification of the nature of any particular cataract. To this end the extensive use of illustrations should prove helpful. In a book of this dimension, full coverage cannot be given to every aspect of the lens and it has not been possible to cover the biochemistry of cataract in the same depth as in the recent book, *Cataract: Biochemistry, Epidemiology and Pharmacology*, by our colleague John Harding. We feel that the two books will complement one another.

We are much indebted to the help that we have received from others who have supplied material, and in particular (and in no special order) to Gijs Vrensen and Ben Willekens and also to Gerry Kuszak, who have contributed their wonderful electron micrographs, and in addition have given most helpful advice on the text. Margaret Travers has also presented us with beautiful electron micrographs from her thesis on lens form and accommodation. We are also indebted to Jane Koretz, whom we were privileged to receive in Oxford on her sabbatical year, and with whom we have a long standing co-operation in the field of measurement of the lens of the eye and its accommodation. John Harding has kindly given advice on lens biochemistry. We are indebted to Prof. David Pickwell and his associates at the Department of Optometry, University of Bradford, from whom we have learned much about the nature of vision in cataract and with whom we enjoy a continuing working relationship. We are indebted to all those past and present personnel of the Clinical Cataract Research Unit who have contributed in many areas, and particularly to Adrien Shun-Shin, who supplied several illustrations. Many of the illustrations would not be possible without the engineering skill of Tim Dawson of Marcher Enterprise, who builds our cameras.

There are many others who have given time in discussion or supplied material and whose contributions are acknowledged in the figures or tables which they have generously supplied. We extend fullest thanks to them also. Particular thanks are due to George Duncan, Dr Mary Lyon, Mr David Taylor, Professor Robert Weale and Dr Alfred Wegener.

This book is dedicated to
Antoinette Pirie and Ruth van Heyningen
for their teachings and for their contributions
to the study of the lens.

1

Early studies of the lens

Grom (1975) has summarized the earliest knowledge of the crystalline lens. It is thought that Aristotle (circa 384–322 BC) conceived the lens as a post-mortem artefact due to a pathological accumulation of 'phlegm'. The first scientific description is ascribed to Herophilos (344–280 BC) and this description was preserved by Claudius Galen (AD 129–201) who referred to the lenticular and crystalline tunics of the lens (Polyak 1957).

Aurelius Cornelius Celsus (first century AD) noted that the lens (crystalloid) was situated in front of the hyaloid, and consisted of a drop of liquid (humour) resembling the white of an egg. It was believed to be the site of visual function (Figure 1.1).

For some time this view held sway, and drawings of the eye, such as those by Witelo (*ca.* 1220–1280), Ruff (1541) or Vesalius (1514–1564) located the lens at the centre of the eye (Figure 1.2). Girolamo Fabricius of Aquapendente (1537–1619) was the first to depict the lens in its proper place.

Ibn Rushd (Averroes) (1126–1198) suggested that the retina and not the lens was the site of vision, and the mathematician Francisco Maurolycus of Messina (1494–1575) announced in his book *Photoisme de Lumine et Umbra* (1554) that the role of the lens was to form an image, much as a convex lens converges rays of light to a focus.

Felix Platter (1536–1614) suggested in his book *De Corporis Humani Structura* that the lens was the spectacle of the optic nerve and this was further affirmed by the astronomer, Johannes Kepler (1571–1630), in 1604. Christoper Scheiner (1575–1650), a Jesuit from Bavaria and author of *Oculus* (1619), demonstrated the role of the lens by cutting away the sclera from the posterior pole to observe image formation upon the retina in the animal and human eye. This had earlier been demonstrated by Aranzi (1595) in his book *De Humano Foetu Anatomicarum Observationem Liber*, but it received little attention.

Purkinje (1787–1869) described the catoptric images of the refringement surfaces of the lens,

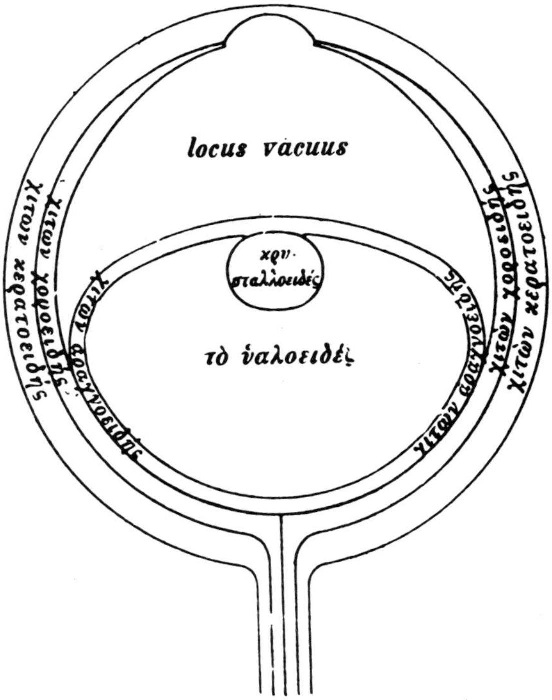

Figure 1.1 The anatomy of the eye after Celsus (reconstructed by Hugo Magnus, *Die Augenheilkunde der Altern*, Breslau, 1901). (From Grom 1975 with permission.)

suggesting their location *in vivo,* and this was further demonstrated by Sanson (1838).

The epithelium of the lens was described by Werneck of Salzburg in the first half of the nineteenth century. The capsule was described by Valentin, and its fibrillar structure was observed by Leeuwenhoek and Hunter, and later by Reil of Halle. The greatest contribution to the study of the anatomy and embryology of the lens was by Rabl of Leipzig, (1898).

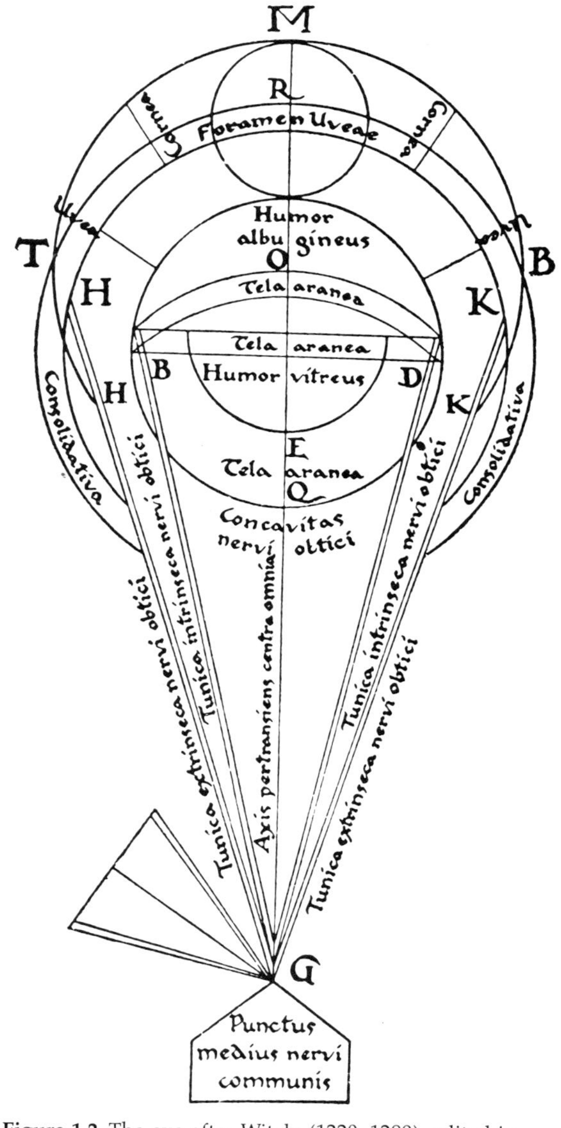

Figure 1.2 The eye after Witelo (1220–1280), edited in 1535. (From Grom 1975 with permission.)

The suspensory ligament of the lens was first described by Antoine Maître-Jan (1707) and later in great detail by Johann Gottfried Zinn (1717–1759) who recognized its relationship to the ciliary body.

Von Jaeger measured the diameter of the lens in 1861 and its weight in 1900. The radii of curvature were measured by von Helmholtz (1856), Tscherning (1898) and Gullstrand. Allvar Gullstrand received the Nobel Prize in 1911 for his studies on the refractive power of the lens. The refractive index was measured by Freytag (1907).

The nature and mechanism of accommodation was an enigma for many years. In 1619 Scheiner demonstrated the existence of accommodation by observing a needle through two holes in a sheet of paper separated by less than one pupil diameter. Albrecht von Haller (1763) considered that the phenomenon of accommodation was explained by the accompanying miosis, and the reduction in confusion circles which it brought about. Other observers considered that altered refraction could be brought about by the effect of extraocular muscle contraction on the length of the globe (e.g. Sturm 1697, Hosack 1794 and Listing 1853).

Thomas Young (1801) excluded a change in globe length as a factor by placing two rings upon his eye to produce phosphenes during the act of accommodation. He also showed that accommodation was not abolished if the eye is immersed in water, thereby excluding a change in corneal shape as its basis.

Kepler (1811), and others later, believed that the lens changed its position to achieve a change in focus. Rene Descartes (1596–1650) suggested that the lens changed shape. This was confirmed by Porterfield in 1759 and John Hunter (1728–1793) and by Langenbeck (1849) who studied changes in images. Hensen and Volckers (1873) showed, with needles inserted into the ciliary body, that the muscle moved forward during accommodation.

Between the period 1853–1856 von Helmholtz evolved the theory that the unaccommodated lens was normally under tension, and that this was relaxed during accommodation by ciliary muscle contraction, so that the lens was restored to a more curved shape by its own elastic recovery. He showed that the curvature of the lens increased during accommodation by observing the reflection of two luminous spheres. Tscherning opposed this view, and proposed that ciliary contraction increased zonular tension and resulted in a flattening of the lens periphery and an increase in central curvature as a result of vitreous pressure. Ultimately von Helmholtz's theory was upheld.

In 1911 Gullstrand ascribed the elastic recovery of the lens during accommodation to the properties of the lens capsule, and Fincham attributed the characteristic shape of the accommodated lens to the moulding effects of the capsule.

Thus we have been brought by a number of steps to our current state of knowledge, and the story is not yet finished.

2

Development of the lens

The following chapter is inspired by Ida Mann's *Development of the Human Eye* (1964) which the reader is encouraged to read in full. Until recently it was believed that the lens was induced by the optic vesicle, on the basis of observations that absence of the optic cup, as in anophthalmia, or separation of the cup from surface ectoderm, was noted to lead to an absent lens (Herbst 1901). It was also shown that, after ablation of the cup, both eye and lens failed to develop (Spemann 1901), while, conversely, transplantation of the optic vesicle beneath an ectopic, non-ectodermal site still induced lens development (Lewis 1904).

The stages of lens development are presented in Table 2.1.

Recent studies suggest that the process is more complicated, and precedes the appearance of the optic vesicle. Four stages may be recognized:

1. In the lower vertebrates (e.g. *Xenopus*) there is a brief period during gastrulation in which head ectodermal cells become *competent* to form the lens. The signal appears to arise from the anterior end of the neural plate, perhaps potentiated by neighbouring mesoderm (Grainger *et al.* 1992). In other species, other tissues may be the source of the signal.
2. For a limited period, a large area of head ectoderm takes on a *lens bias* in response to these inductive signals. That is, it can be stimulated to grow lens cells *in vitro*.
3. By the time of neural tube formation, 'lens specification' has occurred, and lens ectoderm is capable of forming undifferentiated lens tissue *in vitro*, in the absence of other tissue (Slack 1991).
4. The optic vesicle arises from the forebrain at the 2.6 mm stage of the human embryo. Signals arising from the vesicle cause the specified lens tissue to differentiate while other signals, possibly from mesoderm or neural crest, suppress lens formation in adjacent regions of head ectoderm. The lens plate (or placode) is induced in head ectoderm at about the 4 mm stage of development, when the forebrain is a closed tube, and the optic vesicle, which arises from it, is in direct contact with the undifferentiated surface ectoderm (Figures 2.1, 2.2).

The precise details of the signalling from the optic vesicle, and later the retina, to the developing lens are not fully established, but β-FGF (fibroblast growth factor) is thought to be an important stimulus to fibre differentiation throughout the intrauterine period and postnatally (Chamberlain and McAvoy 1987; Rieck *et al.* 1992; Lubsen *et al.* 1992). It is known to be synthesized by the retina, and there are receptors for both FGF and IGF (insulin-like growth factor) on the lens epithelium. IGF 1 is also a growth factor for the lens and it may be surmised that this and other plasma-borne factors would be delivered to the vitreous compartment at this time (Beebe and Hyatt 1992; Beebe *et al.* 1987). IGF 1 is also synthesized by developing lens epithelial cells themselves (De Pablo *et al.* 1992). The lens capsule, like other basal laminae, may function as a reservoir for growth factors, allowing their action to be prolonged in relation to specific target organs.

The cells of the placode proliferate and become columnar and the multiple nuclei give a pseudostratified appearance. With further growth, the plate buckles below its centre to form the lens pit at a time when the optic vesicle is converted into the optic cup (Figures 2.3, 2.4, 2.5). Cytoplasmic processes may be observed between the contiguous surfaces of the plate and the optic vesicle (Figure 2.6).

At the 5 mm stage flattened epitrichial cells, which elsewhere will form the epidermis of the embryo, line the lens pit. Once the lens pit has formed into a lens vesicle, the epitrichial cells within it break down and disappear by the 16 mm stage.

Table 2.1 The stages of lens development

Length of embryo	*Condition of the eye*
2.6 mm	The optic pits are visible as depressions in the floor of the wide open neural plate.
3.2 mm	The optic pits have been converted into optic vesicles by the closure of the anterior end of the neural tube. The optic vesicles are in vesicular contact with the surface ectoderm which is beginning to thicken to form a lens plate.
4.5 mm	The lens plate is more defined and the outer wall of the optic vesicle is thickening. Vascular mesoderm is the first sign of the hyaloid artery, which begins to insinuate between lens plate and optic vesicle.
5.0 mm	The optic vesicle begins to invaginate and form the optic cup, and the inner and outer walls are established. Pigment granules are in the outer wall. The primitive choroid forms. The pit appears in the lens plate.
7.00 mm (end 4th week)	The optic vesicle is fully invaginated. The fetal fissure is recognizable and open throughout its length. The lens vesicle is still in continuity with surface ectoderm. The posterior part of the tunica vasculosa lentis (TVL) begins to form. It is definite by the 9 mm stage.
10.00 mm	Pigment is present in the outer cup. The fetal fissure is still open. The lens vesicle separates from surface ectoderm, retaining epitrichial cells in its cavity. The posterior wall cells are slightly elongated. The lateral part of the TVL is seen and an annular vessel is developing. The optic axes are set at 160°.
12.00 mm	The fetal fissure is closing centrally. The posterior wall of the lens vesicle forms the primary lens fibres – a cavity is still present. The primary vitreous forms. The posterior and lateral elements of the TVL are more advanced.
13.00 mm (6th week)	The fetal fissure is closed, apart from an inferior notch. The lens vesicle is almost filled by primary lens fibres. The lens capsule has appeared.
17.00 mm	The cavity of the lens vesicle is obliterated by primary lens fibres. The anterior part of the TVL forms.
18.00 mm	The anterior chamber (A/C) starts to form.
20.00 mm	The A/C is present as closed space. The anterior part of the TVL is more advanced. The vasa hyaloidea propria are present.
26.00 mm	Secondary fibres begin to form sutures. The TVL and vasa hyaloidea propria are at their peak. The optic axes make an angle of 72°.
70.00 mm (3rd month)	There is forward growth of the margin of the optic cup to form the epithelium of the ciliary body and iris. The vasa hyaloidea propria atrophy. This coincides with the formation of the secondary vitreous. The central retinal artery begins to branch on the disc. The outer layer of choroid appears. The suspensory ligament begins to form.
4th month (110 mm)	The sphincter pupillae begins to differentiate from the margin of the ectodermal iris; it separates the anterior TVL from the lens. The TVL begins to regress especially posterolaterally. The ciliary body forms, and the middle layer of choroid.
5th month	Four sets of superimposed vessels are visible in the mesodermal iris.
6th month	The circular fibres of the ciliary muscle are formed.
7th month	The main trunk of hyaloid artery shrinks considerably, and the pupillary membrane atrophies centrally.
8th month	The macula begins to develop; the retinal layers are fully developed elsewhere.
9th month	The pupillary membrane and the hyaloid artery have practically disappeared.

From Mann 1964 with permission.)

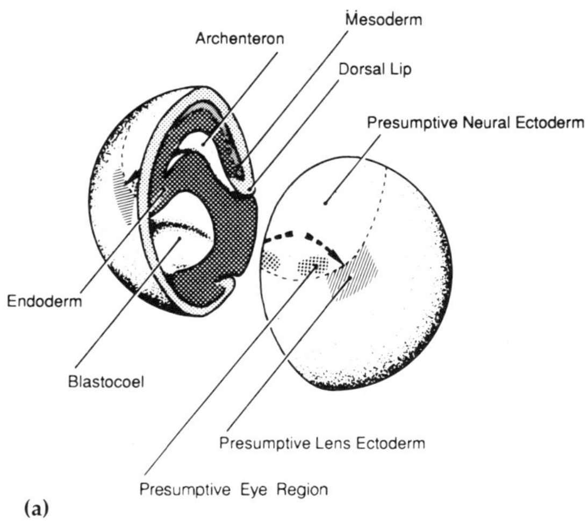

(a)

Figure 2.1(a) Mid to late gastrula stage. Lens induction is presumed to be underway at this stage. At this point the lens-forming competence of ectoderm is still high. During this stage the presumptive lens ectoderm first contacts the tissue which has involuted the farthest during gastrulation, the presumptive foregut endoderm, which may act as an early lens inducer. Experiments with *Xenopus* embryos indicate that an important interaction with the presumptive neural plate and presumptive lens ectoderm occurs at this stage (arrows). The presumptive eye regions are also denoted, and may be the source of this early inductive signal. (From Grainger *et al.* 1992 with permission.)

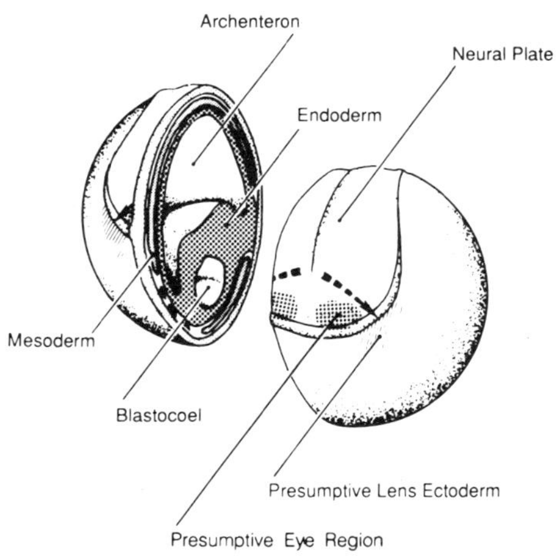

(b)

Figure 2.1(b) Neural plate stage. The boundaries of neural tissue are delineated at this stage by the neural folds, with the presumptive eye regions just inside the folds, and the presumptive lens ectoderm just outside of them. At this stage the presumptive lens ectoderm is underlain by mesoderm which contributes to the lens-forming response in *Xenopus*. The continued inductive influence of the anterior neural plate at this stage is indicated by the arrows. (From Grainger *et al.* 1992 with permission.)

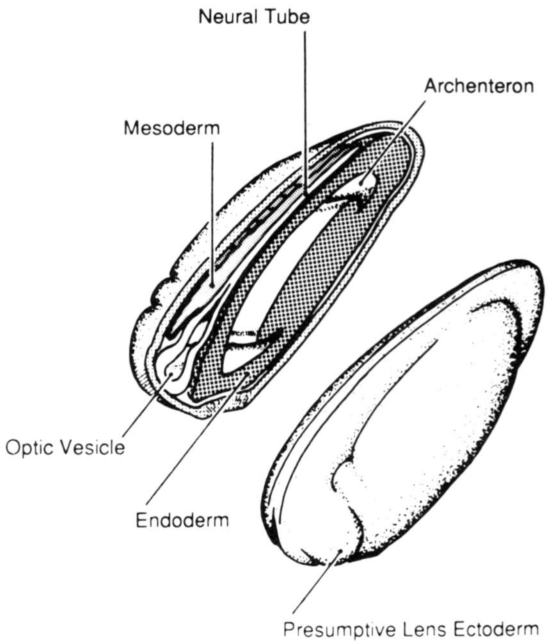

Figure 2.2 Neural tube stage. At this time the presumptive lens ectoderm first comes into contact with the newly formed optic vesicles. Inductive interactions between these tissues result in enhanced differentiation of the lens. Surrounding tissues may at this point inhibit any lens-forming bias in ectoderm adjacent to the lens region. (From Grainger *et al.* 1992 with permission.)

By the 7 mm stage of the embryo, the lens pit has enlarged into a sac-like structure open at the surface by the lens pore. The pore is closed off rapidly by an encircling neckfold, while the stalk of attachment to the surface ectoderm is finally pinched off by the 8 or 9 mm stage. This creates a spherical lens vesicle about 0.2 mm in diameter whose wall is about 40 μm thick. The vesicle is separated from the surface ectoderm, but in protoplasmic continuity with the cells of the optic cup (Figure 2.6).

Formation of the lens vesicle is rapidly followed at the 10 mm stage by a remarkable elongation of the cells of its posterior wall, resulting in the obliteration of the cavity of the vesicle by 18 mm. These cells are destined to be the primary lens fibres. Their nuclei assume an anterior location, either by active migration, or differential growth of

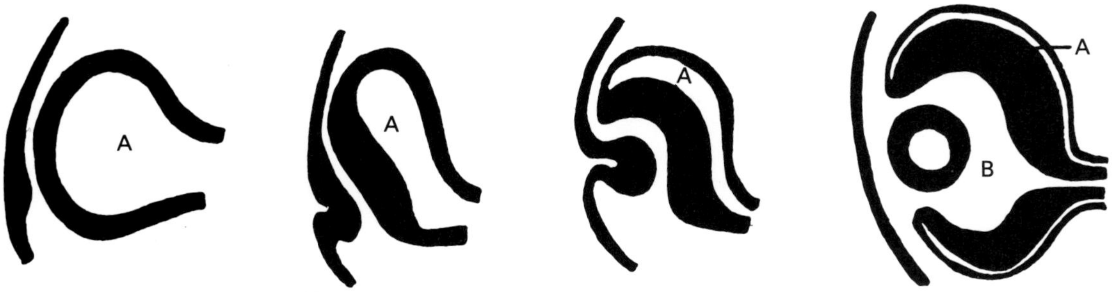

(a)

Figure 2.3(a) Scheme showing the increasing apposition of the superficial and deep walls of the optic vesicle during the process of invagination. The first three diagrams show vertical sections through the invaginated area, the last gives a horizontal section. A, cavity of primary optic vesicle. B, cavity of secondary optic vesicle. (From Mann 1964 with permission.)

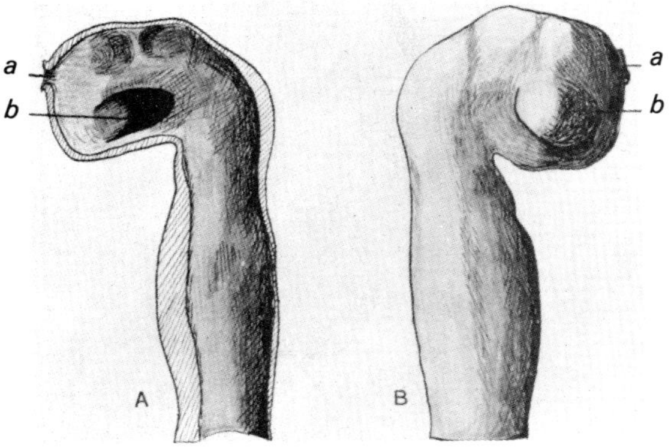

(b)

Figure 2.3(b) Reconstruction of the brain of a 3.2 mm human embryo (after His) shows the exterior of the neural tube. *a*, anterior neuropore: *b*, optic outgrowth. The upper flexed portion is the fore-brain and the optic outgrowth projects from this. The fore-brain is connected by a short curved mid-brain with an elongated hind-brain. (From Mann 1964 with permission.)

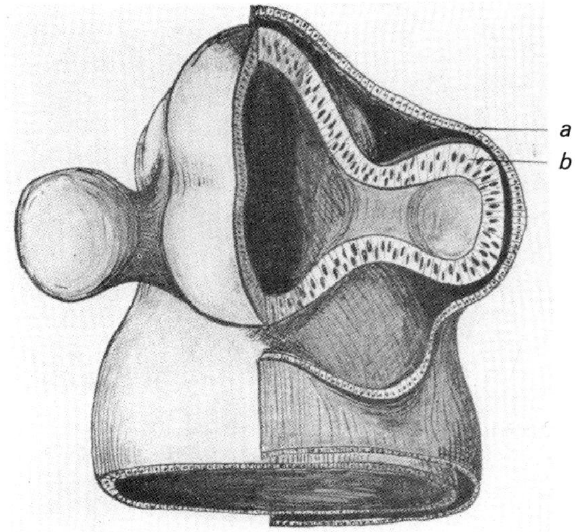

(c)

Figure 2.3(c) Model of fore-brain and optic vesicles of a 4 mm human embryo seen from the front. The optic vesicle on the left of the embryo is represented in section *a*, surface ectoderm; *b*, neural ectoderm.

the cell. The cells of the anterior wall, which are unchanged in appearance, will become the lens epithelium. At the 17 mm stage of the embryo, the lens diameter is about 350 μm in the anteroposterior plane and 300 μm in the equatorial diameter (Table 2.2).

The presumptive primary fibres elongate further, reaching nine times their original height (in the lens pit) in the 25 mm embryo. Formation of the definitive primary fibres is signalled by a progressive nuclear pyknosis, which spreads centrifugally from the centre of the fibre mass. Meanwhile, the anterior sheet of epithelial cells becomes less crowded and cells revert to a cuboidal shape. The sheet is expanded by mitotic activity. With the addition of secondary fibres by division of the equatorial cells of the vesicle the primary fibre mass becomes separated from the epithelial cells anteriorly and the capsule posteriorly. It becomes compressed initially into a tear shape, and later into a spheroid. This occurs in the 26–30 mm embryo. The primary fibre mass comes to occupy the centre of the definitive lens as the embryonic nucleus. In the postnatal lens, this is its most transparent part, when viewed in the fine beam of a slit lamp.

Secretion of the lens capsule begins by the 13 mm stage of the embryo, by cells at the equator as well as those of the posterior wall. The anterior capsule is secreted more slowly, so that the lens is said not to be fully encapsulated until mid-term. However, synthesis of the anterior capsule ultimately overtakes that of the remainder, so that, at 2 years, the ratio of thickness between anterior and posterior poles is 4 to 1. At 35 years, it is reduced to 7 to 2.

The lens capsule has features of particular interest, partly as the basal lamina of the lens, and partly because it must undergo a process of remodelling which is quite different to that required of the lens fibres themselves. It is obliged to remodel throughout the life of the lens because of its continuous increase in volume. As has been noted, the posterior capsule initially grows more

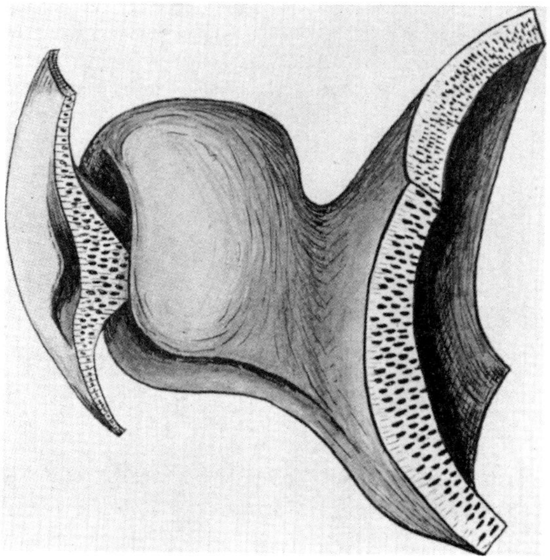

Figure 2.4 Model of optic cup and lens thickening of a 5.5 mm human embryo showing invagination of the optic vesicle to form the optic cup, and the deepening of the lens pit. (From Mann 1964 with permission.)

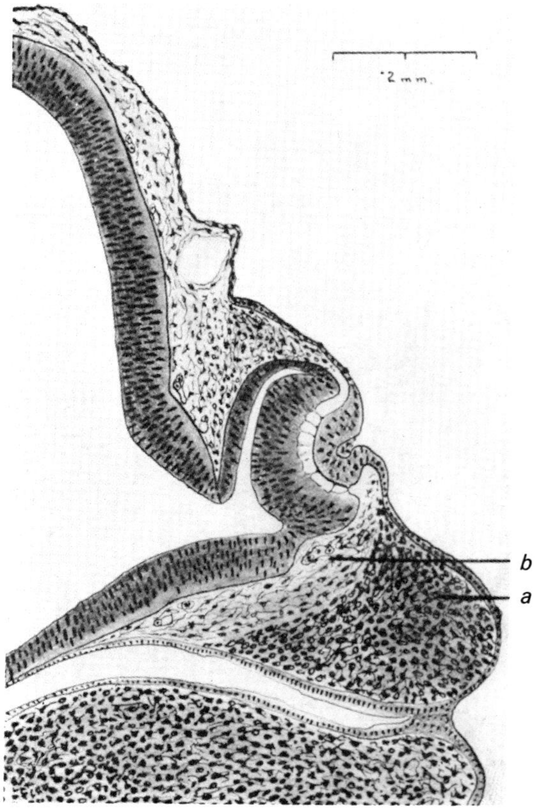

Figure 2.5 Transverse section through the optic vesicle and maxillary process of a 5 mm human embryo. *a*, visceral mesoderm of maxillary process; *b*, paraxial mesoderm.

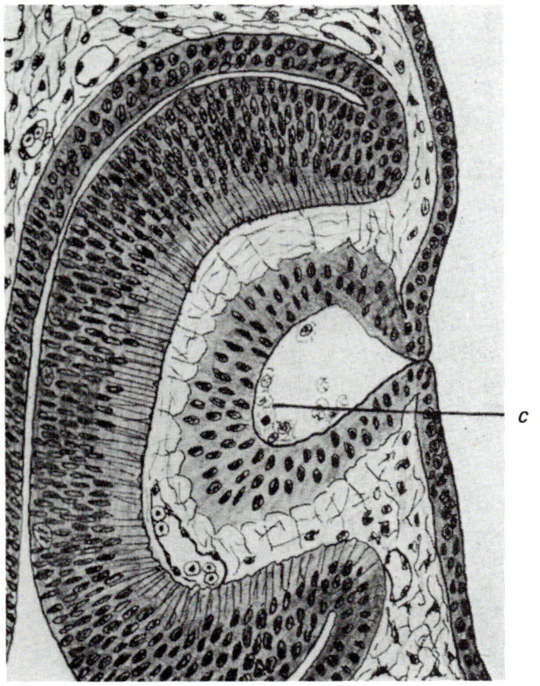

(a)

Figure 2.6(a) Section through the lens vesicle of a human embryo of 7 mm. (After Bach and Seefelder.) *c*, cells in cavity of lens vesicle. (From Mann 1964 with permission.)

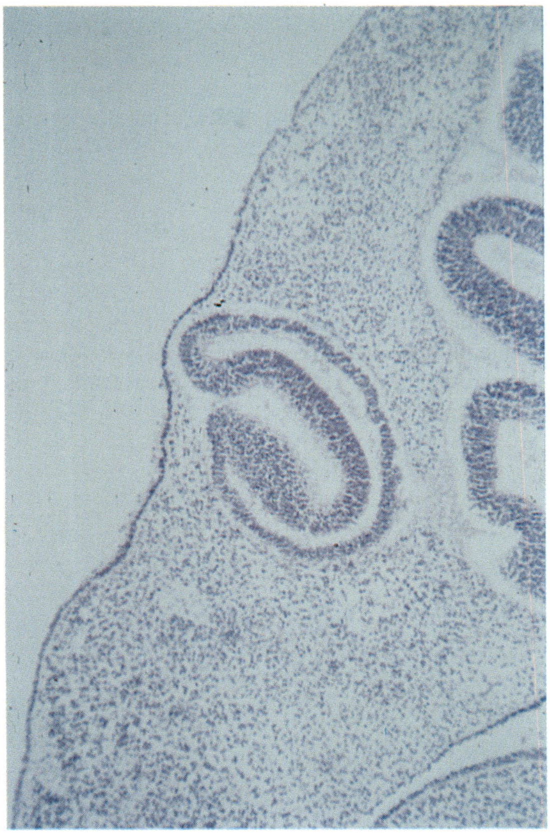

(b)

Figure 2.6(b) Human embryo 7.8 mm (× 100). (Courtesy M. England.)

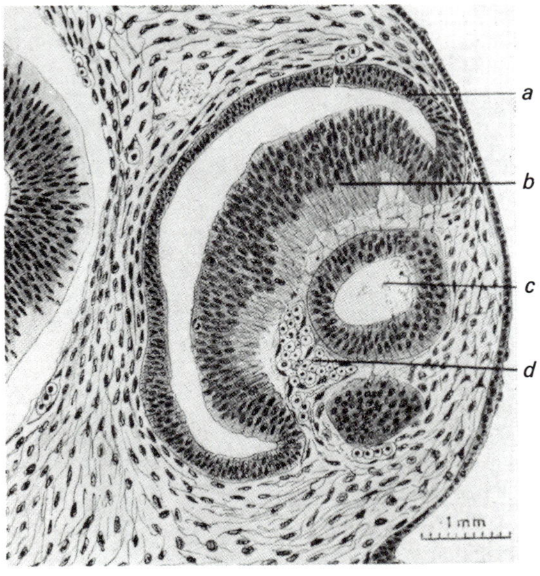

(c)

Figure 2.6(c) Section through the eye of a human embryo of 10 mm. *a*, outer layer of optic cup; *b*, inner layer of optic cup; *c*, lens vesicle; *d*, blood vessel. (From Mann 1964 with permission.)

vigorously than the anterior in fetal life, but postnatally its synthesis by the posterior parts of the lens fibres is negligible, while the lens epithelium anteriorly continues to secrete anterior capsule. This view has arisen from studies in the rat (Young and Ocumpaugh 1966), but there is a strong inference that it applies to the human lens, since there is little evidence for growth in thickness of the posterior capsule postnatally, while the anterior capsule shows a steady increase with age. The interaction between lens fibres and the capsule has been studied in detail in the rat by Parmigiani and McAvoy (1991), who demonstrated that, in early fetal life when the rat capsule contains both laminin and fibronectin, both will act as effective substrates for the growth of differentiating lens fibres. In later life only fibronectin will serve this purpose and, at this stage, laminin is no longer present in the capsule in the rat.

After the 25 mm stage of development new fibres are added to the primary fibre mass which arise from the division of pre-equatorial epithelial cells. These are the secondary lens fibres (Figure 2.7) (Table 2.2). At the 65 mm stage, shortly before the end of the embryonic period, the lens is approximately 1200 μm in the sagittal width, and 1800 μm in equatorial diameter. It can be seen that the embryonic nucleus of the lens contains both primary and secondary lens fibres within it.

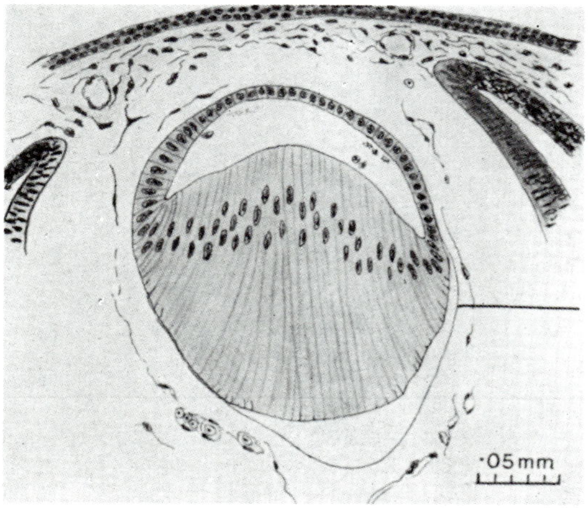

(a)

Figure 2.7(a) The lens of a 13 mm human embryo. Note the appearance of the hyaline capsule *H*. (From Mann 1964 with permission.)

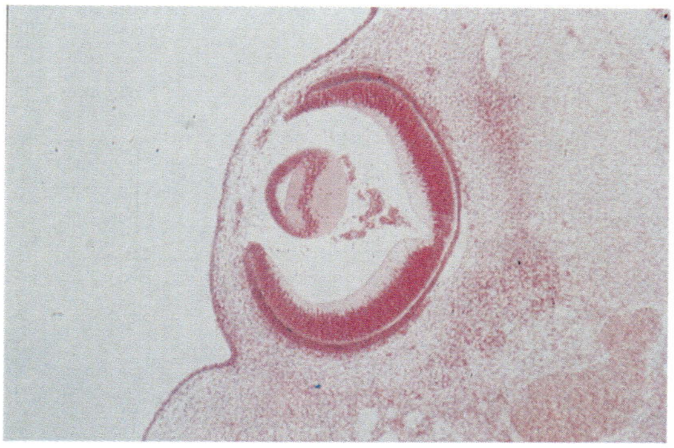

(b)

Figure 2.7(b) Human embryo 12 mm (× 100). (Courtesy of M. England.)

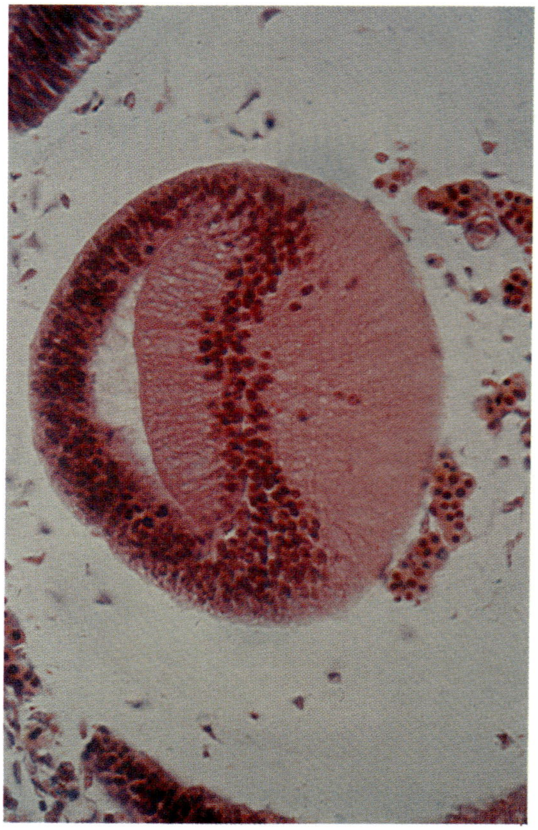

(c)

Figure 2.7(c) Human embryo 12 mm (× 400). (Courtesy of M. England.)

Table 2.2 Growth of the lens in utero

Age at end of period[a]	*Size of embryo at end of period*[a]	*Stage of development*	*Lens measurements*[b]	
			Sagittal width μm	*Equatorial diameter μm*
3–4 weeks	3 mm	Optic pit transforms into optic vesicle		
end of 4th week	7 mm	Optic vesicle invaginates to form optic cup		
6th week	13 mm		200	190
	14 mm	Lens separated from surface; primary fibres form		
	16 mm	Lens vesicle obliterated	350	300
	26 mm	Secondary lens fibres begin to form	420	410
	35 mm		600	700
	48 mm		841	1107
9–10 weeks	60 mm	Secondary vitreous and Cloquet's canal form		
	65 mm		1231	1758
3 months	70 mm	End of embryonic life		
4 months	110 mm	Fetal period		

[a]Approximate
[b]Data from Mann (1964) from fixed material

The taller cells at the periphery of the epithelial sheet exhibit a proliferative capacity in the pre-equatorial region and become the germinative zone of the lens. Mitosis here gives rise to ordered parallel rows, lying in the meridia of the lens which give rise to the secondary lens fibres. In meridional section it can be seen that the cells alter their orientation as they elongate, so that the basal end of the cell (next to the capsule) comes to lie posteriorly to its apical end. This facilitates the insinuation of the anterior tips of the newly forming secondary lens fibres as they elongate forwards between the lens epithelium and, initially, the primary fibre mass. The posterior ends of the new fibres elongate posteriorly between the lens capsule and the primary fibre mass. The process of elongation is accompanied by differentiation into typical secondary lens fibres whose nuclei migrate forwards as each successive generation of lens fibres is laid down. The process of superficial accretion of lens fibres proceeds rapidly in fetal life and then at a decreased rate. New fibres are added throughout life. It has been estimated that the number of fibre generations exceeds 2000 in the adult.

The secondary lens fibres arch over the lens equator to form the anterior and posterior lines of junction termed the lens sutures. Their detailed features are described elsewhere (p. 43). According to Mann (1964), the fibre lengths are sufficient to encompass the lens hemisphere and the sutures comprise a horizontal anterior and a vertical posterior suture. With growth of the lens, fibre elongation no longer accommodates the formation of such line sutures, and a triradiate Y suture is formed at mid-term which is erect anteriorly and inverted posteriorly. Postnatally more complex branching occurs leading to the typical nine-point star of the adult lens (Kuszak and Brown 1991; p. 44).

With the formation of the secondary lens fibres, there is a change in shape of the lens, which is

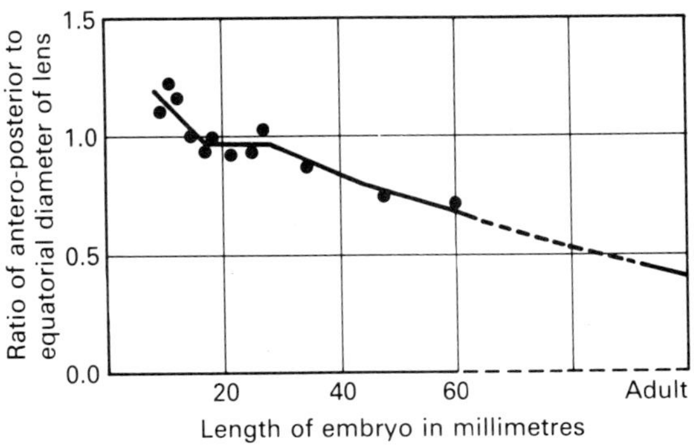

Figure 2.8 Graph showing the effect on shape of the lens of the addition of secondary lens fibres. (From Mann 1964 with permission.)

initially slightly longer in the anterposterior plane and now becomes broader in the equatorial plane (Figure 2.8). This is indicated in Table 2.2.

The suspensory ligament

After the third intrauterine month, and following the formation of the secondary vitreous, the fibres of the suspensory ligament develop as fibrils which pass across from the presumptive ciliary region of the neuroectoderm to the lens equator. They pass through a forward prolongation of the secondary vitreous at the lens margin (the *fasciaeu isthmique*) at a time when the lateral part of the tunica vasculosa lentis has almost disappeared. The zonular fibrils are first recognized extending towards the lens at the 65 mm stage of the embryo and show the adult arrangement by 110 mm (Figure 2.9). The zonular fibrils are composed of fibrillin (Sakai *et al.* 1991).

The tunica vasculosa lentis

At the 4.5 mm stage two vascularized mesenchymal masses are present: a paraxial one around the optic vesicle and a visceral (maxillary) one below this which will supply the maxillary region (Figure 2.10).

From these systems, most developed at the lower part of the optic cup near to the fetal fissure, one vascularized mesenchymal mass passes up on either side to create an annular vessel around the cup margin. The annular vessel is initially incomplete above, and anastomoses with derivatives of the hyaloid vascular system over the cup margin (Figure 2.11).

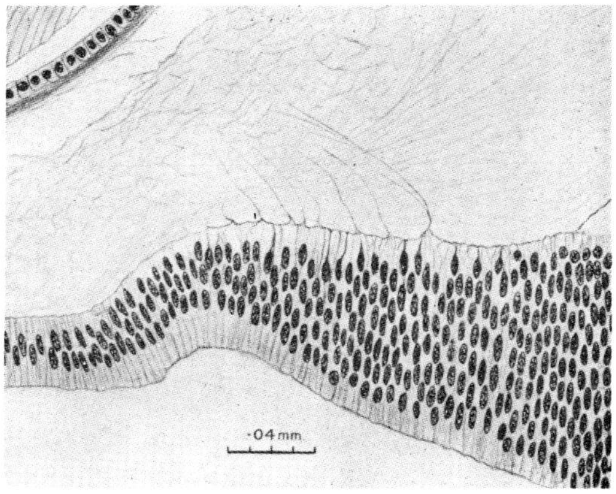

(a)

Figure 2.9(a) Section showing the developing suspensory ligament of the lens in a 65 mm human embryo. Fibrils forming it are seen passing at right angles across the 'faisceau isthmique' towards the lens. This portion of the 'faisceau' will subsequently disappear. (From Mann 1964 with permission.)

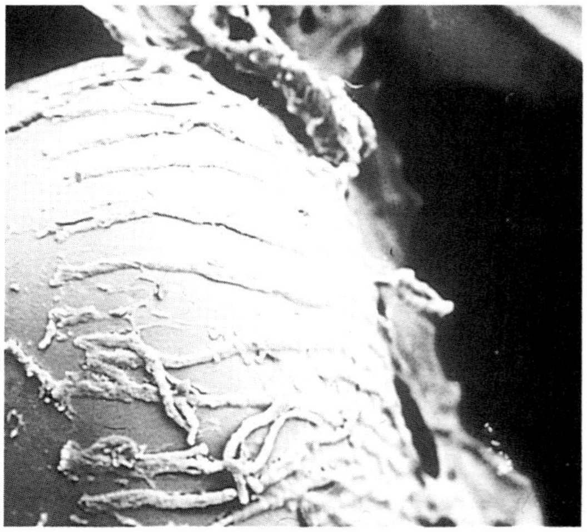

(bi)

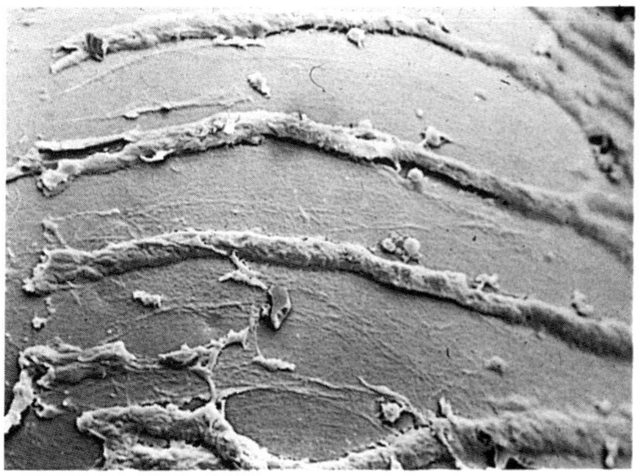

(bii)

Figure 2.9(b) SEM of the human lens equator at the 60 mm stage of fetal life, showing the regular arrangement of the zonular fibres. **(i)** original magnification × 98; **(ii)** original magnification × 263. (Courtesy of M. England.)

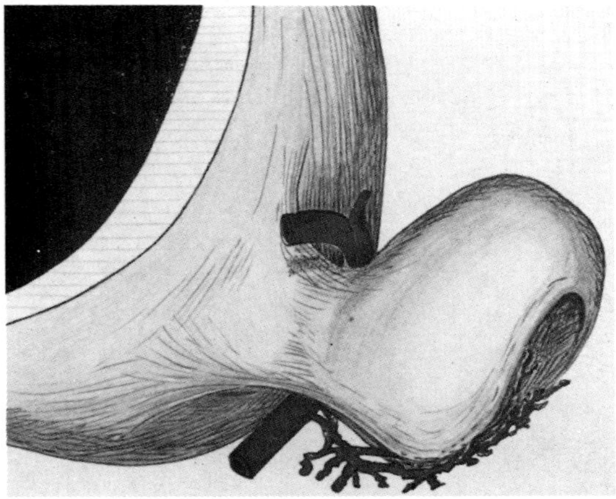

Figure 2.10 Reconstruction of the optic cup of a 5 mm human embryo seen from the front. The large vessel passing up behind the optic stalk and curving forwards above this is the internal carotid. Two main vessels can be seen below the cup: one, the future hyaloid artery, is already penetrating into the interior of the cup, the other is vascularizing its margin. (From Mann 1964 with permission of the BMA.)

The other vessel, the hyaloid artery, at first a continuation of the dorsal ophthalmic artery and later (at 16 mm) becoming a discrete branch in its own right, enters the optic cup from below, through the fetal fissure, and is responsible for the fetal intraocular vascular system. Initially this forms the posterior and lateral elements of the vascular capsule of the lens (the tunica vasculosa lentis (TVL)); later it is supplemented by a branching system within the primary vitreous, the vasa hyaloidea propria (Figures 2.12, 2.13).

Shortly after the 10 mm stage a distinct 'extra-ocular' vascular system arises outside the optic vesicle, supplying the orbit and the choriocapillaris, and the system (hyaloid and TVL) (Figure 2.14).

The choriocapillaris begins to appear at 5–6 mm, at about the time of the appearance of the retinal pigment epithelium. It communicates with the annular vessel, which in turn communicates with the hyaloid artery, enclosed within the optic cup by closure of the fetal fissure.

The hyaloid artery enters the optic cup at the 5 mm stage, along the groove which becomes the

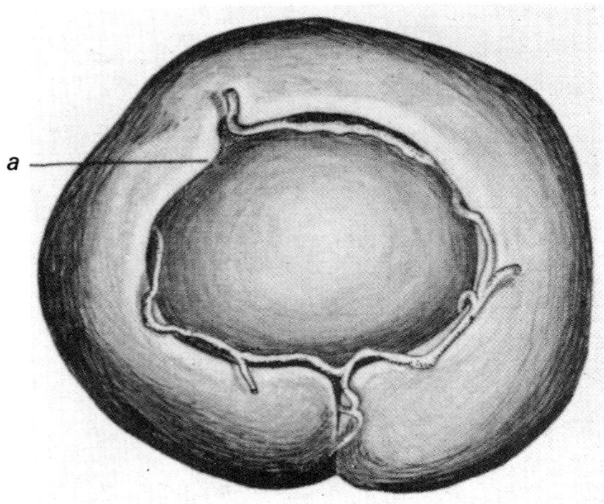

Figure 2.11 Model of the eye of a 10 mm human embryo seen from the front. The annular vessel is seen around the margin of the cup, and vessels are seen passing from this between the margins of the cup and the lens to join the hyaloid artery behind the lens. The fetal fissure is seen below. *a*, gap in annular vessel. (From Mann 1964 with permission.)

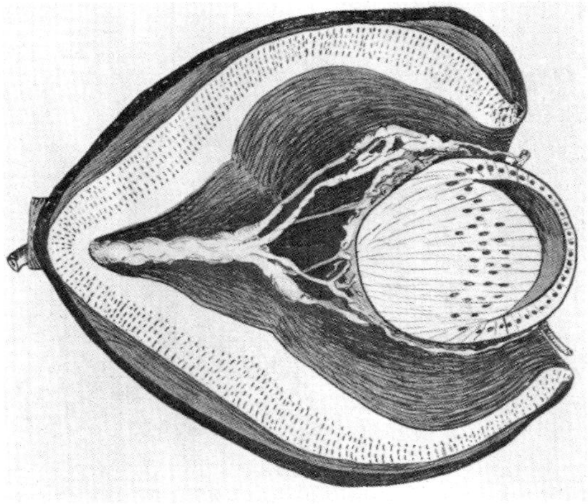

Figure 2.12 Reconstruction of half the optic cup and contents in a 13 mm human embryo. The hyaloid artery is seen breaking up into branches which pass to the back of the lens. Small channels (capsulo-pupillary) unite these with the annular vessel which can be seen cut at the margin of the cup on either side of the lens vesicle. (From Mann 1964 with permission.)

fetal fissure. It retains connections with the choroidal network on the outside of the optic vesicle until the fissure closes, from its proximal to its distal end.

At 6–7 mm, the vascular termination of the hyaloid artery vascularizes the tissue (comprising mesenchyme and ectoderm of the primary vitreous), close behind the lens plate. This becomes the capsula perilenticularis fibrosa when the vesicle separates from surface ectoderm. Within this meshwork the hyaloid artery develops a vascular network over the posterior lens surface at the 8–9 mm stage. This is the posterior part of the TVL, which communicates initially with the choroidal system through the fetal fissure, and later with the developing annular vessel at the margin of the optic cup. At the 10 mm stage, these connections form the lateral part of the TVL, or its capsulo-pupillary portion, made up of a series of parallel vessels. The posterior part is supported by branches of the vasa hyaloidea propria after the 16 mm stage, and these reach a maximum by 40 mm. By 13 mm, the posterior and lateral aspects of the TVL are well developed (Figure 2.15).

At the 17 mm stage the anterior part of the TVL develops, starting as small loops or buds which pass centripetally within a vascular mesoderm

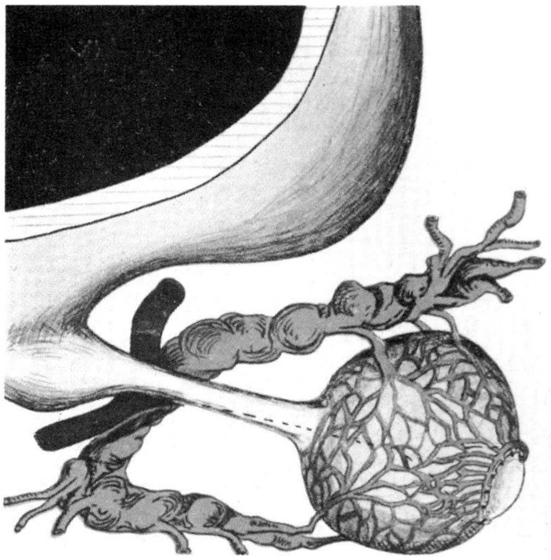

Figure 2.14 Reconstruction of the eye and part of the fore-brain of a 13 mm human embryo, seen from the front. The internal carotid artery is seen passing up behind the optic stalk giving a branch, the hyaloid artery which passes along the under surface to enter the eye. The venous plexuses above and below the eye drain the choroidal net which is connected anteriorly with the annular vessel and so with the terminal branches of the hyaloid artery passing round the margin of the cup. (From Mann 1964 with permission.)

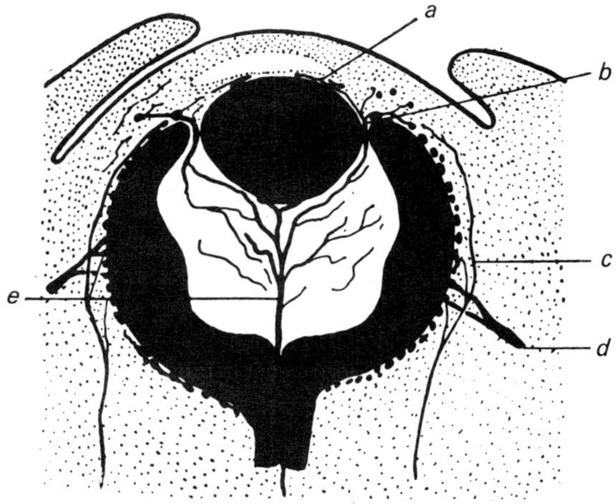

Figure 2.13 Diagrammatic representation of the intra- and extraocular blood systems at 25 mm, stage. *a*, pupillary membrane; *b*, annular vessel; *c*, choroidal vessel; *d*, hyaloid artery; *e*, vortex vein. (From Mann 1964 with permission.)

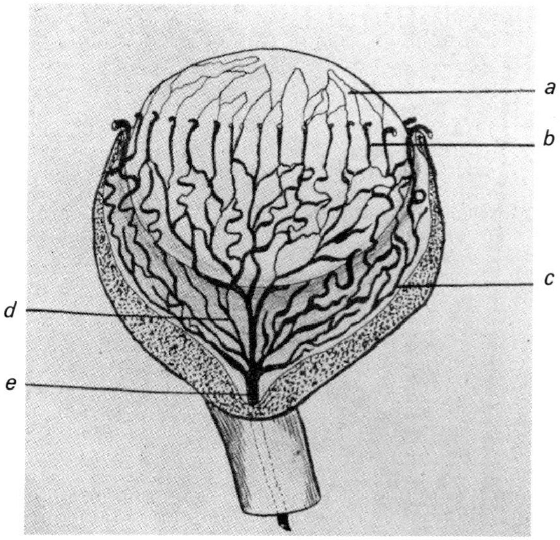

Figure 2.15 Reconstruction of the hyaloid artery and its connections in a 40 mm human embryo (after Versari). *a*, pupillary membrane; *b*, capsulo-pupillary vessels; *c*, outer set of vasa hyaloidea propria; *d*, inner set of vasa hyaloidea propria; *e*, main trunk of hyaloid artery. (From Mann 1964 with permission.)

lying between the lens and the surface ectoderm. They extend across the anterior surface of the lens vesicle and, by the 25 mm stage, they complete the anterior investment of the lens by the TVL. The anterior and posterior systems are in continuity through the annular vessel, into which they drain (Figure 2.16).

At 26 mm, with the formation of the anterior chamber, the anterior vascular loops occupy the presumptive iris mesoderm and stretch across the optic cup; together they compose the pupillary membrane. At first, before the inward extension of the margin of the optic vesicle to form the iris ectoderm, the aperture encompassed by the pupillary membrane is wider than the lens diameter.

As the iris ectoderm grows inwards, the overlying mesoderm thickens and becomes more vascular, and the pupillary membrane becomes separated from the developing lens. Two or more layers of vessels are formed within the mesoderm and although the central part remains thin, it gives rise to multiple vascular arcades.

This process reaches a peak by the fifth month with the formation of three or four tiers of vessel arcades. Sets of deeper vessels appear within the peripheral pupillary membrane derived from the ciliary artery system and give rise to the straight or 'rete' vessels of the iris stroma. The ciliary system supplies the arcades of the pupillary membrane, and the iris stroma and the ciliary region via recurrent vessels. The rete vessels pass in with the ectodermal iris to vascularize the sphincter and sub-sphincteric tissues.

The process is complete at the seventh month, when the vasculature comprises:

1. A superficial supply to the vascular arcades of the central pupillary membrane.
2. A deep supply to the iris stroma.
3. The inter- and sub-sphincteric supply.

Vascular regression

The vessels of the posterior network of the TVL become stretched and elongated as lens growth proceeds. After the 50 mm stage there is a decrease in the number and calibre of the vessels, which is preceded by a regression of the vasa hyaloidea propria which contribute to it. Gradually the calibre of these vessels decreases until, ultimately, their proximal origins close and detach. Their distal ends persist in continuity with the posterior network as corkscrew-like threads suspended in the vitreous. The process starts at the periphery and by

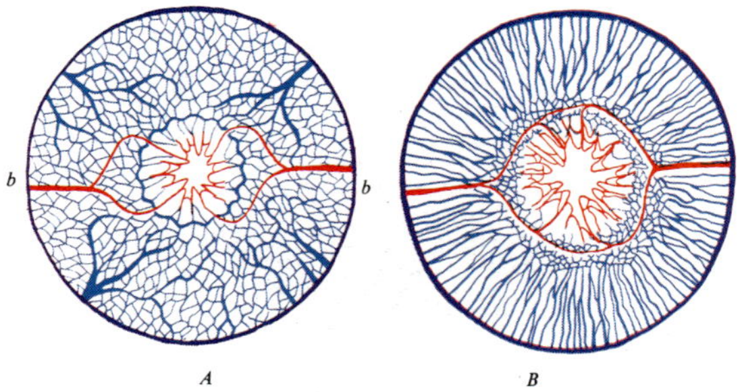

Figure 2.16 *A*, the anterior portion of the choroid and pupillary membrane at 25 mm stage, after the appearance of the long ciliary arteries but before their anastomosis. The annular vessel is seen in blue in the centre and the long ciliary arteries at *b*, *b*. The large radial veins are tributaries of the venae vorticosae. *B*, the same region after formation of the anastomosis between the long ciliary arteries. The annular vessel is no longer distinct. (From Mann 1964 with permission.)

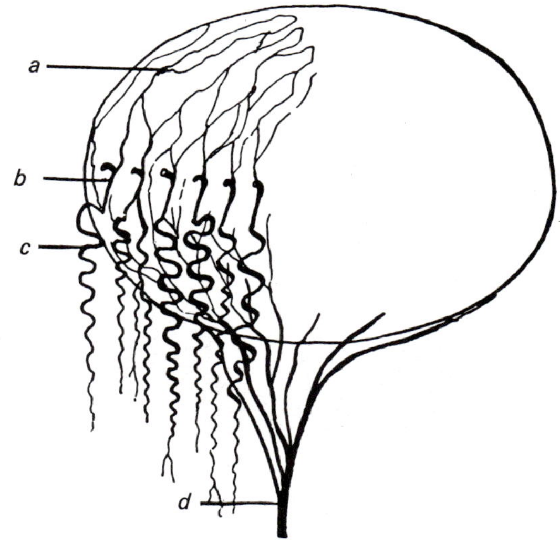

Figure 2.17 The vessels on the lens as the vasa hyaloidea propria starts to atrophy. *a*, anterior vascular capsule (pupillary membrane); *b*, capsulo-pupillary vessels; *c*, remains of vasa hyaloidea propria; *d*, main trunk of hyaloid. (From Mann 1964 with permission.)

160 mm the peripheral branches cannot be identified. Atrophy of the central branches is practically complete by 8.5 months. Occlusion of the main trunk of the hyaloid artery also occurs in the twenty-eighth month, with separation of the artery from its origin proximally, leaving it to float free in Cloquet's canal (Figure 2.17).

The parallel channels of the capsulo-pupillary part of the TVL (lateral) begin to atrophy at about 50 mm, when the margin of the optic cup moves inward over the anterior surface of the lens vesicle, to form the iris ectoderm. This coincides with the regression of the vasa hyaloidea propria, and a reduced need to drain blood from this source via the annular vessel to the choroid. They shrink centrally first, and by the fourth month cease to be visible at the edge of the ectodermal margin (Mann 1964).

Their disappearance coincides with, and may facilitate, the development of structures lying at the lens equator, such as the suspensory ligament and the ciliary processes. During the seventh month (between 28 and 34 weeks) the process of atrophy affects the anterior TVL, or pupillary membrane. This vascular network is supplied ultimately by the long ciliary arteries and the major arterial circle of the iris, which explains its persistence beyond the initial period of regression of the hyaloid system. Only the central region of the pupillary membrane atrophies and this affects the superficial tiers of vascular arcades. The presence of a pupillary membrane in a premature infant may be a guide to its gestational age. Occasionally, a few threads of the pupillary membrane running from the iris collarette to the central lens capsule may persist as a congenital pupillary remnant.

3

Lens growth

The human lens is exceptional in that its growth continues throughout life (Figure 3.1) whereas in other species, such as the rat, rabbit or dog, or in the bovine lens, growth plateaus in the latter part of the life span (van Heyningen 1977).

A description of human lens growth has been complicated by the limited age groups and small sample sizes studied, and because of methodological problems and differences between studies. These problems have been addressed in part by Weale (1963, 1982a) and are summarized as follows:

1. Early work involved excised lenses studied in the fixed or fresh state. When lenses are fixed *in situ* in the globe and then removed, the ciliary

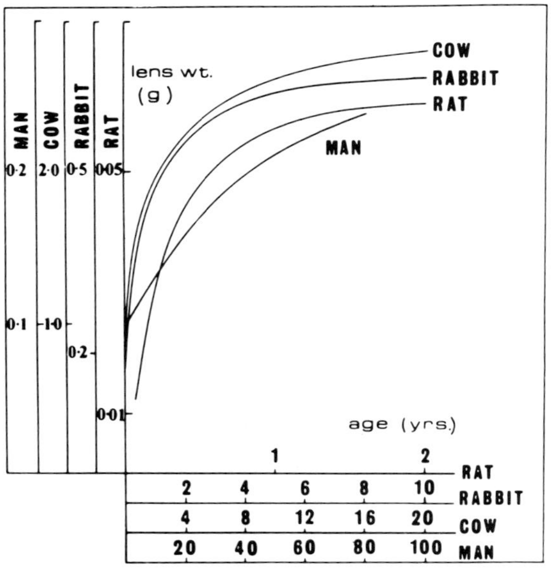

(a)

Figure 3.1(a) Lens weight plotted against age. Life span occupies the same distance along the abscissa and maximum lens weight approximately the same distance along the ordinate, for man and three species of animals.

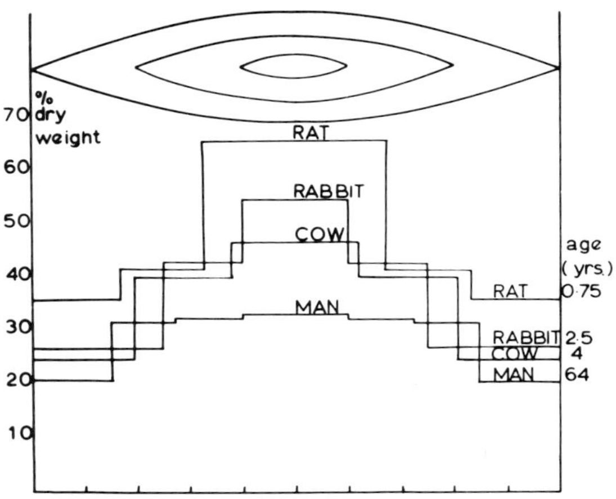

(b)

Figure 3.1(b) Per cent dry weight (largely protein) of the various layers of the lens of man, compared with that of rat, rabbit, and cow. (From van Heyningen 1976 with permission.)

muscle is in the relaxed state, and the lens is consequently unaccommodated, more flattened, and thinner anteroposteriorly. If the lens is removed from the eye before fixation it assumes an accommodated profile and a thicker sagittal section. These events do not affect lenses systematically, since they will be least in the infant lens, which is almost spherical at birth, and in the late adult lens (after the age of 40 years) which is least deformable.

2. Fixation of excised lenses may give rise to swelling (Smith 1883) or shrinkage of the lens, according to the fixative used, while immersion in aqueous solutions such as aqueous humour or Ringer's saline induces swelling, in a time-dependent manner (Pau 1951). Many older studies gave little information about the time elapsed after removal of the lens, thus raising the possibility of drying and shrinkage. In other studies lenses were immersed in water for the purpose of optical measurements (Smith 1883).
3. Measurements of the sagittal and equatorial dimensions of the freshly excised lens resting on a surface is likely to underestimate the true value, owing to the flattening of the lens under its own weight (Smith 1883, Weale 1982a). This would have the greatest effect on the softer young lens, and least on the older stiffer lens (Pau 1990). Weale (1963) suggested that this problem might be resolved by flotation of the lens, but noted that other problems might be introduced.
4. Optical and photographic methods which have been used to measure the sagittal width of the lens, are influenced by the angle of observation, and the constants used to calculate magnification factors. It has been customary to measure sagittal width with the eye in cycloplegia, and the lens therefore in the unaccommodated state. Such values will therefore be lower in the lower age groups.
5. Similar considerations influence the calculation of lens thickness using ultrasound, which relate to the values adopted for the velocity of ultrasound passing through the ocular media, and in particular through the lens itself. Such measurements are usually made without cycloplegia, so that the degree of accommodation, and hence the effect of accommodation on thickness, may vary.

Despite the potential variables in measurement listed above, a coherent account of lens growth can be given which indicates that growth is not linear over time, as was once thought, but goes through distinct phases. The prenatal period has the most rapid growth. The lens at birth is almost spheroid, with a slightly shorter sagittal than equatorial axis. After birth the growth rate slows down. In the first two decades there is an important shape change in which most of the growth is equatorial while sagittal growth is relatively static. The final phase of growth is concentrated in the sagittal axis, while equatorial growth is limited. This latter restriction leads to an increased curvature of the anterior, and to a lesser extent the posterior curvature of the lens.

Lens growth may now be considered in terms of mass and volume, and sagittal and equatorial dimensions.

Growth in lens mass and volume

A few authors have weighed lenses harvested at various stages of intrauterine life, and several have reported the weight of the lens at birth (Table 3.1). If this value is taken to be about 65 mg (Scammon and Hesdorfer 1937) and the lens placode assumed to appear at about 6 weeks of intrauterine life, then an average growth rate can be calculated to be roughly 181 mg/year. After birth the rate of increase in mass of the lens is much slower, and has been estimated to be 1.32 mg/year by Spencer (1976) using data from several sources. Other figures are given in Table 3.2. The compilation of data from the literature presented by Weale (1982) suggests a flattening of the growth curve in the prepubertal period.

Table 3.1 Weight of the newborn lens

		Weight mg
W Collins	1894	120
Heine	1898	78.5
Imachi Tadahiko	1934	65.6
Scammon, Hesdorfer	1937*	65 ± 1.9

*Calculated values
From Spencer 1976 from several authors

Table 3.2 Rates of increase of lens weight from fetal to adult life

State	*Period*	*Rate of growth*
fetal	119–242 days	181 mg/year[1]
fetal	13–39 weeks	181 mg/year[2]
newborn	7–150 days	63 mg/year[2]
newborn	0–11 months	24 mg/year[2]
newborn–juvenile	0.01–10 years	2.8 mg/year[2]
juvenile–adult	10–90 years	1.43 mg/year[2]

From regression equations presented by Bours and Fodisch, 1987: 1. Their own study, 2. Data from the literature. See Bours and Fodisch for references.

Measurements of lens volume are presented in Table 3.3. Priestly Smith (1883) devised a precise instrument to measure lens volume, and showed a steady increase across most decades, while specific gravity remained fairly constant (Table 3.3). Other workers have demonstrated that protein represents a relatively fixed fraction of the wet weight of the lens over a wide age span, with the dry weight of the lens being about 33–34% of the wet weight. As is noted elsewhere, protein is not distributed homogeneously across the thickness of the lens. The concentration is lowest in the first 50–200 μm of the superficial cortex, and then rises steeply to a

Table 3.3 The weight and volume of the human lens in postnatal life

Age range	*No. of lenses*	*Mean weight Mg ±*	*No. of lenses*	*Mean volume mm³ ±*
Birth	10	65.6 ± 1.9	–	72
1 to 3 months	24	92.9 ± 1.2	–	–
4 to 5 months	4	109.0 ± 6.1	–	–
10 to 11 months	2	124.5	–	–
1 to 10 years	1	146.8	–	–
10 to 20 years	6	152.8 ± 2.1	–	–
20 to 30 years	24	172.0 ± 2.0	21	162.9 ± 1.8
30 to 40 years	31	190.3 ± 1.5	22	177.3 ± 1.7
40 to 50 years	34	202.4 ± 1.9	23	188.1 ± 2.1
50 to 60 years	25	223.3 ± 2.5	22	205.4 ± 2.7
60 to 70 years	41	230.1 ± 3.1	32	213.0 ± 3.0
70 to 80 years	22	237.1 ± 3.4	21	218.3 ± 2.9
80 to 90 years	15	258.2 ± 2.8	15	238.7 ± 3.0

From Scammon and Hesdorfer 1937; collated from: Becker 1883; Clapp 1913; Collins W.J. 1984; Engel 1850; Heine 1898; v. Jaeger 1861; P. Smith 1883a,b.

Table 3.4 The newborn lens

Author		*Sagittal width mm*	*Equatorial diameter mm*	*n*
von Jaeger	1861	4.5	6.35	70
Merkel and Orr	1892	5.0	6.0	–
W. Collins	1891	4.3	–	3
E. T. Collins	1894	–	4.3	3
Diekmann	1896	–	6.29	–
von Hippel	1898	6–6.5	–	–
Heine	1898	3.5	6.25	–
Stadfelt	1898	3.93	–	11
Seefelder	1908	–	6.4	7
Hess	1910	–	7.2	–
von Pflugk	1911	3.76	7.4	7
Larsen	1971	3.95	–	86

Radii of curvature: anterior 5mm; posterior 4mm; (von Pflugk 1909)
From Spencer 1976 and Larsen 1971.

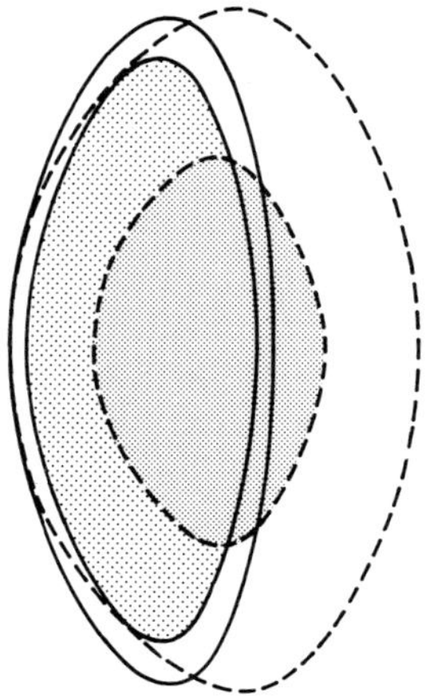

Figure 3.2 The superimposed outlines of nucleus and cortex of lenses aged 8 and 80 years (80-year-old lens shown with interrupted lines; 8-year-old nucleus cross-hatched; 80-year-old nucleus, single hatch).

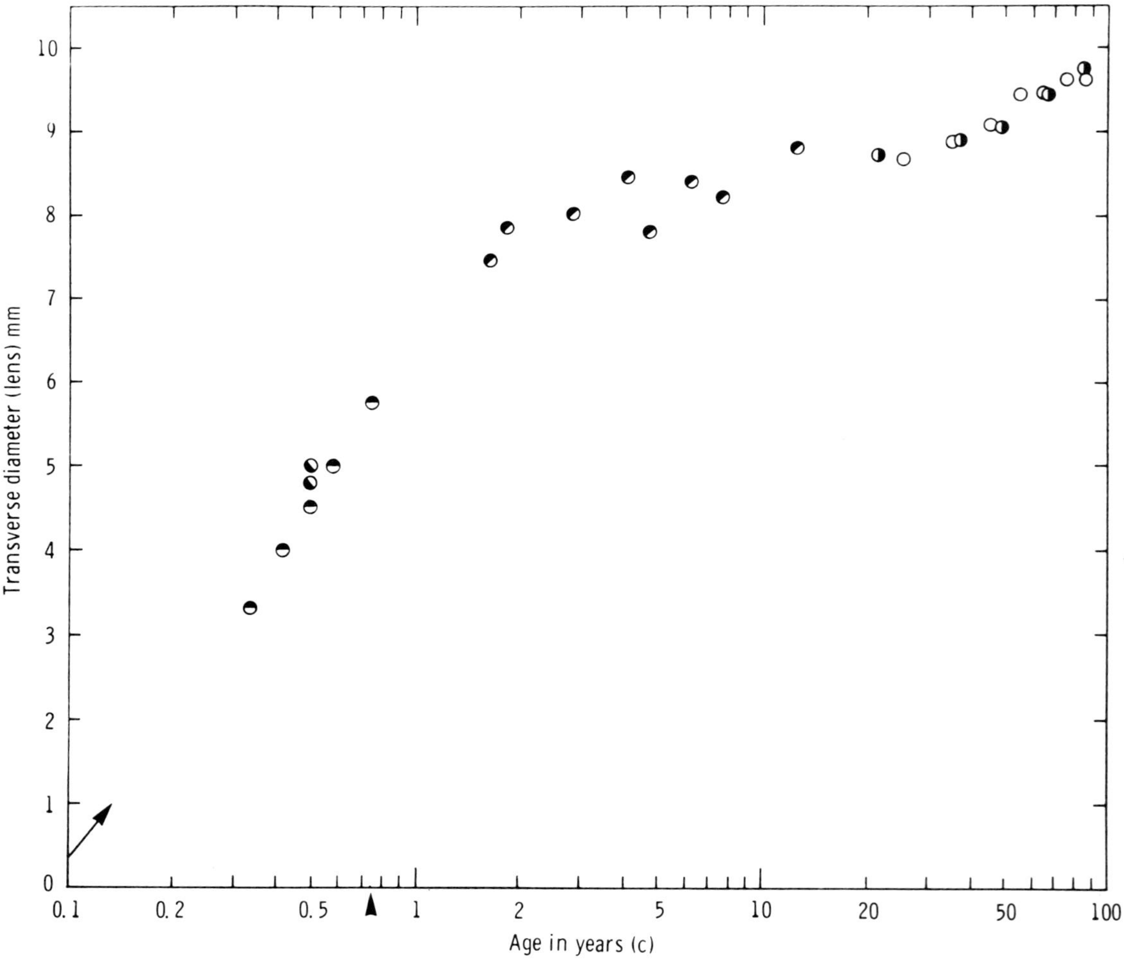

Figure 3.3 The transverse diameter of the lens as a function of age. Collins (1894): ◓; Dub (1891): ◐; Johansen (1947): ◑; Smith (1883): ○; Weale (1982): ◒.

level which is maintained in the deeper cortex and nucleus (p. 27; Siebinga *et al.* 1990). Nordmann's data suggests that the growth rate of the lens decreases in the older age groups (Nordmann *et al.* 1974) and Kuwabara (1975) has reported that epithelial mitotic rate falls in late age.

Growth in equatorial thickness

There is little information about equatorial diameter of the lens during prenatal life. Initially equatorial growth keeps pace with sagittal growth, so that the lens is perfectly spherical in early fetal life. Towards the end of fetal life, equatorial growth outstrips the sagittal so that the lens begins to take on an ellipsoidal shape (p. 11; Figure 2.8; Mann 1964). The diameter of the lens is about 6.5 mm at birth (Table 3.4). Equatorial growth continues postnatally, so that in the first one or two decades, while net sagittal growth is minimal, the characteristic shape of the mature lens becomes established. There is some disagreement about whether the equatorial diameter continues to increase after the third decade, as suggested by Smith (1883) and Johansen (1947) or remains relatively static. Willekens *et al.* (1987) found the diameter to be unchanged after the age of 30 years (Figure 3.2). Fisher (1969a) found most values to lie between 8.8 and 9.2 mm between the ages of 30–60 years. Scammon and Wilmer (1950) reported a value of 9.0 mm in subjects aged 20–40 years, and Pierscionek (1990) found the same figure over the age span 16–84 years (Figure 3.2).

Growth in sagittal thickness

A few authors have measured the prenatal sagittal growth of the lens and their findings are plotted in Figure 3.3a (Dub 1891; Collins 1894). If the sagittal width of the lens at birth is taken to be about 4.0 mm, then an average rate of sagittal growth *in utero* can be estimated to be 5.78 mm / year, which is

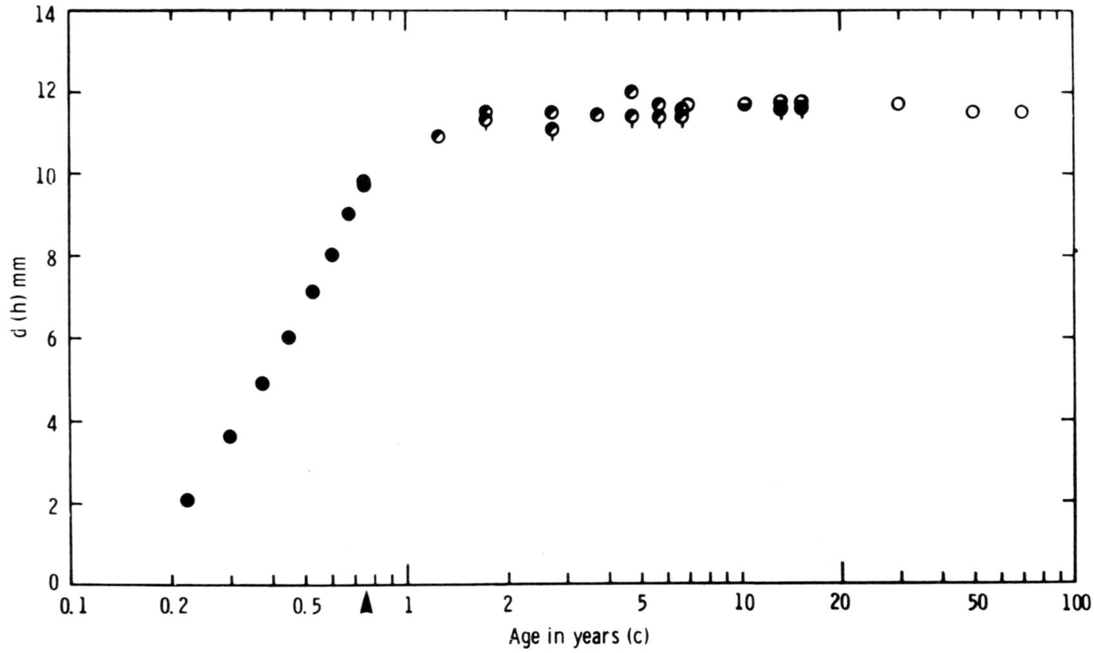

Figure 3.4 The horizontal corneal diameter as a function of age Kaiser (1925): ◐; Peters (1924): ◒; Scammon and Armstrong (1925) ●; Smith (1883) ○; sample data from women are marked with a tail. (From Weale 1982, with permission.)

about 200 times the sagittal growth rate in the adult. The picture becomes even more remarkable in early life (e.g. the first two decades after birth), where it has been demonstrated by ultrasound (Luyckx 1966; Manzitti *et al.* 1994), and by slit-image assessment (Forbes *et al.* 1992), that sagittal width does not increase over this period and may even decrease. Figure 3.5 shows the sagittal lens growth in a group of children and young adults aged 3–20 years. This surprising finding is explicable partly as an effect of zonular tension on lens growth, and partly on the basis of central compaction, a process in which the volume of the central parts of the lens diminish with time (see below). Weale (1982) suggested that, with the continued (saggital) growth of the eye postnatally, chiefly over the first 3–5 years of life, zonular tension acting in the equatorial plane might encourage a redistribution of volume towards the equator, while constraining sagittal growth. However, there is little significant coronal growth of the anterior segment after the age of 2 years (Figure 3.4). Slit-image photography demonstrates that, although the sagittal width of the lens is relatively stationary over this period, there is vigorous cortical growth, and this is accommodated by a progressive reduction in nuclear width (i.e. by nuclear compaction) at a rate of about 46 μm/year. Reduction in nuclear width has been noted in earlier studies by Brown (1976).

The sagittal growth of the adult lens has been measured by several techniques, including ultrasound, slit-image photography and direct measurement in the excised lens. From the ages of 20–80 years, the axial width of the lens increases at a steady rate of approximately 25 μm/year (Brown 1976; Figures 3.6, 3.7). This figure varies considerably from author to author (Figure 3.8; Table 3.5). This growth is cortical, with no increase in nuclear width (Figure 3.2). The disproportionate sagittal versus equatorial growth of the lens results in an increase in curvature of the lens surfaces (Figure 3.9; Brown 1974). This would be expected to

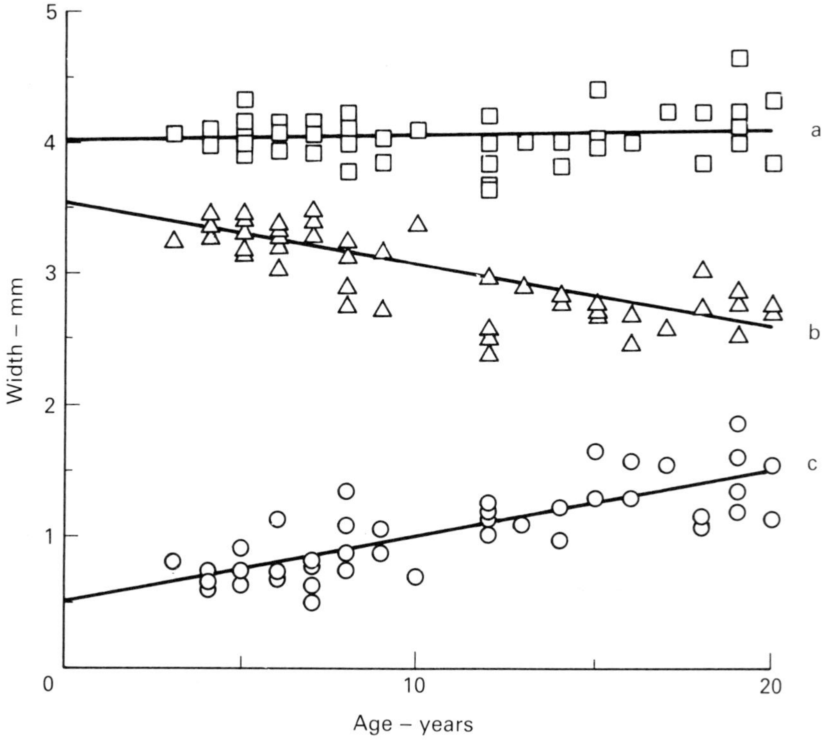

Figure 3.5 Linear regression curves of (a) total axial lens width, (b) nuclear width and (c) combined cortical width, against age. (From Forbes *et al.* 1992 with permission.)

produce an increase in the effective lens strength and thus a shift in vision towards myopia. In fact the opposite occurs, and the healthy ageing lens progresses in the direction of hypermetropia (Brown and Hill 1987).

Lens size is increased in diabetes (Huggert 1953) and there is also widening of the zones of discontinuity, i.e. the scattering zones which interface between the clear zones (Figure 3.10) (Huggert 1946a, b; Brown and Hungerford 1982). It is not yet known to what extent increased lens size reflects accelerated growth, and to what extent it is due to increased hydration or cell hypertrophy.

Lens growth in the adult is associated with a steady rate of shallowing of the anterior chamber (Figure 3.11) but not with a reduction in the length of the posterior segment, since there is little movement of the posterior pole of the lens (Figures 3.2 and 3.12) (Koretz *et al.* 1989). This is reflected by the redistribution of the zonular insertion into the lens capsule which occurs with age.

The zones of discontinuity

The zones of optical discontinuity of the lens develop from childhood to reach the fully developed pattern in middle age (Figure 3.13) (Niesel 1982). Various classifications of the lens zones have been presented in the past, which include the presumption that various regions can be labelled with their time of occurrence, using such terms as 'juvenile and adult' nucleus. Such a nomenclature is confusing since the same sets of lens fibres would be regarded as 'cortex' at one period, and 'nucleus' at a later date when they occupied a deeper position in the lens. We prefer a simplified classification which is as follows (Figure 3.14):

The term *nucleus* is used here to describe that part of the lens which is present at birth. Thus, at birth, only nucleus is present. The nucleus is

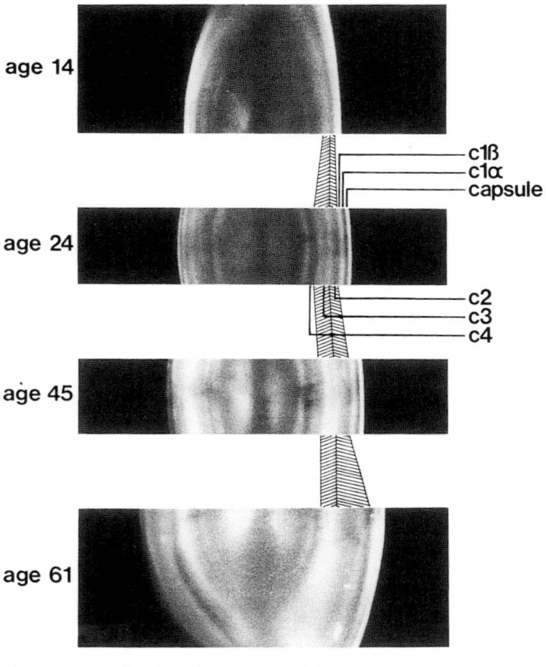

Figure 3.6 The development of the zones of discontinuity with age. The anterior cortical zone C2 is not present at birth and is identified by the age of 7 years. It is this zone that then undergoes the largest expansion with age.

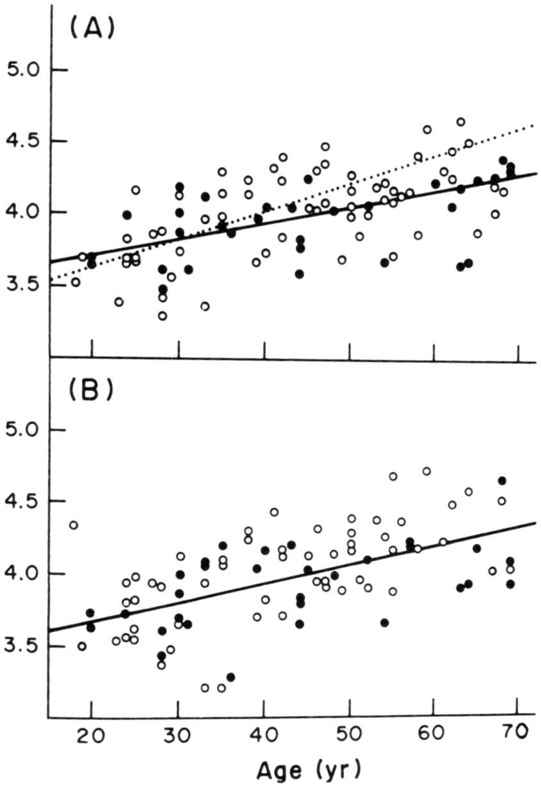

Figure 3.7 Increase in lens width with age comparing (A) ultrasound and (B) slit-image photography (Courtesy of J.F. Koretz).

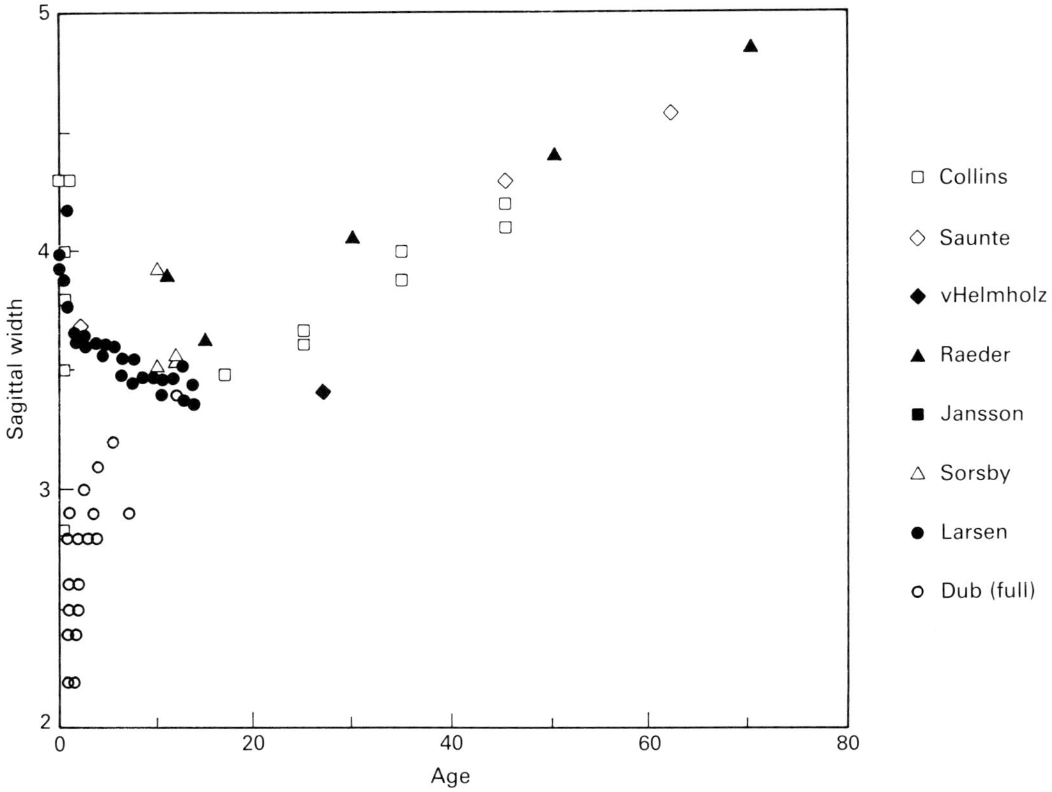

Figure 3.8 Combined data from the literature – sagittal width : age. (From Forbes *et al.* 1992 with permission.)

Table 3.5 The rate of sagittal growth of the lens

Rate microns/year	*Author*	*Year*
13.0	Koretz *et al.*	1992 (corrected*)
14.0	Huggert *et al.*	1945
20.5	P. Smith	1883
21.0	Koretz *et al.*	1992 (uncorrected*)
21.0 F	Alsbirk	1977
23.4	Alsbirk	1977
23.5	Weekers *et al.*	1974
24.0	Goldmann, Niesel	1964
29.0	Brown	1976
30.0 F	Jansson	1963
35.0 M	Jansson	1963

*for magnification; F = female; M = male

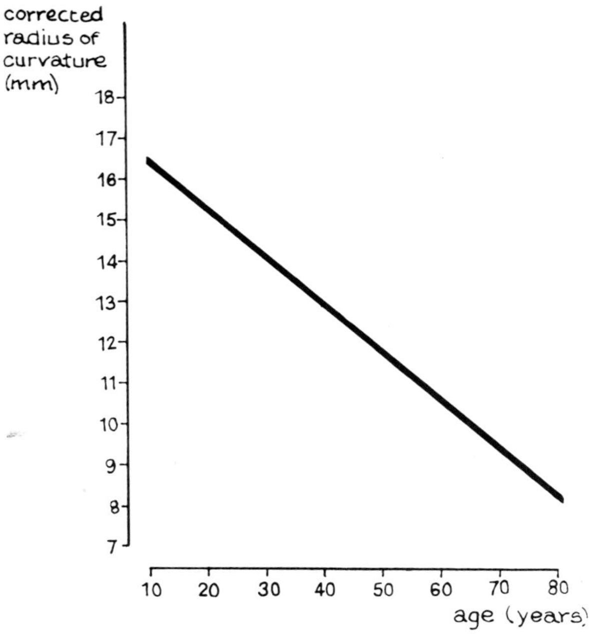

Figure 3.9 The reduction in radius of curvature of the anterior lens surface with age.

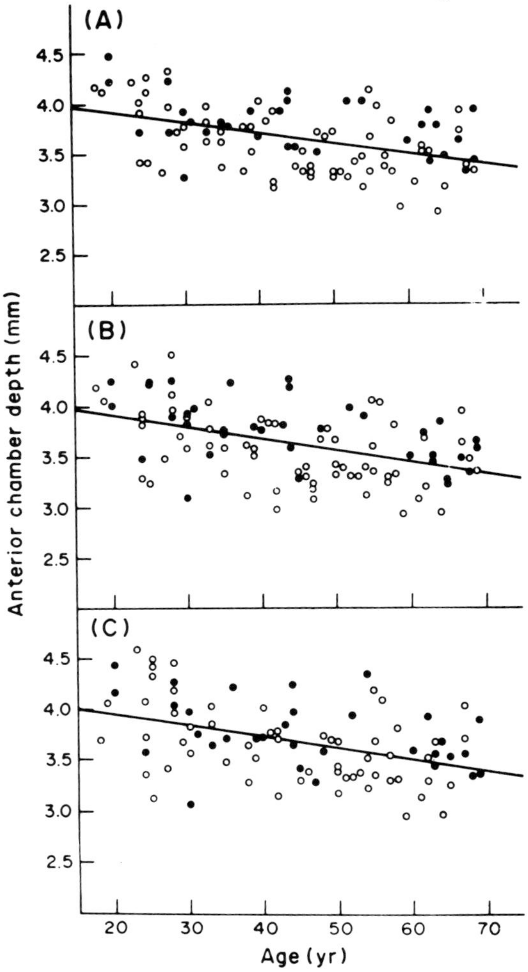

Figure 3.11 Anterior chamber depth shallowing with age. (A) pachymetry, (B) ultrasound and (C) slit-image photography. (Courtesy of J.F. Koretz.)

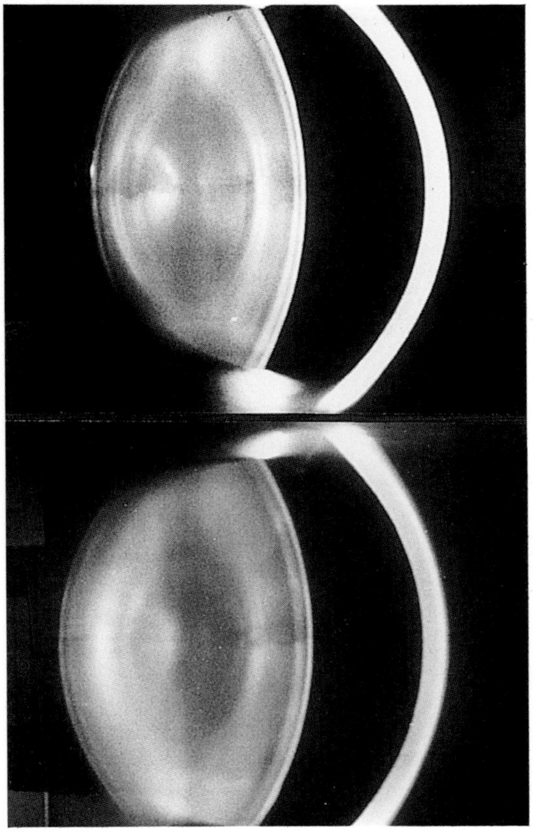

Figure 3.10 The difference in size between a normal lens (above) and a diabetic lens (below) each from a subject aged 48 years. (From Brown and Hungerford 1982 with permission.)

approximately 6–8 mm in equatorial diameter and about 4.00 mm in sagittal width and contains the embryonic nucleus (about 0.3 mm in diameter), surrounded by the fetal nucleus.

Postnatally the cortical layers are added and an anterior clear zone (cortical zone 1α or C1α) is defined. A narrow light-scattering zone of discontinuity separates C1α from the deeper cortex as fibres are added to the lens (C1β). With the appearance of a new scattering zone of discontinuity (C3) within the cortex in childhood, deep to C1, the mature zone system of the lens can be said to be established, with C2 superficial and C4 deep to C3. (For convenience C1 and C2 are then described as the *superficial cortex*, and C3 and C4 the *deep cortex*) (Figure 3.14).

The scattering properties of the brighter zones of discontinuity increase with age, particularly C3, which is absent at birth and during early childhood, and which becomes conspicuous, increasing in width and scattering properties (Smith *et al.* 1990b; Eckerskorn *et al.* 1989a). The growth in width of the cortex with age is accomplished by the expansion of C2. It is considered that the degree of scatter is related to the refractive index (Huggert 1946a) which in turn is related to protein concentration (Pierscionek and Augusteyn 1991). Most of the

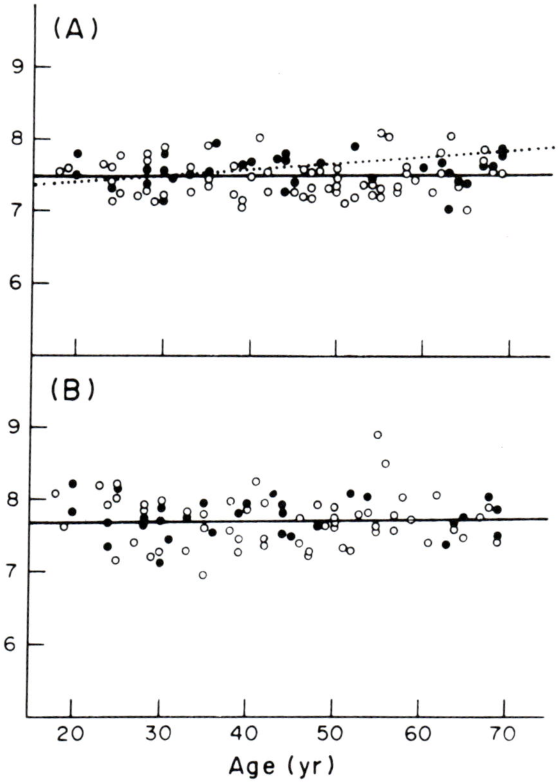

Figure 3.12 The posterior pole position with age. (A) ultrasound. (B) slit-image photography. (Courtesy of J.F. Koretz.)

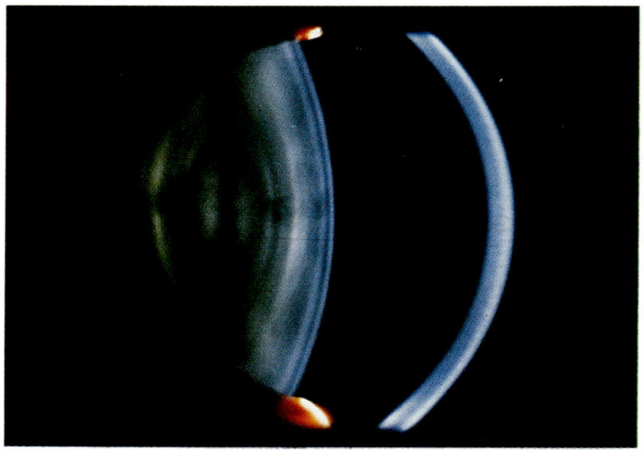

Figure 3.13 The normal human lens at age 45 years. The shorter wave lengths are scattered preferentially making the anterior cortex appear blue. (Brown slit-image camera.)

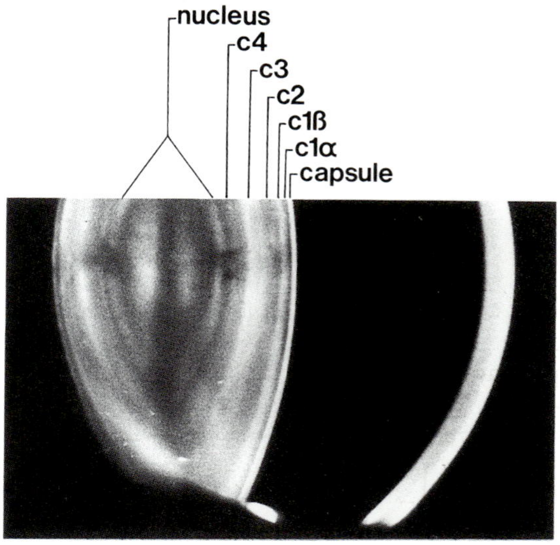

Figure 3.14 The classification of the zones of discontinuity of the lens by the Oxford system. (From Sparrow *et al.* 1986 with permission.)

light scatter is thought to arise from the fibre cell membranes, which have a higher refractive index than the surrounding cytoplasm (Bettelheim 1985). The separation between the lens fibre membranes is probably also important in determining whether destructive interference of the scattered light occurs (Trokel 1962). Thus the axial width of the lens fibre is likely to be important in determining the brightness of the zone in which they lie. Several studies have shown that protein concentration rises on passing from the cortex to the nucleus of the lens. The change is fairly acute, whether measured by microdensitometry (Fagerholm *et al.* 1990) or Raman spectroscopy (Siebinga *et al.* 1991) or derived from the refractive behaviour of the lens (Pierscionek 1990). The water content of the lens is shown to be high in the immediate subcapsular region and to drop very rapidly in the surface layer of 0.05–0.2 mm thickness (Siebinga *et al.* 1991) (Figure 3.15), which corresponds roughly in width to the anterior subcapsular clear zone (C1α) (see below). The high water content of this zone may be an explanation of its transparency. But at deeper levels the water content remains constant and so fluctuations in water content cannot explain the occurrence of the other zones of discontinuity.

The lens grows by the surface accretion of new lens fibres. At the same time central compaction of lens fibres occurs, as witnessed by the reduction in diameter of congenital nuclear cataracts with age (Brown *et al.* 1988) which reflects compaction of the nucleus, and by the behaviour of superficial opacities, such as traumatic cataracts and glaucoma flecks, which are seen to sink into the lens at twice the rate of lens growth (Brown 1976). On the basis of studies of sagittal lens thickness with age, the net, or apparent growth rate of the lens is 25 μm per year in the adult, while the true growth rate is much greater than this. It appears that nuclear compaction only occurs during the first 20 years of life, while cortical compaction occurs throughout the life span. Its location is not yet established. The subcapsular clear zone (C1α) (Figure 3.14) is approximately 125 μm in width, reducing slightly with age. It can be calculated, assuming that there is no compaction within the zone itself, that this represents about 2 years' true growth.

As noted earlier, central compaction would account for the lack of growth in the sagittal width of the lens in early life (approximately 3–20 years) if the compaction at this age fully balanced the growth by surface accretion. In this case, the increase in weight during this period (Harding *et al.* 1977) would be compatible with growth in equatorial diameter or with an increase in specific gravity, both of which might occur. However, little or no increase in specific gravity occurs with age in the adult lens (Scammon and Hesdorffer 1937; van Heyningen 1972). This implies that some degradation of the protein content of the lens fibres must take place whilst they sink in and compact. Protein synthesis in the lens does not decline with age (de Vries *et al.* 1991).

The creation of the lens zones by the accumulation of layers of lens fibres suggests a resemblance to the formation of tree rings. This resemblance is purely superficial, since the zones of discontinuity of the lens are not fixed bands, as in the tree, but are made up by a shifting population of lens fibres.

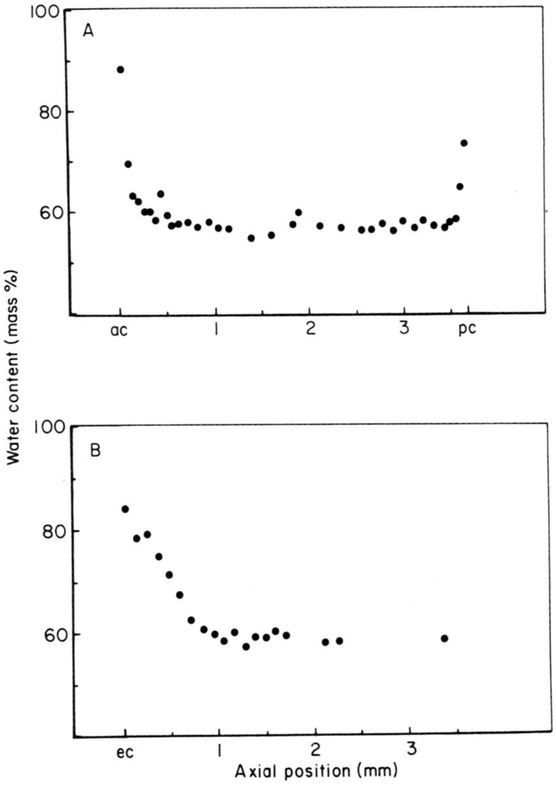

Figure 3.15 Absolute water content along (A) the visual and (B) equatorial axis of an eight-year-old human lens. ac = anterior capsular side; pc = posterior capsular side; ec = equatorial capsular side. (From Siebinga *et al.* 1991 with permission.)

Thus C1β (Figure 3.14), which is the first bright band of the cortex, is composed of recently formed lens fibres, which with time occupy a deeper position in the lens, to form the less scattering C2 zone. It is a closer analogy to compare the formation of this zone of discontinuity with standing waves in a stream, where the wave remains at the same site, but the water that makes it is continuously on the move (Brown and Hungerford 1982).

Capsular and zonular forces evidently play a significant part in determining the shape of the lens and the form of the zones of discontinuity. The zones show peripheral divergence, so that in the adult they are conspicuously wider at the periphery (Figure 3.13). When the zonule is deficient as in lens dislocation the growth of the lens is spherical and there is lack of divergence of the zones of discontinuity (Figure 3.16).

Changes in optical properties with age

The hypermetropia of the young child declines towards emmetropia in the young adult, which is followed by a gradual hypermetropic shift in middle age (Figure 3.17). The average shift in the aged is in the direction of myopia, but this is due to the frequent development of changes proceeding to nuclear cataract (page 220). If these subjects are omitted, then the healthy ageing lens is seen to have a continuing hypermetropic shift (Brown and Hill 1987).

The maintenance of emmetropia, or increasing hypermetropia with age, in spite of the increase in curvature of the lens, has been described by Brown

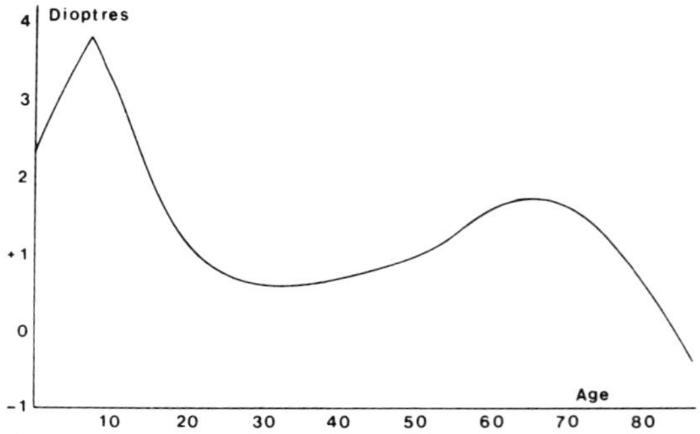

Figure 3.17 Change in refraction with age. (After Slataper 1950).

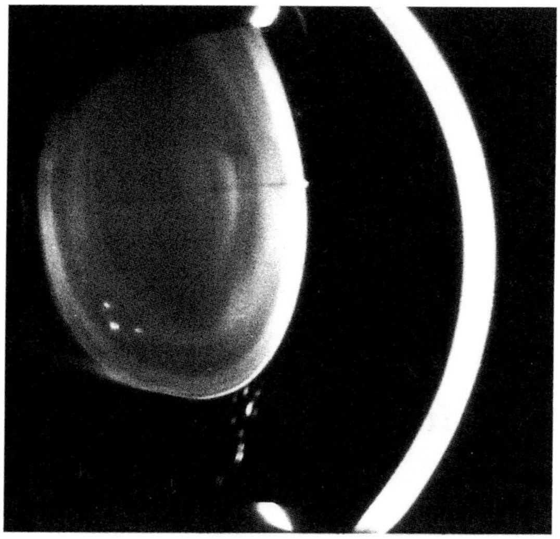

Figure 3.16 Upward subluxation of the lens in Marfan's syndrome. The lens shows lack of divergence of the zones of discontinuity.

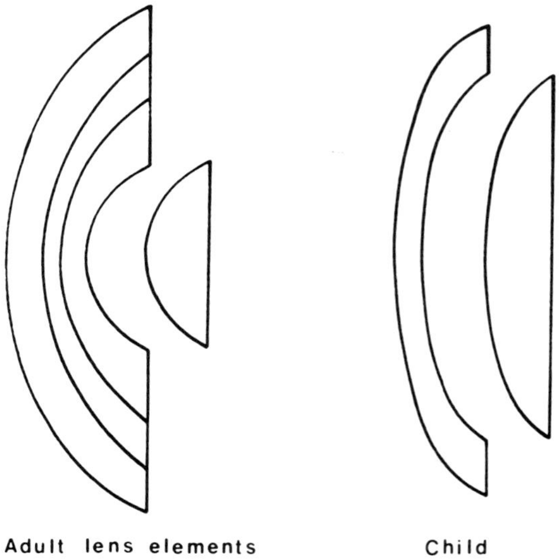

Figure 3.18 The lens nuclear and cortical shells of a child and of an old person. The cortex can be regarded as a concavo-convex element. Refractive index changes are needed to explain the maintenance of emmetropia on ageing.

as the lens paradox (Koretz and Handelman 1986). For the hypermetropic shift to occur, there must be changes in refractive index between the nucleus and the cortex. The cortex (Figure 3.18) can be regarded as a concavo-convex negative lens element and the nucleus as a biconvex positive element. In youth it appears that the nucleus has the higher refractive index and that the situation becomes reversed in the aged, with the cortex assuming the higher refractive index of the two (except in senile nuclear cataract (p. 152)). An increase in the refractive index of the cortex with age can be explained on the basis of increased light scatter (Huggert 1946a, b). A reduction in refractive index of the ageing nucleus can be explained on the basis of a reduction in the protein concentration in the nucleus which has been demonstrated by Raman spectroscopy (Siebinga 1991). Additionally the ageing of lens protein leads to the formation of an increasing proportion of insoluble protein, which no longer contributes to the refractive index of the cytoplasm (Cook *et al.* 1994).

The light transmission of the lens is reduced progressively with age (Figure 3.19) (Lerman and Borkman 1976) and this particularly affects the blue end of the spectrum. The reduced light transmission is due both to absorption and to scattering, each of which increase with age and further increase if cataract develops. In particular there is a large reduction in blue transmission with the development of nuclear brunescence (p. 222).

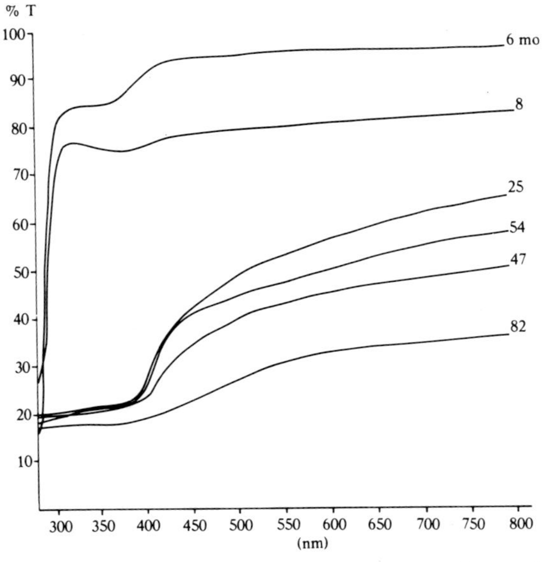

Figure 3.19 Transmission characteristics (%T) of normal human lenses ranging in age from 6 months to 82 years. (From Lerman 1980.)

The healthy adult lens emits green fluorescence at around 520 nm when stimulated by blue light of 420–430 nm. The fluorescence is concentrated in the nuclear and perinuclear regions. Fluorescence is first identifiable after the age of 20 years and increases at a linear rate with age. A more rapid rate of increase is seen in the diabetic (Sparrow *et al.* 1992).

Changes in mechanical properties with age

The lens substance becomes harder with age. In youth the nucleus is the more flexible, but becomes less flexible than the cortex at the age of 40 years (Fisher 1971) and thereafter the nucleus becomes progressively harder (Pau and Krantz 1992). In the phenomenon termed 'the relief pattern of the adult nucleus' (Figure 3.20) radial corrugations are demonstrated on the surface of the nucleus by specular illumination. It appears to result from uneven compaction of the nucleus with the 'ribs' of the pattern lying at the locations of the lens sutures and implying that compaction is hindered in the suture region. The relief pattern is seen at the front surface of C3.

The increased hardness of the nucleus with age is not explained by changes in the lens proteins because the reduction in protein content with age (Siebinga 1991) would have the reverse effect. It may be that the compaction of fibre membranes into the nucleus provides an explanation or that crystallin cross-linking is an important factor. However this is negligible in the absence of cataract.

The refractive profile of the lens

The refractive state of the lens is dependent on the curvature of its surface and upon its refractive index. The latter is dependent on its protein content. Thirty-three per cent of the wet weight of the lens is due to protein and this fraction is relatively constant over most of the age span (Nordmann 1966; van Heyningen 1972; Bours 1987; Bours and Fodisch 1986; Bours *et al.* 1987). Since 90% of the dry weight of the lens is contributed by the crystallins, changes in crystallin concentration reflect changes in protein concentration as a whole, and are indicative of the level of hydration of the lens.

A number of studies indicate that there is little equatorial growth of the lens in adult life. Fisher (1969a) found that most equatorial diameters over the age of 30–60 years lay between 8.8 and 9.2 mm. Scammon and Wilmer (1950) reported a diameter of 9.0 mm over the age group 20–40 years, while Pierscionek (1990) reported the same figure over the age range 16–84 years. After the plateau period of growth in sagittal width, there is a steady rate of sagittal growth at the rate of about 25 μm/year. Continued sagittal growth from the age of roughly 20 years, in the presence of stationary equatorial growth, is associated with an increase in anterior and, to a lesser extent, posterior curvature (Lowe and Clark 1972a,b; Brown 1974). This age-related change on its own would be expected to result in a steady increase in lens power (i.e. an increasing lenticular myopia). However, this does not occur and it may be inferred that, with ageing and the continued growth of the lens, there is an associated decrease in the average refractive index. This is supported by direct and indirect evidence.

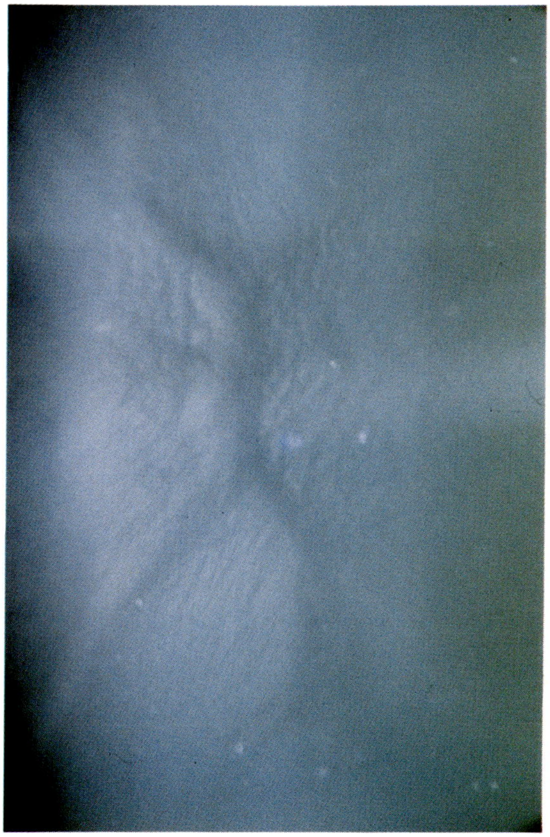

Figure 3.20 Relief of the adult nucleus seen in specular illumination.

The contribution of refractive index to the refractive power of the lens depends on the refractive and therefore protein gradients across the lens, from surface to centre. There is now substantial information about the distribution of crystallins in the lens and refractive gradients at different ages. In fetal life there is relatively little difference in crystallin concentration across the lens, from anterior to posterior pole, from which it may be inferred that the lens is optically homogeneous at birth (Bours *et al.* 1990). In an infant of 18 months a gradient of protein will already have developed across the lens, with a lower concentration of protein in the cortex (Fagerholm *et al.* 1981). Fagerholm *et al.* (1981) using a microdensitometric technique, Bessems *et al.* (1990) using iso-electric focusing and Siebinga *et al.* (1991) using Raman spectroscopy, have demonstrated this profile throughout adult life. Protein concentration is highest in the centre of the lens, and plateaus for approximately 4.0 mm in the equatorial plane before dropping more acutely towards the lens capsule (Figure 3.21). This more acute gradient would be expected to equate with a higher lens hydration, and a lower refractive index. Although refractive index can be derived from a knowledge of protein concentration (Fagerholm *et al.* 1981), the refractive increment for each crystallin is not identical. Thus gamma crystallin, which predominates in the nucleus of the lens, has the highest refractive increment, and beta the lowest. Although this contributes to interspecies differences in refractive index, with the rat lens (high in gamma crystallin) having a much higher refractive index than bovine or human lenses, it appears to have only a minor influence on the refractive profile of the human lens (Pierscionek and Augesteyn 1991).

Pierscionek has carried out ray-tracing studies in excised human lenses and used the findings to

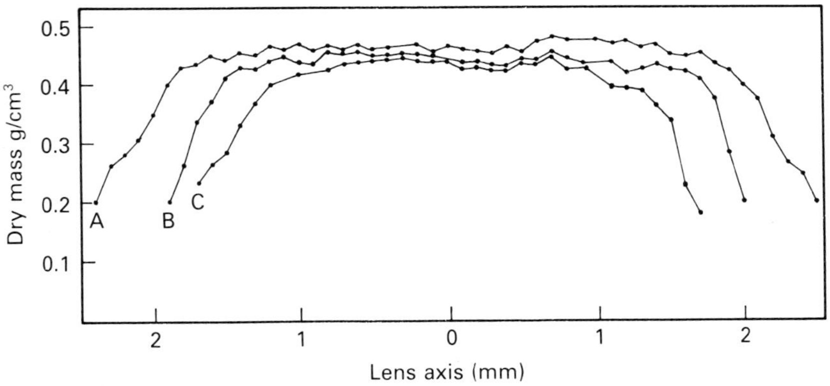

Figure 3.21 Graph showing the dry mass distribution along the lens axis in three normal lenses of different ages: (A) 62 years; (B) 24 years; (C) 1–5 years. In the subcapsular cortex there is an increase in dry mass concentration up to about $0.4\,g/cm^3$. The central part of the lens represents a core of homogeneous mass distribution. (From Fagerholm *et al.* 1981.)

construct refractive profiles across the lens in the equatorial plane, subsequently transforming these to refractive profiles in the sagittal plane (Pierscionek *et al.* 1988; Pierscionek and Chan 1989; Smith *et al.* 1991; Pierscionek 1990). These profiles resemble the protein profiles, showing a higher refractive index at the centre of the lens (1.40/1.41), with a refractive plateau which declines gradually towards the cortex and then more acutely to reach a value of about 1.34 in the peripheral cortex. The point of inflexion, 3.0–3.5 mm from the centre of the lens in the equatorial plane, is said to represent the diameter of the newborn lens (Pierscionek 1990); however, this does not appear to take nuclear compaction into consideration, and it is likely that the deep cortex is included in this figure.

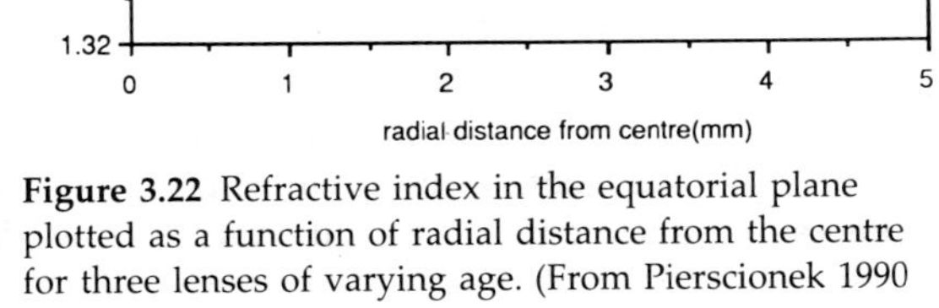

Figure 3.22 Refractive index in the equatorial plane plotted as a function of radial distance from the centre for three lenses of varying age. (From Pierscionek 1990 with permission.)

An important aspect of this study was the demonstration that with age, the refractive gradient in the peripheral cortex shallows (Figure 3.22). The effect of this is paradoxical, in that a rise in cortical refractive index, by reducing the refractive gradient, reduces the average refractive index of the lens. Siebinga *et al.* (1991) have reported a fall in protein concentration in the lens nucleus, which would reduce refractive index further. This reduction in refractive index compensates for the increase in curvature of the lens referred to earlier so that there is no increase in lenticular power with age. Pierscionek (1990) has estimated that the rise in refractive index, at 4.0 mm peripheral to the centre of the lens in the equatorial plane, is from 1.34 to 1.36 between the ages of 16–56 years and represents a decrease in water content of 10%.

4

Lens structure

Capsule

The lens capsule is an unusually thick basal lamina which surrounds the lens. It is secreted *in utero* by the lens epithelium. After formation of the primary lens fibres, only the anterior epithelium persists, so that future thickening of the capsule is chiefly anterior, although the posterior lens fibres have a limited capacity to secrete new lamina (Parmigiani and McAvoy 1991). The capsule is thus thickest anteriorly and increases in thickness throughout life; it is thicker towards the insertion of the zonule.

Like other basal laminae, the capsule is rich in type IV collagen. It also contains type I and III collagens in addition to a number of extracellular matrix components including, laminin, fibronectin, heparan sulphate proteoglycan and entactin (Marshall *et al.* 1991) (Figure 4.1). Electron microscopy shows a homogeneous appearance, with fibrillar features in the more superficial layers (Seland 1974) (Figure 4.1). Linear densities are also found, which may be granular or contain coarse filaments parallel to the surface. They have been identified to contain laminin and are not found in the posterior capsule. Zonular fibres are received into the fibrillar zone of the capsule anterior and posterior to the equator. At the equator itself is a thin superficial zone, the zonular lamella (pericapsular membrane) which stains metachromatically.

Human capsular permeability has been investigated by Hess (1911), Friedenwald (1930), Francois and Rabaey (1958), Fisher (1969b, 1973) and Hockwin *et al.* (1973). The capsule is freely permeable to water, ions and other small molecules, and to protein, offering a barrier to molecules greater than the size of albumin (Mr 70 kDa; molecular diameter 74 Å) and haemoglobin (Mr 66.7 kDa; molecular diameter 64 Å). Neither Friedenwald (1930) nor Fisher (1973) noted a difference in permeability of capsules between normal and cataractous lenses, but Fisher noted a correlation between permeability and cortical water content.

Zonule (suspensory ligament)

The ciliary zonule consists of a series of fine fibres passing between the ciliary body and the lens. They transmit a force from the ciliary muscle to the lens in the unaccommodated eye. The force is relaxed during accommodation. The fibres consist of an elastin-associated glycoprotein called fibrillin, which is found ubiquitously in vascular and other connective tissues (Dietz *et al.* 1991; Lee *et al.* 1991; Sakai *et al.* 1991; Pereira *et al.* 1994). Weakness of the zonule leads to lens subluxation in the Marfan syndrome, due to a fibrillin gene mutation (15 q 15–21.3).

The fibres arise from the pars plana and ciliary valleys of the ciliary body, and are distributed to the anterior, equatorial and posterior parts of the lens margin. Between the ciliary processes they form a flattened ciliary plexus whose fibres are firmly attached to the bases of the ciliary valleys. More anteriorly they are angulated, according to Rohen (1979), to form a 'zonular fork' through which a more equatorial force is exerted on the lens (Figure 4.1b). Farnsworth and Burke (1977) and Farnsworth *et al.* (1979) describe a more complex attachment, (Figure 4.1c) with zonules from the lens attaching posteriorly to the ciliary body, those from the equator attaching perpendicularly to the lens equator, and zonules from the anterior lens attaching posteriorly near the ora seratta, and also more anteriorly. With age, the boundaries of the zonular attachment become more diffuse and the anterior and posterior attachments diverge, while the equatorial attachment is unchanged (Farnsworth and Shyne 1979; Stark and Streeten 1984). This must be assumed to be in part due to the remodelling process which must occur in the lens capsule with growth.

The zonular fibres are elastic in behaviour (Fisher 1971). They are not renewed after injury.

Epithelium

The epithelium forms an anterior subcapsular monolayer extending to the equator. Its cells are cuboidal in sagittal section, but polygonal in

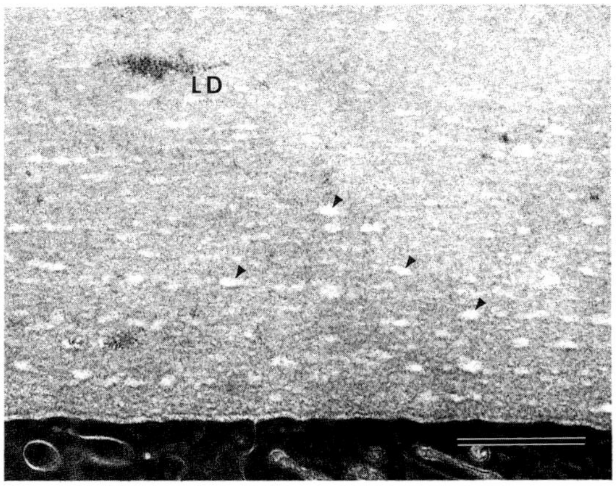

(b)

Figure 4.1(b) Higher power of lens capsule. The linear density (LD) exhibits a periodicity of about 60 nm due to axial banding of its constituent fibrils. Electron lucent 'bubbles' (arrowheaded) occur between adjacent lamellae. Bar indicates 1 μm. (Courtesy of G.E. Marshall and S. Cameron.)

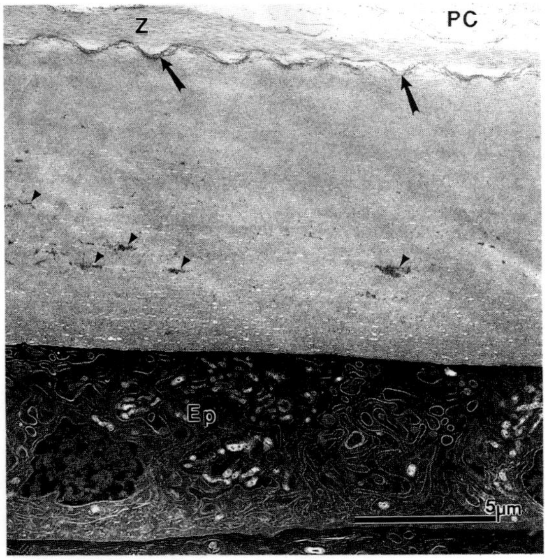

(a)

Figure 4.1(a) Transmission electron micrograph of anterior equatorial lens capsule in a 13-year-old girl. Linear densities (arrowheads) are scattered throughout the substance of the capsule. The interface of the capsule with the posterior chamber (PC) is bounded by a pericapsular membrane (zonular lamella) [arrows], above which lies a zonular process (Z). Note the smooth interface between the single layer of lens epithelial cells (Ep) and the lens capsule. (Courtesy of G.E. Marshall and S. Cameron.)

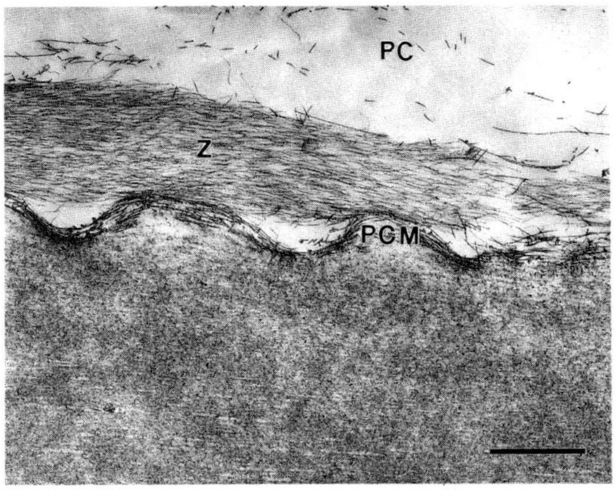

(c)

Figure 4.1(c) Superficial portion of human lens capsule. The pericapsular membrane (PCM), also referred to as the zonular lamella, is composed of fibrils morphologically indistinguishable from those of zonules (Z). Note the faint fibrillar nature of the capsule. PC = posterior chamber of eye. Bar indicates 1 μm. (Courtesy of G.E. Marshall and S. Cameron.)

surface view (Figure 4.2a,b). There are about 500 000 cells in the mature lens (Young 1991) with a central density of about 5009/mm^2 in men, and 5781/mm^2 in women (Guggenmoos-Holzmann *et al.* 1989), and an increased density towards the periphery (Hogan *et al.* 1971, Figure M001). Density decreases with age (Figure 4.3a). Kuszak and Brown (1991) have estimated the average epithelial and fibre number based on average lens dimensions (Table 4.1).

The cells show large indented nuclei with two nucleoli and a moderate number of organelles including small mitochondria, Golgi apparatus, smooth and rough endoplasmic reticulum, ribosomes and polysomes, lysosomes, dense bodies and glycogen particles. Cytoskeletal proteins include actin, vimentin (intermediate filaments), microtubular protein spectrin, alpha-actinin and myosin.

There are prominent actin networks subjacent to the apico- and baso-lateral membranes ('geodomes') which presumably perform a structural function (Figure 4.3b) (Rafferty and Scholz 1984, 1989; Yeh *et al.* 1986). Alpha crystallin is present, but not beta or gamma crystallin.

The cells show extensive lateral interdigitation and are attached by desmosomes (Figure 4.4). Gap junctions are present between contiguous cells which permit the free movement of small molecules between cells (Kuwabara 1975) (Figures 4.5a,b). The gap junctions are of liver type, that is their intra-membranous particles show tight packing, and the inter-membranous gap is 2–4 nm. The type is infrequently found among the lens fibres.

There are infrequent gap junctions between the epithelial cells and the underlying cortical lens fibres. This is in keeping with the findings among other epithelia, where apico-apical gap junctions are uncommon. In the lens, the apical face of the epithelial cells (away from the capsule) makes contact with the apical face of the fibres (Kuszak *et al.* 1992). Although tight junctions were reported to be present between epithelial cells in the lens (Lo *et al.* 1983, 1986), their presence has been denied by Kuszak and Brown (1991) or said to be infrequent (Vrensen – personal communication). In keeping with this view, there appears to be no significant barrier to extracellular flow between lens epithelial

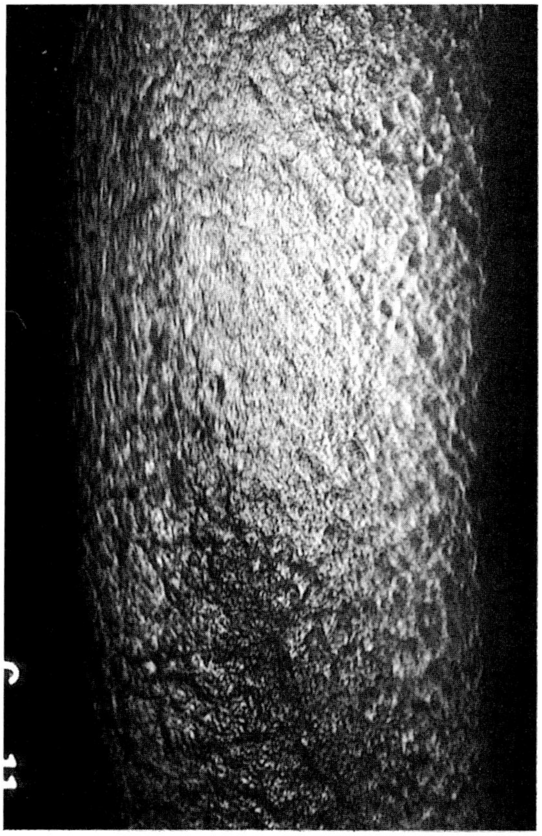

(a)

Figure 4.2(a) Lens epithelium by specular reflex photography in the living eye: a marked lens shagreen is visible.

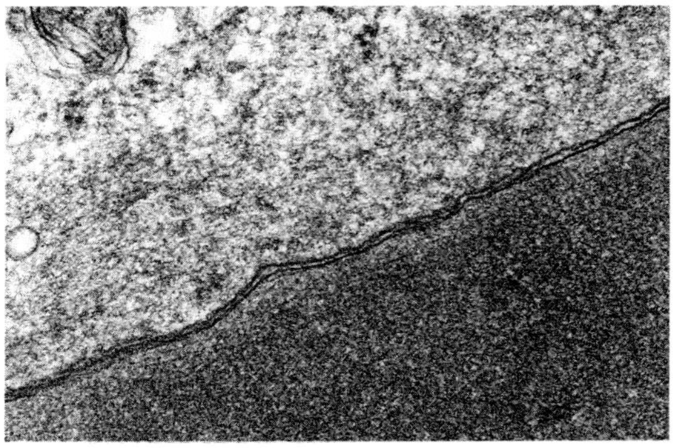

(b)

Figure 4.2(b) Epithelial-fibre cell interface of a primate lens. Note the absence of any well defined intercellular junction. (Courtesy of J.R. Kuszak.)

cells (Rae and Stacey 1979, Goodenough *et al.* 1980).

Although epithelial cells are coupled ionically to underlying elongating fibre cells, they are not coupled using tracer dyes (Rae and Kuszak 1983).

Various membrane specializations have been noted in the epithelial cells, such as the presence of 'square array' membrane in the apicolateral regions, and of protrusions and clathyrin-coated pits at the epithelial–fibre interface (Figures 4.5c,d,e,f). The latter signify the occurrence of receptor-mediated endocytosis (Brown *et al.* 1990), and reflect the presence of a number of defined receptors in the epithelium (e.g. to insulin, growth hormone and beta-adrenergic agonists) and their likely involvement in epithelial metabolism and traffic between the fibres and epithelial cells.

Few mitoses occur in the central region of the lens epithelium. The germinative zone is pre-equatorial and mitoses here give rise to the highly

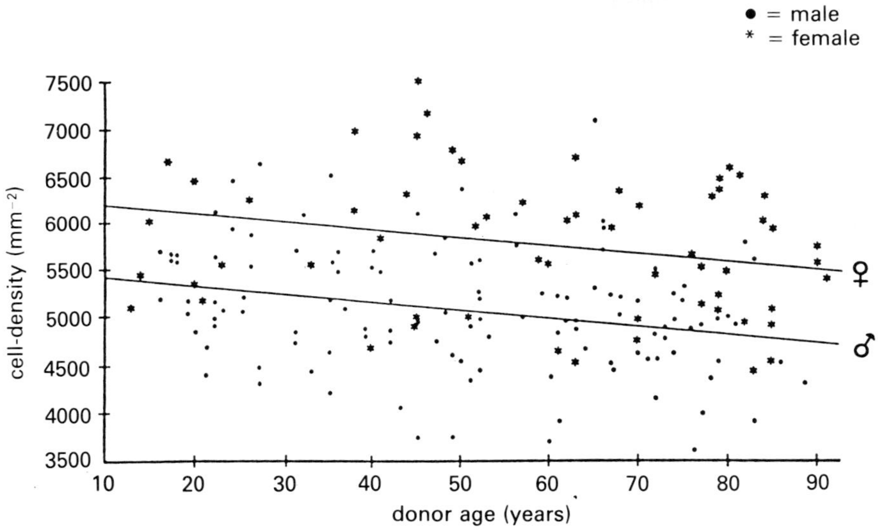

(a)

Figure 4.3(a) The density of the lens epithelium decreases with age. (From Holzmann *et al.* 1989 with permission.)

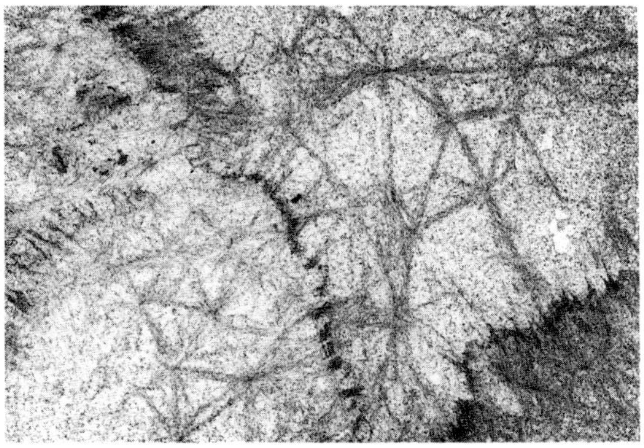

(bi)

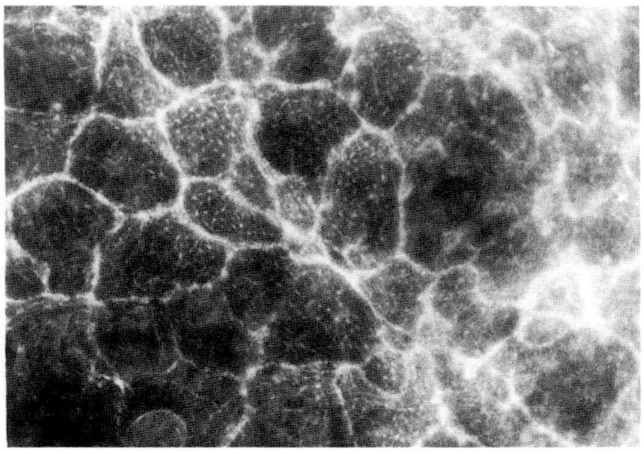

(bii)

Figure 4.3(b) Polygonal arrays demonstrated at the apical ends of lens epithelial cells. **(i)** rabbit TEM (magnification ×6600) (bar = 0.5 μm); **(ii)** human, rhodamine-phalloidin fluorescence microscopy (magnification ×750) (bar = 10 μm). (From Rafferty and Scholz 1989 with permission.)

Table 4.1 Estimates of lens epithelial and fibre cell number based on average lens dimensions as a function of age (adapted from Kuszak and Brown 1991)

Lens age	*No. of epithelial cells**	*No. of fibre cells***
At birth	402 595	1 662 010
Young lens (20 yr old)	761 184	3 045 100
Old lens (80 yr old)	1 009 312	3 546 100

*Estimates of the number of lens epithelial cells as a function of lens age are based on dividing the average cell diameter (280 μm^2) into the total surface area of the anterior lens. For the purposes of these estimates no allowance has been made for the fact that lens epithelial cells of the pre and germinative zones are smaller than average. In this manner, estimates of the total number of lens epithelial cells are purposely underestimated.
**Estimates of the number of growth shells in lenses at different ages are calculated by dividing the lens radius by the average thickness of fibres (2 μm). Estimates of the number of fibres/growth shell are determined by dividing the circumference of a growth shell by the average width (10 μm) of a fibre. Estimates of the total number of fibres/lens at different ages are the result of summating the number of fibres in all growth shells.

ordered meridional rows of cells (Figure 4.6). These differentiate posteriorly into secondary lens fibres, rotating through 180° while elongating anteriorly and posteriorly. The new lens fibres retain their polarity, so that the posterior (basal) part of the fibre remains in contact with the capsule (basal lamina) while the anterior (apical) part is separated from it by the epithelium.

Epithelial mitosis is associated with DNA synthesis, while fibre elongation involves increased

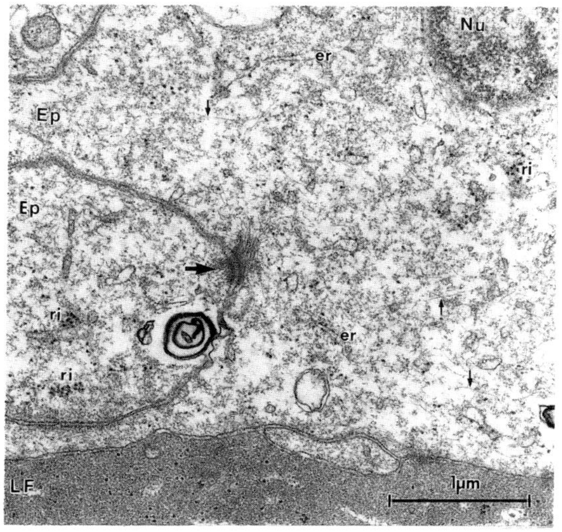

(a)

Figure 4.4(a) Lens epithelium showing two epithelial cells (Ep) and adjacent lens fibre (LF). A desmosome (arrow) is present between the two epithelial cells. The cells contain a nucleus (Nu), fibrils (small arrows), ribosomes (ri) and endoplasmic reticulum (er). (Courtesy of G. Vrensen.)

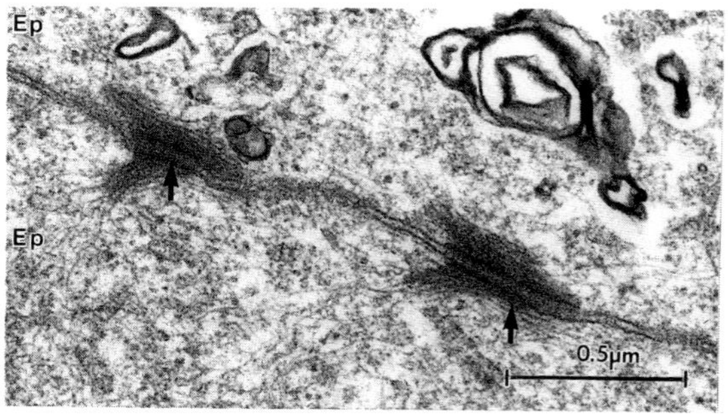

(b)

Figure 4.4(b) The desmosomes (arrows) have filaments extending into the cytoplasm. (TEM). (Courtesy of G. Vrensen and B. Willekens.)

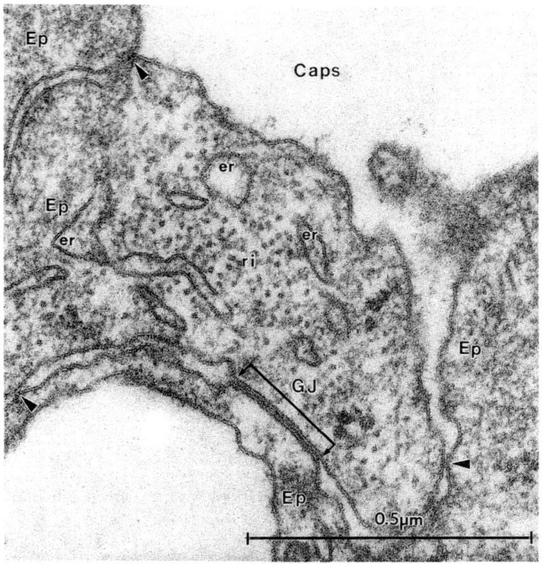

(a)

Figure 4.5(a) Junctions between epithelial cells (Ep). A gap junction (GJ) is present. In addition the membranes are confluent at three sites suggesting the presence of tight junctions. Within the cells are ribosomes (ri) and endoplasmic reticulum (er) (TEM). (Courtesy of G. Vrensen and B. Willekens.)

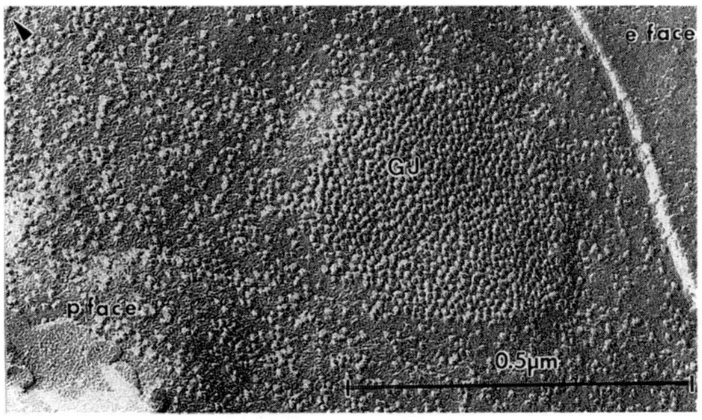

(b)

Figure 4.5(b) In freeze fracture the gap junction (GJ) is marked by 90 nm particles. The cytoplasmic face (p face) surface has many isolated intramembranous particles. These are scarce on the extracellular surface (e face). Arrow indicates direction of platinum shadowing (SEM). (Courtesy of G. Vrensen and B. Willekens.)

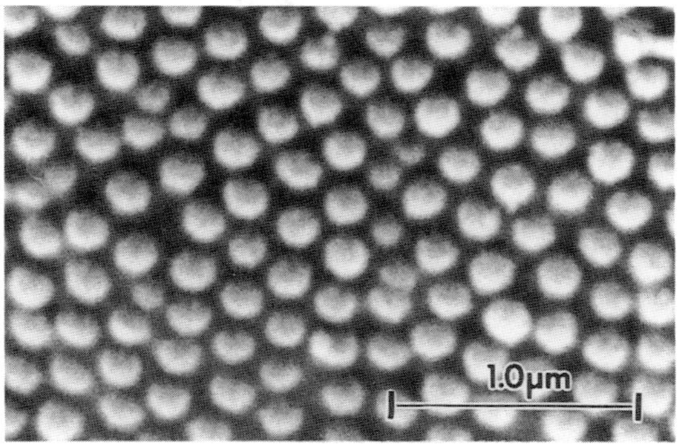

(ci)

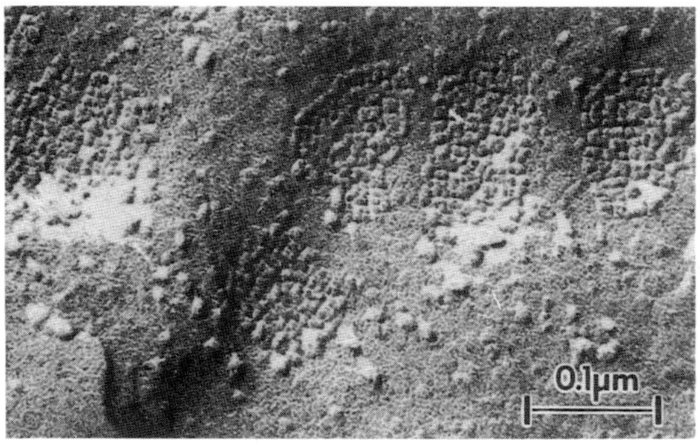

(cii)

Figure 4.5(c) **i** High power SEM of the aberrant membrane of a spoke opacity showing globular elevations of the surface. **ii** Freeze fracture transmission electron micrograph. The globular elements of i are seen as agglomerates of orthogonally organized intramembrane particles, the so-called square arrays. (Courtesy of G. Vrensen and B. Willekens.)

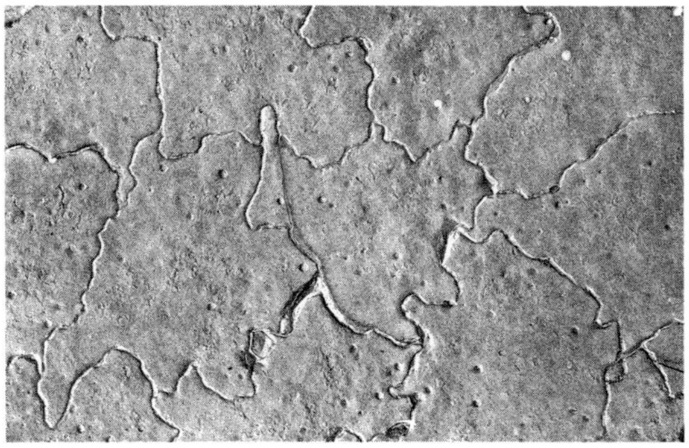

(d)

Figure 4.5(d) Low power SEM of lens epithelium.

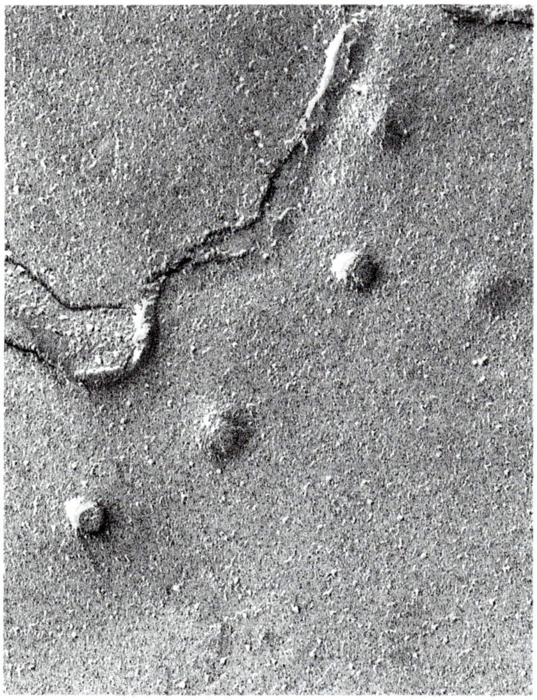

(e)

Figure 4.5(e) High power SEM of lens epithelial cell membrane showing protrusions.

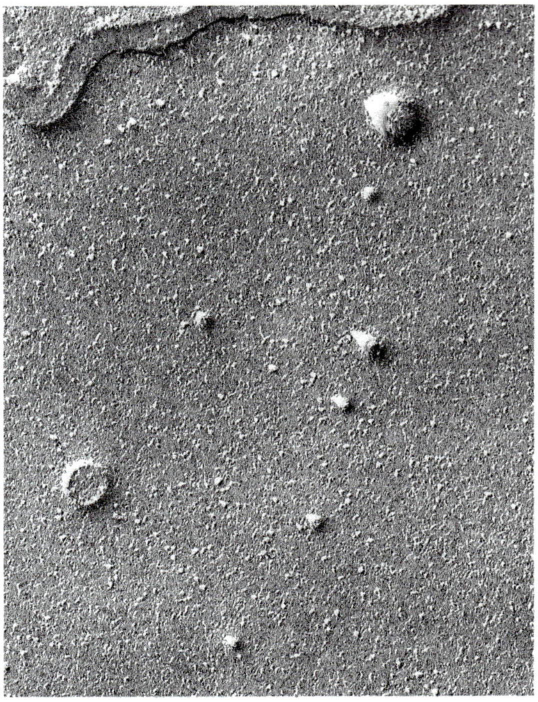

(f)

Figure 4.5(f) High power SEM of lens epithelial cell membrane showing clathycin-coated pits. (Courtesy of G. Vrensen and B. Willekens.)

transcriptional activity and RNA synthesis as specific structural, membrane and other proteins are formed. The fibres undergo a process of terminal differentiation, in which the nuclei become pyknotic and finally disappear, and the cell organelles are lost. Loss of nuclear DNA is preceded by increasing evidence of DNA strand scission (Figure 4.7) (Modak 1972).

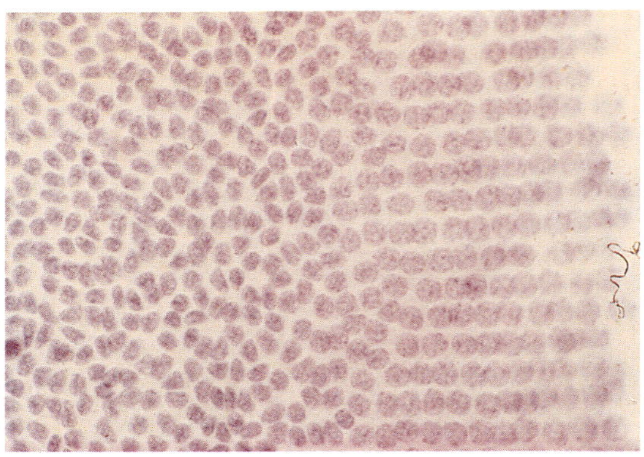

Figure 4.6 Meridional rows of epithelial cells near equator (rat).

Lens fibres

The tips of the new fibres grow over the surface of established fibres to reach the sutures anteriorly and posteriorly. Growing fibre tips have a ruffled border by confocal microscopy (B. Masters – personal communication). The suture branches lie at varying distances from the lens poles; the distance of anterior or posterior growth varies accordingly. As successive new generations of fibres are laid down, the older fibres come to lie further from the lens capsule and their nuclei move anteriorly to form the lens bow (Figure 4.8). The means by which the lens bow is formed is not known, but it is unlikely to involve fibre elongation alone since this will have ceased in the deeper regions; a significant participation by cytoskeletal proteins may be assumed.

With age, the fibre nuclei become elongated and the chromatin breaks into clumps as the nuclear envelope disintegrates. As noted, the nuclear material eventually disappears. The superficial fibres contain a sparse endoplasmic reticulum and few mitochondria. These are absent from the deep cortex and lens nucleus.

The lens fibres are ribbon-shaped with a hexagonal cross-section. The acutely angled short faces connect the parallel broad faces, and form the lateral membranes of the cells. Their average width is 10–12 μm and their average thickness is 1.5–2.0 μm at the adult equator. The primary fibres of the embryonic nucleus are less than 250 μm in length, while those of the adult lens may be over 7 mm long. The fibres are thinner posteriorly, which explains the asymmetrical shape of the lens in sagittal section (Kuszak *et al.* 1986, 1992; Kuszak and Brown 1991, 1993).

Fibres are intimately joined to one another by ball and socket joints at their lateral angles and to some extent over the broad faces of the fibres

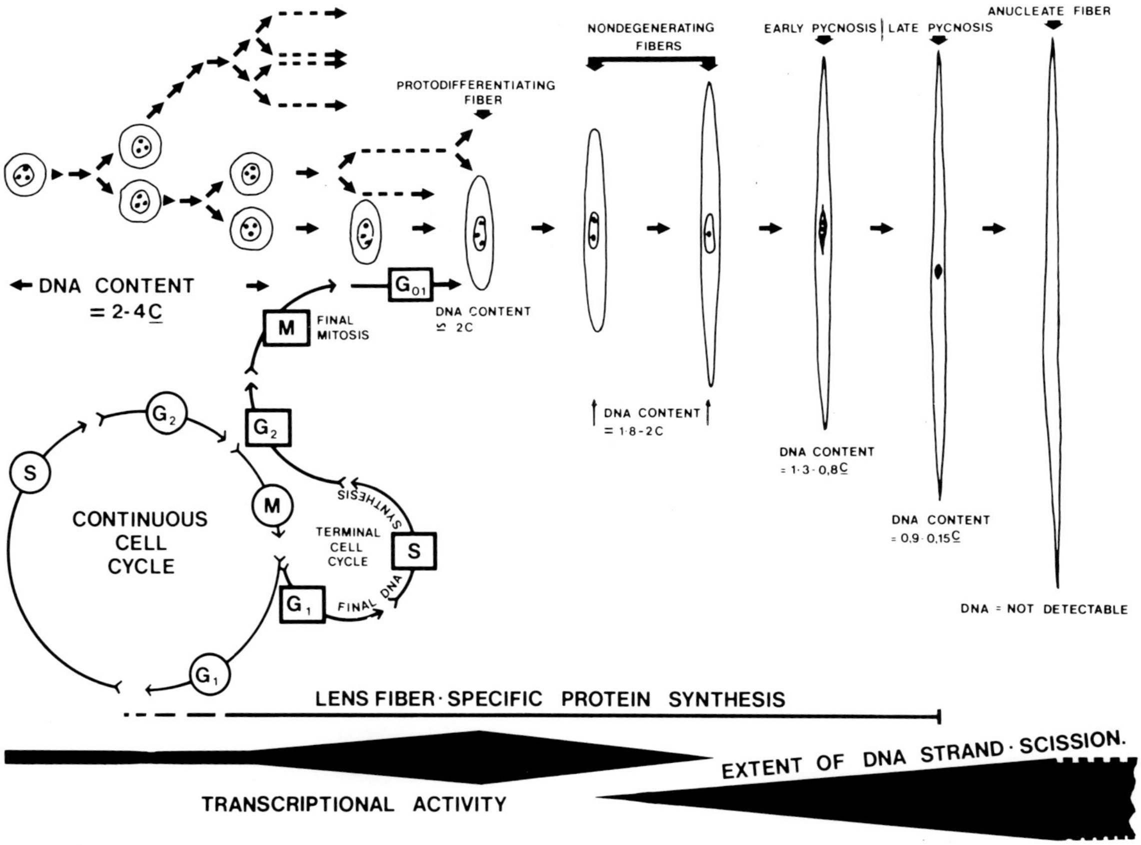

Figure 4.7 A schematic representation of terminal lens fibre differentiation. (From Modak 1972.)

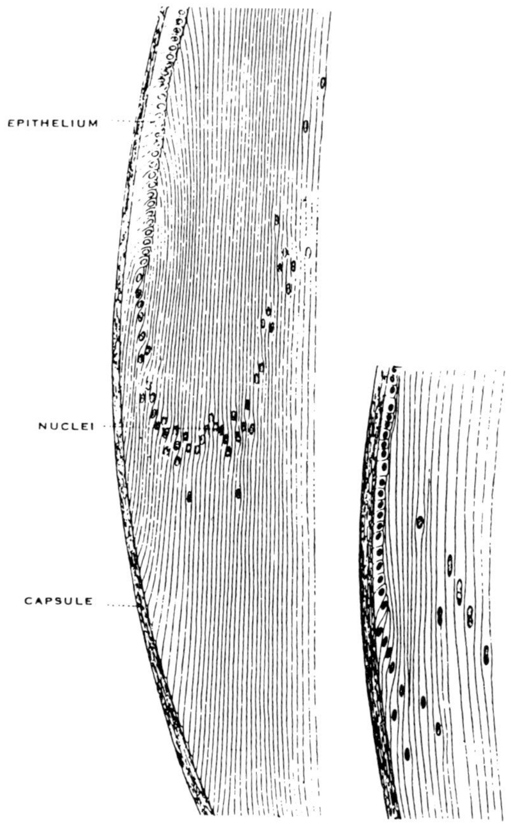

Figure 4.8 The lens fibre nuclear bow. (After Otto Becker.)

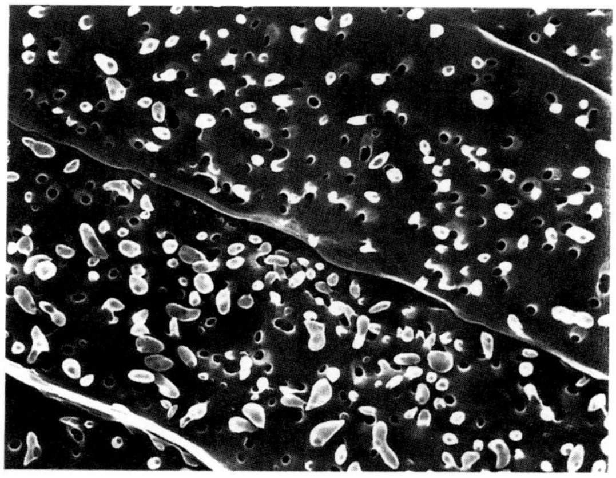

Figure 4.10 The ball and socket junctions of cortical fibres (EM). (Courtesy of M. Travers.)

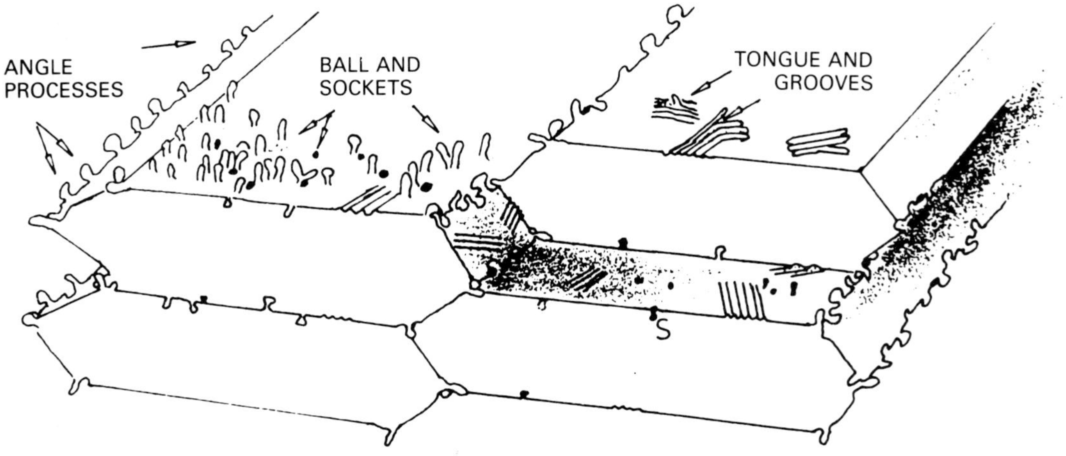

Figure 4.9 The form and junctions of the primate cortical fibres. (Courtesy of M. Travers.)

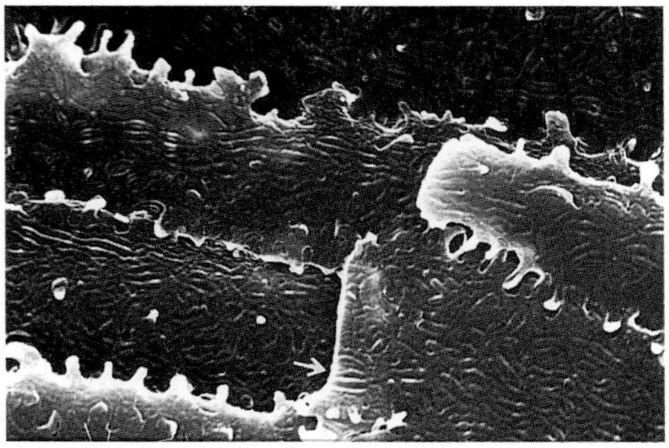

(a)

Figure 4.11(a) Angle processes joining the angles of the fibres in the primate cortex (EM). (Courtesy of M. Travers.)

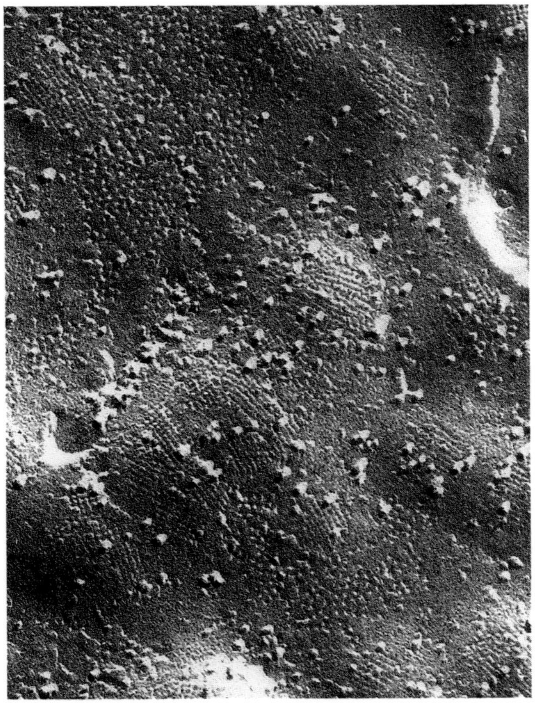

(b)

Figure 4.11(b) Scanning electron micrograph of an E-face freeze-etch replica showing the ultrastructure of superficial cortical fibre cell apico- or baso-lateral membrane. Note the numerous sites of orthogonal arrays of proteins or 'square array membrane' and the less frequent gap junctions (magnification × 150 000). (Courtesy of J.R. Kuszak.)

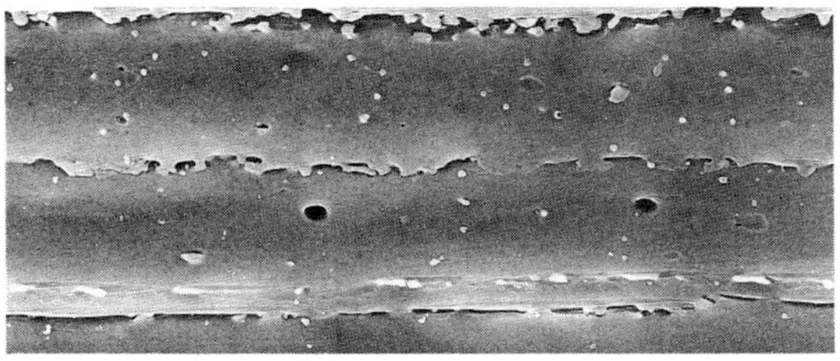

(c)

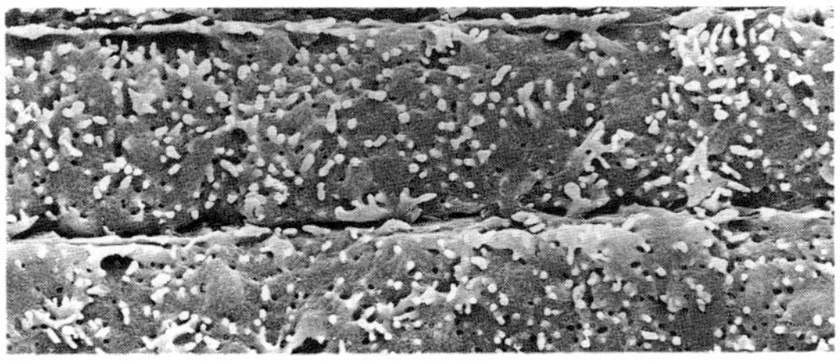

(d)

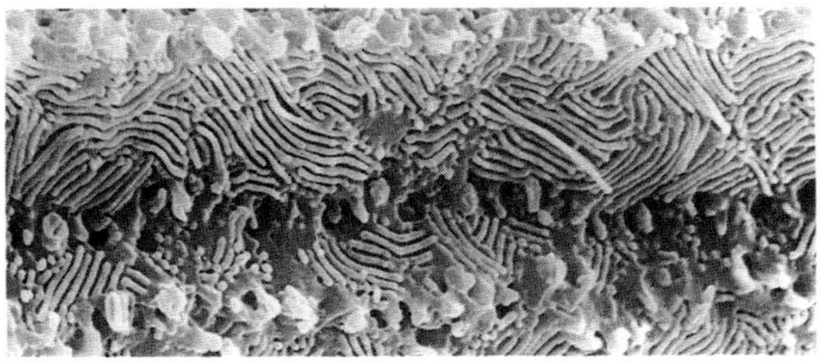

(e)

Figure 4.11(c–e) Series of scanning electron micrographs showing the dramatic transition in the surface membrane morphology of fibre cells as a function of development, maturation and growth: **(c)** the surface morphology of newly formed fibres is relatively smooth with developing lateral interdigitations (magnification × 12 000); **(d)** as fibres mature, their smooth surfaces are altered by the development of numerous microplicae (magnification × 10 000); **(e)** mature primate fibres feature polygonal domains of furrowed membrane, many with overlying microvilli (magnification × 10 000). (Courtesy of J.R. Kuszak.)

(Figures 4.9 and 4.10). Tongue and groove joints are seen as surface corrugations at the narrow lateral faces of the fibres (Kuwabara 1975) and the angles of the fibre interfaces are also joined by such processes (Willekens and Vrensen 1982; Vrensen *et al.* 1990; Travers 1990) (Figure 4.11). Deep in the nucleus of the primate lens, Kuszak and others have demonstrated polygonal domains of 'furrowed membrane' borne by the primary lens fibres, the oldest fibre cells of the lens, which exhibit numerous, elongated microvilli (Lo and Harding 1986; Kuszak *et al.* 1988). Thus the entire lens structure must flex in accommodation as the fibres cannot slide over one another. These attaching structures are not evenly distributed throughout the lens. The most superficial fibres are relatively featureless. The ball and sockets are characteristic of the cortex and in the primate lens are more prevalent in the mid-periphery of the cortex, which is the appropriate position to resist zonular stresses in accommodation (Travers 1990). Each fibre extends from an anterior to a posterior suture (Figure 4.12). The sutures are regions of complex overlap and interdigitation of fibre tip membranes (Figures 4.13, 4.14).

Earlier textbooks depicted the fibre tips as tapering towards the suture. This does occur in lower vertebrates (Kuszak *et al.* 1986), but not in animals with star-shaped sutures, including primates. It has been shown *in vivo* by specular microscopy (Figure 4.13) and scanning microscopy (Figure 4.14) that the fibres flare in width, and also curve as the suture is approached (Brown *et al.* 1987b, Kuszak *et al.* 1986) (Figure 4.15).

Kuszak has studied the geometry of the lens sutures in great detail. In the fetal lens there is an anterior Y suture and an inverted, posterior Y. With further growth, there is additional, symmetrical branching of the suture, ultimately to form the nine-point star of the mature cortex. Later, in senescent lenses, there is further, irregular subbranching (Figure 4.16).

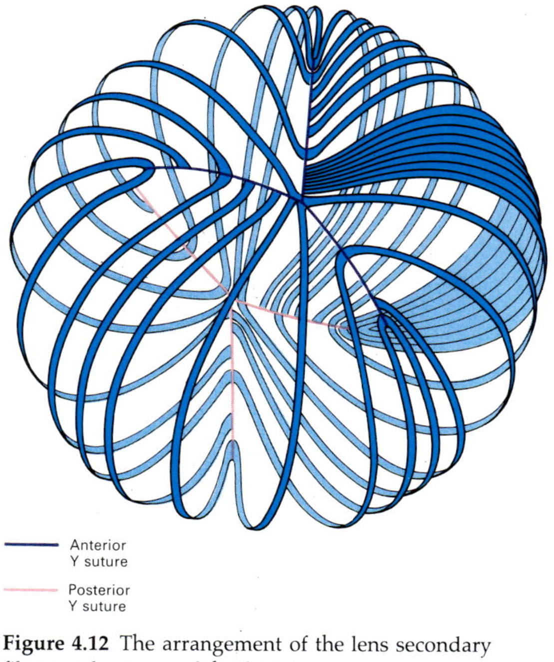

Figure 4.12 The arrangement of the lens secondary fibres and sutures of the fetal lens.

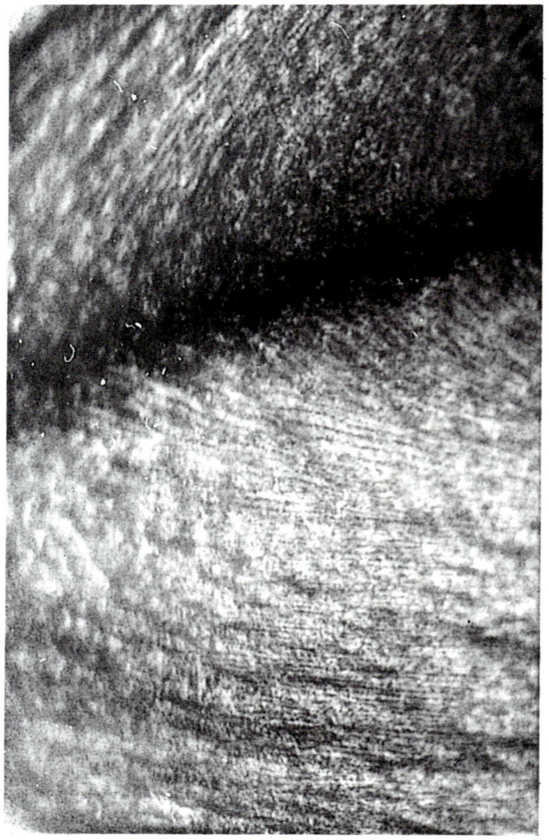

Figure 4.13 Lens fibres converging on a suture, seen by specular reflex photography in the living eye.

The manner in which the lens fibres are arranged with respect to the sutures is as follows: 18 fibres are found to run precisely in the meridia at 20° apart. Half of these originate at the anterior pole and end slightly posteriorly (at 10° latitude), while the other half start at the posterior pole and end slightly anteriorly (at 10° latitude). On either side of these straight fibres the fibre tips curve away from the polar axis as they insert into their respective sutures. This end curve is in an opposite sense anteriorly compared with posteriorly. Because the equatorial circumference of the fibres is shorter than the length of the sutures into which they insert, the fibre tips are expanded as well as curved. (Thus in a nine-star suture, the group of fibres occupying 20 longitudinal degrees of the equator inserts over greater than 75° at the suture).

This situation is different at the lens nucleus since fibres arising over a span of 60 longitudinal degrees insert into suture branches measuring 30 latitudinal degrees. These fibres are thus wider at the equator than at the sutures (Kuszak *et al.* 1986). Because there are only six branches associated with the Y sutures, the end curves are more pronounced.

Also in relation to the Y suture, since fibre length varies only slightly with meridian, the overlap of fibre cells within successive growth shells produces ordered meridional columns (of Rabl 1900). In the fetal nucleus, there is also superimposition of the suture zones, which is visible as a suture plane during biomicroscopy because of the light-scattering behaviour of the overlapping membranes within the sutures. In the postnatal lens, where fibre length is not a function of radial location, the sutures do not lie in perfect register but are offset, so that continuity of the suture plane is more difficult to see.

The radial columns of fibres of the lens (Rabl 1900) (Figure 4.17) are demonstrated in histological sections at a normal to the surface. It has been pointed out that as the lens grows, an increase in equatorial circumference can be achieved in two ways, either by an increase in fibre width, or an increase in number of rows. Although the former

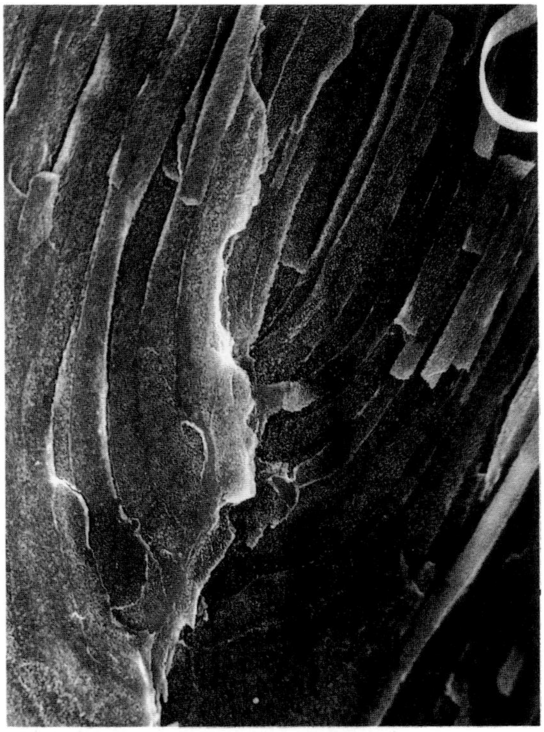

Figure 4.14 The flare and curve of cortical fibres in the region of a lens suture (TEM). (Primate lens – courtesy of M. Travers).

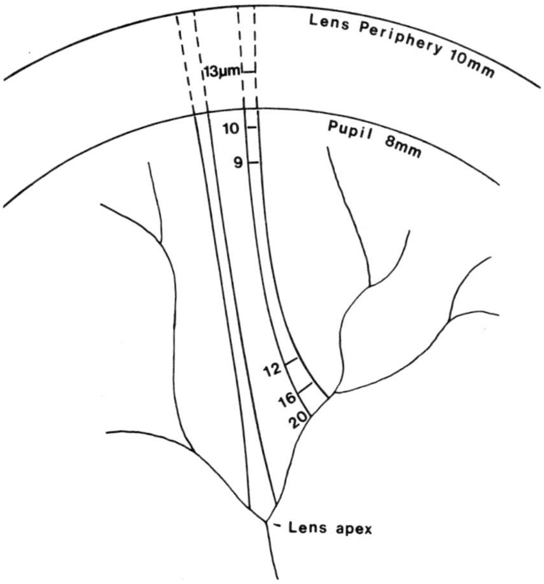

Figure 4.15 The shape of the human lens fibre. Since it is not possible to draw a single fibre, the figure shows a group of 20 fibres.

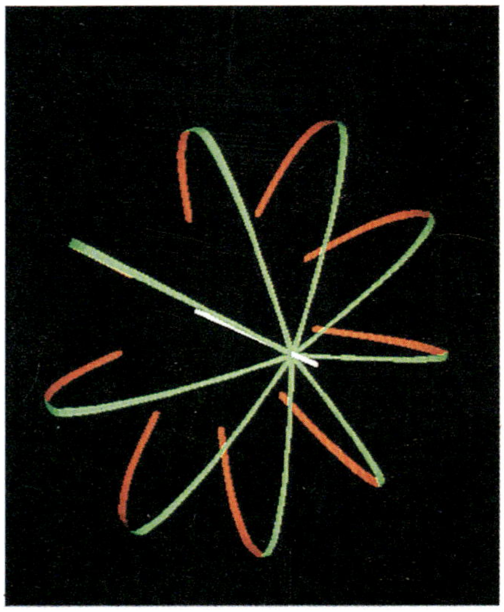

(a)

Figure 4.16 Three-dimensional computer assisted drawings depicting the essential suture parameters that result in the construction of a symmetrical 'star' suture in young adult primate lenses. **(a)** the positions of the nine straight fibre cells that extend to confluence at the anterior pole.

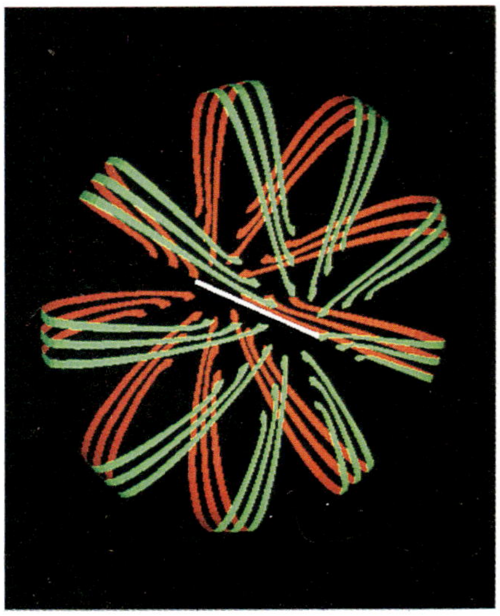

(c)

Figure 4.16(c) The positions of the groups of fibre cells with clockwise anterior end curvature and counter-clockwise posterior end curvature in a single growth shell.

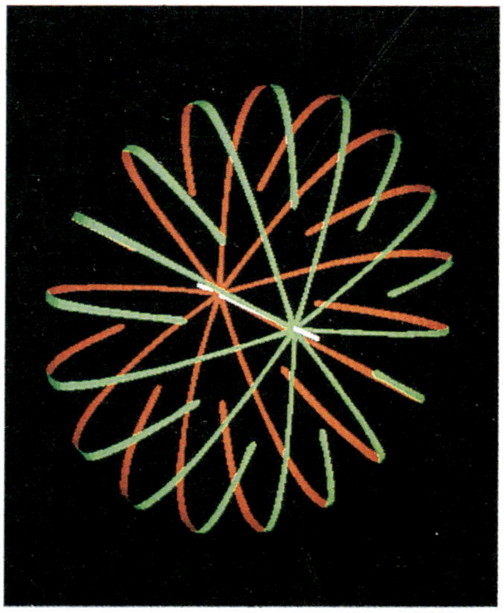

(b)

Figure 4.16(b) The positions of the eighteen straight fibre cells that extend to confluence at the anterior and posterior poles.

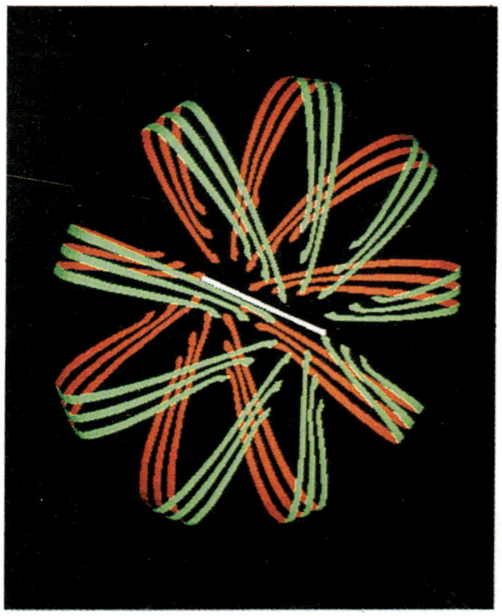

(d)

Figure 4.16(d) The position of the groups of fibre cells with counter-clockwise anterior end curvature and clockwise posterior end curvature in a single growth shell.

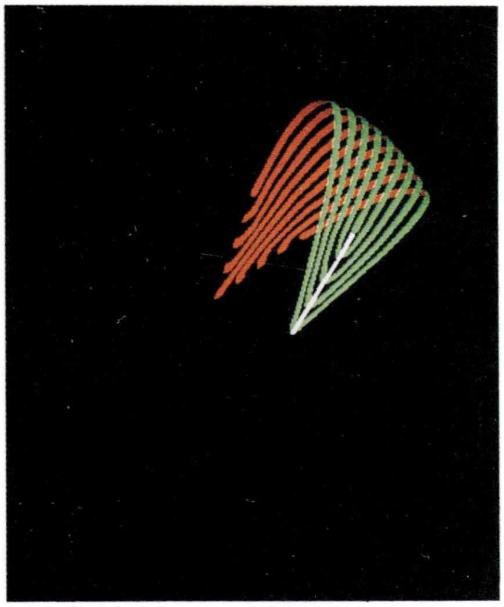

(e)

Figure 4.16(e) One of the nine anterior suture branches. Note that as a result of opposite end curvature the groups of fibre cells that overlap to form an anterior suture will not overlap with the same fibre cells to form a posterior suture. Rather, they overlap with two different groups of fibre cells to form two different posterior sutures.

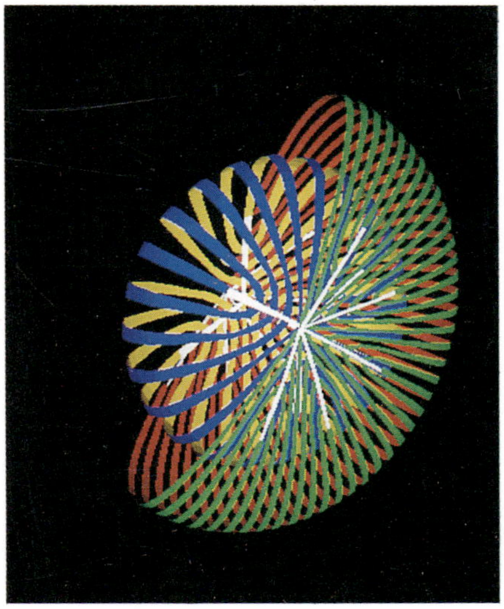

(g)

Figure 4.16(g) The position of the Y suture characteristic of primate lenses at birth exposed by removing several sutural branches of the star suture.

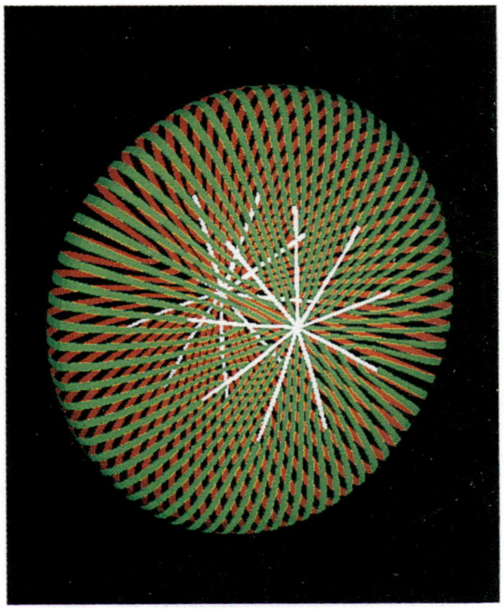

(f)

Figure 4.16(f) The symmetrical crystalline latticework formed by exactly offsetting anterior and posterior star sutures.

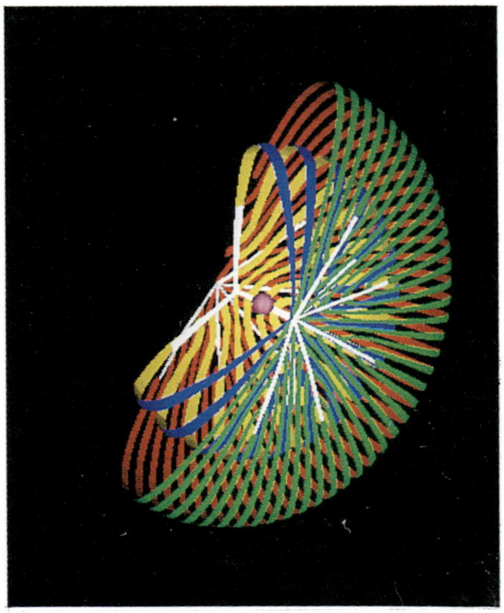

(h)

Figure 4.16(h) The position of the embryonic nucleus, a portion of the fetal nucleus and a portion of the adult nucleus (deep cortex according to the nomenclature used in this book) shown schematically. (From Kuszak, Peterson and Brown 1991, with permission.)

has been demonstrated in lower vertebrates (Bron and Lambert 1984) it appears that in the primate lens this is achieved by an increase in the number of rows. It has been noted that the increase in row number occurs at sites of fibre cell fusion. These fused cells are pentagonal in cross-section instead of hexagonal, and are thought to possess positional information which directs the formation of the additional radial columns (Kuszak *et al.* 1989) (Figure 4.18). Fibre cell fusions are found throughout the superficial and deep cortex and also in the nucleus. SEM examination reveals that, as secondary lens fibre cells elongate towards their sutural terminations, a number of cells fuse. This exerts a fine control on the direction and extent of fibre cell end curvature (Kuszak *et al.* 1984, 1985, 1989).

Gap junctions are present between the lateral faces of contiguous fibre membranes as in other epithelia (Figure 4.19). Less numerous gap junctions are found within the interdigitating processes (ball and socket, tongue and groove) and more sparsely along the broad faces of the fibres. In the human lens only 5% of the lateral fibre membrane is specialized in this way. (Kuszak *et al.* 1978, 1985). The gap junctions of the fibres differ from those of the liver (and from those of the lens epithelium) in that their intramembranous particles are less densely packed, and the intermembranous gap is narrower (i.e. <2 nm) (Figure 4.19). Gap junctions are not found at the anterior and posterior tips of the fibres, and therefore not within the sutural zone. Their density increases towards the lens equator and thus their location along the fibre will vary according to the meridional position of the fibre.

The apico-lateral border of the superficial fibre cell is comparable to the apico-lateral border of the

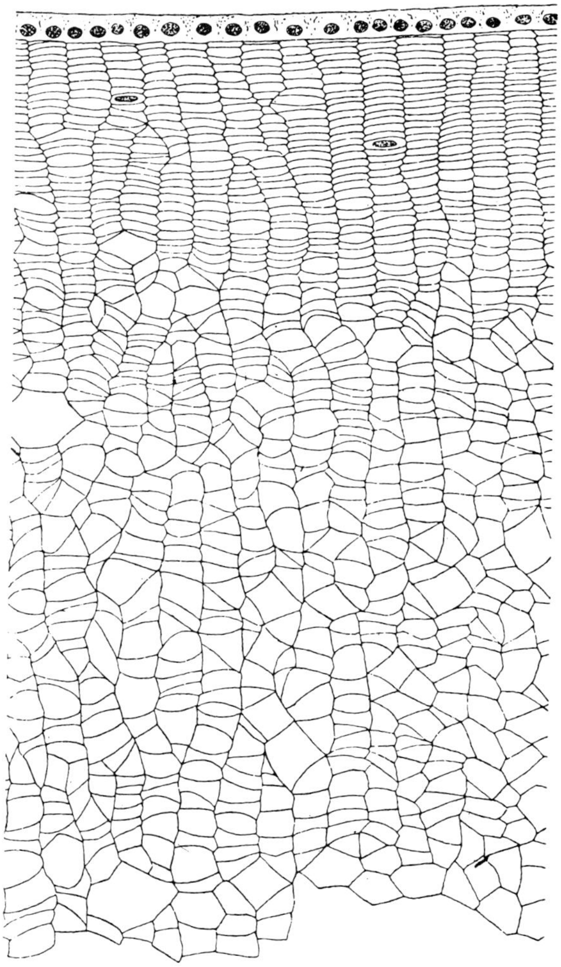

(a)

Figure 4.17(a) Peripheral portion of an equatorial section of the human lens to show the radial lamellae. (From Rabl 1900.)

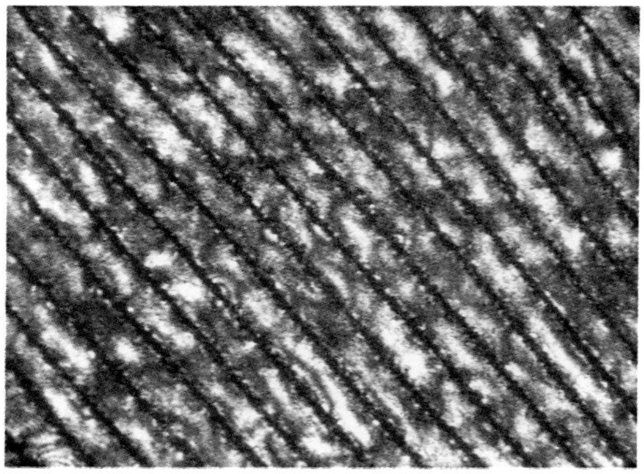

(b)

Figure 4.17(b) Confocal reflected image of the *in situ* crystalline lens. The spacing between the lenticular fibres is 7 μm. The image is back scattered light in the confocal mode. Reflected light confocal microscope image of the enucleated *in situ* rabbit eye. BioRad MRC 600 confocal microscope. Light wavelength 488 nm, objective Leitz 25x, 0.8 NA water objective. (Courtesy of B.R. Masters.)

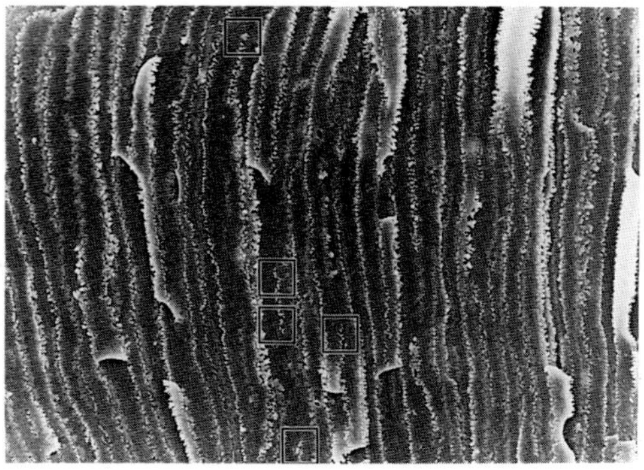

Figure 4.18 Fibre fusion and its effect on row number. (From Kuszak *et al.* 1989.)

lens epithelial cell. Both share endocytotic processes and pits, square array membrane and an absence of gap or tight junctions. The square array membrane is more prominent in the fibre (Figures 4.11b–e). Endocytotic events and square array membrane are also typical of the basal membranes of lens epithelial and superficial fibre cells. Square array membrane is also found in relation to the ridges and microvilli of the primary lens fibres. Zampighi *et al.* (1989) have suggested that they provide a unidirectional channel system. Kuszak suggests that they might provide a route of egress for materials passing from the fibres to the sutures, and hence towards the capsule posteriorly and the regions of transcytotic endocytosis anteriorly.

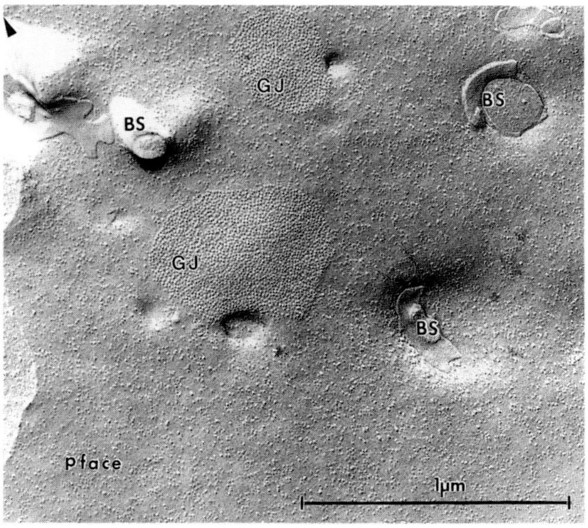

(a)

Figure 4.19(a) Cytoplasmic surface (p face) of superficial cortical fibre showing gap junctions (GJ) and fractured ball and socket joints (BS).

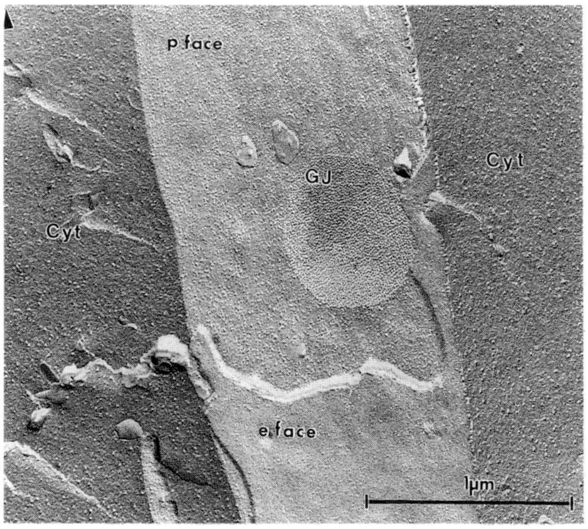

(b)

Figure 4.19(b) Intramembranous particles are common on the cytoplasmic surface (p face) and scarce on the extracellular surface (e face). Fibre cytoplasm (Cyt). Arrow indicates direction of platinum shadowing (SEM). (Courtesy of G. Vrensen and B. Willekens.)

5

Accommodation and presbyopia

Accommodation

Accommodation is the process by which the refraction of the eye is changed in order to focus an image on the retina. The term is used to imply focusing on a near object. In primates, including man, this is achieved by a change in shape and thickness of the highly deformable lens.

In the young emmetrope, when the eye is focused on infinity, the lens is at its flattest and thinnest as a result of the tension residing in the suspensory ligaments. Focusing for near involves contraction of the ciliary muscle and relaxation of zonular tension. The controlled elastic recovery of the lens allows it to 'round-up' and increase its refractive power.

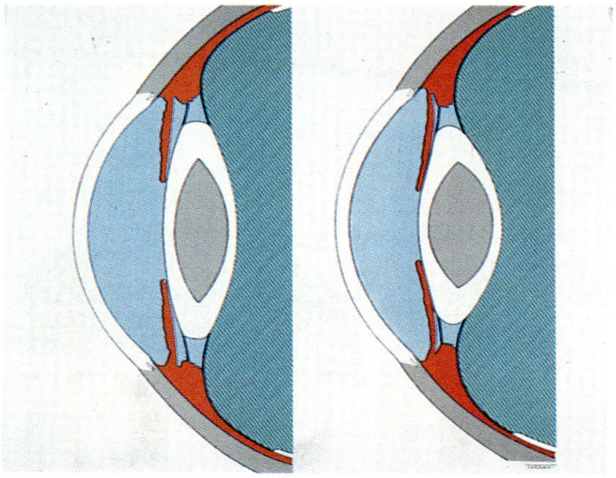

(a) (b)

Figure 5.1 The changes in the eye on accommodation: **(a)** unaccommodated state and **(b)** accommodated. The figure attempts to show all the recognized changes. Note constant location of posterior pole – see text for details.

The observed changes in the young adult lens during accommodation are shown diagrammatically in Figure 5.1 (Brown 1973):

1. There is an increase in curvature of the anterior lens surface which becomes more cone-shaped. The radius of curvature falls centrally and lengthens peripherally, while the parabolic contour is maintained. The coning is maximal at age 30 years and absent in the child. Changes are less posteriorly.
2. The lens centre and the anterior pole move forwards, while the posterior pole moves slightly posteriorly, or not at all (Brown 1973).
3. The lens nucleus is thickened and bowed forwards, while the overlying cortex is unchanged in thickness.
4. Lens equatorial diameter is reduced.
5. There is a reduced angulation of the lens capsule periphery at the line of insertion of the zonule.
6. The anterior chamber angle is widened peripherally and shallowed centrally (Figures 5.2).

The form of curve of the accommodated lens is age-dependent. It is close to being spherical under the age of 20 years and becomes increasingly conoid above this age, most marked by about the age of 30 (Figure 5.3).

Accommodation is brought about by contraction of the ciliary muscle, which moves inwards and forwards, so relaxing the zonule. The capsule then supplies the force to mould the lens into the accommodated state. The capsule is thicker in the region of the zonular insertion, but it appears that the differences in elasticity between the cortex and nucleus account for the conoid change on accommodation and that it is not the form of the capsule which accounts for the cone. In youth, the nucleus is the more flexible and, since the nucleus accounts for the main volume of the lens under 20 years, the change is spherical. By the age of 30, the nucleus is confined to the central region and, in accommodation, carries the central region of the cortex forward, thus causing the central region of the anterior capsule to cone. The change in form of the lens substance requires a redistribution of the cytoplasm within each fibre, since the fibres cannot slide over one another (Travers 1990). The cytoplasm is assumed to flow in an axial direction as the lens accommodates. The speed of accommodation is extraordinarily rapid and has been studied by Koretz using a video adaptation of the Oxford CCD slit-image camera. She demonstrated that accommodation occurs within 0.1 secs and disaccommodation over a similar period. The limiting factor is assumed to be the movement of cytoplasm within the lens fibres.

The vitreous has been cast in an active role by some authors, but would appear to have at the most a minimal effect in stabilizing the position of the posterior pole, since accommodation still takes place after vitrectomy. The vitreous volume must remain constant during accommodation (Figure 5.1) but it has yet to be established whether it plays a part in determining the position of the posterior lens surface. The volume of the aqueous in the anterior chamber does not change at the time when

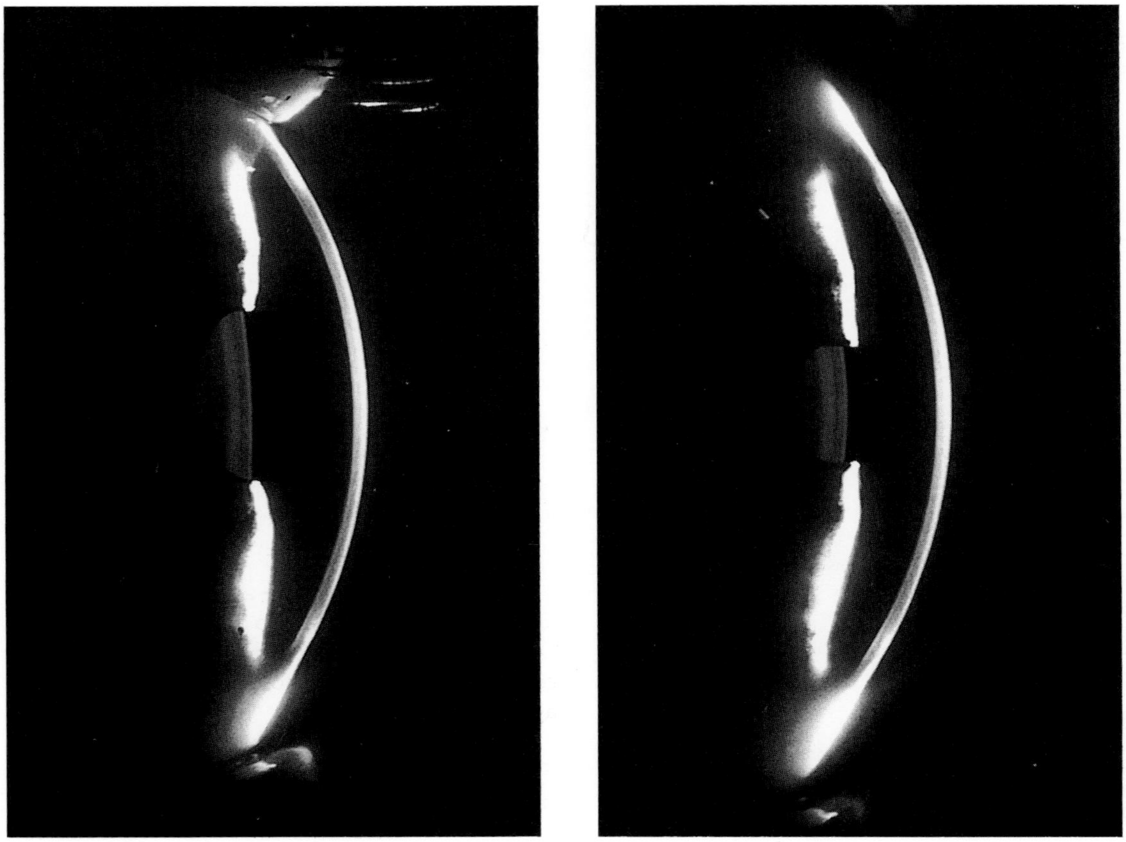

(a) (b)

Figure 5.2 The change in shape of the anterior chamber on accommodation: **(a)** relaxed and **(b)** accommodated. The iris is seen to bow back in the periphery with widening of the angle on accommodation.

the eye accommodates rapidly and so the aqueous is driven forward and causes the widening of the AC angle (Figure 5.2). This widening becomes reduced on prolonged accommodation.

Presbyopia

Presbyopia is the loss of accommodative range which occurs with age. The far point remains unchanged, while the near point recedes towards it. By the age of about 40 years the accommodative amplitude is as low as 2 dioptres, and even this may simply reflect the effect of miosis on depth of field (Figure 5.4) (Koretz *et al.* 1989). The process of presbyopia proceeds roughly linearly with age, and creates difficulty in the fifth decade for near vision in the emmetrope.

The events leading to presbyopia are not straightforward. The lens grows throughout life by addition to its cortical layers. There is a shift forwards of the lens centre, and an increase in both its anterior and posterior curvatures. Rohen (1952) has reported a forward movement of the internal apical region of the human ciliary body with age. This would decrease the zonular tension, and account for some of the increased curvature of the lens with age, the rest being due to lens growth. It would also be responsible for a loss of accommodative reserve.

With age, degenerative changes appear in the primate ciliary muscle, which include the appearance of membranous whorls, or 'fingerprints' within the muscle fibres, similar to those seen in denervated human striate muscle. Increasing

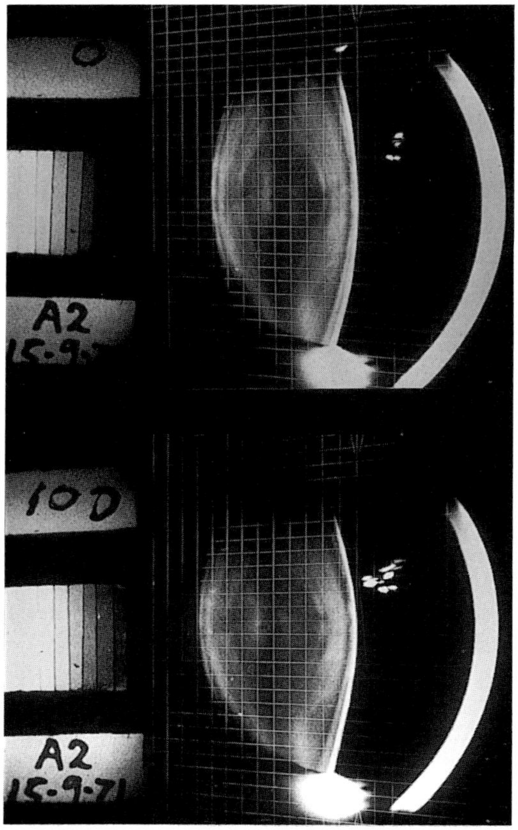

Figure 5.3 The change in form of the lens on accommodation in a 29-year-old: relaxed above; accommodated below. (Grid squares 0.4 mm.)

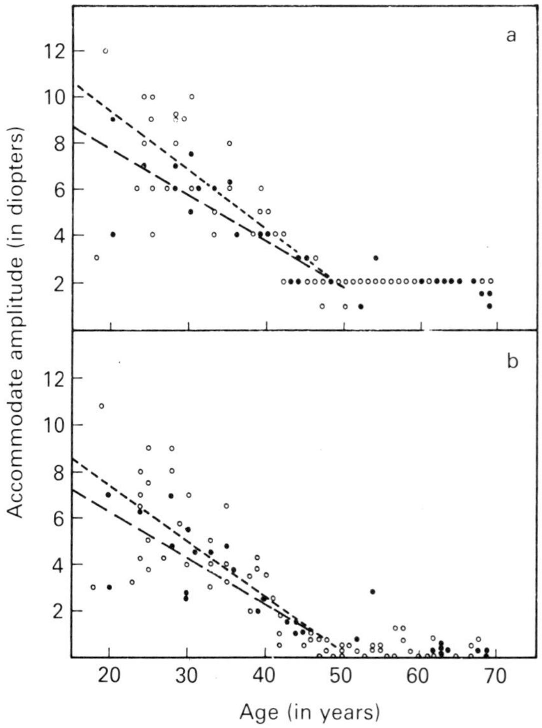

Figure 5.4 Decline in amplitude of accommodation with age measured subjectively and objectively. (Courtesy of J.F. Koretz.)

numbers of lysosomes and lipofuscin inclusions are also noted in human muscle fibres with age (van der Zypen 1970), and myelin figures are found within the nerve axons and terminals, just as have been described in striated muscle (Miller 1975). These changes have also been described in human ciliary muscle. Notwithstanding this, Fisher (1969) has calculated that the amount of force that could be exerted by the human ciliary muscle should be sufficient adequately to change the shape of the newly presbyopic lens. He estimated that at about 50 years of age the ciliary muscle 'is some 50% more powerful than in youth'. This estimate was based on measurements of lens deformability *in vitro*, where the directions of forces acting on the lens are not precisely known. Bito and Miranda (1989) have also queried the relevance in such studies of estimating ciliary muscle forces as opposed to the forces required to counteract the recoil of the extralenticular elastic components. Therefore the functional state of the presbyopic human ciliary muscle may still be regarded as unclear. In the monkey, it seems certain that ciliary muscle responsiveness, even to neural stimuli, is diminished (see below).

A significant event which has been established in both the monkey (Nieder *et al.* 1990) and the human eye with age (Hollins 1974; Enoch 1976) is the reduced or absent forward movement of the ciliary body on accommodation. The reduction in ciliary muscle area in meridional section which occurs in the monkey might indicate a loss of contractile cells, but although degenerative changes occur both in ciliary muscle cells and nerves, these are not of marked degree, and have been discounted as the major factor in primate presbyopia. Of possibly greater relevance, at least for the loss of accommodative ability in the aged monkey and probably in the human, is the thickening and alterred morphology which occurs in the posterior elastic tendons, consisting of a pronounced increase in the collagenous and microfibrillar content of the tendons. The tendons become almost completely ensheathed by collagenous fibrils, and the homogeneous part of the elastic tissue takes on an electron-lucent fibrillogranular appearance under electron microscopy, and contains abnormal scattered microfibrils (Tamm *et al.* 1990). Lutjen-Drecoll and Rohen have postulated that this structural change causes a loss compliance of the posterior insertion of the ciliary muscle in the monkey and limits the critical anterior-inward movement of the muscle during contraction which is essential to achieve zonular relaxation. Bito and colleagues lay emphasis on the decline and eventual loss of disaccommodative capacity (resumption of a flattened lens profile), and of the forces necessary to overcome the elastic components of the accomodated lens in presbyopia (Bito *et al.* 1987, Bito and Miranda 1989). They point out that, with the development of presbyopia in the monkey, the speed of disaccommodation declines more rapidly than the speed of accommodation. (Nieder *et al.* 1986, Bito *et al.* 1987). This is in keeping with the current knowledge of structural changes within the ciliary muscle, but it is important not to give undue weight to the disaccommodative step and neglect events which affect accomodation itself. The act of acommodation depends most on ciliary muscular contraction, while disacommodation depends on recoil generated by elastic tissue within the ciliary muscle and neighbouring choroid. Both are probably affected by the structural changes observed and are influenced by age-related changes in the intrinsic viscosity of these tissues.

These age-related ciliary muscle changes not only parallel a progressive decline in accommodative amplitude (Bito *et al.* 1982; Kaufmann *et al.* 1983), but are associated with a decreased responsiveness to pilocarpine (Lutjen-Drecoll *et al.* 1988) or to electrical stimulation of the Edinger-Westphal nucleus (Bito *et al.* 1987). This is unassociated with any change in muscarinic receptor affinity or density, or in the muscle content of choline acetyl transferase or acetylcholinesterase (True-Gabelt *et al.* 1987).

Presbyopia may result from a change in properties of the ciliary muscle, zonule or lens or a combination of all three. Those factors which are thought to be important are:

1. There is a forward shift of the internal apical region of the ciliary body with age, which reduces the reserve and therefore amplitude of accommodation (Rohen 1952).
2. There are relatively minor changes in ciliary muscle structure with age which could decrease the strength of ciliary muscular contraction and hence the speed of the accommodative step. Muscle innervation is unaltered but muscle responsiveness to pilocarpine or to neural stimulation, is reduced.
3. There is a major increase in the connective tissue content of the ciliary muscle with age

particularly in the region of the posterior elastic tendons. This is thought to decrease the compliance of the posterior insertion and limit anterior inward movement of the muscle during contraction and presumably disacommodative relaxation.

4. Reduction in size of the lens nucleus relative to the cortex, reducing the effect of changing nuclear curvature on the surface curvatures of the lens.
5. Increase in the modulus of elasticity of both nucleus and cortex so that they both become stiffer.
6. Increase in the stiffness of the nucleus relative to the cortex, with the nucleus eventually becoming the more stiff.
7. Reduction in the elasticity of the capsule.
8. Increased diameter of the lens, relocation of ciliary and lenticular attachments of the zonule, and increase in size of the ciliary body, all tending to reduce zonular tension in the unaccommodated eye.
9. Increased curvature of the lens surface. The nearer the lens becomes to a sphere, the less effect can the capsule have in further increasing curvature. It is as if the old lens becomes stuck in the accommodated posture.

The relative importance of these factors has not yet been adequately resolved.

Presbyopia occurs earlier in areas of high ambient temperature and the onset of presbyopia is more clearly related to the temperature level than it is to the light level (Weale 1981).

6

Biology of the lens

The chief role of the lens is to provide an optical component of high transparency and refractive index, which assures that objects may be focused upon the retina without excessive globe length. The additional function of accommodation enables near objects to be brought into focus by the relaxation of the suspensory ligaments. The speed of accommodation and its relaxation will depend in part on the elastic properties of the lens, which decrease with increasing age. As has been noted earlier growth of the lens proceeds throughout life, continuing well beyond the time at which ocular growth finally ceases, at about the twelfth year of life. Thus other factors must operate than those which control the growth of the globe as a whole. It is tempting to suggest that the 'need' for continued growth relates in part to the limited survival of DNA in the superficial cortical lens fibres and of the requirement to maintain a complement of lens fibres with a full metabolic capability throughout the life span.

The lens environment

The chemical composition of human aqueous and vitreous given in Tables 6.1, 6.2 and 6.3 shows that there is an ample supply of glucose for energy requirements (2.7–3.9 mM), although the level is lower than that in the plasma (about 76%, decreasing to 64% in the aged (Pohjola 1966)). Amino acids provide an additional source of energy. The levels of amino acids in the aqueous are lower than those encountered in the lens but are higher than those in the vitreous. Differing entry and utilization rates by the lens account for marked variation in plasma/aqueous ratios (Riley 1983). The pO_2 in human aqueous is about 60 mmHg, while the pCO_2 is 39 mmHg. The high lactate content of the aqueous (4.5 mmol) reflects its origin in part from the lens, whose metabolism is chiefly anaerobic, although it is derived also from the ciliary body (Cole 1984).

Cations such as Na^+, K^+ and Mg^{2+}, and HCO^{3-} and Cl^- ions are present in the aqueous at concentrations similar to those in plasma, while the concentration of Ca^{2+} is markedly less.

Ascorbate is actively secreted into the aqueous by the ciliary epithelium and aqueous levels are 10–20 times those in the plasma. Ascorbate plays an important role in protecting the lens from oxidative damage. Notwithstanding this, the H_2O_2 also found in the aqueous in low levels is thought to be derived from the oxidation of ascorbic acid in the presence of molecular oxygen (Pirie 1965). There is a direct relationship between aqueous ascorbate and H_2O_2 in the rabbit and guinea pig (Giblin *et al.* 1984) but not in human aqueous (Spector and Garner 1981). Glutathione, over 99% in the reduced state, is found at low concentration in the aqueous where it helps to protect against damage from H_2O_2 and other reactive species. A co-operative scheme involving glutathione, ascorbate and H_2O_2 has been proposed (Riley *et al.* 1980; Riley 1983) in which H_2O_2 is detoxified to water by a continuous low level supply of reduced glutathione.

Other constituents of the aqueous include steroid hormones, prostaglandins and catecholamines, whose roles in relation to the lens are not fully known (Berman 1991). Noradrenaline, for instance, is present at a concentration of about 0.8 ng/ml in patients with cataracts (Cooper *et al.* 1984; Trope and Rumley 1985). It is of note that beta receptors have been detected in the lens epithelium, linked to the cAMP system (Osborne 1991), but their role is unknown.

Insulin, which has no action on glucose entry into the lens, is found in the aqueous, as is insulin-like growth factor, both of which can act as growth factors for the lens. It is probable that other growth factors, such as β-FGF, reach the lens from the retina, and are important in the maintenance of growth throughout life. Receptors for each of these factors are found in the lens.

Proteins, chiefly albumin, are found in the aqueous in low concentration, at about 1/500 of the plasma levels, with a mean value of 12.4 ± 0.2 mg/dl (Tripathi *et al.* 1989). Hyaluronic acid is also present in the aqueous and imparts a viscosity which influences the outflow resistance. It has a concentration under 1/100 of that in the vitreous, and its wider average range of Mr suggests an origin additional to the vitreous, probably the ciliary epithelium.

Lens permeability

The capsule of the lens is freely permeable to water, ions and other small molecules (Hess 1911). The capsule is also permeable to protein molecules the size of albumin (Mr 70 kDa; molecular diameter 74 Å) and haemoglobin (Mr 66.7; molecular diameter 64 Å) (Fisher 1969a,b, 1973). Neither Friedenwald (1930) nor Fisher (1973) noted a difference

Table 6.1 Composition of human aqueous humour

Property or constituent	*Value*	*Remarks*	*Reference*
Volume	350 μl		Mestrezat and Magitot 1921
Ascorbate	1.06 ± 0.31 μM/g H_2O	Plasma + 0.042 μM/g H_2O	de Bernadinis *et al.* 1965
B_{12}	29.9 pg/ml	Plasma 271.9	Phillips *et al.* 1968
Bicarbonate	19.64 ± 1.4 μM/g H_2O	Plasma 26.47 2.64 μM/g H_2O	de Bernadinis *et al.* 1965
Carbon dioxide	pCO_2 = 38.6 mmHg	16 cataract patients	Thiel 1967
Chloride	134 ± 22.4 μM/g H_2O	Plasma 109 μM/g H_2O	de Bernadinis *et al.* 1965
Glucose	3.00 ± 2.04 μM/g H_2O	Plasma 6.33 μM/g H_2O	de Bernadinis *et al.* 1965
	3.70–4.78 μM/g H_2O	Plasma 4.72–6.66 μM/ml	Pohjola 1966
Glycoprotein	63–75 μ/ml		Cardia and Coriglione 1962
Hexosamine	14.9–18.3 μg/g		Meyer *et al.* 1938
Lactate	4.28 μM/g H_2O	Plasma 1.78 μM/g H_2O	de Bernardinis *et al.* 1965
Oxygen	pO_2 59.7 mmHg	Cataract patients, 64–90 yrs	Thiel 1967; Becker 1957
pH	7.21		
	7.38 (7.31–7.42)	Cataract patients, 60–94 yrs	Thiel 1967
Protein	Total protein 31 1000 mg/100 g		Kronfield *et al.* 1941
Sodium	162.9 μM/g H_2O	Serum 176.4 μM/g H_2O	Cagainut 1957
Magnesium	1 mM	Plasma 0.71–1 mM	
Potassium	4 mM	Plasma 3.5–5.0 mM	
Calcium	1.2 mM	Plasma 2.0–2.6 mM	
H_2O_2	0.024–0.069 mM	Plasma 0.02–0.10 mM	
Glutathione	1–10 × 10^{-3} mM	Plasma 0.1 mM	
Citrate	0.1 mM	Plasma 0.1 mM	
Urea	4.1 mM	Plasma 3.3–6.5 mM	

From Cole (1984) and Berman (1991) with permission.

in permeability comparing normal with cataractous lenses but Fisher noted a correlation between cortical water content and capsular permeability.

Leakage of the smallest crystallins, the gamma crystallins (Mr 20 kDa) through the lens capsule was suggested by Francois and Rabaey (1958) and others, and the presence of crystallins in human aqueous has been confirmed in normal eyes by a number of authors (Maisel 1963; Little *et al.* 1965; Sandberg 1976). Levels were found to be less than 50 ng/ml in non-cataractous post-mortem eyes, and raised in the presence of cataract. Alpha crystallins have been demonstrated in normal aqueous humour using antisera against native crystallins. This implies breakdown of fibre membranes and, given the permeability characteristics of the capsule, it is likely that it is some fragment or subunit component of alpha crystallin which is released. (Mehta and Lerman 1972; Manski and Spector 1972; Zouzias and Manski 1972). In cataractous patients, breakdown of the fibre membrane can release crystallin subunits or proteolytic frag-

Table 6.2 Biologically active substances and protein in human aqueous

Component	*Aqueous humour*	*Plasma*
Prostaglandins	2 μg/ml	
Cyclic AMP	8 μg/ml	
Catecholamines		
Norepinephrine[ab]	0.8, 1.14 μg/ml	0.311 μg/ml
Epinephrine	0.0–0.13 μg/ml	0.0–0.97 μg/ml
Dopamine[c]	0.12;0.32 μg/ml	0.037 μg/ml
Steroid hormones		
Testosterone		
Oestrogen		
Corticosterone		
Aldosterone		
Basic fibroblast growth factor[d]		
Protein[e]	12.4 ± 2.0 μg/ml	7000 μg/ml
Albumin[f]	5.5–6.6 mg/dl	3400 mg/dl
Transferrin[f]	1.3–1.7 mg/dl	
Prealbumin[f]	0.3–0.4 mg/dl	
Orosmoucoid		
α-$_2$-acid glycoprotein		
Enzymes		
Carbonic anhydrase		
Lysozyme		
Diamine oxidase		
Plasminogen activator[g]		
Fibronectin	0.25 mg/dl	29 mg/dl
Immunoglobulins	3.0 mg/dl	1270 mg/dl
IgG		16–218 mg/dl
IgE (iu/ml)		
Complement C2–C7[h]	< 0.745 mg/dl	

[a]Cooper *et al.* 1984
[b]Trope and Rumley 1985
[c]Nil detected by Trope and Rumley 1985, measurable quantities by Cooper *et al.* 1984
[d]Tripathi *et al.* 1988
[e]Tripathi *et al.* 1989
[f]Inada *et al.* 1984
[g]Geanon *et al.* 1987
[h]Mondino and Rao 1983a,b
From Berman (1991) with permission.

ments of appropriate size including monomeric gamma crystallin.

Estimations of the extracellular space of the lens have varied, there being general agreement that it is small. Tracer studies by Yorio and Bentley (1976), after removal of the capsule, gave a value of 1.3%.

It is likely that this small extracellular space limits the rapid diffusion of substances between the cells of the lens and there is some uncertainty as to the integrity of the extracellular space of the lens nucleus, particularly in old age. The absence of tight junctions between the lens epithelial cells also suggests that there is no major barrier across the epithelium and into the extracellular spaces between the lens fibres. This is of potential importance to the effects on the lens of drugs delivered topically to the eye, and could influence both their toxic and therapeutic potential.

Ion pumps and channels in the lens

The relative permeability of the lens membranes to Na^+ and K^+ ions varies from species to species. As in other cells, the intracellular K^+ levels are high (about 120 mmol) while Na^+ levels are low (about 20 mmol) in both the epithelium and fibres. This situation is maintained by the activity of a Na^+K^+ATPase pump concerned with the outward movement of $3Na^+$ ions coupled with the inward movement of $2K^+$ ions with each cycle (Figure 6.1). Electron histochemical studies have demonstrated the enzyme in the apical and apicolateral part of the epithelial membranes and in the superficial cortex along the fibre cell margins, but not in the posterior cortex along the basal (capsular) borders of the fibres, e.g. in the rat (Gorthy and Anderson 1980). A calmodulin-dependent Ca^{2+}-activated ATPase is also present in the epithelium and superficial cortex whose activity is about one fifth that of Na^+K^+ATPase (Iwata 1985; Iimuro *et al.* 1987; Borchman *et al.* 1989a,b). It is engaged in driving Ca^{2+} out of the lens cells. Na^+K^+ATPase but not Ca^{2+}ATPase activity is said to be detectable in the cortex and the nucleus.

The sodium and, to a lesser extent, calcium content of the lens, the sodium influx and potassium efflux, and the electronic conductance all increase with age and there is evidence that this is due to an increase in membrane permeability. (Duncan *et al.* 1989). These changes are seen in an exaggerated form in cortical cataract.

Total calcium in the transparent human lens is in the region of 0.2–0.5 mmol, while free calcium in the fibre cells is less than 1% of this. Free calcium is

Table 6.3 Composition of human vitreous humour

Property or constituent	*Value*	*Remarks*	*Reference*
Volume	3.9 ml		Mestrezat and Magitot 1921
Ascorbate	2.21 μM/ml		van Heyningen 1961
CO_2 (total)	24.1 μM/g H_2O	Plasma 35.2 μM/g H_2O	Davson and Luck 1956
Chloride	114 μEq/ml		Naumann 1959
Collagen	286 μg/ml		Balazs 1960
Glucose	3.44 μM/ml		Naumann 1959
Hexosamine	36 μg/g		Meyer *et al.* 1938
Lactate	7.78 μM/ml		de Vincentiis 1951
Mucopolysaccharide	240 μg/ml		Balazs 1960
Phosphate	1.2 μEq/ml		Naumann 1959
Potassium	7.7 μEq/ml		Naumann 1959
Pyruvate	0.81 μM/ml		de Vincentiis 1951
Sodium	144.0 μEq/ml		Naumann 1959

From Cole (1984) with permission.

maintained at a low level in the cells partly by the Ca^{2+}ATPase pump, and partly by a carrier based regulatory process linked to the transmembrane sodium gradient, through a coupled Na^+/Ca^{2+}ATPase. Calcium is sequestered in part in the endoplasmic reticulum. It is released in response to the action of several mediators, such as IP_3 (inositol, 1,4,5-triphosphate). Activation would lead to a rise in intracellular calcium. (Duncan *et al.* 1991). Increased calcium also occurs if internal cell sodium is raised by ouabain poisoning (Marcantonio *et al.* 1986) reducing external sodium concentration (Duncan *et al.* 1991), or oxidation of membrane thiols with *p*-chloromercuribenzoic acid (*p*-CMB), which appear to act by opening non-specific cation channels (Duncan *et al.* 1988a) (Figure 6.2). Much of the lens calcium is found in this sequestered form.

Experimental cataracts, such as those caused by naphthalene, 8-methoxy psoralen and selenite, and diabetic cataracts (Duncan 1981; Duncan and Hightower 1986) are associated with significant rises in lens calcium, accompanied by increased light scatter. In the diabetic rat lens, the regions showing greatest light scatter show the greatest increase in free calcium (Hightower *et al.* 1989). The formation of high molecular weight aggregates or proteolysis resulting from the action of calcium-activated calpain II (Shearer *et al.* 1987) may account for these opacities.

These findings are mirrored by those in human cataracts. Sodium and calcium levels are increased in cortical cataract, while both ions are normally distributed in nuclear cataract (Maraini and Mangili 1973). Both free and total calcium levels increase in cortical cataract, with total calcium rising from 0.1 mM to over 20 mM. Those regions of the cortex scattering most light have the highest internal calcium levels. Total sodium in such cataracts rises from 20 mM to over 200 mM (Duncan and Jacob 1984).

Removal of Ca^{2+} from the incubating medium *in vitro* causes a fall in lens potential and a twofold rise in K^+ efflux, which is entirely attributable to an increase in Na^+ permeability (Dellamere and Patterson 1978). When the anterior and posterior surfaces of the lens are isolated, Ca^{2+} lack in the incubating medium appears to cause changes in the anterior lens due to increased Na^+ permeability, and at the posterior lens face due to a more generalized increase in ion permeability.

The asymmetrical distribution of ions inside and outside the cell creates a membrane potential across the lens, which is negative inside, generated in part by electrogenic means and in part in response to the ion gradients created by the pumps. The potential (and hence the relative permeabilities to K^+, Na^+ and Cl^- ions) varies from species to species and also with age. Thus the resting voltage is about −90 mV in amphibia and fish (Duncan *et al.*

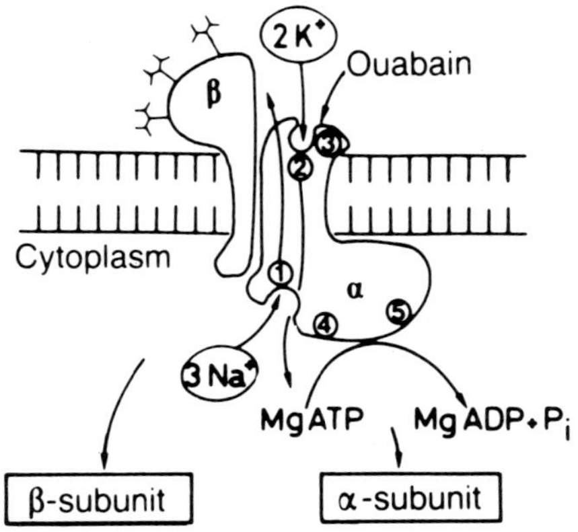

(a)

Figure 6.1(a) Model of Na^+K^+ATPase in cell membranes. There are binding sites for sodium (1), potassium (2), ouabain (3), phosphorylation (4) and ATP (5). (From Rossier *et al.* 1987 with permission.)

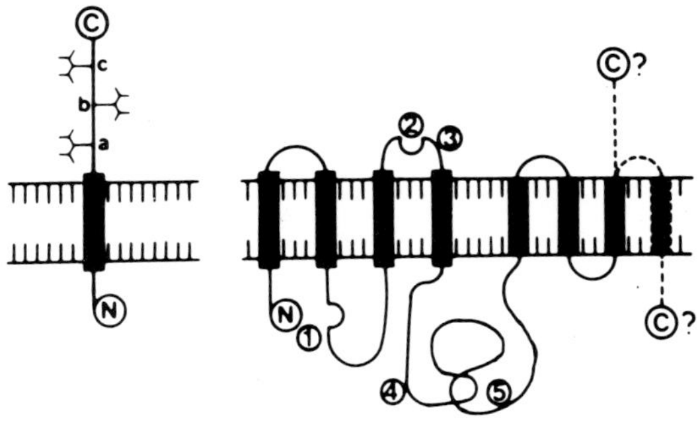

(b)

Figure 6.1(b) Model for membrane insertion of the β-subunit (left), and α-subunit (right). (From Bron after L. Rossier *et al.* 1987 with permission.)

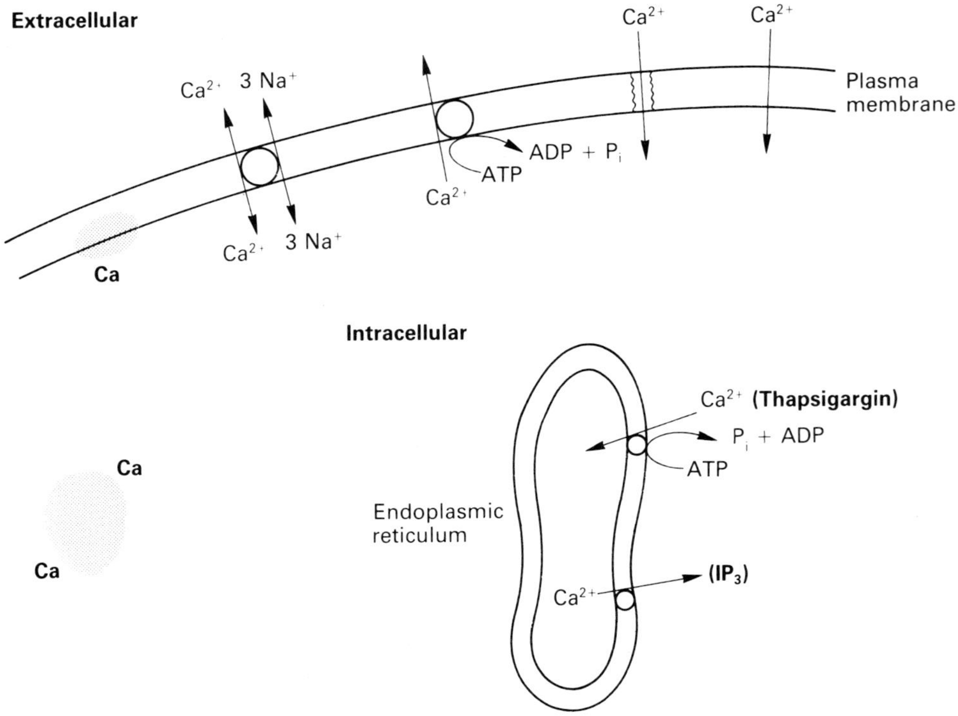

Figure 6.2 Outline of mechanisms for the regulation of lens internal calcium. These include influx through different types of channel and efflux via two carrier mechanisms. Calcium sequestration could occur through binding proteins in the membrane and cytosol and also by incorporation into a dynamic cytoplasmic store. (From Duncan *et al.* 1991 with permission.)

1988a, 1988b; Fraser *et al.* 1990), but only −20 mV in the older human lens. However, in the young human lens the voltage is about −50 mV (Duncan *et al.* 1989).

Since the size of the membrane potential is independent of the position of the electrode in the lens, it has been concluded that the lens behaves as a syncytium, with the epithelial and fibre cells in free contact ionically and electrically (Duncan 1969 a, b). Duncan attributed this electrical coupling to the presence of gap junctions between cells. Rae clearly demonstrated the movement of tracer dyes from fibre to fibre, which supports this view (Rae 1974; Rae and Stacey 1979).

The structural and functional features of gap junctions and their regulation differ between species and also with the age of the lens (Lo and Harding 1983). The coupling between neighbouring epithelial cells is very efficient and that between epithelial cells and fibres is poor. That between neighbouring fibres is age dependent. Thus in the frog lens studied by dye transfer methods, fibre–fibre coupling is poor for newly formed fibres, improves with fibre elongation, and is poor again once the suture is attained (Duncan *et al.* 1991).

Kinsey and his colleagues demonstrated an asymmetrical movement of Na^+ and K^+ ions across the lens, determined by the distribution of ion pumps and differential ion permeability. In this view the net outward pumping of sodium by the epithelium and cortex is forwards at the anterior surface of the lens, and is accompanied by a net inward movement of Na^+ posteriorly. Potassium is pumped inwards anteriorly and diffuses out posteriorly into the posterior chamber (Figure 6.3). This process, termed the 'pump–leak' system (Kinsey 1973) is generally accepted, but Duncan has pointed out that the hypothesis implies a low resistance of the posterior membrane of the 'syncytium' compared with the anterior, actively transporting, membrane while in fact the posterior is more highly resistant (Davson 1990).

Studies of the human lens *in vitro* show a small translenticular potential of 7 mV, which is reduced to 5.7 mV by application of ouabain (an inhibitor of Na^+K^+ATPase) to the anterior face of the lens (Platsch and Wiederholt 1981). The short circuit current, which was found to be dependent on the presence of bicarbonate in the medium of the human lens, was also found to be reduced, by about 30% but restored by removal of Na^+ from the medium. Duncan *et al.* (1988b) could find no difference in membrane potential between frog lens epithelium and whole lens, nor in sensitivity to K^+, and concluded that the channels are of the same nature in epithelial and fibre cells, but that their density is much higher in the epithelium. The bow region appears to have a higher density of Ca^{2+} activated K^+ channels (also voltage sensitive), and this sets up a circulating current. The major asymmetry in the lens is thus *not* anterior to posterior, but rather from the equator to the anteroposterior axis.

Studies by Robinson and Patterson (1983) and Parmalee (1986) suggest that the central zones of the lens fibres are relatively more polarized than their tips, explaining the steady current flow from the equator to the poles, with an outward K^+ current at the equator and an inward Na^+ current at the poles in relation to the fibre tips (i.e. at the sutures). Current was increased in a Ca^{2+}-free medium (which would tend to increase Na^+ permeability), suggesting a greater tendency of the fibre tips to depolarize through high permeability to Na^+ (Parmalee *et al.* 1985).

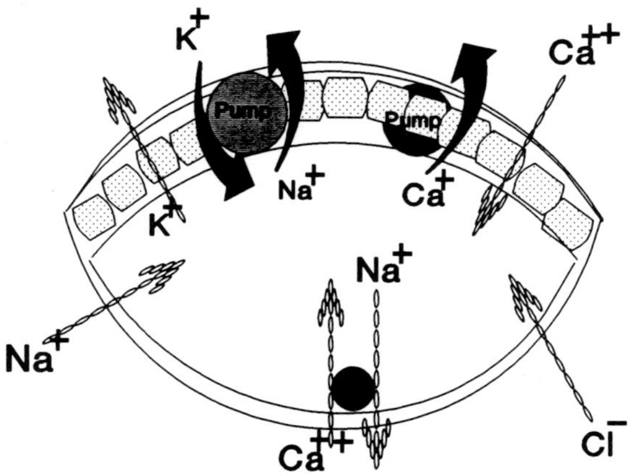

Figure 6.3 Schema for ion movement across lens membranes. (After Kinsey and Hightower 1977.) The presence of Ca^{++} activated K^+ channels at the equator introduces an asymmetry in ion movement which is not shown in the figure. See text for details.

The lens must continually extrude protons (H^+) for two main reasons. First, in common with most cells the lens has a relatively high negative resting potential, so that there is an inwardly directed electrical gradient for mobile positive charge. Secondly, since lens metabolism is chiefly anaerobic, there is a continuous production of protons from lactic acid (Williams *et al.* 1992). A number of systems exist to regulate the internal pH of cells. These include Na^+–H^+, Cl^-–HCO_3^- and the quadruple Na^+–Cl^-–H^+–HCO_3^- exchangers. The pH of the outermost cells of the rat lens is about 7.0 (Bassnett and Duncan 1985). The Na^+–H^+ exchanger plays a major role in pH regulation in the amphibian lens (Wolosin *et al.* 1988) and chick epithelium, and a Cl^-–HCO_3^- exchange system has been found in the rat lens (Bassnett *et al.* 1988). Further studies by Duncan *et al.* (1992) have provided evidence for the Na^+–Cl^-–H^+–HCO_3^- exchanger in the rat lens. The mechanism does not discriminate between Cl^- and HCO_3^-. Anion exchange is coupled to the external Na^+ gradient to provide an energetically feasible transport and a high intracellular pH. Although the system may use cAMP to modulate Cl^- efflux, the manner by which the system senses pH is not known. Similar evidence has been adduced for these transporters in the bovine lens epithelium, in which a lactate–H^+ cotransporter has also been demonstrated (Williams *et al.* 1992). In the amphibian lens epithelium the Na^+–H^+ exchanger is activated by a change in lens volume (Wolosin *et al.* 1988), but the bovine exchanger does not exhibit this sensitivity (Williams *et al.* 1992) (Figure 6.4). The principal intraepithelial buffer is bicarbonate (Williams *et al.* 1992).

Experimental oxidation of lens membrane thiols by *p*-CMP causes an increase in membrane permability similar to that encountered in the ageing lens and, more dramatically, in cortical cataract (Duncan *et al.* 1989; Tomlinson and Duncan 1991). In the human lens there is evidence for oxidation of membrane thiols both with age and cataract (Garner and Spector 1980). Membrane changes are associated with a rise in internal cell sodium and calcium concentration due to the activation of a non-specific cation channel which is the most abundant channel demonstrated by the patch clamp technique (Rae 1985). This channel predominately conducts Na^+ in the physiological situation, but Ca^{2+} is also able to pass (Cooper *et al.* 1986). Tomlinson and Duncan (1991) have also shown that Ca^{2+} influx into the lens in the *p*-CMB experiments is inhibited by the voltage gated L-type Ca^{2+} channel antagonist diltiazem, but by amiloride only at high concentration (1 mmol) where it acts as an L and T type blocker. Two antagonists which will block K^+ channels, quinine and EIPA, were also effective in reducing Ca^{2+} influx.

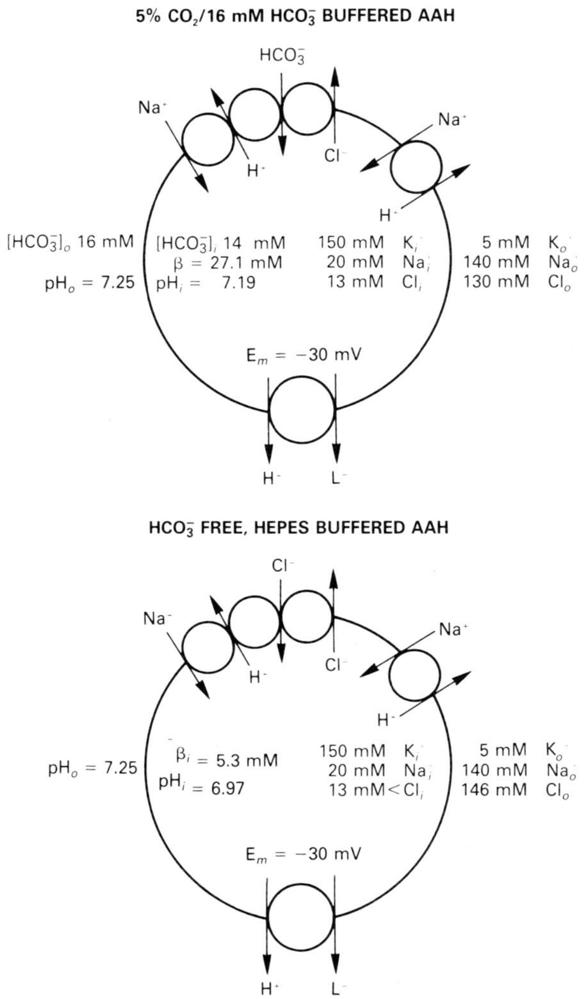

Figure 6.4 Summary of acid-regulating systems present in bovine lens cells together with relevant membrane potential and ionic data. The internal concentrations of Na^+, K^+, and Cl^- are whole bovine lenses, (recalculated from data given in Duncan and Bushell 1976, while the membrane potential data are taken from Jentsch *et al.* 1985.) The internal bicarbonate concentration in control artificial aqueous humour (AAH) has been computed assuming $pH_i = 7.19$ and that internal $CO_2 = 5\%$. No Cl^- values are available for mammalian lens cells incubated in HCO_3^- free media and so the value in B has been assumed to be greater than 13 mM. (From Williams *et al.* 1992 with permission.)

Amino acids

Amino acids are transported into the lens coupled to the influx of sodium, and concentrations are higher than in surrounding fluids (Duncan 1974). The concentration ratio is particularly high for the acidic amino acids, glutamic and aspartic acids, e.g. glutamic acid is 17× the aqueous and 35× the vitreous concentration in rabbit lens (Reddy and Kinsey 1962). The basic amino acids lysine, histidine and arginine scarcely reach twice the aqueous level, while other amino acids reach levels which are intermediate.

Despite their high lenticular concentration, glutamic and aspartic acids are least readily taken up by the lens (Kern and Ho 1974). They are preferentially taken up as their amides glutamine and aspargine.

Gap junctions and MP26, MP70

Gap junctions constitute about 5% of the fibre membrane surface in the human lens. MP26 (main intrinsic polypeptide – 26 kDa), is the principal intrinsic protein of the fibre cell membrane and originally was localized to the gap junctional domain using monoclonal antibodies (Sas *et al.* 1985). It is not found in the lens epithelium, whose gap junctions are morphologically different from those of the fibres (p. 33), and is only synthesized by differentiating fibre cells, appearing first in the secondary lens fibres, (Alcala and Maisel 1985; Revel *et al.* 1985, 1987). The gene for MP26 has been assigned to the long arm of chromosome 12 (cen–q14).

Early evidence suggested that MP26 was the lens fibre gap junctional protein but recently it has been suggested that it may serve as a volume regulating channel.

In the model proposed for MP26 by Gorin *et al.* (1984) the hydrophobic parts of the polypeptide span the membrane six times, while its hydrophilic part could operate as an aqueous channel (aquaporin). The terminal regions may offer a potential proteolytic cleavage site (Figure 6.5a).

Reconstituted lens junctions containing chiefly MP26 form voltage dependent channels in planar lipids (Zampighi *et al.* 1985), while incorporation into liposomes creates channels which are gated by Ca^{2+}/calmodulin (Peracchia *et al.* 1985). Lens calmodulin binds to MP26 (van den Eijnden-van Raaij *et al.* 1985). Within liposomes, freeze fracture studies and immunogold labelling show organized domains in the lipid bilayer similar to junctional complexes seen *in situ* (Dunia *et al.* 1987).

It is not known whether gap junctions in the normal lens are constantly open or whether this is regulated on a moment-to-moment basis, but it is likely to differ between cortex and nucleus of the lens, since there are morphological and biochemical changes which reflect this.

MP26 may be modified by two post-translational reactions which could modulate its functional activity; it is phosphorylated by two Ca^{2+}-dependent systems (chiefly at a serine residue), either through a cAMP system involving calmodulin and a G protein (Louis *et al.* 1987), or by a system involving protein kinase C (Lampe and Johnson 1989). Both phosphorylating systems are known to alter junctional permeability in other tissues, and

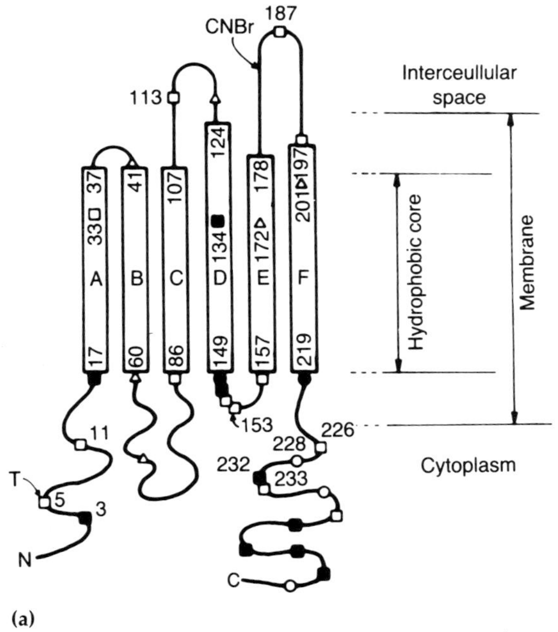

(a)

Figure 6.5(a) Diagrammatic representation of MIP based on the deduced amino acid sequence. The six putative transmembrane helices, labelled A to F, are shown as boxes with the amino acid of origin and termination indicated. Transcore regions of the protein are considered to have an α-helical configuration with a rise of 1.5 Å per residue. For the segments of polypeptide outside the membrane core, a rise of 3.3 Å per residue (β-sheet configuration) has been assumed to show the maximum possible length. All charged residues are indicated. T denotes a tryptic site identified by Edman sequencing. CNBr represents the site of cleavage that yields CB1. Arg, □; Lys, ○; His, △; Glu, ■; Asp, ●. (From Gorin *et al.* (1984) with permission.)

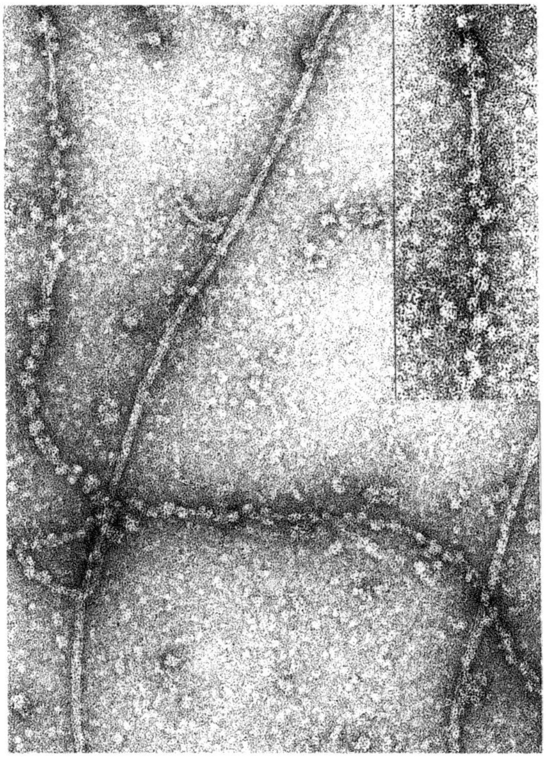

(b)

Figure 6.5(b) Beaded filament protein (From Ireland and Maisel 1984 with permission.)

could therefore influence the permeability of gap junctions in the lens.

Proteolytic cleavage of MP26 to MP22 appears to occur with age, and is responsible for the higher content of MP22 in the human lens nucleus than the cortex, and of its increase in older lenses (Roy *et al.* 1979; Broekhuyse and Kuhlmann 1980). Incorporation of the related proteolytic cleavage product MP21 in liposomes suggests that the carboxy-terminal part of MP26 could function as the gate which closes the gap junction and that, as a corollary, MP21, which has lost this tail, maintains an open channel (Peracchia *et al.* 1985). Thus the increase of MP22/21 polypeptide with age could render the lens fibre system vulnerable to injury, since damaged fibres would be less able to shut down communications between neighbouring cells. This would favour the spread of ionic and other metabolic instability to normal fibres and hasten fibre breakdown and loss of transparency.

More recently, another protein, MP70, has been thought to play a role as a gap junctional protein. It is confined to the superficial cortex, but its cleavage product, MP38, is found more deeply in the lens (Kistler *et al.* 1985; Kistler and Bullivant 1987). It is possible that MP70 provides a junctional role confined to the superficial lens fibres.

Other fibre membrane components (Table 6.4)

The membrane contains many other proteins, including two glycosylated proteins (33 and 35 kDa) which are bound to the membrane by Ca^{2+} and are EDTA-extractable (EEP). These proteins bind to actin and spectrin of the cytoskeleton (van den Eijuden-van Raaij *et al.* 1987). They may be endonexins (I and II); the 33 kDa component may be the core protein of the actin-associated protein calpactin I (Russell *et al.* 1987). The ability of these proteins to undergo phosphorylation suggests that they may play a role in regulating the cytoskeleton. Adrenergic stimulation can lead to phosphorylation of a number of membranous and cytoskeletal

Table 6.4 Proteins of the human lens fibre membrane

Membrane component	*Identification*	*Species*
MP 200, 250	Spectrin	All
MP 220–225	Fibronectin	All
MP 96–130	α-actinin	All
MP 90–107	Na^+K^+ATPase[a]	All
MP 86–95	Beaded-chain filament protein	All
MP 54–57	Vimentin	All
MP 43	Extrinsic protein	Human
MP 40	Actin	All
MP 32, 35	EEP[b]	All
MP 26	MIP[c]junction protein	All
MP 22–23	MIP junction protein	Mammals
MP 22	Extrinsic protein	Human
MP 20–22	Unknown[d]	Mammals
MP 17–18	Unknown	Mammals
MP 12	Unknown	Human

Adapted from Alcala and Maisel (1985).
[a]Sodium potassium activated adenosine triphosphatase
[b]EDTA extractable protein
[c]Main intrinsic polypeptide
[d]Lens-specific calmodulin-binding protein
From Harding (1991).

proteins (involving a cAMP-mediated protein kinase), such as vimentin or beaded filament protein, with the translocation of protein from cytoplasm to membrane. This presumably has implications for regulation of the cytoskeleton (Ireland and Maisel 1987, 1988). Cadherin, a protein which binds to actin, is also present in human lens membrane. Various receptor proteins are found in lens membranes, including beta receptors in the lens epithelium (Elena *et al.* 1987; Ireland and Jacks 1989).

Membrane lipids

The major lipid of the lens membrane is cholesterol (50–60%) with phospholipids making up the remainder. The ratio of cholesterol to phospholipid is 2:1 in the chick lens membrane, and higher in the gap junctions, 3:1, where sphingomyelin content is also enriched (Alcala *et al.* 1982; Alcala and Maisel 1985). Sphingomyelin is the most abundant phospholipid, and imparts rigidity to the membrane where cholesterol supplies fluidity. In human and primate lenses, phosphatidyl choline levels are low. Levels of phosphatidyl inositol (PI) are also low but this phospholipid performs an important role in supplying the key intermediates of the PI second/messenger system. Activation of the system can be stimulated by epidermal growth factor, glucagon and serotonin; it is activated in the developing chick lens (Zelenka 1980).

Choline is transported into incubated rabbit lenses by a special transporter, after which it is rapidly phosphorylated and can rapidly be incorporated into phospholipid (Kador *et al.* 1980b; Jernigan *et al.* 1981).

The cytoskeleton

The cytoskeletal proteins of the lens cells play an essential role in determining fibre shape, differentiation (especially elongation) and the organization of proteins and organelles within the cells. The three main classes of cytoskeletal proteins are found within the lens.

Microtubules, which are important elsewhere in the formation of mitotic spindles and, in neurons, in axonal transport, are found both in the lens epithelium and cortex, but not in the lens nucleus. The intermediate filament protein, vimentin, is also present in the cortex and is absent from the lens nucleus, while the vimentin-associated protein, plectin, is found in the membrane. Actin microfilaments are present in epithelial cells and fibres (Alcala and Maisel 1985).

Beaded chain filaments (composed of 86–95 kDa and 47–49 kDa proteins) appear to be unique to the lens and have been found in the fibres of a number of species. They are thought to provide attachment sites for crystallins (Ireland and Maisel 1984a) (Figure 6.5b). Another protein, termed band 4.1 protein (87–175 kDa), has been detected in the bovine lens (Aster *et al.* 1984). In the red cell, this protein forms stable complexes with actin and spectrin and also binds to tubulin. It forms a latticework which lines and is anchored to the red cell membrane. The proportion of 4.1 protein increases in the lens after differentiation, and it is presumed that this stabilizes the fibre membrane (Aster *et al.* 1985).

Messenger RNAs for the proteins α and β spectrin and α fodrin have also been identified in the lens (Yoon *et al.* 1989).

Lens water and water soluble components of the cytoplasm

About half of the lens water is in the bound (non-freezable) state which decreases throughout the lens with age. There is a parallel increase in free water. This release of water from the bound state is termed syneresis and is associated with an increase in the turbidity of the lens (Bettelheim 1985; Bettelheim *et al.* 1986).

Water soluble components of importance to the lens include ascorbate, glutathione and the lens crystallins.

Lens ascorbate

Ascorbate is present in the lens in as high a concentration as it is in the aqueous (1–2 mM). It has been suggested that it is transported into the lens in an oxidized form, as dehydroascorbate, and reconverted to the reduced form within the lens, where it may function as a powerful antioxidant. It may also have a pro-oxidant role, giving rise to active oxygen species, including H_2O_2 (Garland *et al.* 1986; Wolff *et al.* 1987).

Glutathione

Glutathione is present in high concentration in the lens cytoplasm (i.e. 1.43 μg/g wet weight) mainly in its reduced form. It acts co-operatively with ascorbate in:

1. Maintaining protein sulphydryls.
2. Scavenging free radicals and other reactive oxygen species.
3. Removal of toxic substances (xenobiotics).
4. Participation in amino acid transport as the γ-glutamyl donor, for example to cysteine or glutamine.

Glutathione is a tripeptide, γ-glutamyl-cysteinyl-glycine and is maintained in a steady state concentration in the lens by the operation of the γ-glutamyl cycle (Figure 6.6). Synthesis involves transport of the requisite amino acids into the lens, formation of γ-glutamyl cysteine, and the addition of glycine to form Glutathione, two of the steps requiring ATP and Mg^{2+}. About 12% of the total ATP produced by the lens is used in this way. The lens membranes are impermeable to reduced glutathione (GSH) but are permeable to its oxidized form (GSSG) whose concentration in the lens is consequently low.

The reduction of H_2O_2 to water by GSH is catalysed by glutathione peroxidase, and the resynthesis of GSH from its oxidized state is catalysed by glutathione reductase (Figure 6.6) with the necessary NADPH being generated by the pentose shunt pathway (Figure 6.7). Glutathione reductase is the rate-limiting enzyme in the glutathione redox cycle.

In the human lens there is a steady decrease in concentration of GSH with age; the decline in synthesis resulting from a reduction in γ-glutamyl

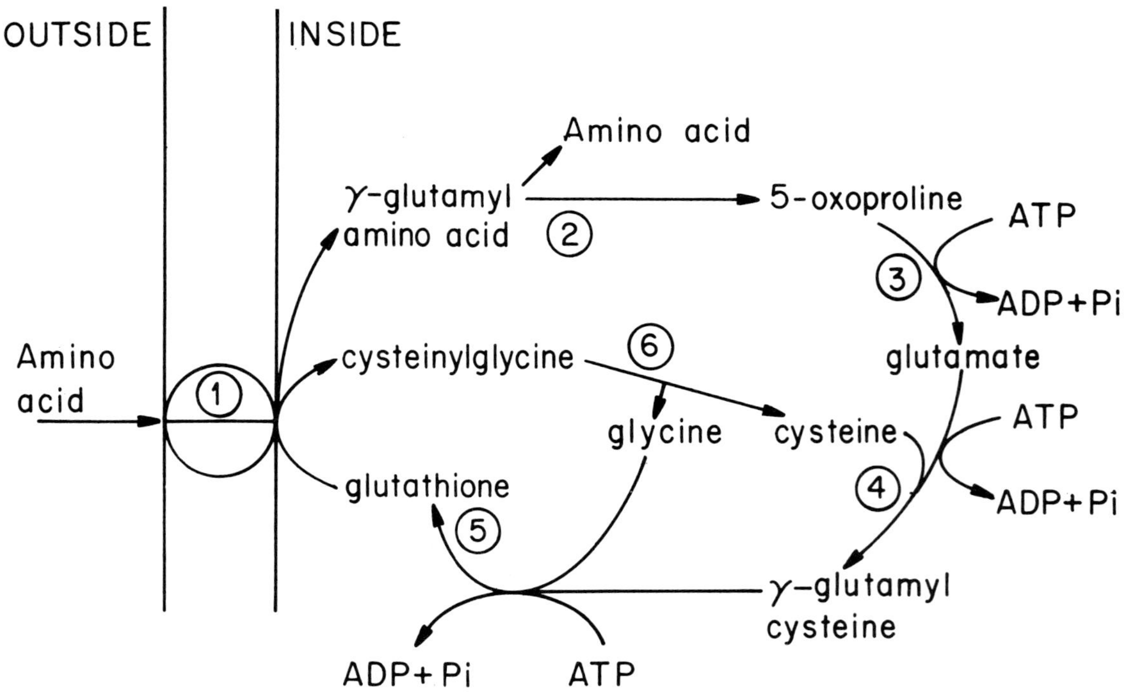

Figure 6.6 The γ-glutamyl cycle. The enzymes in encircled numbers are: 1, membrane-bound α-glutamyl transferase; 2, γ-glutamyl cyclotransferase; 3, 5-oxoprolinase; 4, γ-glutamylcysteine synthetase; 5, glutathione synthetase; 6, dipeptidase. (From Harding and Crabbe 1984 with permission.)

cysteine synthetase activity (Rathbun 1984). In the monkey, glutathione peroxidase activity is low at birth, increases until adulthood and then declines, while glutathione reductase falls from birth until juvenile life and then steadies (Rathbun *et al.* 1986). Detoxification of H_2O_2 probably also involves catalase in some species (Bhuyan and Bhuyan 1977) (Figure 6.8).

Glutathione is also involved in the detoxication of various hydrophobic compounds by a reaction involving glutathione-S-transferase and a series of steps leading to the formation of mercapturic acid (Figure 6.9).

Harding and Crabbe (1984), Harding (1991) and Berman (1991) may be consulted for further details.

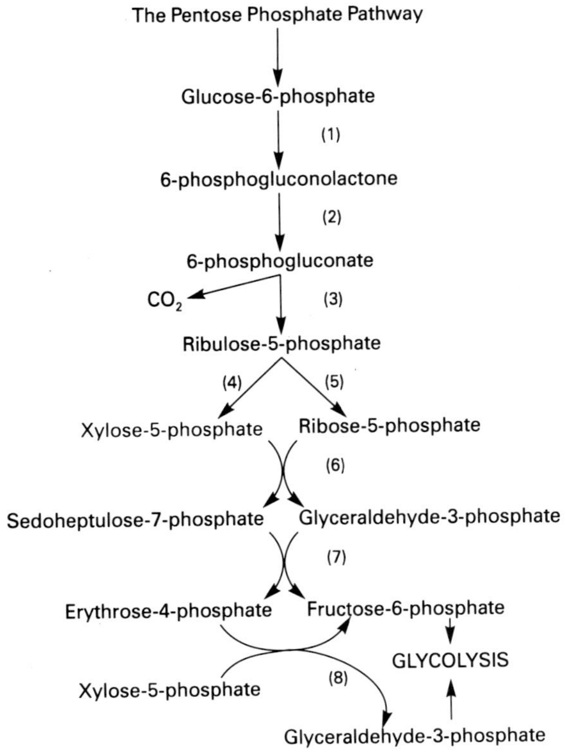

Figure 6.7 The pentose phosphate pathway. Enzymes: (1) glucose 6-phosphate dehyrogenase, (2) lactonase, (3) 6-phosphogluconate dehydrogenase, (4) ribulose-phosphate-3-epimerase, (5) ribosephosphate isomerase, (6) transketolase, (7) transaldolase, (8) transketolase. All these enzymes have been found in the lens. (From Harding and Crabbe 1984 with permission.)

The lens crystallins

The protein content of the lens is about 33% of its wet weight, and of a similar order to that of the liver. About 90% of this consists of the lens crystallins, proteins which were at one time thought to be specific to the lens, but which are now known to exist in other tissues (αB and to a lesser extent αA, but not the βγ crystallins), in some species such as the heart and lung (Wistow and Piatigorsky 1987). Their concentration in the lens provides the high refractive index necessary for the lens's optical function. In the human lens there is an increase in concentration of crystallins centripetally in the peripheral cortex which results in a graded increase in refractive index and probably serves to diminish spherical aberration. The crystallins have an important role in the transparency of the lens. Many of the genes controlling human crystallins are known (Table 6.5).

Until recently there were thought to be three major classes of mammalian crystallins, α, β and γ. It is now recognized that the β and γ genes are homologous and have arisen by gene duplication of an ancestral βγ gene, to produce the family of β crystallin subunits and closely related γ gene monomers. (Wistow and Piatigorsky 1988; Lubsen *et al.* 1988; Bloemendal *et al.* 1989). Two 'superfamilies' of crystallins thus exist, α and βγ, each showing a varying degree of peptide and three-dimensional homology within a family (Bloemendal 1985).

Alpha crystallins

Alpha crystallins are the product of two genes giving rise to the αA and αB subunits (Figure 6.10). αAp and αBp are phosphorylated forms (Voorter *et al.* 1986; Chiesa *et al.* 1987). Of the major crystallin classes, only alpha is found in the epithelium, and while phosphorylation of B chains only occurs in the epithelium, A chains are only phosphorylated in differentiating lens cells and not in deeper cortex or nucleus. This is presumed to have a functional significance.

There is remarkable homology (60%) between the A2 and B2 polypeptides and it has been proposed that they have arisen from a single duplication of an ancestral crystallin gene (Figure 6.10).

Alpha crystallin has a molecular weight of 600–900 kDa and is the largest of the crystallins.

One view of its tertiary structure is as a three-layer model accommodating up to 51 subunits (Bindels *et al.* 1979) (Figure 6.11). A and B subunits generally interact covalently, but a 43 kDa aggregate exists in which A and B chains are covalently cross-linked by non-reducible bonds (Spector 1984). Until recently, it has not been known what role the lens crystallins and their different subtypes provide, in addition to their contribution to refractive index and transparency. However, it has now been shown that α crystallin performs a chaperone role in relation to other crystallins and probably certain lens enzymes. This resembles the role of the heat-shock proteins (e.g. Groel) which prevent the denaturation and facilitate folding of other proteins in other systems (Horwitz 1993; Carver *et al.* 1994). It has been demonstrated that certain well conserved peptide regions in the α crystallins are homologous to a non-lenticular, heat-shock protein, or to the p40 protein of *Schistosoma mansoni* (Ingolia and Craig 1982; Nene *et al.* 1986).

In various species homology has been demonstrated between the lens crystallins and certain enzymes, such as the ε crystallin of duck lens which is homologous with duck lactic dehydrogenase (Wistow and Piatigorsky 1987). Other examples are given in Table 6.2. However, such structural homology is probably functionally incidental, simply reflecting an evolutionary recruitment of non-lenticular proteins to the lens, perhaps because of an innate thermodynamic stability (Wistow and Piatigorsky 1987).

Beta/gamma crystallins

The evolutionary relationship between the β/γ crystallins is shown in Figure 6.11. The beta crystallins exist as aggregates (except βs or γs,

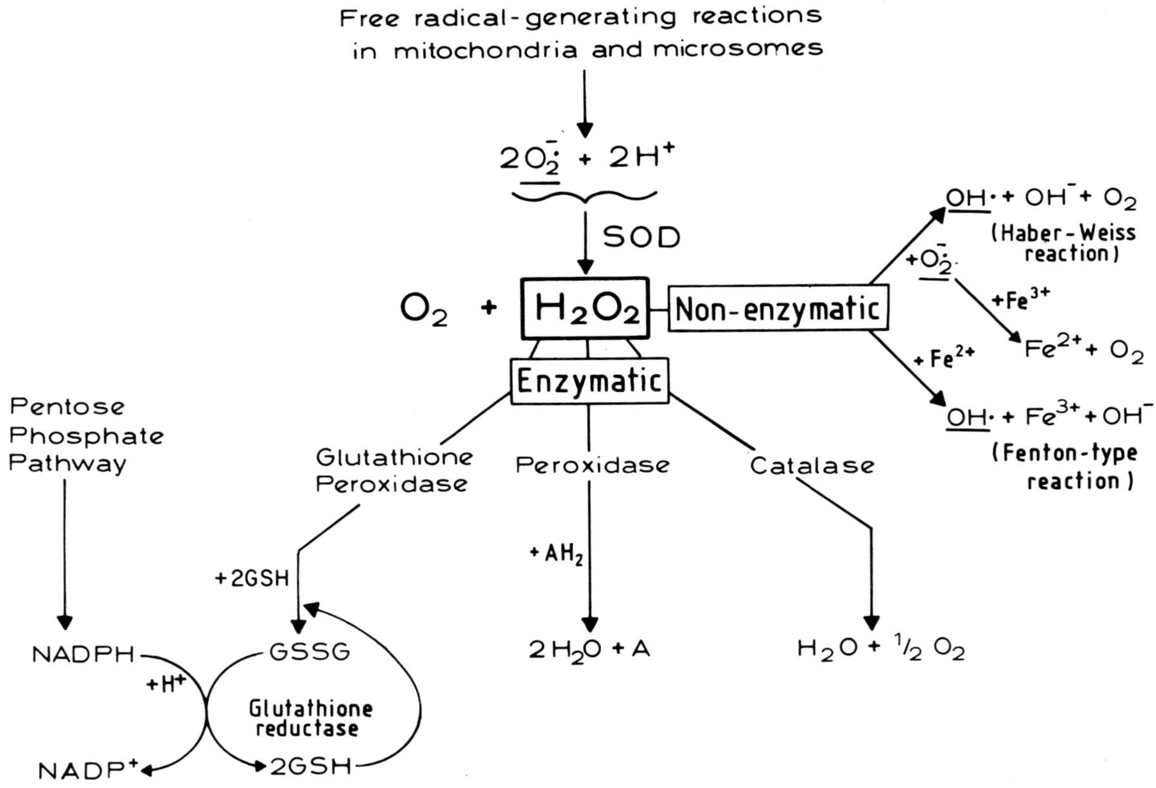

Figure 6.8 Degradation of H_2O_2 by enzymatic and non-enzymatic pathways. The free radical species are underlined. Maintenance of reducing conditions for the continuous generation of GSH depends on an adequate supply of NADPH from the pentose phosphate pathway. (From Berman 1991 with permission.)

which are monomeric). Their subunits are the products of 8–10 genes, and range in mass from 20–35 kD.

Their basic summits have C- and N-terminal extensions and some insertion sequences, while the 'acidic' subunits (βA) have multiple insertions but less prominent N-terminal extension segments. All beta crystallin polypeptides are none the less longer than the gamma. Thiol groups are at the surface of the subunits rendering them vulnerable to oxidation and available for cross-linking, while charge networks are also extensive at the surface of the polypeptides.

There is strong sequence homology between βB2 (formerly βBp) and the gamma crystallin γB (formerly γII). βB2 is a duplicated protein with two symmetrical halves and a fourfold repeat sequence within each half (Figures 6.10, 6.11b, 6.12, 6.13).

βs crystallin is most closely related to the gamma crystallins. It is monomeric, has a molecular weight of 21 kDa and, unlike the gammas, has a blocked N-terminal region and similar electrophoretic mobility. For these reasons, it has been renamed γs.

As noted above, the gamma crystallins are monomeric, with each subunit of molecular weight about 20 kDa. Five of the six crystallin genes are on the long arm of chromosome 2 (p3.3–3.6) (den Dunnen *et al.* 1985). The γ crystallin genes are labelled A–F. Two of the human genes are not expressed, and two are expressed at a low level, leaving γC and γD as the major crystallins in the young human lens (Siezen *et al.* 1987). γC and γD genes account for 81% of the γ crystallin transcripts in the human 'embryonic' lens, γA contributing 14% and γB only 5%; a gene gragment, γG, is also present (Brackenhoff *et al.* 1990). γE and γF have been regarded as pseudogenes by virtue of an in-frame stop codon, but it appears that the ψγE gene is transcriptionally active and does yield a properly processed and translatable mRNA although in low

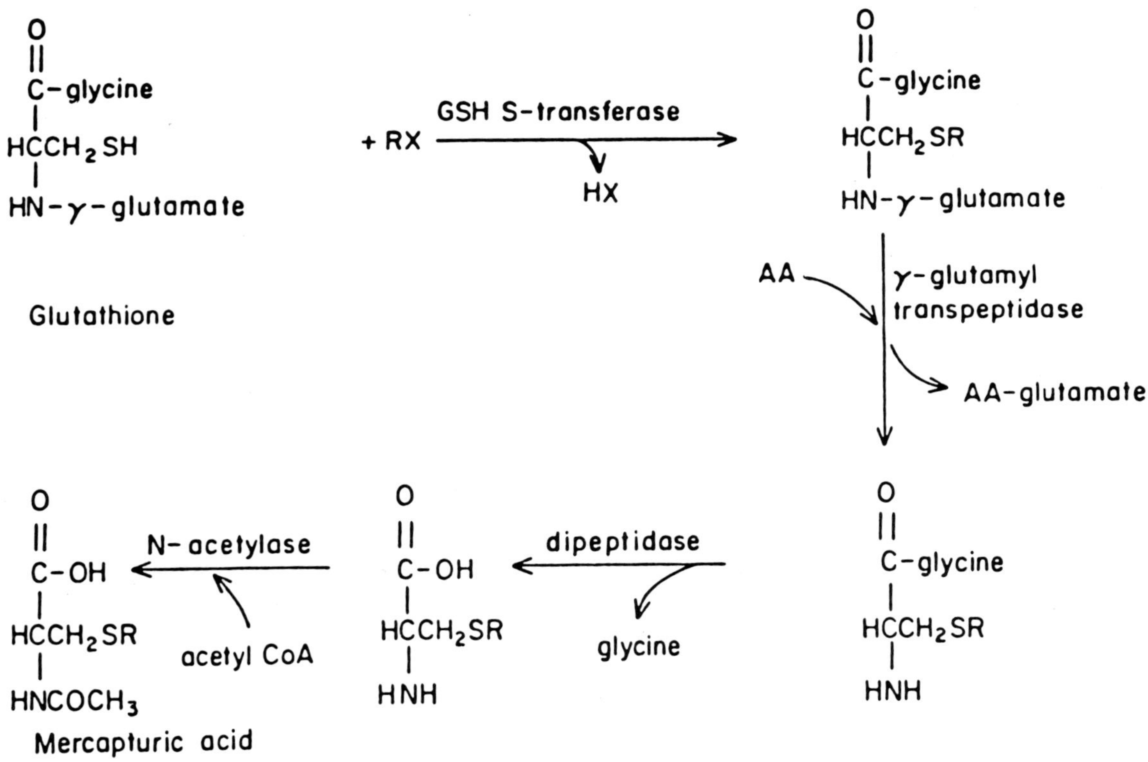

Figure 6.9 Proposed mechanism for the conjugation of xenobiotics and other substances with glutathione and the production of mercapturic acids. RX is a hydrophobic compound having an electrophilic group; AA is an acceptor amino acid. (From Harding 1991 with permission, after Awasthi *et al.* 1980.)

Table 6.5 Some properties of the lens crystallins

Property	α	β	γ
Molecular form	Aggregate	Aggregate	Monomers
Molecular weight	Over 5×10^5	$4–20 \times 10^4$	2×10^4
Thiol content	Low	High	High
N-terminal amino acid	Masked	Masked	Gly or Ala
Known sequences	A2, B2 Many species	Bovine βBp; a murine β	Bovine γ(II); a murine γ
Secondary structure			
α helix	None	None	None
β pleated sheet	Some	Some	Mostly

Modified from Harding (1991).

yield. In the dominantly inherited Coppock cataract (p. 168) mutation within the promoter region of the γE gene leads to an increased expression of γE, which is responsible for the embryonic/fetal cataract (Brackenhoff *et al.* 1994).

Brackenhoff *et al.* (1990) have commented on the decreased expression of the γ crystallins with hominoid evolution, both in quantity and complexity, a change correlated with an increased water content of the lens. The decreased expression is

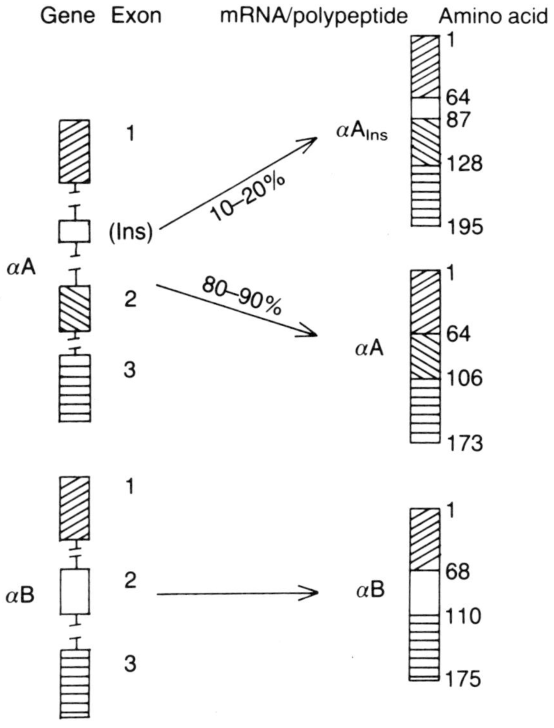

Figure 6.10 Diagram depicting the action of the αA- and αB-crystallin genes. (From Harding 1991 with permission.)

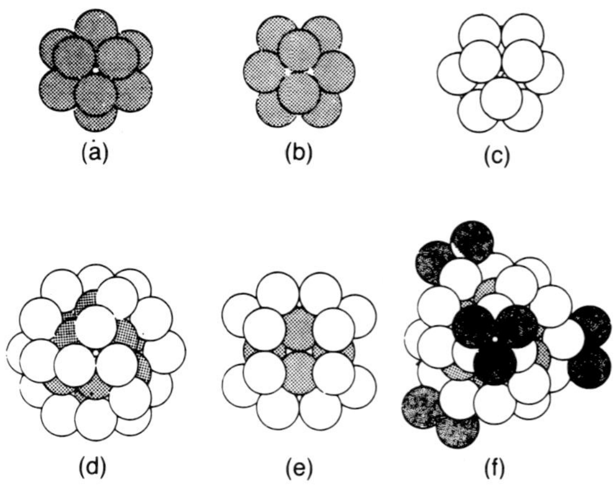

Figure 6.11 Schematic representation of the three-layer model of α-crystallin where the subunits have been modelled by spheres. (a) First layer seen from a three-fold axis. (b) First layer seen from a two-fold axis. (c) First layer of the model proposed by Bindels *et al.* (1979), seen from a three-fold axis. (d) First and second layer seen from a three-fold axis. (e) First and second layer seen from a two-fold axis. (f) First, second and third layer seen from a three-fold axis; only 12 equivalent sites were filled to yield a 48-subunit particle. (From Tardieu *et al.* 1986.)

attributed to various factors: gene loss (γG), inactivation of coding sequences (ψγE and ψγF), decreased rate of transcription (γA), increased rate of RNA turnover (γB) and a delay in the onset of transcription duing development. γD is a cryoprotein (γB was formerly γII and was the first ocular protein to be sequenced (Croft 1972)). The γ crystallins are rich in thiol groups and, in contrast to the beta crystallins, most of these are buried within the protein. It has been suggested that they may have a role in redox reactions or electron transfer within the fibres.

As noted earlier, it has been suggested that alpha crystallins perform a chaperone role with respect to the beta and gamma crystallins, by regulating protein folding during synthesis and protecting these proteins from denaturation (Horwitz 1993; Nicoll and Spector 1994; Rao *et al.* 1994; Wang *et al.* 1994; Carver *et al.* 1994).

Some features of the crystallins are listed in Table 6.5.

The weight of the lens increases steadily in utero, and is about 65 ± 1.9 mg at birth (Scammon and Hesdorfer 1937 and see Bron and Brown 1994). Bours and Fodisch (1987) calculated a prenatal growth rate of approximately 181 mg/year. Further growth rates have been estimated to be 181–24 mg/year in the early and late newborn period, 2.8 mg/year in the newborn-juvenile period and 1.43 mg/year in the juvenile-adult period. The dry mass of the lens also increases steadily, chiefly due to the synthesis of each of the lens crystallins (alpha, beta and gamma), in addition to the cytoskeletal and membranous proteins. At this stage the crystallins are readily distinguished from one another by a variety of analytical techniques, while, postnatally, separation is less distinct as they undergo post-translational modification. The core of the fetal lens is more hydrated than its outer part throughout fetal life. Studies of the protein and water content of the fetal lens, using a microdissection technique, have shown a steady dehydration of the lens core (Table 6.6) which, however, is of a much lesser degree than that exhibited in other species, such as the mouse,

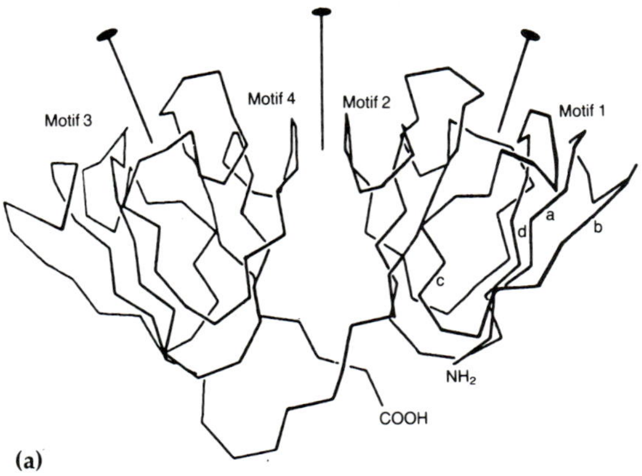

(a)

Figure 6.12(a) The three-dimensional structure of γB-crystallin showing two domains of similar structure, related by a pseudo dyad. The two motifs of each domain are related by a pseudo dyad. (From Summers *et al.* 1984 with permission.)

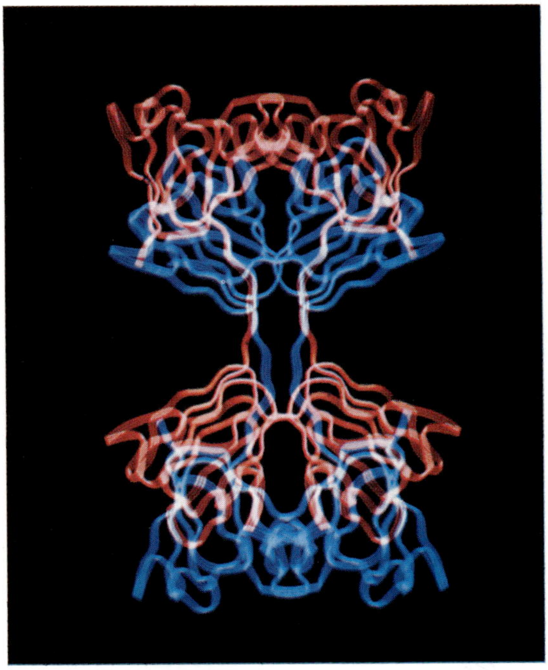

(b)

Figure 6.12(b) The three-dimensional structure of the major eye lens protein βB_2-crystallin determined by X-ray crystallography. There are four subunits, each of molecular mass 23 000, depicted by red and blue ribbons showing the conformation of the polypeptide backbone. The protein tetramer is very symmetrical, being intersected by three mutually perpendicular twofold axes. Note that there are two sets of four interacting globular domains separated by space that will be occupied by water. (Courtesy of C. Slingsby.)

rat, rabbit, dog and bovine lens (Bours 1987). The fetal lens becomes the nucleus of the postnatal lens. There is continued dehydration of the nucleus postnatally, but of much lesser degree than prenatally, so that dehydration is said to be increased by as little as 2% between the ages of 18–84 years (Bours *et al.* 1987). A gradient of protein density nonetheless persists throughout adult life (p. 31).

Bessems *et al.* (1990), have calculated the rates of synthesis of the lens crystallins during the period 112–231 days of fetal life. During this period, there is an increase in the proportion of gamma crystallins present, including gamma s, and a fall in the proportion of alpha crystallin (see Table 6.7). Total beta crystallin concentration remains the same, although there is a fall in high molecular weight beta crystallins (β1 and β2) and a rise in the remaining fractions (β3 and β5). Postnatally, gamma crystallin synthesis ceases. Thomson and Augestyn (1985) suggest that this occurs at or before birth, while Bours *et al.* (1980) reported that gamma crystallin synthesis ceased at about 5–6 years of age. Loss of gamma synthesis is probably gradual, with a preferential loss of 21 kDa gamma preceding that of 19 kDa gamma. The role of gamma crystallin for the fetal lens can only be

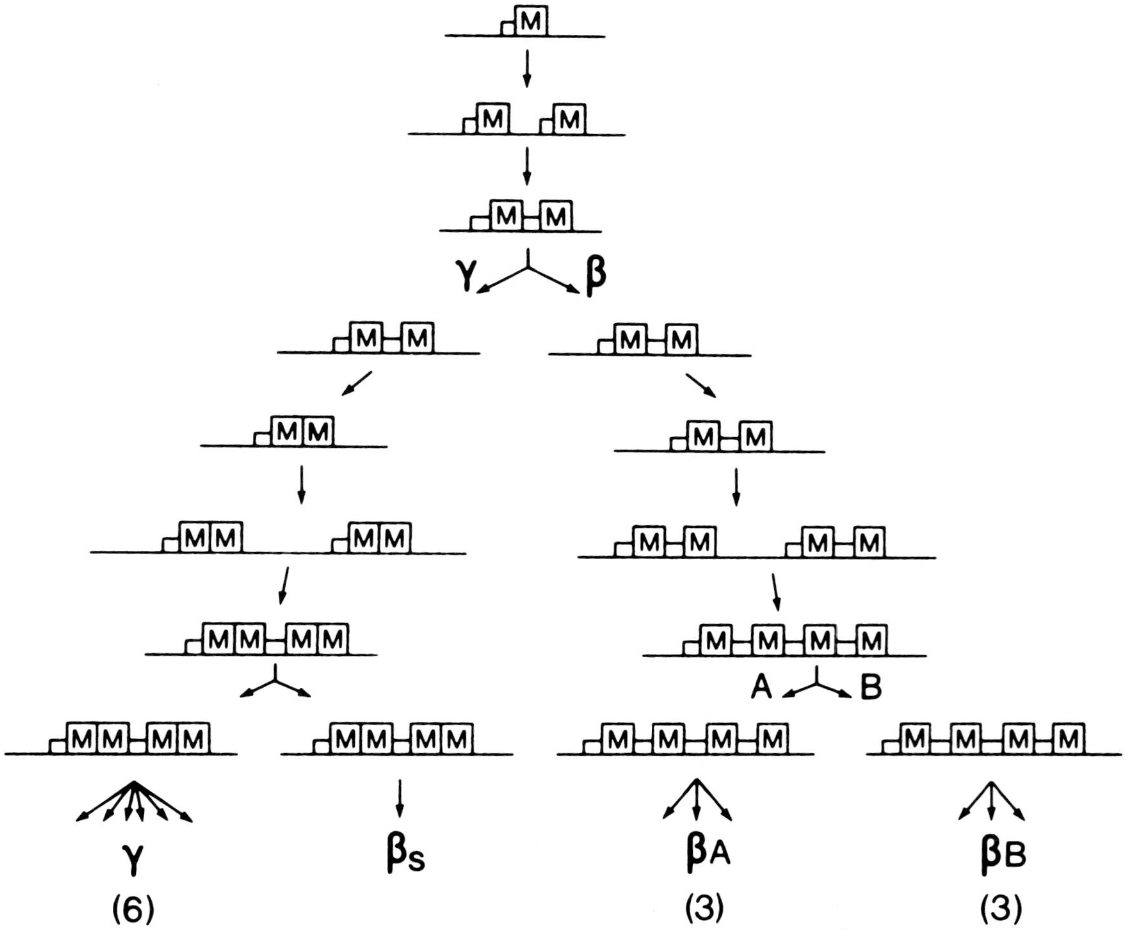

Figure 6.13 Schematic view of the evolution of the present β- and γ-crystallin gene families from an ancestral one-motif sequence. The region encoding a single motif is shown as a boxed M. The numbers between brackets at the bottom of the figure indicate the number of members of a particular gene family. (From Lubsen *et al.* 1988 with permission.)

Table 6.6 Dry mass and hydration of the fetal and adult lens

**	*f175 days*		*f285 days*		*62 years*		*68 years*	
	OUTER	*CORE*	*OUTER*	*CORE*	*CORTEX*	*NUC*	*CORTEX*	*NUC*
Dry mass	10.6%	15.6%	19.2%	25.1%	6.4%	28.7%	21.2%	45.0%
Hydration*	8.5	5.4	4.2	3.0	–	2.5	–	1.2

$$\text{*Quotient} = \frac{\text{WATER}}{\text{DRY WEIGHT}}$$

**From Bours, Födisch and Hockwin (1987).
f = fetal

speculated. It is the most ordered and most stable of the crystallins, with the lowest molecular size, and the greatest rigidity. It is possible that it performs a special function in relation to the differentiating fetal lens fibres in the special environmental of the fetal eye, or that its role relates to the maintenance of transparency of the lens nucleus in adult life. However, it must be noted that the concentration of gamma crystallin in the nucleus falls postnatally, due to post-translational modification and to uptake into high molecular weight (HMW) aggregates. Its concentration in the fetal lens is about 22.5% while that in the adult lens (at 74 years) is about 2.6% (Bours *et al.* 1989).

Although the crystallins are found in the soluble protein fraction during fetal life, an HMW crystallin fraction can be detected by the 119th day of fetal life, which is composed chiefly of low molecular weight alpha crystallin, with small amounts of beta and gamma crystallin incorporated. After birth, the relative amount of beta crystallin incorporated increases. The incorporation of crystallins into HMW aggregates within the lens nucleus is most striking between the ages of 35 and 45 years, although it proceeds beyond this time. It has been suggested that, since change in nuclear shape is important to the accommodative process, an increase in viscosity of nuclear crystallins, due to an accumulation of HMW aggregates might contribute in a major way to the loss of accommodation after the age of 45 years.

Table 6.7 Change in fetal crystallin concentration with age

Crystallin	*Percent*	
	f119 days	*f231 days*
Total alpha	23.5	19.6
Total beta	49.3	42.6
Gamma (1,2,3)	25.6	29.1
Gamma S	6.1	7.2

From Ahrend *et al.* (1987). f = fetal

The energy and carbohydrate metabolism of the lens

Glucose is the chief source of energy of the lens (van Heyningen 1969a) and although fatty acids can be metabolized in a similar way, entering the tricarboxylic acid cycle at the level of acetyl CoA, the supply of triglyceride or free fatty acid from the aqueous does not provide significant energy from this source. Some amino acids can also be metabolized, with the production of energy after decarboxylation and deamidation and the flux through this pathway *in vitro* can be increased when the availability of glucose is reduced (Trayhurn and van Heyningen 1972, 1973a, 1973b; van Heyningen and Linklater 1975).

Glucose enters the lens by a facilitated transport mechanism which is stereo specific for D-glucose and blocked by cytochalasin B. The transporter has been shown to be located primarily in membranes of the cortical and nuclear lens fibres of the monkey lens with very little in the epithelium. It occupies about 0.5% of total membrane protein in the monkey (Lucas and Zigler 1987, 1988).

Glycolysis and the tricarboxylic acid cycle

Transparency of the incubated lens cannot be maintained in the absence of glucose but, if adequate glucose is present, it will remain transparent in the absence of oxygen (Reddy and Kinoshita 1962). This reflects the fact that ATP generation in the lens is predominantly an anaerobic process, occurring in its metabolizing, cortical fibres. Aerobic breakdown of glucose through the tricarboxylic acid (Krebs) cycle also takes place in the lens, mainly in the epithelium, but also in the superficial lens fibres, which are sparsely equipped with mitochondria. Because aerobic metabolism generates higher amounts of ATP per molecule of glucose than anaerobic glycolysis, it transpires that one-third of the energy production by the lens is produced aerobically, chiefly by the epithelium, from only 3% of the glucose consumed by the lens (about 3–5 mg/day in the rabbit) (Kleifeld and Hockwin 1960; Sippel 1962).

The ATP generated in the epithelium and superficial cortex is presumably of particular importance in providing the energy for ion pumps, and mitosis in the epithelium, and the major synthetic requirements of differentiating cells. In general, in the cortical lens fibres it is required for the synthesis of the crystallins, cytoskeletal proteins, enzymes, membrane proteins and lipids, and for various housekeeping activities within the cells such as transport. Metabolic activity in the nucleus of the lens is at a low level, although mRNA for lens crystallins has been detected.

Glucose enters the lens cells by facilitated transport, using energy generated by the sodium gradient across the cell membranes. This arises from the activity of the Na^+K^+ATPase pump. Within the cells it enters the first stage of glycolysis in which each glucose molecule is converted to two pyruvate molecules (Figure 6.14). This takes place in the cytosol and does not involve molecular oxygen.

All of the intermediates of glycolysis are phosphorylated. Phosphorylation of glucose itself to form glucose-6-phosphate involves the enzyme hexokinase and provides a rate-limiting step in glycolysis. ATP is generated during glycolysis by the transfer of high energy phosphate bonds from phosphorylated intermediates to ADP. This process of substrate level phosphorylation, occurs in the cytosol and yields a net gain of two ATP molecules for each molecule of glucose converted to pyruvate. With the formation of pyruvate, four hydrogen atoms are produced (four protons, four electrons) during the phosphorylation of glyceraldehyde-3-phosphate:

$$\underset{\text{glucose}}{C_6H_{12}O_6} \rightarrow \underset{\text{pyruvate}}{2C_3H_4O_3} + \underset{\text{hydrogen}}{4H}$$

Four electrons and two protons are transferred to two molecules of NAD^+, to produce two molecules of NADH.

In the relatively anaerobic conditions of the cortical lens fibres, pyruvate is converted to lactate by the action of lactic dehydrogenase using NADH as a cofactor. The availability of NADH may regulate the production of lactate by the lens; it is also influenced by the level of intracellular calcium (Hightower and Harrison 1987). Lactate released from the lens makes a major contribution to aqueous lactate levels (Table 6.1).

In the lens epithelium, where aerobic conditions obtain, pyruvate in the cytosol is transported across the mitochondrial membrane. The complete oxidation of pyruvate to CO_2 and H_2O occurs in the mitochondrion using molecular oxygen as the final electron acceptor (Darnell *et al.* 1990).

Pyruvate passes across the membranes of the mitochondria to enter the matrix. Here it reacts with coenzyme A to form acetyl CoA, which may then enter the citric acid cycle (Figure 6.15). Acetyl CoA provides a route also for the oxidation of fatty acids and many amino acids, and is involved as an intermediate in biosynthetic reactions such as the acetylation of histone lysine or of the N-terminal of many proteins.

Oxidation of pyruvate to CO_2 in the citric acid cycle is associated with the process of oxidative phosphorylation, in which about 30 ATP molecules are generated for each glucose molecule (two pyruvate) oxidized. The reactions involve the transfer of electrons from certain intermediates to coenzymes NAD^+ and FAD^+, and subsequently from their reduced forms NADH and $FADH_2$, via the electron transport chain, to molecular oxygen. This process occurs in the inner mitochondrial membrane and is coupled to the generation of an electrochemical proton (H^+) gradient. This provides the motive force for ATP synthesis, involving the complex F_0F_1 ATP synthase enzyme also located on the inner membrane. The electron transport chain itself involves a series of 12 or more electron carriers grouped into four complexes which span the inner mitochondrial membrane

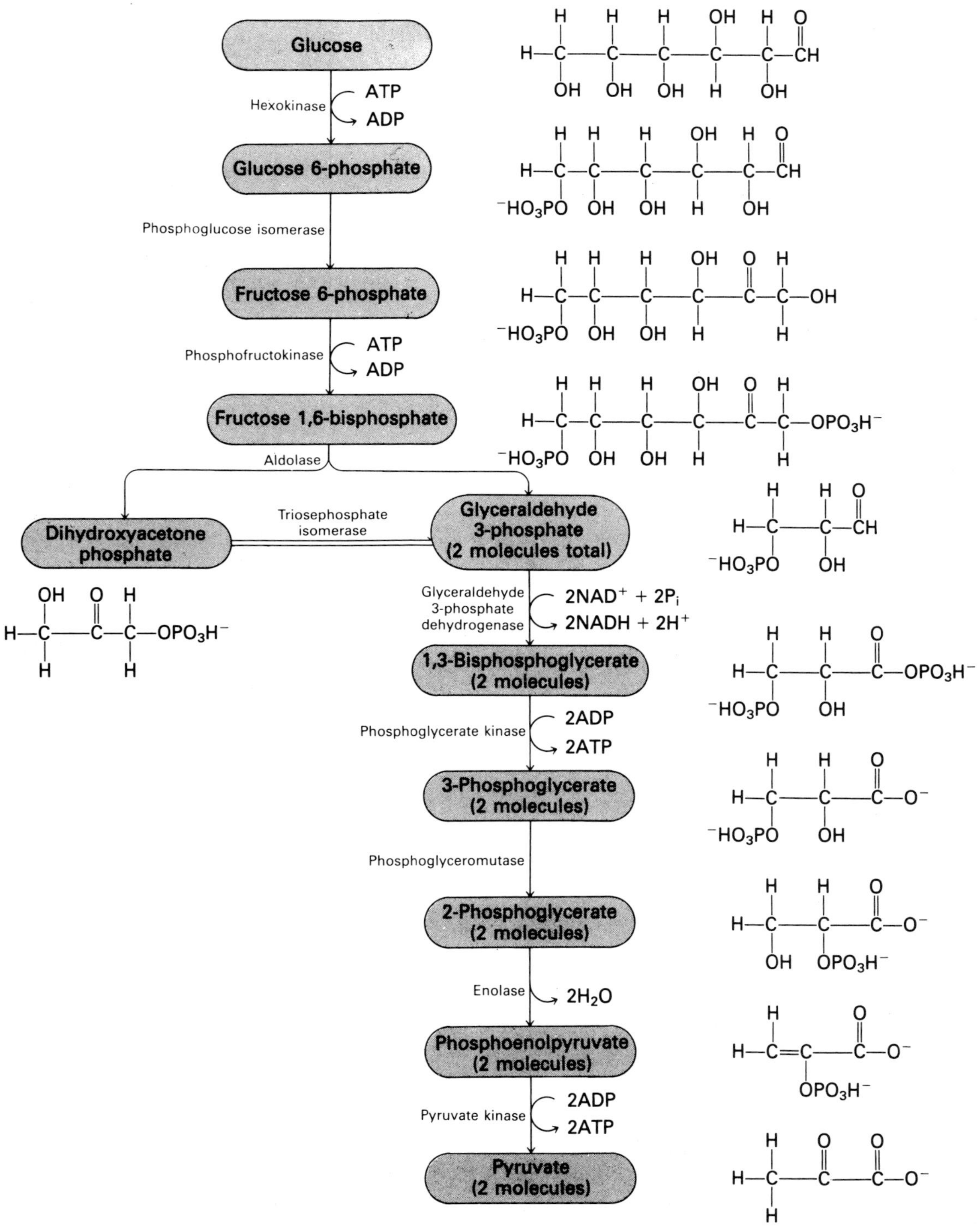

Figure 6.14 The Embden–Meyerhoff glycolytic pathway, by which glucose is degraded to pyruvic acid: the enzymes catalysing the reactions are as follows: 1, hexokinase; 2, phosphoglucose isomerase; 3, phosphofructokinase; 4, aldolase; 5, triosephosphate isomerase; 6, glyceraldehyde 3-phosphate dehydrogenase; 7, phosphosoglycerate kinase; 8, phosphoglyceromutase; 9, enolase; 10, pyruvate kinase; (From Darnell *et al.* 1986 with permission.)

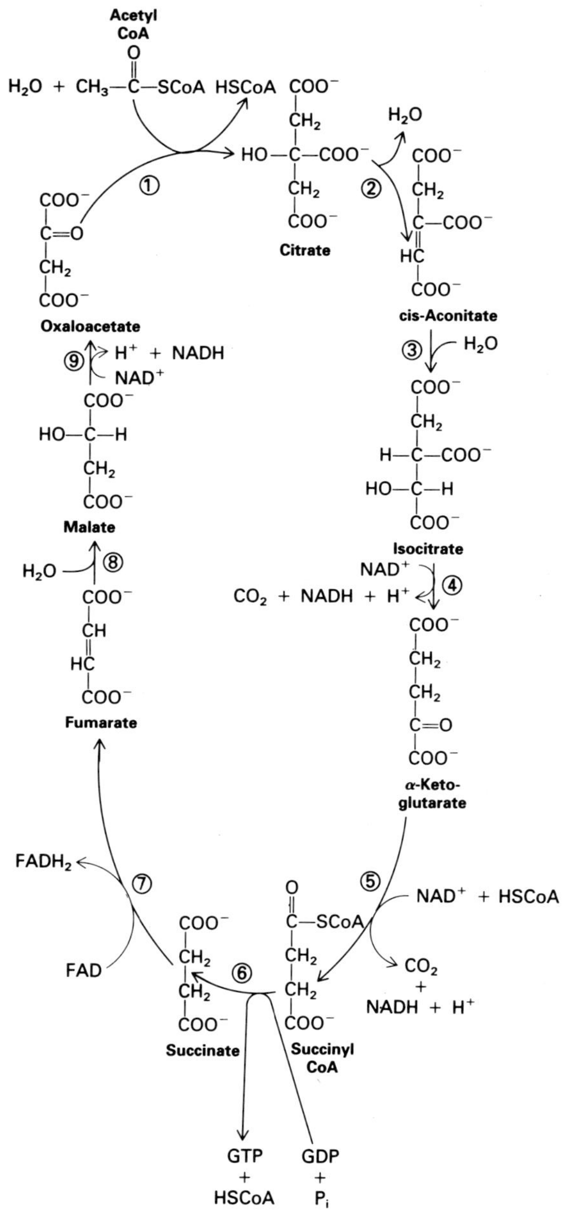

Figure 6.15 The citric acid cycle. First, a two-carbon acetyl residue from acetyl CoA condenses with the four-carbon molecule oxaloacetate to form the six-carbon molecule citrate. Through a sequence of enzymatically catalysed reactions (2–9), each molecule of citrate is converted to oxaloacetate, losing two CO_2 molecules. In four reactions, four pairs of electrons are removed from the carbon atoms: three pairs are transferred to three molecules of NAD^+ to form $3NADH + 3H^+$; one pair is transferred to the acceptor FAD to form $FADH_2$. The enzymes involved are: 1; 2; 3; 4; 5; 6; 7; 8; 9. (From Darnell *et al.* 1986 with permission.)

(e.g. NADH-Co Q reductase; succinate-Co Q reductase; Co QH_2-cytochrome *c* reductase; cytochrome *c* oxidase) (Darnell *et al.* 1990).

The pentose phosphate pathway

(Figure 6.7)

Ten to twenty per cent of lens glucose is metabolized by the pentose phosphate pathway (the pentose shunt, or hexose monophosphate shunt). In this, glucose-6-phosphate is converted to ribulose-5-phosphate and provides pentose sugar for nucleic acid synthesis. This pathway is the major source of lens CO_2, and produces two reducing equivalents of NADPH per molecule of glucose oxidized, which is an important source of NADPH for nucleotide, fatty acid and sterol synthesis, for the maintenance of glutathione in its reduced state (GSH) and for the reduction of hexose sugars to sugar alcohol, in the polyol pathway. Since GSH is a major free-radical scavenger in the lens, its regeneration is a critical event; it is known that hyperglycaemic states (which lead to NADPH consumption through the action of aldose reductase) and oxidative stress (such as *in vitro* exposure to H_2O_2, which oxidizes GSH to GSSG), both stimulate pentose shunt activity and the generation of NADPH.

In the lens epithelium two NADP-dependent mitochondrial enzymes, isocitrate dehydrogenase and malic enzyme, have a significant NADPH generating potential.

The polyol pathway

The polyol (or sorbitol) pathway involves the conversion of glucose to fructose in two stages. Glucose is reduced to its sugar alcohol sorbitol, catalysed by the enzyme aldose reductase (AR) with NADPH as coenzyme (Figure 6.16). Sorbitol is then oxidized to fructose by the enzyme polyol dehydrogenase (PD) with NAD as coenzyme. The reactions would favour formation of fructose, since NADPH is usually found in the reduced form and NAD chiefly in the oxidized form in the lens (van Heyningen 1969a), but the kinetics of AR are too slow to encourage this.

AR also catalyses the formation of dulcitol from galactose, or xylitol from xylose, but of these, only xylitol can be further oxidized by polyol dehydrogenase. This enzyme has a high ability to convert sorbitol to fructose in human lenses. The activity of AR in the human lens is 16–30% of that present in the rat or rabbit lens (Jedziniak *et al.* 1981). AR has been localized to the epithelium of the human lens.

Glyceraldehyde-3-phosphate is an effective substrate for AR with the production of glycerol-3-phosphate, which has been proposed as a precursor for the synthesis of membrane phosphoglycerides (Harding and Crabbe 1984).

The kinetics of AR are such that, in the human lens, little sorbitol formation would be expected although some formation might arise in poorly controlled diabetics. For this reason the role of AR in the lens has been questioned, particularly by

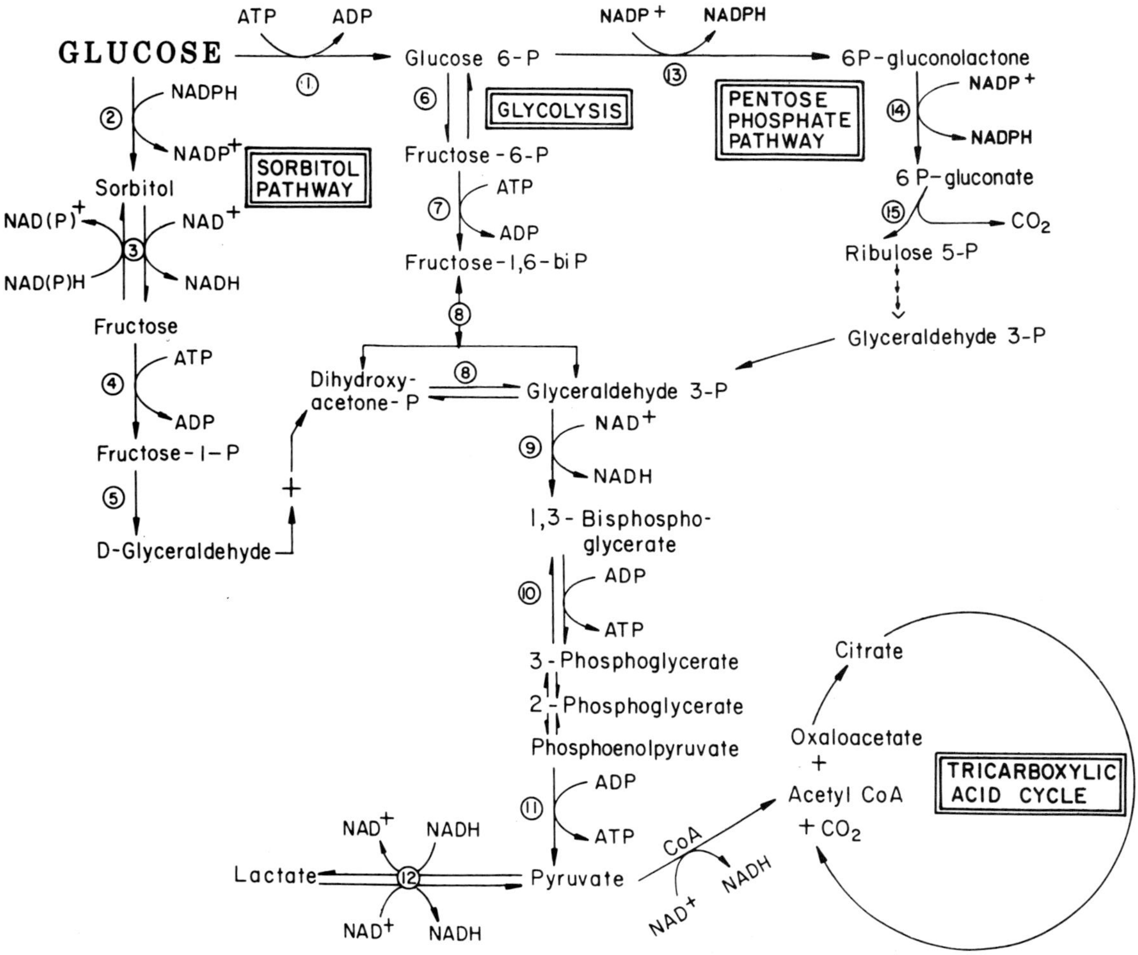

Figure 6.16 An overview of glucose metabolism in the lens. The major pathways shown are glycolysis, pentose phosphate pathway, sorbitol pathway, and tricarboxylic acid cycle. The enzymes shown in encircled numbers are: 1, hexokinase; 2, aldose reductase; 3, polyol dehydrogenase; 4, ketohexokinase; 5, aldolase; 6, phosphoglucose isomerase; 7, 6-phosphofructokinase; 8, aldolase and triosephosphate isomerase; 9, glyceraldehyde 3-phosphate dehydrogenase; 10, phosphoglycerate kinase; 11, pyruvate kinase; 12, lactic dehydrogenase; 13, glucose 6-phosphate dehydrogenase (G6PD); 14, lactonase; 15, 6-phosphogluconate dehydrogenase (6PGD). The pentose phosphate pathway and glycolysis are linked by two enzymes (not shown): transketolase and transaldolase. (From Berman 1991 with permission.)

Harding and Crabbe (Harding and Crabbe 1984; Harding 1991). It has been pointed out that the catalytic activity of the enzyme is so low as to suggest that it is not a true enzyme. Its molecular structure shows a hydrophobic cleft which would not provide an adequate binding site for glucose (Wilson *et al.* 1994). Its fourfold ability to enhance the reaction rate is tiny compared with most enzymes (e.g. over one million-fold), it shows poor substrate specificity and no control mechanisms. The efficiency of AR as judged by K_{cat}/K_m values is less than that of other enzymes by a factor of 100 000 or more (Harding 1991).

Human lens AR has been cloned and partially sequenced and shows some sequence homology with a frog lens crystallin and liver AR. Harding has suggested that human lens AR is an NADPH binding protein with minimal catalytic properties, which is ancestrally related to the frog crystallin and to a primordial aldehyde dehydrogenase. Synthesis of sorbitol by the purified enzyme has not been demonstrated.

Transparency

The transparency of the lens results from the optical homogeneity of its parts and this depends on its microscopical structure and upon its chemical constituents.

There are many interdependent factors responsible for the maintenance of lens transparency. Interference with some, such as ion pumps or membrane permeability, respiration, and structure or concentration of crystallins, has been shown experimentally to cause cataract.

There is a regular arrangement of the fibres with minimal extracellular space. The total lens extracellular space is only 1.3%. Increased separation of the fibres would cause light scatter. Only the superficial fibres are nucleated.

The high concentration of the major lens proteins (crystallins), at 33% of the wet weight of the lens, minimizes scatter from the cytoplasm/membrane interface. The lens protein molecules have a short range order similar to that of glass, which explains the transparency of the cytoplasm (Delaye and Tardieu 1983). There are small spatial fluctuations in the number of protein molecules over the dimensions comparable to the wave length of light and, due to the high concentration of these molecules, none scatter light independently of one another (Benedek 1971). Turbidity of a solution of lens crystallins decreases as the protein concentration increases towards that found in the lens.

An increase in molecular size or separation causes scatter. Modification of the lens proteins leads to their aggregation into light-scattering macromolecules. Alternatively, excessive water entry separates lens cells or cytoplasmic constituents and causes light scattering. These mechanisms have each been demonstrated in the development of cataract. The lens metabolism fulfils the task of maintaining the health of lens fibre membranes and the lens proteins, and also in expelling water.

Light-scattering occurs in the normal ageing lens after 50 years of age, and results in a sense of glare in certain conditions (Carter 1982). This is likely to be the result of the increase in lens thickness which occurs with age, causing the light to traverse more fibres, and with the increase in lens crystallin molecular size (Spector 1982).

The lens transmits light throughout the visible spectrum but absorbs heavily in UV at below 400 nm (Figure 3.19) while the cornea transmits freely from 300 nm (Lerman and Borkman 1976; Lerman 1980) so that the band of 300–400 nm is largely absorbed by the lens. This may be significant in cataract causation (p. 205). With increasing age there is absorption in the visible blue spectrum, which is exaggerated in the presence of nuclear brunescence (p. 222).

Protective mechanisms

The lens possesses repair mechanisms, both at a cellular and at a molecular level and it has the ability to isolate damaged fibres (Bron and Brown 1987) and the histology of this has been shown (Vrensen and Willekens 1988).

At a molecular level, a number of scavenger molecules are present that protect against oxidative stress. Lens membranes contain vitamin E which protects against lipid peroxidation. GSH, a potent free-radical scavenger, is synthesized in the lens from amino acid precursors (L-glutamic acid, L-cysteine, and L-glycine). It is present in high concentration in the cortex and in the epithelium, and at a low concentration in the nucleus (Pau *et al.* 1990). It is probably important in maintaining lens protein thiols in the reduced state, such as that of Na^+, K^+ATPase or of the lens crystallin thiols. It maintains ascorbate in the reduced state and scavenges peroxides and radiation-induced free-radicals. Vitamin C, already in high concentration in the aqueous, is actively transported into the lens, where it is at a high concentration. Like GSH it is an effective reducing agent. Other compounds, carotenoids, choline, taurine and thioredoxin-T have been ascribed similar roles.

7

Examination of the lens and evaluation of lens changes

Examination of the lens

It is assumed that the reader is familiar with the various methods of illumination available at the slit-lamp. Focal illumination shows opacities in the lens, partly because they scatter, and partly because they reflect light, according to the angle of view (Weale 1986). Focal illumination is particularly useful in estimating the width of C1α, the anterior subcapsular clear zone of the lens, which may be thinned in relation to cataract development or expanded in diabetes (Brown and Tripathi 1974). Retro-illumination with the dilated pupil is the most useful single form of illumination to observe the entire lens and its contained opacities. The illumination should be offset and the beam directed close to the pupil margin on one side to give indirect retro-illumination. It is then swept to the other side. Specular illumination is used to define the nature of surfaces including the capsule anteriorly and posteriorly, the epithelium and the superficial lens fibres. In older subjects this illumination also demonstrates an uneven face on the surface of the nucleus called the relief pattern of the adult nucleus (Figure 3.20) (Vogt and Lüssi 1919).

Evaluation of lens changes

Objective qualitative and quantitative evaluation of the lens is essential to any epidemiological or therapeutic study of cataract and in studying the natural history of cataract types. This has assumed recent importance because of the arrival of drugs that may have a beneficial influence on cataract. There is also concern that newly introduced drugs may be cataractogenic.

Subjective methods of visual assessment are also needed in a clinical study of the lens, including visual acuity testing with high contrast optotypes and contrast sensitivity testing using low contrast targets. A glare light source may be included to demonstrate the effect of the cataract on visual function by demonstrating a loss of contrast sensitivity in the presence of the glare source (see 'Vision in Cataract', Chapter 14). There is a considerable lack of correlations between the subjective and objective methods (Holden *et al.* 1994), which makes it important to use both these approaches to the evaluation of the patient.

No single objective method can adequately evaluate the status of cataract, so that the worker in this field needs to use a number of methods in conjunction. The available methods are:

1. Clinical cataract classification and grading.
2. Resolution test target projection ophthalmoscope.
3. Photography and other forms of image capture.
   - Slit-image (scheimpflug).
   - Retro-illumination.
   - Specular.
   - Image analysis of photographs.
4. Ultrasound.
5. Light-scattering analysis.
   - Tyndallometry.
   - Laser quasi-elastic light-scattering.
6. Fluorimetry.

Clinical cataract classification and grading

The morphological classification of cataract must precede any system of measurement. For most studies there is concern with those types of cataract that are progressive. Non-progressive or relatively stationary types, which include congenital nuclear, sutural and coronary, may be recorded, but not necessarily quantified. The progressive types fall into the three major categories: cortical, subcapsular and nuclear.

The morphological classification is best determined *in vivo* by the clinician at the slit-lamp microscope. It is possible to classify cataracts by the examination of photographs, but photographs necessarily present a limited view of the lens and do not demonstrate all of the features seen biomicroscopically.

Clinical classification can be performed without grading, but it takes very little extra time for the clinician to perform grading of a cataract at the same time and this is worthwhile, even if photography is to be used for measurement. The Oxford Clinical Cataract Classification and Grading System (Sparrow *et al.* 1986) and LOCS Systems II and III (Chylack *et al.* 1989, 1993) have been devised for this purpose.

The Oxford system is performed at the slit-lamp microscope and the observer is guided by a booklet fixed to the head frame of the microscope (Figure 7.1). The booklet provides standards with which to compare the features in the lens. Geometric diagrams are provided for grading the extent of a feature. The features that are provided for grading are: anterior subcapsular clear zone thickness, anterior subcapsular opacity, posterior subcapsular opacity, cortical spoke opacity, water clefts, vacuoles, fibre folds, retro-dots, focal dots, nuclear brunescence and white nuclear scatter. Most features are graded on a 0–5 scale; the results are recorded on a standard chart (Figure 7.2) and other features, such as polychromasia and pseudoexfoliation, are recorded but not quantified.

A clinical grading system is capable of being used on its own for the quantitative evaluation of cataract and, in some field studies in remote areas,

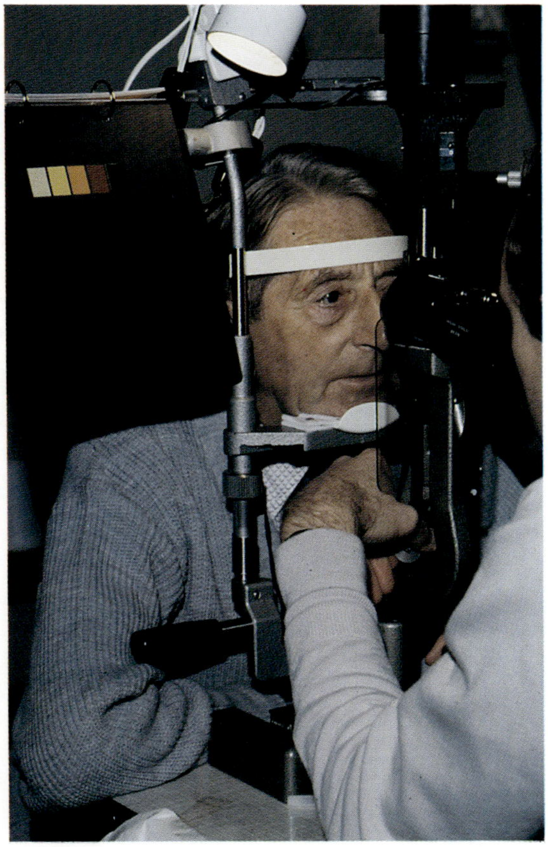

Figure 7.1 The Oxford clinical cataract classification and grading system. The grading book, here showing the colour standards for nuclear brunescence grading, is fixed to the microscope head stand.

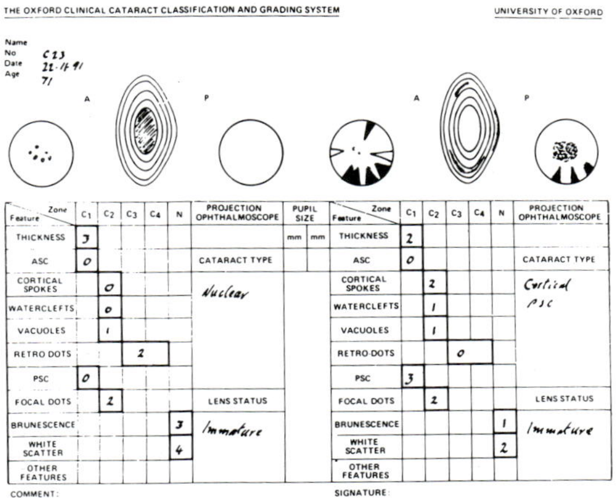

Figure 7.2 The Oxford clinical cataract and grading system recording chart.

a clinical grading system may be all that is practical. However, photographic methods are better suited to measurement.

LOCS III uses colour slides as standards for subjectively quantifying cortical (CC), nuclear (NC) and posterior subcapsular (PSC) cataract. It has evolved from LOCS II which had the following limitations: 1) the scale for nuclear colour was small and coarse; 2) the early stages of NC and PSC were under-represented; 3) the scaling intervals for all types of cataract were unequal; and 4) integer grading of features was not sensitive at detecting small changes in cataract. Efforts have been made to solve these problems in LOCS III. The number of slides, used for LOCS III, has been increased for the grading of nuclear opalescence (NO), nuclear brunescence (NB), and posterior subcapsular cataract (PSC), in order to overcome limitations 1 and 2. Equal scaling intervals between standard slides of cataract have been acheived by using objective techniques to measure NO, NB, CC and PSC. The grading for LOCS III has been converted from an integer to decimal system. This has increased the sensitivity of LOCS at the expense of some reduction in repeatability which still remains very good (Chylack *et al.* 1993).

Resolution test target projection ophthalmoscope (acuityscope)

The image degrading effect of cataract can be assessed objectively with a resolution test target project ophthalmoscope (Cotlier 1981). The Cotlier instrument contains a standard USAF three-bar resolution test chart. The image of the chart is projected via the dilated pupil on to the patient's retina, where it is observed. The smallest three-bar group in which both the vertical and horizontal elements can be separately discerned is identified and recorded. The projected image occupies the central 3 mm of the pupil, so that it is affected by cataract within this region of the lens; this is also the region of the lens where cataract is most relevant to degrading the patient's vision. Cataract degrades the observed image, both in the projection and in the visualization stages.

The Cotlier principle has been developed into the Keeler acuityscope (Brown *et al.* 1991) in which the target has been rearranged with the sizes of the bar groups arranged in logarithmic progression (Figure 7.3) for better statistical assessment.

Photographic methods

Photographic methods of lens measurement compare well with clinical observation for the measurement of the lens and for the estimation of the amount of cataract. Slit-image and retro-illumination photography each have their own advantages and limitations and neither is to be regarded as superior to the other. Ideally, the two systems are used in combination. Slit-image photography to date has been shown to have the better repeatability, but this can now be equalled by retro-illumination cameras with fixation lights for alignment, supported by a software program capable of compensating for the inevitably uneven illumination.

Slit-image photography

Scheimpflug slit-image photography (see Figures 3.6, 3.13) (Brown 1972; Hockwin and Dragomirescu 1981) is effective in giving information on the dimensions (widths and curvatures) of the lens and on the optical densities of the non-cataractous regions. The slit-image is effective in measuring nuclear cataract (Chylack *et al.* 1984), but is inefficient in measuring cortical cataract, which may be

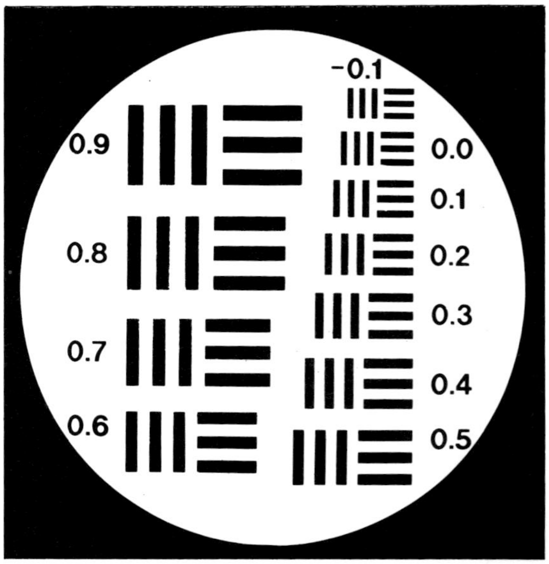

Figure 7.3 The acuityscope resolution chart.

missed altogether if the opacity does not lie on the axis of the slit-beam. This information loss can be reduced by making multiple images with the slit-beam, but even so it cannot give a statement of the total amount of cortical cataract that is present. Trigonometrical alignment ensures that the optical axis section of the lens is imaged on each occasion for reliable repeatability (Harris *et al.* 1991). The Brown slit-image camera has been used for the slit-image pictures in this book.

Retro-illumination photography

In current methods of retro-illumination photography the optical axes of the camera and of the illumination are made to coincide by a glass plate acting as a partial mirror. The corneal reflex is eliminated with crossed polarizing filters. The Oxford retro-illumination camera (Brown and Dawson 1987) has been used for the reflex-free retro-illumination pictures in this book (Figure 7.4). Retro-illumination photography produces a silhouette picture of the cataract from which it is possible to measure the total area of the dilated pupil that is occupied by cataract. In practice, the depth of field is inadequate, so that two separately focused exposures are needed to measure the cataract in a lens that has both cortical and posterior subcapsular cataract. A fixation light ensures alignment and repeatability (Harris *et al.* 1994). This method is unsatisfactory with nuclear cataract, which is best assessed with the slit-image. It is also unsatisfactory for measurement purposes with retro-dot cataracts, which tend to appear bright by birefringence (Figure 7.5) (see p. 156). Indirect retro-illumination, in which half of the background is illuminated (Brown 1971), is used to show objects differing in refractive index from the substance of the lens. Vacuoles and retro-dots are well demonstrated, but simple water clefts (p. 142) do not show.

Specular

Images of the lens surfaces are made possible with a specular camera designed for corneal use (Laing and Bursell 1981) or with a macro camera (Figure 4.2a, 7.6) (Brown 1970 and Brown *et al.* 1987). Refractive interfaces within the lens, such as those caused by retro-dots, are also demonstrable (Figure 7.7).

The specular image of the anterior surface of the lens is adjustable to produce images of the lens shagreen, of the lens epithelium, or of the lens fibres. From these images the dimensions of the lens epithelial cells or the lens fibres can be determined. The images are better seen in the normal lens, so this technique has not so far produced information about changes in the lens epithelium and fibres in cataract.

Specular examination is used to show refractive interfaces, such as the relief of the adult nucleus,

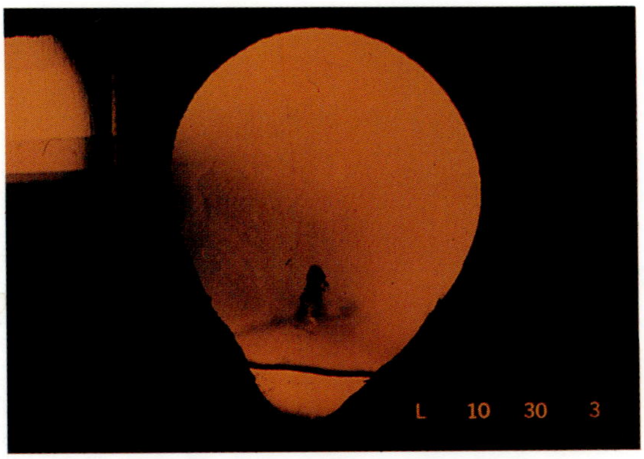

Figure 7.4 Coloboma of lens and iris. A small cortical cataract is related to the coloboma. (Oxford retro-illumination camera.)

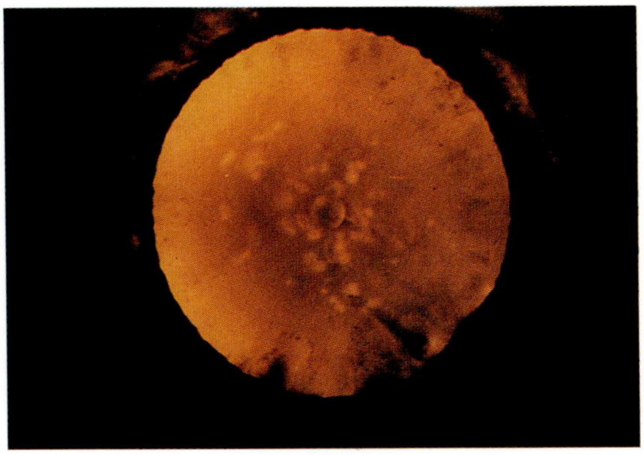

Figure 7.5 Retro-dots by retro-illumination in polarized light appear bright by birefringence against a dark nuclear cataract.

the posterior face of water clefts, the anterior face of retro-dots and of vacuoles. The posterior capsule is examined by specular reflex to show polychromatic lustre.

Image analysis

The images produced by photographic techniques are translated into numerical scores by image analysis techniques. Scanning densitometry was the first technique to be used in this field for the analysis of slit-images (Hockwin *et al.* 1982). This technique is time consuming and is limited to single line scans through the image. The computerized systems of image analysis have the greatest versatility (Sparrow *et al.* 1990) and speed in operation. The use of a CCD (charge coupled device) (Mayer and Irion 1985) to read the negative has an advantage over video negative readers in that the CCD has a linear response and the image is digitized by the CCD itself without the need for a separate digitizer. A system using a CCD input coupled to an image-analysing personal computer has been developed at Oxford for reading existing negatives and the images stored on optical discs. The computer analysis of the slit-image picture is relatively straightforward, but the retro-illumination images require a sophisticated algorithm to allow for the variability in the background illumination (Harris *et al.* 1993). Once this has been done, the percentage area of the lens that is occupied by cataract is measurable (Figures 7.8–7.10). The Oxford modular system has been extended to

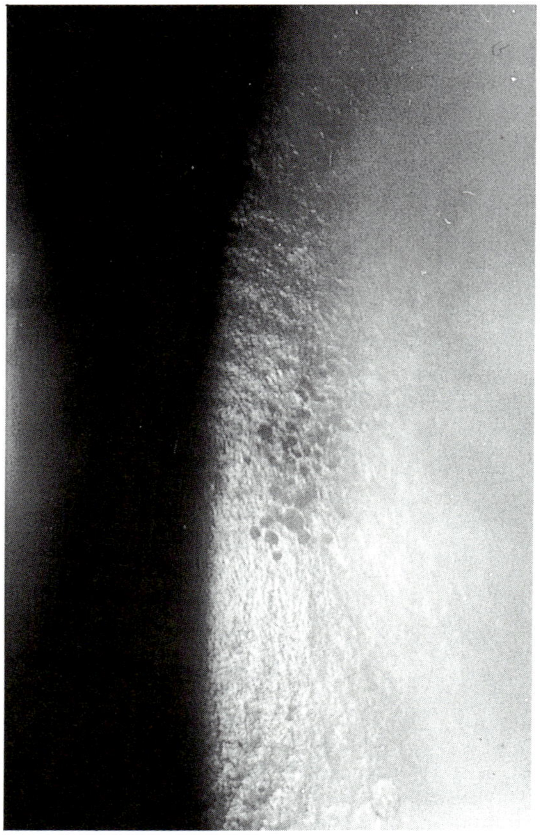

Figure 7.6 Capsular bleb-like disorder by specular photography (magnification × 10).

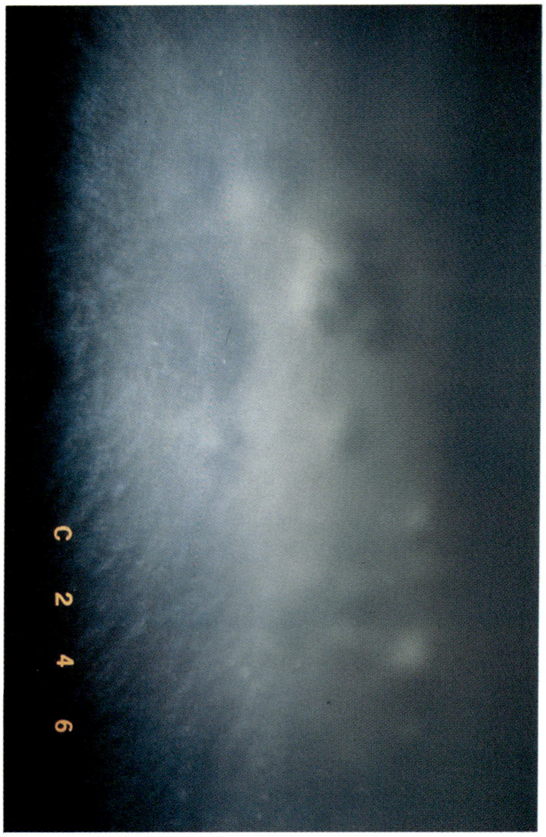

Figure 7.7 Retro-dot cataract appears raised by specular illumination (magnification × 10).

include CCD slit-image and retro-illumination cameras (Figure 7.11) that take the image directly from the patient to the computer (Sparrow *et al.* 1990) (Figures 7.8, 7.12). The all-electronic camera systems have the advantage of eliminating the vagaries and storage problems of film.

Ultrasound

Ultrasound has been used extensively to measure the lens of the eye (Weekers *et al.* 1973a,b). It is capable of measuring the position of the lens and

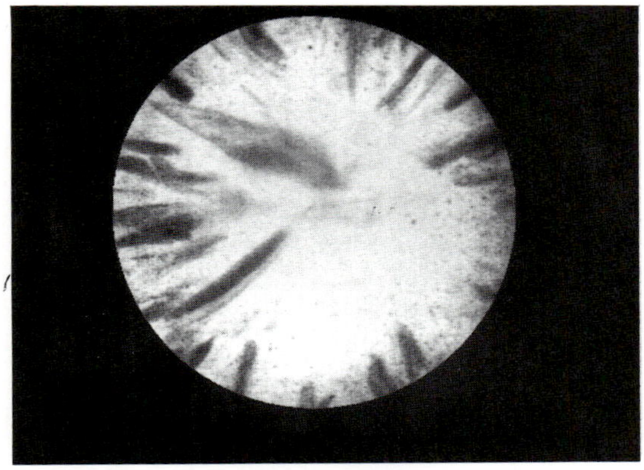

Figure 7.8 Retro-illumination picture of cortical cataract generated by a CCD camera.

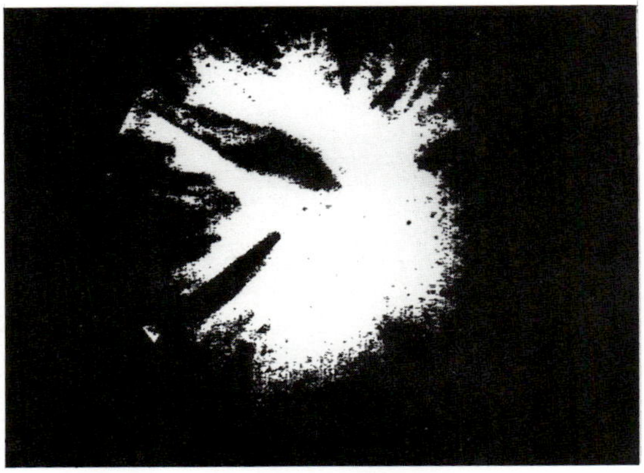

Figure 7.9 The simple binarized picture of Figure 7.8. The computer cannot fully distinguish the cataract from the background.

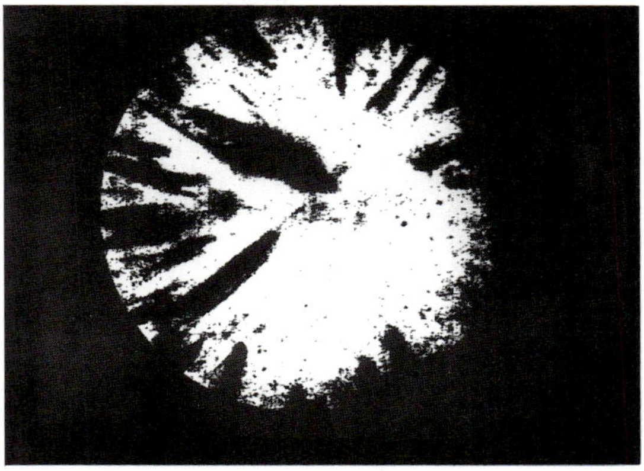

Figure 7.10 The binarized picture after applying a brightness algorithm differentiates all the cataract from the background and allows the amount of cataract to be measured.

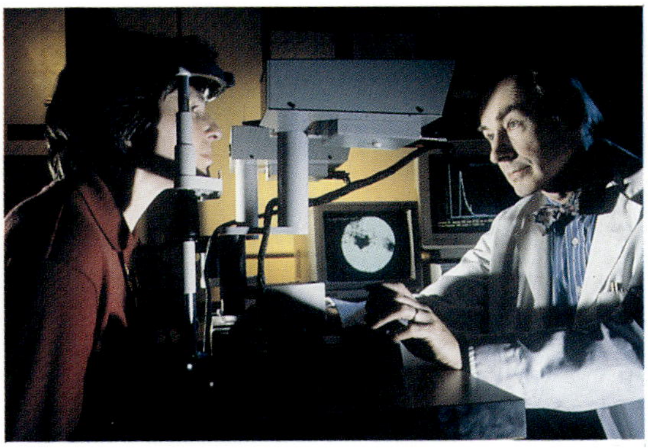

Figure 7.11 The Oxford modular CCD cameras and computer image analysis system.

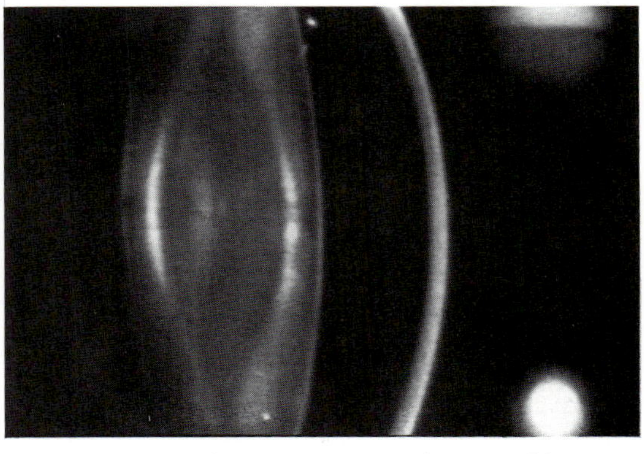

Figure 7.12 CCD slit-image picture of a normal lens.

its width, even when the lens is densely opaque. Ultrasound is also capable of demonstrating the growth of the normal lens, and measuring the lens dimensions in accommodation (Koretz *et al.* 1984), but the change in curvature must be measured photographically (Brown 1973) (Figure 7.13).

Light-scattering analysis

The densities that are present in a slit-image negative relate to the intensity of light-scattering in the lens produced by the Tyndall effect and by scattering from membrane interfaces. Some of the light returned from a cataract appears to have been reflected, rather than scattered, since it is interrupted by a polarizing filter (Weale 1986). The light-scattering can be measured by photometric methods without photography (Ben-Sira *et al.* 1980). These methods have the advantage of giving an instant numerical reading, but lack the ability to measure the different scattering properties of the various regions of the lens. There is a commercially available instrument that measures the average value of the lens scattering.

Laser quasi-elastic light-scattering

Laser light differs from ordinary light in being coherent and in phase, so that differences in phase between the ingredient light and scattered light can be measured. This technique has the potential for estimating the size of the lens protein molecules (Benedek *et al.* 1987) and it is considered that the more slowly diffusive particles represent protein molecular aggregates. A computer is used to analyse the shift in phase of the reflected laser light from the eye compared with the ingredient laser light. This technique can be expected to give correct estimates of the sizes of the protein molecules that are present in a solution *in vitro*, but *in vivo* the reading will be affected by other events in the lens such as changes in cytoplasmic viscosity, or fibre breakdown, which invalidate such calculations. Even so, this technique may well be valuable in demonstrating changes in the lens proteins.

Fluorimetry

The adult lens contains chromophores that exhibit autofluorescence. This phenomenon can be elicited at various wavelengths, some in the visible spectrum (Occhipinti *et al.* 1986; Mosier *et al.* 1986) and some in the UV spectrum. Excitation and emission wavelengths can be studied *in vivo* by the use of pairs of narrow pass filters placed appropriately in the illuminating (excitation) light path and in the emission light path (the barrier filter). For example, when the lens is stimulated within the visible range

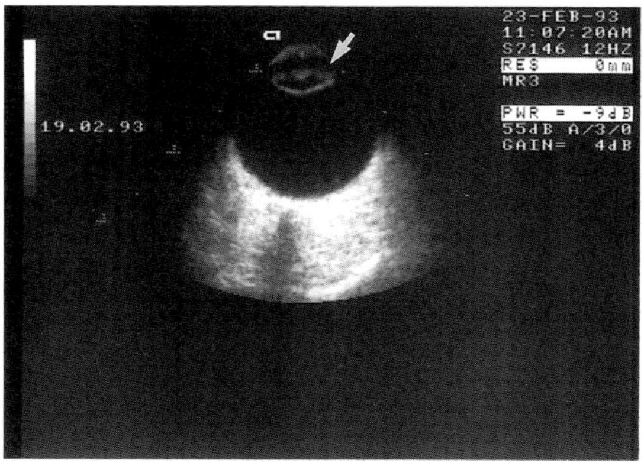

(a)

Figure 7.13 B-mode ultrasound images. **(a)** Central transverse sector B-mode image of normal eye to show the lens in meridional section.

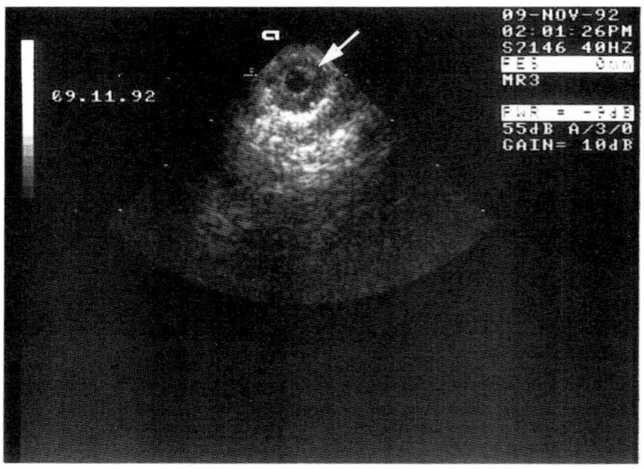

(b)

Figure 7.13(b) Transverse sector B-mode image with the eye in depression. The cataractous lens is seen in coronal section and therefore has a spherical profile. (Courtesy of M. Restori.)

with light of around 490 nm, the fluorescence is emitted at around 530 nm. Using appropriate narrow pass filter combinations, the intensity of the fluorescence can be recorded either with a photometer (fluorimeter) or photographically.

The nucleus and the perinuclear cortical regions of the lens show the most intense fluorescence. Lenticular fluorescence has been shown to increase with age and to be increased in lenses of diabetics (Sparrow *et al.* 1992) and in cataractous lens nuclei. As diabetics have an increased risk of developing a cataract, changes of this nature are important to an overall understanding of the cataractogenic process.

Colour

Lens nuclear colouration may be assessed subjectively in the Oxford and LOCS grading systems. Photographic assessment uses colour film and spectroscopy of the transparencies (Khu and Kashiwagi: 1993). Further developments are likely to replace film with CCD technology.

8

Lens malformations and displacements

Aphakia

Primary aphakia is rare and occurs with gross malformations such as microphthalmia (Baker 1887; Cherryholmes 1902; Adams *et al.* 1915). In Vogt's cases congenital aphakia was associated with microphthalmia, microcornea and nystagmus (Vogt 1931). Bilateral, dense corneal opacities were attached by a tissue strand to irregularly developed zonular fibres and the iris was defective in part. A primary defect in surface ectoderm (Manschott 1963) or in formation of the optic cup has been proposed (Mann 1957). (Mann 1921) described bilateral primary aphakia in a human embryo at the 13 mm stage. The optic cup was otherwise normal and it would appear from this that the defect lay in an earlier stage of induction (p. 4). Rabl described unilateral aphakia in the axolotl embryo with accompanying unilateral underdevelopment of the neural ectoderm, including the optic vesicle, occurring on the same side. A plaque of thickened ectoderm was present, separated from the defective but invaginated optic vesicle, which might have represented an abortive lens plate (Mann 1957) (Figure 8.1).

Secondary aphakia is due to partial or complete absorption of the lens, which may follow congenital cataract due to rubella (Smith *et al.* 1990a) (Figure 8.2), or be associated with developmental abnormalities, such as microcornea. Some remnant of lens tissue or capsule distinguishes this condition from primary aphakia.

Duplication of the lens

Duplication of the lens is described in association with corneal metaplasia and coloboma of the iris and choroid. It has been ascribed to a metaplastic change in surface ectoderm preventing the invagination of the lens placode to form a single vesicle (Lyford and Roy 1974).

Microspherophakia

The formation of small spherical lenses in this bilateral condition is due to defective development of the zonule. It may occur as an isolated defect and be familial, or occur in association with other defects in the Weill–Marchesani syndrome (Figures 8.3, 8.4) and in hyperlisinaemia.

The condition results in lenticular myopia. The lens zones of discontinuity (Figure 3.16) lack the peripheral divergence seen in the normal lens and run parallel with the surface. Lens dislocation, which is usually downwards, and pupil block glaucoma are common complications.

Lenticonus and lentiglobus

In each of these conditions there is an abnormality of the curvature of the central part of the lens surface associated with thinning of the affected part of the capsule and deficiency of the subjacent epithelium. In lenticonus (Figure 8.5a) the protrusion of the lens surface is conoid and in lentiglobus it is spherical. Each may occur anteriorly or posteriorly, the latter being the more common. Each may cause lenticular myopia with irregular astigmatism and an oil droplet effect is seen with the retinoscope (Figure 8.5b). The lens defect may be an isolated event, inherited as an autosomal recessive trait, or associated with Alport's syndrome (familial haemorrhagic nephritis). Posterior lenticonus is reported in Lowe's syndrome (p. 179).

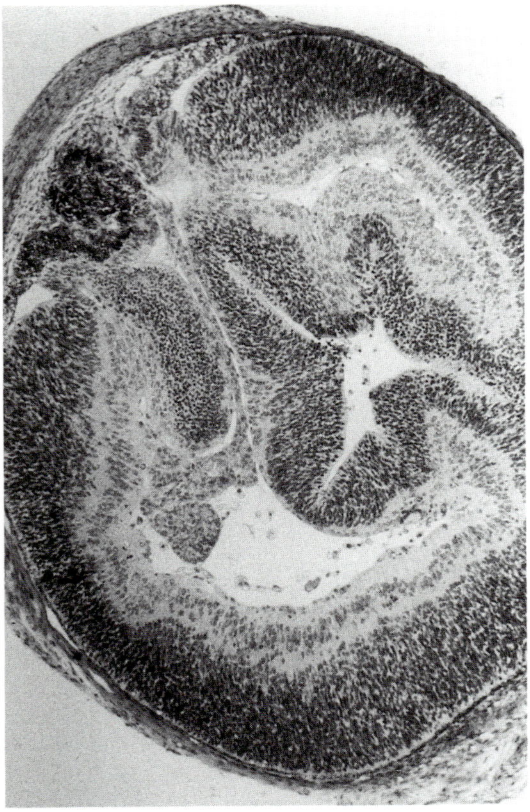

(a)

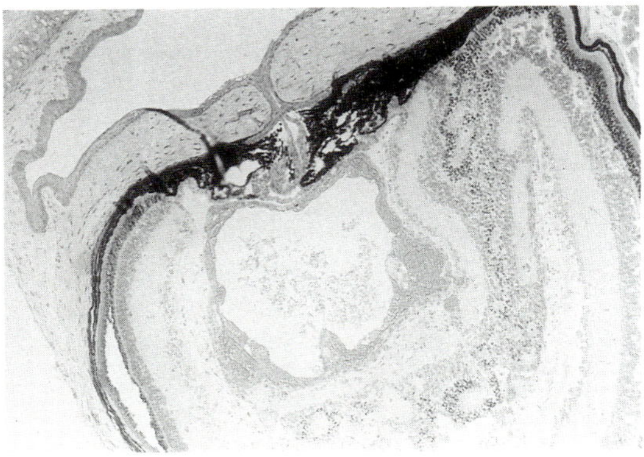

(b)

Figure 8.1 **(a)** and **(b)** Aphakic mutant mouse embryo. (Johan Zwaan with permission.)

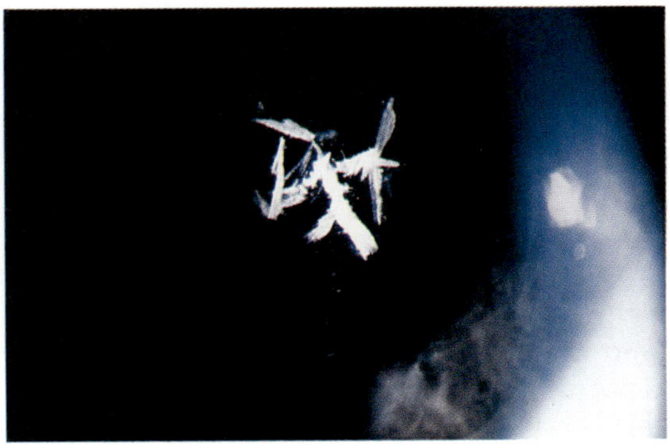

(a)

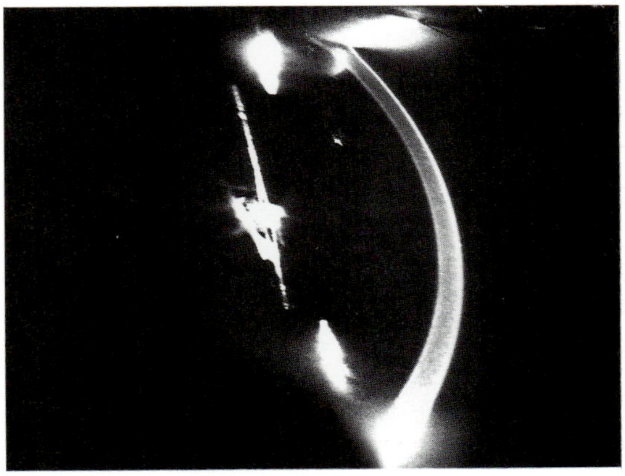

(b)

Figure 8.2 Secondary aphakia in congenital rubella. **(a)** *en face* view of intracapular calcification. **(b)** Slit image. (From Smith *et al.* 1990a with permission.)

The posterior defect is more often uniocular. The posterior pole fibres subjacent to the defect commonly opacify (Figure 8.6), and the opacification may extend into the nucleus, indicating that the defect began in fetal life. A suggested cause is weakness of the capsule, and in Alport's syndrome (p. 180) there is a generalized weakness of basement membranes. Spontaneous rupture of the capsule is an occasional complication.

Internal lenticonus is a rare defect in which the contour of the capsule is normal, but the curvature of the nucleus forms a cone anteriorly, posteriorly, or in both directions. This may be seen as a developmental defect in the child, or acquired in the adult (Figure 8.7).

Coloboma

This is a congenital indentation of the lens periphery which is usually a uniocular defect. It is due to

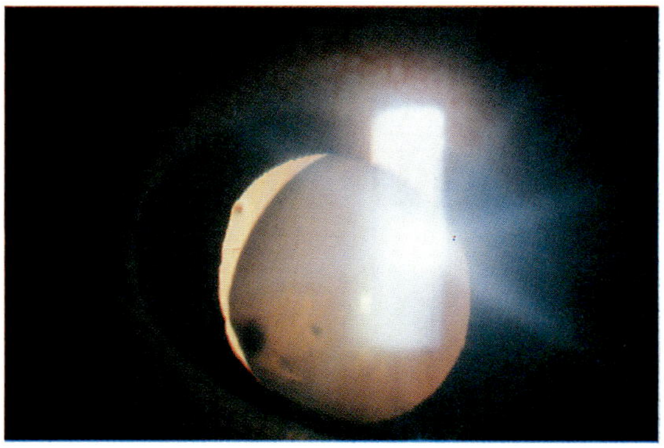

Figure 8.3 Downward subluxation of the lens in Marchesani's syndrome.

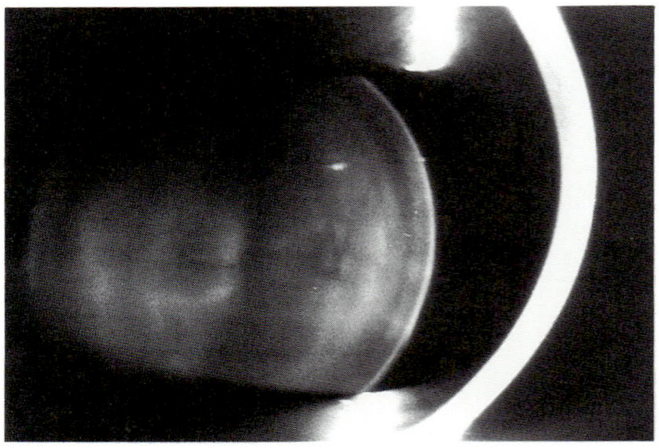

Figure 8.4 Spherophakia in Marchesani's syndrome.

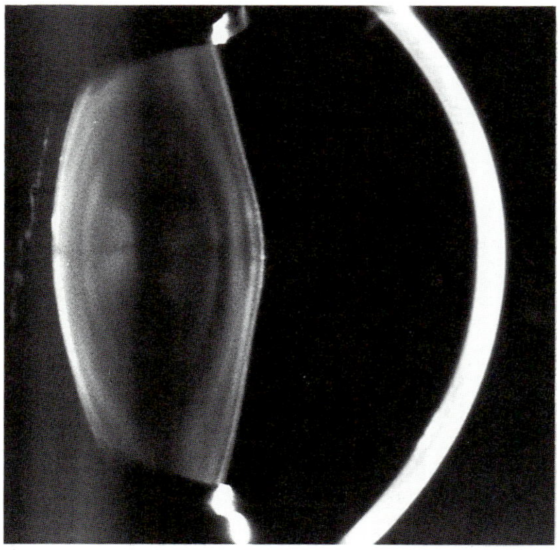

(a)

Figure 8.5(a) Anterior lenticonus in Alport's syndrome.

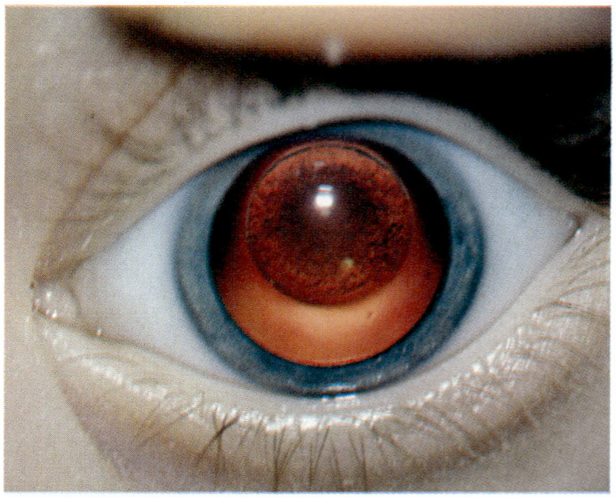

(b)

Figure 8.5(b) Posterior lenticonus seen in red reflex

a localized absence of the zonule and may be associated with coloboma of the iris, ciliary body and choroid (Figure 7.4).

Ectopia lentis (subluxation/dislocation)

A partial displacement of the lens is termed subluxation (Figure 8.8), and a complete displacement in which there is total loss of all zonular attachment is termed dislocation or luxation (Table 8.1).

Table 8.1 Causes of dislocated lens

Familial (Fig 8.9) familial associated	*Secondary to eye disease*
Marfan's syndrome	Uveitis Buphthalmos
Weill–Marchesani's syndrome Homocystinuria Sulphite oxidase deficiency Hyperlisinaemia Ehlers Danlos syndrome Osteogenesis imperfecta	Tumours Hypermature cataract Concussion injury

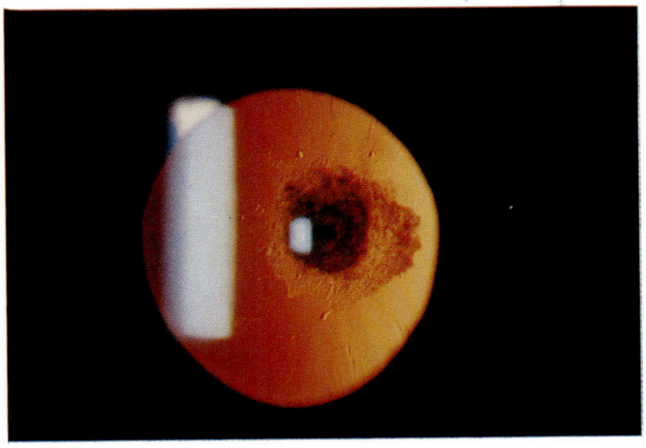

Figure 8.6 Posterior polar cataract secondary to posterior lenticonus.

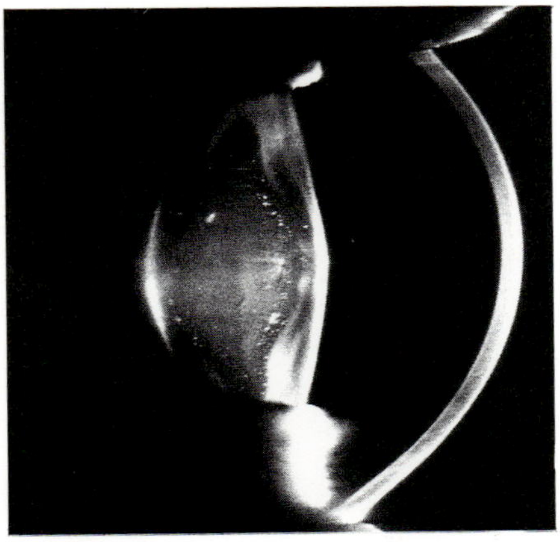

Figure 8.7 Anterior internal lenticonus, which has formed in relation to thinning of the cortex in a lens developing anterior and posterior subcapsular cataract.

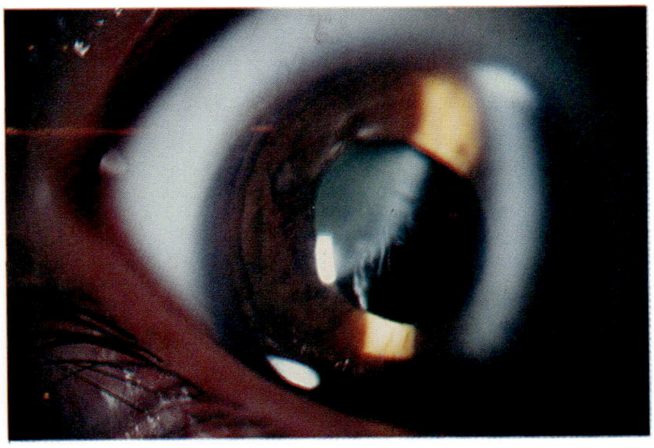

Figure 8.8 Upward subluxation of the lens in a member of a family with dominant inheritance for this condition. Fragmentation of the zonule is seen.

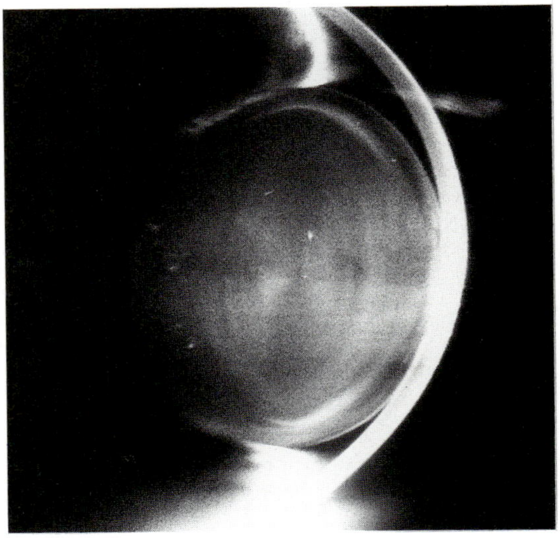

Figure 8.9 Dislocation of a spherophakic lens in Marfan's syndrome.

The causes of lens ectopia are familial and spontaneous, or secondary to eye disease and trauma (Figure 8.10).

In the familial form, which is usually inherited as an autosomal dominant, ectopia may be congenital or develop in youth; it is commonly bilaterally symmetrical (Jaureguy and Hall 1979). Nelson and Maumenee (1971) suggest that there may be a stationary and a progressive form. A recessive form is also described (McKusick 1988). It may occur alone, but other developmental abnormalities of the eye may be associated, such as iris coloboma, microspherophakia, aniridia and ectopia pupillae. Systemic developmental abnormalities are associated in Marfan's syndrome, Weill–Marchesani's syndrome, homocystinuria, sulphite oxidase deficiency and in hyperlisinaemia. The basic cause is deficient development of the zonule, which in homocystinuria is seen as fibrillary abnormal zonular filaments with breakages (Ramsay *et al.* 1972).

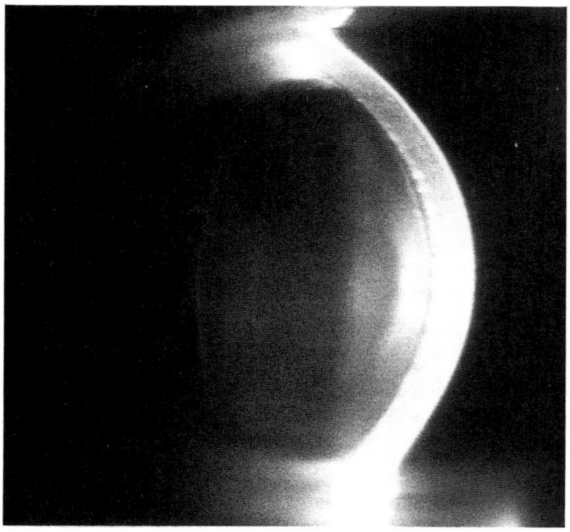

Figure 8.10 Traumatic dislocation.

Spontaneous ectopia may follow weakening of the zonule by uveitis (including syphilitic) and degeneration of the zonule in relation to hypermature cataract, pseudoexfoliation, buphthalmos and in relation to ciliary body tumours.

Traumatic ectopia is the most common cause of the condition. The force required to cause this often causes other damage to the eye including angle recession glaucoma. The possibility of a post-uveitic or familial cause should not be overlooked in the presence of a history of trauma.

The eye with a subluxated lens shows a fluctuating anterior chamber depth and a tremulous iris (iridodonesis). The lens also shows unstable movement (phacodonesis). The lens is commonly displaced vertically upwards in Marfan's syndrome, and downwards in Weill–Marchesani's syndrome and homocystinuria. The vitreous may herniate into the anterior chamber. The internal structure of the lens shows lack of peripheral divergence of the zones of discontinuity (Figure 3.16). Pupil block glaucoma is fairly common and may be due either to the lens or to the vitreous. In traumatic cases, the glaucoma may be due to the associated injury of traumatic iris recession. Subluxation results in progressive myopic astigmatism, reduction of amplitude of accommodation and, in monocular diplopia, in separate phakic and aphakic images. The dislocated lens may pass into the anterior chamber or backwards into the vitreous. The anterior dislocation causes pupil block glaucoma and the posterior displacement may cause lens induced uveitis.

9

Biology of cataract

Cataract is the name given to any light-scattering opacity in the lens, not necessarily with any demonstrable effect on vision. This definition may reasonably be extended to include opacity of the lens capsule and the deposition of opaque material (such as copper) of non-lenticular origin.

Frequency of cataract

Cataract may occur at any age but its incidence is clearly associated with ageing. The Framingham eye study (Leibowitz *et al.* 1980) showed a prevalence of 17.6% in the <65 years age group, 47.1% in the 65–74 years age group and 73.3% in those older than 75 years. The three common types of senile cataract are cortical (spoke), nuclear and posterior subcapsular, in descending order of frequency. When cataract occurs before the age of 55 the posterior subcapsular type predominates (Figure 9.1). Several studies show greater prevalence in the female with a male-to-female ratio of about 3:20.

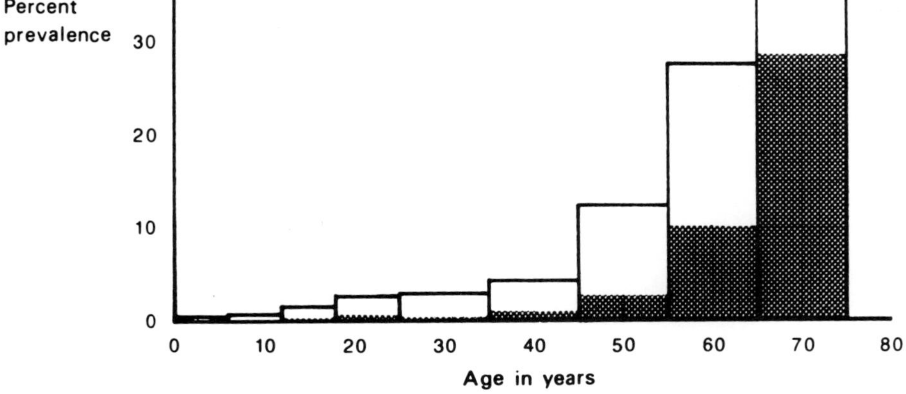

Figure 9.1 Prevalence of cataract with age. (after the National Centre for Health Statistics 1981 – NHANES.)

Basic categories of cataract formation

There are a limited number of ways in which opacification may occur.

Opacification of previously clear fibres

The youngest, most superficially situated fibres, which occupy C1α, are the most sensitive to mechanical and biochemical disturbance, such as concussion, hypocalcaemia, or hyperglycaemia. Thus many acquired cataracts are initially subcapsular and then come to lie at a greater depth with time if the process causing the cataract ceases and healthy fibre growth is resumed (see Chapter 13).

In senile cataract it is the older fibres deeper within the cortex (C2–C3) and the nuclear fibres, which lose transparency. Thus cortical spoke cataract arises in C2 and is confined to this zone until a relatively late stage of evolution, while C1 remains preserved.

When a cataract develops because of opacification of previously clear, mature lens fibres, then there are a limited number of forms that the opacity can take; these forms are determined by the anatomy of the lens fibres and their arrangement within the lens. They have been termed fibre-based cataracts (Bron and Brown 1986). Thus, when fibres within a particular perinuclear fibre shell are affected, often representing a number of fibre generations, a lamellar cataract is formed (Figures 9.2–9.4). When limited groups of fibres are affected, then the appearance is that of a spoke (Figure 9.5). If the tips of the fibres are affected as they enter the suture then the opacity takes on the branching pattern of the suture, as in the typical concussion cataracts (Figures 9.6, 9.7). Such opacities are usually subcapsular, and therefore the complexity of the branching pattern will reflect the degree of complexity of the suture pattern at the age of onset of the cataract. If the length of fibre affected is long then the opacity may take on a floral shape, as in concussion or copper cataracts (see Figure 12.12). In each case the suture line represents the framework for the opacity.

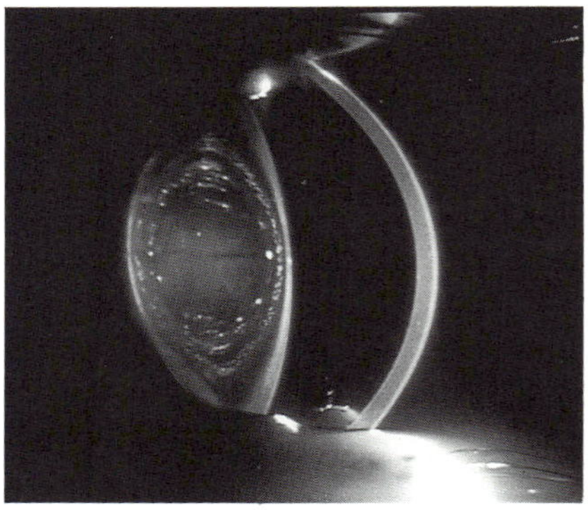

Figure 9.3 Lamellar cataract in a child aged 6.

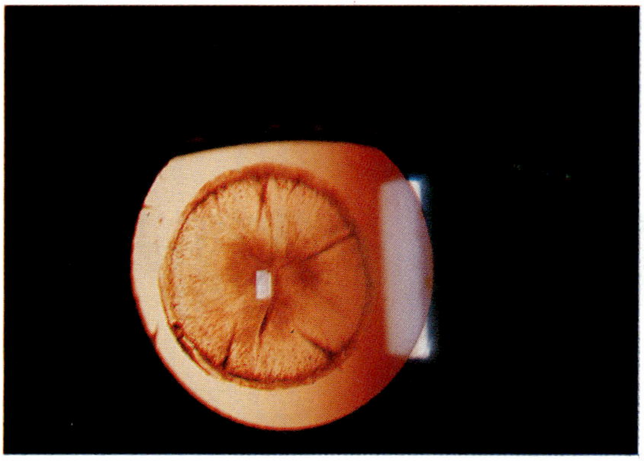

Figure 9.2 A typical congenital lamellar cataract with a relatively clear centre.

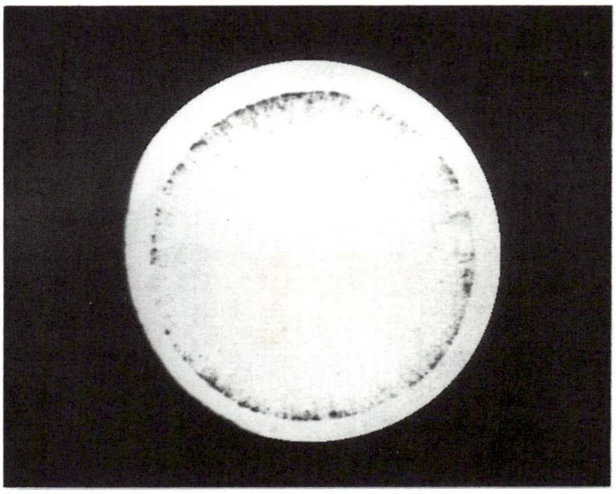

Figure 9.4 Lamellar cataract following an uncontrolled period in a diabetic. (CCD retro-illumination camera.)

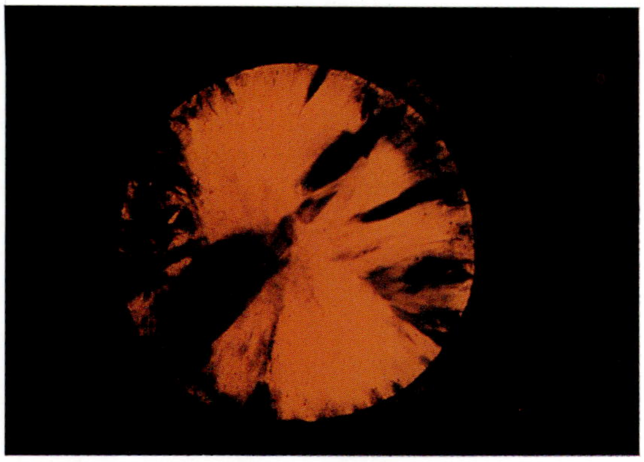

Figure 9.5 A typical senile cortical spoke cataract.

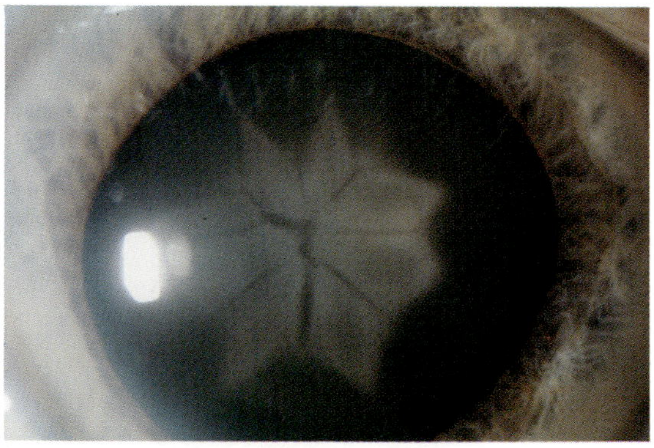

Figure 9.6 Typical flower shaped traumatic cataract. (Courtesy of A. Shun-Shin.)

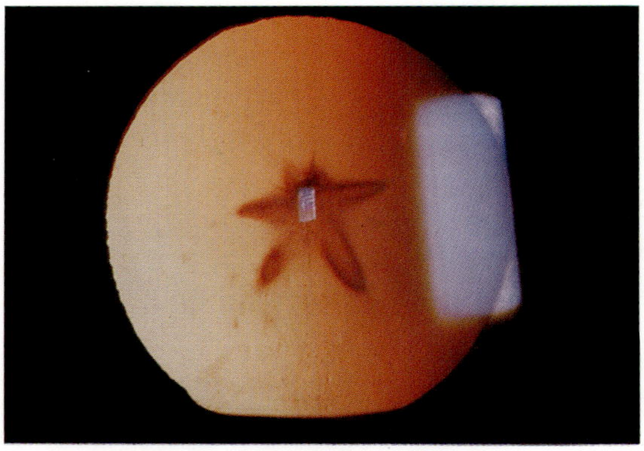

Figure 9.7 Flower shaped traumatic cataract (retro-illumination).

In spoke cataract, the opacity progresses from the periphery along the fibres until the suture is reached, at which point further progress is constrained. In traumatic cataract the suture lines represent the base from which the petal shape forms. In this case the fibre defect may not pass along the full extent of the fibre, which demonstrates that there must be an annealing process present within the lens, which shuts off the healthy remnant of the fibre from the diseased part. Thus the lens is not without its repair mechanisms and further examples will be found in this book (pp. 97, 147).

Formation of opaque fibres

Newly formed fibres that are opaque soon after their formation, a concept introduced by Lowe (1949a), are seen only in congenital (Figure 9.8) and developmental cataracts (Figures 9.9, 10.57, 10.64, 10.65). All the fibres in a lamella, or small groups of fibres, may be opaque and the lens growth otherwise normal.

Formation of material external to lens fibres

Granular material and aberrant epithelial cells are produced by a lens germinal epithelium which has

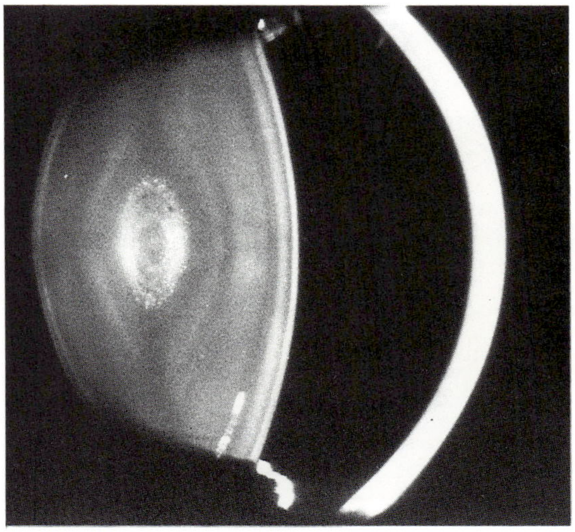

Figure 9.8 Cataracta centralis pulverlenta in an adult lens.

lost the ability to produce normal lens fibres. There is clear evidence for this mechanism in radiation cataract and it is probable that this mechanism also accounts for other posterior subcapsular cataracts including senile (p. 152). The granular material is first seen in the posterior subcapsular region of the lens periphery and the granules then move axially, in the direction normally taken by the growing lens fibres to form a subcapsular cataract around the posterior pole (Figures 9.10, 9.11).

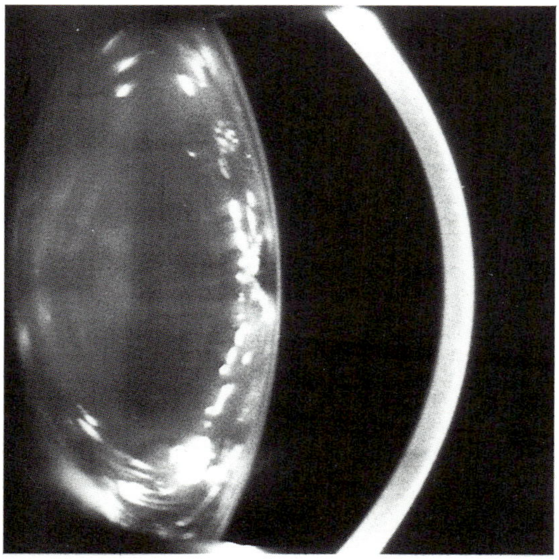

Figure 9.9 Coronary and focal dot opacities in a subject aged 59.

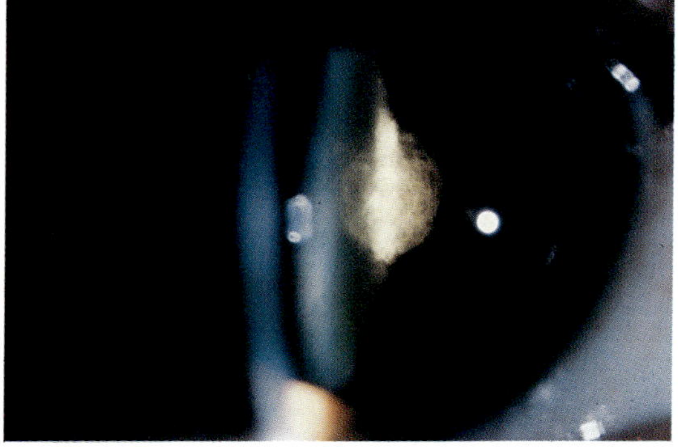

Figure 9.10 Focal illumination picture of posterior subcapsular cataract shows its subcapsular situation and lacy nature.

Fibrous metaplasia

Fibroblastic cells have been shown to be the cause of complicated cataract associated with retinal detachment (Scott 1979). There is evidence that these cells arise by fibrous metaplasia of the lens epithelium. Such fibroblastic cells are also seen following capsular trauma.

Opacification of lens epithelium

Opacification of the lens epithelium is seen typically in glaucoma flecks (*Glaukomflecken*) (Figures 9.12, 9.13) and is attributed to epithelial necrosis (Wistanley 1961). Lens epithelial necrosis due to an acute rise in ocular pressure is probably also responsible for the punctate form of traumatic cataract and also for the epithelial changes seen after chemical injury to the cornea and sometimes in acute iritis (Figure 9.13). Changes to the lens epithelium are also seen in anterior subcapsular cataract, which may add to the light scattering attributable to the cataractous changes in the fibres. Calcification occurs in the epithelium and anterior capsule in hypermature and Morgagnian cataract.

Accumulation of pigment

The human (and primate) lens contains the fluorescent compound 3-hydroxy-L-kynurenine-O-glucoside, which is responsible for the faint yellow colouration of the young lens, and its increase in

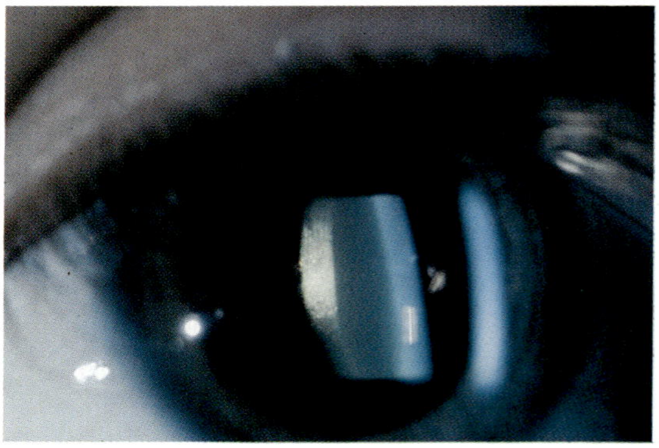

Figure 9.11 Posterior polychromasia.

aging (van Heyningen 1976, 1977). The fluorescence of the lens increases with age and more so in the diabetic and it appears that part of this fluorescence is due to the formation of advanced glycation products. Similar products are formed from the reaction of ascorbate with the lens crystallins (Bensch *et al.* 1985).

Specific chromophores (Pirie 1968) accumulate in the nucleus with the development of senile brunescent cataract and are associated with a highly cross-linked, insoluble fraction of the lens protein.

Extracellular deposits in the lens

Products of abnormal metabolism accumulate in the lens in some storage disorders, such as in Fabry's disease (Franceschetti 1976) and in mannosidosis (Murphree *et al.* 1976a,b) (p. 179).

Various drugs (or their metabolites) and metals may precipitate as fine granules, typically in the superficial cortex and in the capsule anteriorly (Figure 12.12, 12.16) (p. 197).

The physical basis of opacity

Lens transparency (p. 76) depends on the regular arrangement of the lens fibre cells, of their membranes and of the protein molecules that they contain. Loss of transparency is explained on the basis of disorganization of the fibre membranes at a microscopical level or of the lens proteins at a

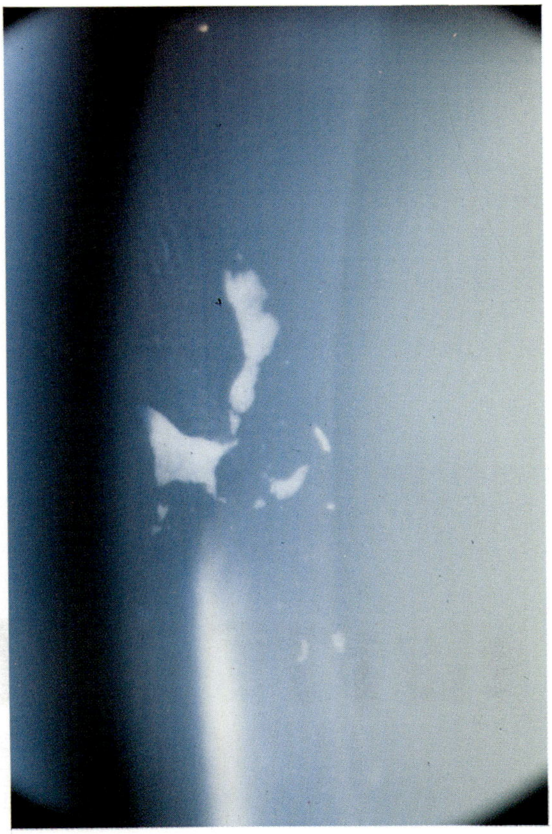

Figure 9.12 Fresh glaucoma flecks (magnification × 10).

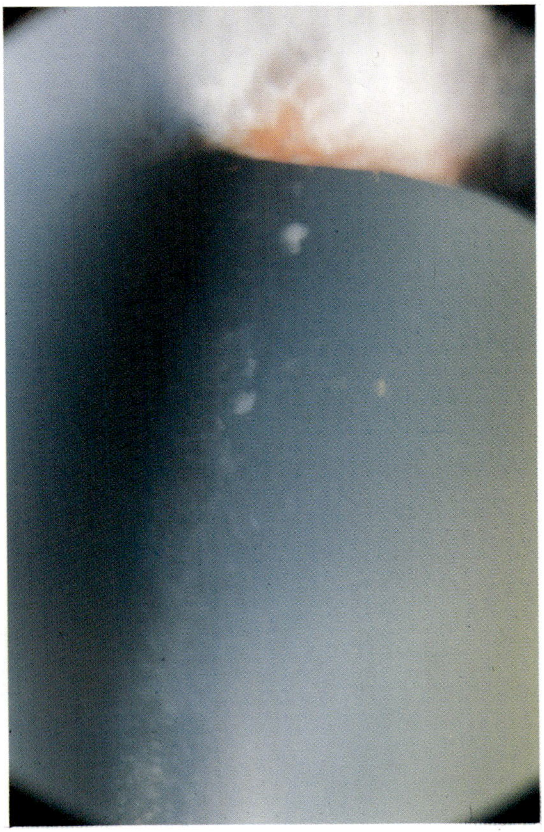

Figure 9.13 Fleck cataract in herpes zoster (magnification × 10).

molecular level. These processes may occur separately, or together, in the various morphological types of cataract.

Within the lens fibres, transparency is explained on the basis of small spatial fluctuations in the number of protein molecules over the dimensions comparable to the wavelength of light. Due to the high concentration of these molecules in the lens, none scatter light independently of one another (Benedek 1971). Turbidity is proportional to the molecular weight of these proteins. Cataract is explained either by the grouping of protein molecules to form large aggregates (Benedek 1971), or by the separation of the molecules due to water entry (Phillipson 1973). Probably both of these mechanisms occur simultaneously in cortical cataract. Also abnormalities of the fibre cell membranes and separation between fibres contribute. Electron microscopic studies of cataract support this view (Philipson 1973; Philipson and Fagerholm 1973), and shows whorls formed by fibre membranes, granularity of the cytoplasm with vesiculation and electron dense inclusions, and enlargement of the extracellular space.

In senile nuclear cataracts, loss of transparency is due to an increase in scattering by the nucleus (Figure 9.14) or increased absorption of light by the development of nuclear brunescence (Figure 9.15). White scatter is accounted for by the accumulation of protein aggregates. Brunescence is due to the accumulation of a yellow-brown insoluble protein pigment (Pirie 1968), which causes loss of transparency by light absorption. It is probable that this also involves aggregates responsible for increased scattering.

In the cortical and subcapsular cataract there is loss of transparency due to both cytoplasmic and membrane changes, whereas in nuclear cataract the changes involve molecular events within the fibre.

The structure of cataract

Epithelium

Degenerative changes occur in subcapsular cataract, which include vacuolation. Electron microscopy shows variations in cytoplasmic density and electron-dense bodies (Brown and Tripathi 1974) (Figure 9.16). At a later stage, proliferation of the epithelial cells may occur, giving rise to bladder cells of Wedl (Yanoff 1975). In association with retinal detachment, the epithelium may undergo fibrous metaplasia (Scott 1979).

Cortical cataract

Cataractous lens fibres become swollen. The nuclei of the superficial fibres degenerate and disappear. Electron microscopy shows a convoluted appearance of the fibre membranes with granularity of the cytoplasm, or reduction in cytoplasmic density and vesiculation (Kuwabara *et al.* 1969; Brini and

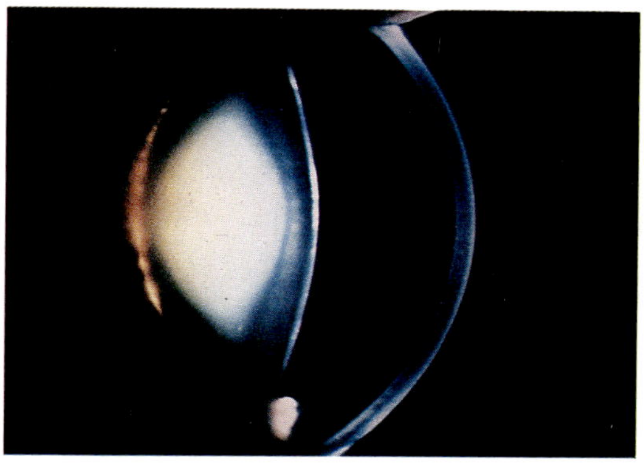

Figure 9.14 Senile nuclear white scatter. The lens also shows posterior subcapsular cataract.

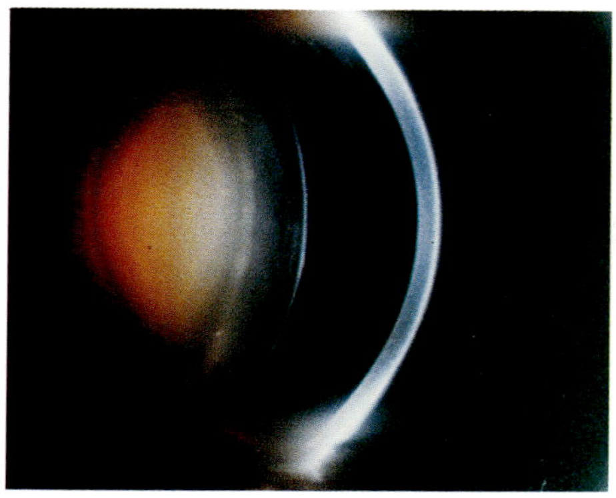

Figure 9.15 Senile nuclear brunescent cataract.

Flament 1973; Philipson 1973; Vrensen and Willekens 1990). Amorphous bodies may form, which, in non-progressive cataract such as coronary opacity, are seen to be separated from the normal lens fibres. These fibres that had previously run through the area of the cataract are shut off by membranes that have developed across them. These membranes lack gap junctions and ball and socket features (Vrensen and Willekens 1988; Vrensen *et al.* 1990) (Figure 9.17).

Water clefts form between the fibres. Electron microscopy shows that the fibres adjacent to the water clefts have an unusual membrane surface, with many sponge-like projections into the clefts (Shun-Shin *et al.* 1991b). Near-equatorial breaks may appear in the fibres and these are associated with fibre folds (Brown *et al.* 1989). Eventually the fibre breaks down to form round Morgagnian globules.

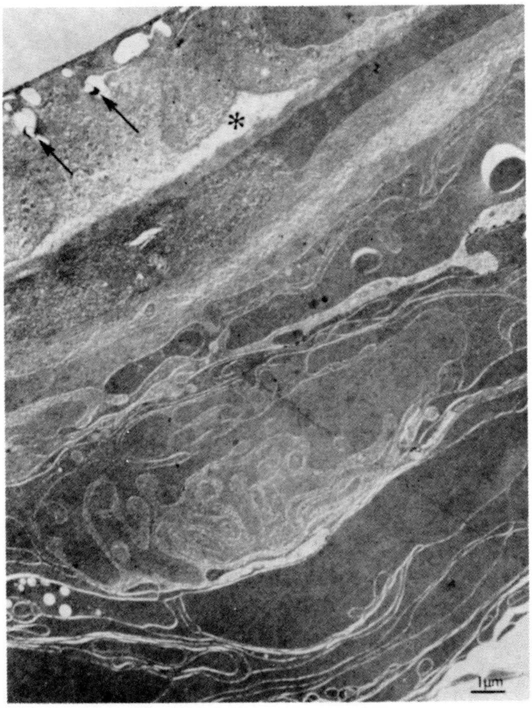

Figure 9.16 EM of the anterior lens cortex and epithelium showing variation in cytoplasmic density with convolution and distortion of the fibre membranes. The epithelium shows electron-dense inclusions (arrows) and loss of cytoplasmic density*. (Courtesy of R. Tripathi.)

Nuclear cataract

Nuclear cataract appears to be the result of light scattering due to the accumulation of high molecular weight protein, without major histological changes.

Posterior subcapsular cataract

The process of swelling and breakdown of lens fibres, as in cortical cataract, has been identified in posterior subcapsular cataract (Nagata *et al.* 1986); there is also an abnormality in the epithelial behaviour, in which cells migrate towards the posterior pole and extracellular granular and fibrillary material is produced (Eshagian and Streeten 1980; Eshagian *et al.* 1980) (p. 203). It is not certain that all posterior subcapsular cataracts result from this process of abnormal differentiation. Many discoid subcapsular cataracts do not appear biomicroscopically to be associated with centripetally migrating cells.

Ageing in the lens

Various regions of the lens are affected differently by the process of ageing. The central epithelial cells undergo limited mitosis and are thus vulnerable to programmed and post-translational ageing events

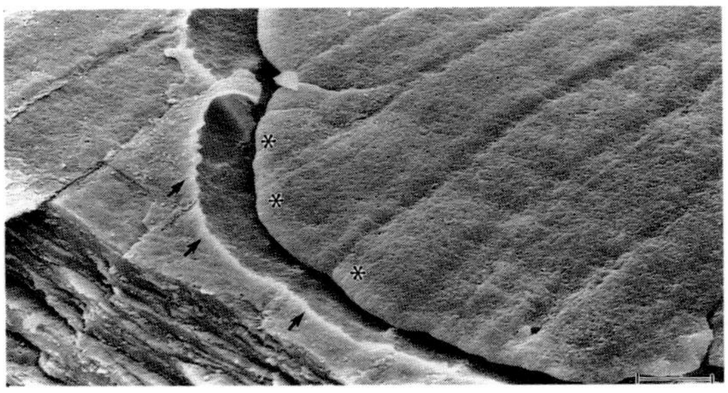

Figure 9.17 A junction between a cortical opacity (asterisks) and healthy fibres (arrows), which shows annealing of their exposed surfaces (scanning EM). (Courtesy of Vrensen and Willekeins 1989 with permission.)

over the lifetime of the individual. This part of the epithelium, exposed in the pupil zone, is particularly at risk of photodynamic stress.

Programmed changes may affect lens protein synthesis in successive generations of fibres. Thus the synthesis of gamma crystallin falls markedly after birth (McFall-Ngai *et al.* 1985) although it is gradually replaced by the homologous gamma s protein (previously called, beta s, see p. 65) in postnatal life.

Differentiation of epithelial cells into fibre cells is associated with the appearance of a beaded cytoskeletal protein (beaded filaments, Maisel 1985; Maisel and Perry 1972; Ireland and Maisel 1984a,b; Quinlan *et al.* 1992) present only in the fibre cells. The cytoskeletal proteins vimentin, actin and spectrin are present in the epithelium, where they persist to the ninth decade. They are present too in the superficial cortical fibres, but their absence from the deeper cortical or nuclear fibres suggests that they are degraded at some interval after fibre differentiation. However, the majority of ageing changes are post-translational, and related to the cumulative effects of exogenous and endogenous insults. Some of the changes which occur in the lens with age may be summarized here.

Lens enzymes show a greater heat lability with age and, in the cortex, an increase in inactive forms occurs (Ohrloff and Hockwin 1983). There is a decrease in the number of nuclear enzymes and in their activity. The activity of epithelial glutathione reductase, important for the regeneration of the reduced form of this free radical scavenger, is decreased in older lenses.

Protein turnover in the nucleus falls with age, and is negligible in the adult lens. Glutathione levels are low in the nucleus of adult lenses compared to cortex. There are dramatic changes in crystallin solubility and aggregate size, with a rise in water insoluble crystallins, and the formation of both soluble and insoluble high molecular weight (HMW) crystallin aggregates, mostly confined to the lens nucleus. There is a fall in gamma crystallin in the nucleus with increasing age. Numerous changes in crystallin structure occur, some of which favour the formation of cross-linked proteins and aggregates.

A major consideration concerns those factors leading to the unfolding of the crystallins which could facilitate protein cross-linking. Harding and Crabbe (1984) listed those age-related changes which could lead to protein unfolding and the mechanisms involved, by altering the charge distribution on the surface of the crystallin molecule (Table 9.1) (Figure 9.18). Thus, removal of an amide group would produce a new negative charge in the crystallin molecule, although this is thought to occur infrequently after the age of 34 years. Oxidation of methionine converts a hydrophobic to a polar group. Glycosylation or carbamylation of the free amino groups of lysine causes loss of a positive charge, while formation of a mixed disulphide (the product of the reaction between oxidized glutathione and a crystallin) introduces three new charges onto the molecule (Figure 9.19). Photo-oxidation of tryptophan generates more

Table 9.1 Non-enzymic post-translational modifications of lens proteins in cataract

Glycation (non-enzymic glycosylation)
Carbamylation
Steroid adduct formation
Mixed disulphide formation
Protein–protein disulphide formation
Methionine oxidation
Racemization
Degradation

From Harding (1991) with permission.

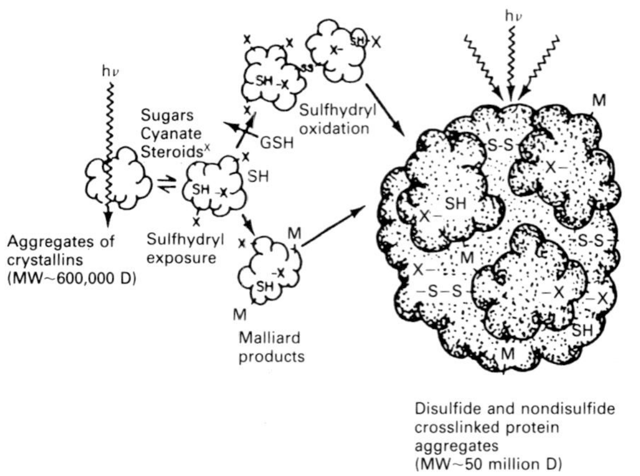

Figure 9.18 A model for crystallin aggregate formation due to post-translational modification. (From Cerami and Crabbe 1986 with permission.)

polar groupings. Glycosylation of lysine amino groups leads to the formation of a Schiff-base compound in which the adduct is stabilized by the so called Amadori rearrangement. The material can then undergo further non-enzymatic browning (or Maillard reactions) to produce brown products which will cross-link proteins. Ascorbate, which is present in the lens in far higher concentrations than glucose, can also react in this way to produce material with the same spectrophotometric and fluorescent characteristics (Bensch *et al.* 1985; Garland *et al.* 1986; Ortwerth and Oleson 1988a). It is the oxidation products of ascorbate, (dehydroascorbic acid [DHA]; 2,3 diketo-gulonic acid [DKG];

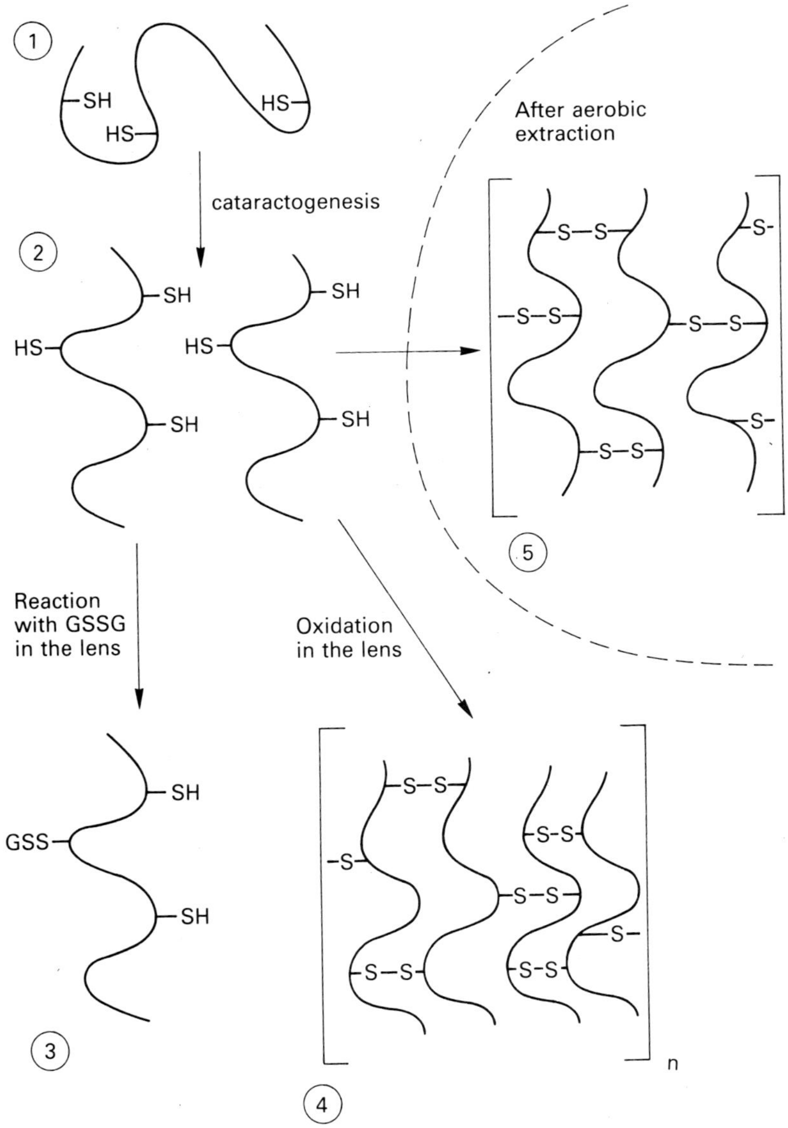

Figure 9.19 Changes in lens proteins in the development of human nuclear cataract: (1) native protein; (2) unfolded protein; (3) mixed disulphide; (4) disulphide-bonded protein of high molecular weight; (5) urea-soluble protein. (From Harding and Dilley 1976 with permission.)

L-xylosone and L-threose) which have been implicated in the process of crystallin glycation (Ortwerth *et al.* 1994) and although they will all cross-link in reducing conditions, threose is the most active (Kwan *et al.* 1972). The low oxygen levels in the human lens (about 20 μM), and other factors, encourage the reduction of DHA back to ascorbate, either non-enzymatically by the action of reduced glutathione (about 2-5 mM) (Khatami *et al.* 1986; Winckler 1987; Ortwerth and Oleson 1988b), or by a glutathione-dependent enzymatic process (Rose and Bode 1992). None the less, both DHA (Lohman *et al.* 1986) and DKG (Kern and Zolot 1987), (intermediates in the formation of xylosone and threose), are found in the human lens, at concentrations ranging from 0.05 to 0.1 mM.

Ortwerth *et al.* (1994) have suggested that the potential for threose to glycate lens crystallins may be offset *in vivo* by reduction of threose to threitol in the presence of aldose reductase. Although, unlike sorbitol, threitol diffuses rapidly from the lens, threitol is found in the human lens at a concentration of greater than 0.1 μmol/g lens tissue, [or 3.4 μg per lens].

Collagen and other proteins undergo cross-linking between pentose, arginine and lysine, with the formation of a yellow fluorescent compound, pentosidine. This compound can also be formed *in vitro* by the fragmentation of pentose sugars, and from ascorbate, which may be an important source of pentosidine (Figure 9.20a). Trioses, tetroses and ketoses are also potential sources (Sell *et al.* 1991). Ribose is the most reactive reducing sugar, while fructose and glucose are 130 and 400 times less reactive (Dyer *et al.* 1991).

Pentosidine levels increase with age in skin collagen and are increased in type I diabetes and in patients with uraemia (Sell *et al.* 1990a,b). The degree of increase correlates with the degree of diabetic complication, such as retinopathy nephropathy and arterial or joint stiffness. (Sell *et al.* 1991a).

An age-dependent accumulation of pentosidine in the human lens has been found by Dyer *et al.* (1991) which is mainly associated with the water soluble rather than the insoluble fraction. The absolute levels are about 2–3 times higher in the water insoluble fractions, so that a contribution of pentosidine to insolubilization has been suggested (Nagaraj *et al.* 1991). There was a dramatic increase in pentosidine in brunescent cataracts compared with normal lenses (Figure 9.20b), and a relationship between the degree of pigmentation and cross-linking in these lenses was suggested by the observation that almost all of the increased pentosidine from cataract crystallins was associated with the alpha crystallin fraction and little with the beta crystallins. In that study, surprisingly, there was no difference in pentosidine levels between non-diabetic and diabetic cataractous lenses, although a significant increase in diabetic cataractous lenses was found by Lyons *et al.* (1991).

A prominent ageing phenomenon of human tissues is the decrease in solubility and elasticity of collagen, with an increase in thermal stability and stiffness due to the progressive formation of cross-links. It also accumulates fluorescent yellow and brown pigments. Reducing sugars can react with non-enzymatically modified amino groups of long-lived proteins to produce both yellow fluorescent adducts and cross-links. This is the non-enzymatic browning, or Maillard reaction, and involves formation of a Schiff-base, which rearranges into a stable Amadori product.

About 2% of the crystallins are glycosylated in the cataracts of normal subjects, and 3% in diabetics. Carbamylation of lens crystallins has been identified in lenses with advanced cataract in Pakistani subjects, which implies adduct formation between crystallin lysine amino groups and cyanate (Harding and Rixon 1980). Cyanate is a hydrolysis product of urea, which is thought to be its natural source. A raised blood urea level has been identified as a risk factor for cataract by a number of groups. Minassian *et al.* (1984) in Raipur, India, found that a history of two or more episodes of severe diarrhoea gave rise to a 21 times higher risk of developing cataract at a relatively young age. About 36% of cataracts could be attributed to this association. It has been suggested that dehydration caused by the diarrhoea, in raising blood urea levels, might contribute to cataract formation; nutritional factors were also in operation.

Whatever the basis for crystallin unfolding, it exposes the protein to the risk of presenting reactive thiols for oxidation, and encouraging the formation of disulphide-linked and other forms of HMW aggregate formation capable of increasing light scatter. It has been noted above that the pigmented products of glycosylation are themselves capable of forming non-disulphide linked HMW aggregates. Ageing is associated with an increase in yellow pigment in the lens for which a

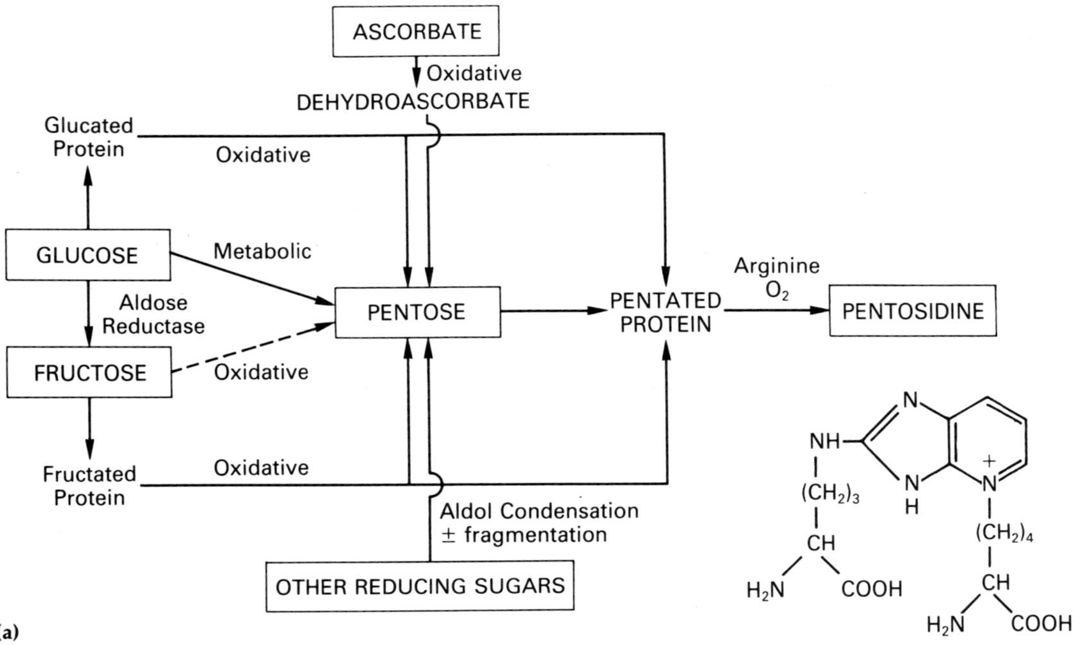

(a)

Figure 9.20(a) Possible biosynthetic pathways leading to pentosidine formation. (From Sells *et al.* 1991 with permission.)

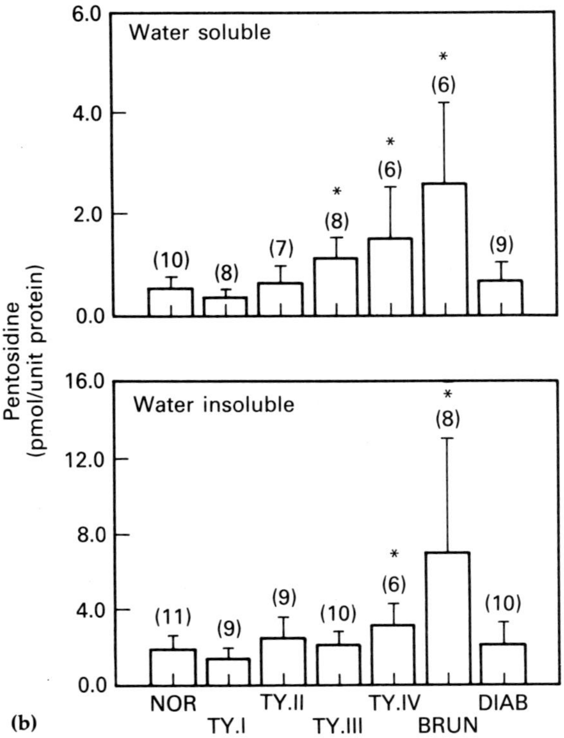

(b)

Figure 9.20(b) Pentosidine level in water soluble and water-insoluble crystallin fractions from cataractous lenses classified on the basis of pigmentation: NOR = Normal; TYI-IV increasing pigmentation in the direction I to IV; BRUN = brunescent lenses; DIAB = diabetic. Number of lenses in brackets. * = significantly different from normal. (From Nagaraj *et al.* 1991 with permission.)

number of candidates have been proposed. It has been suggested that photo-oxidation may give rise to various pigments. Certain membrane components of the lens are disulphide cross-linked in the young lens. The proportion of disulphide cross-linked proteins increases with age and this could interfere with the fluidity of the membrane and also with membrane permeability, since experimental oxidation of membrane thiols causes a selective increase in permeability to calcium and sodium.

Biochemical changes in cataract

Protein and water content

Protein synthesis is continuous in the normal lens partly due to normal protein turnover and partly to the addition of new fibres. The protein content increases with age. In cortical cataract there is a decrease in total protein content and initially the lens is low in weight. This is followed by an increase in the percentage water content as membrane permeability increases and the fibres swell (Maraini and Pescatori 1972; Duncan *et al.* 1989) (Figure 9.21). There is a decrease in soluble proteins and a relative increase in insoluble protein (albuminoid).

In nuclear cataract the water balance remains normal and there is no decrease in protein content, but there is an increase in the insoluble protein at the expense of the soluble (Maraini and Pescatori 1972). Protein molecular aggregates form, causing light scatter. Brunescence is due to the accumulation of specific chromophores. These may be accounted for by brown adducts, formed by the combination of glucose or ascorbate with protein (Bensch *et al.* 1985).

Denaturation of lens proteins leads to unfolding of protein molecules and aggregation to form large molecules, which scatter light. Several agents lead to protein denaturation in the lens (Harding and Crabbe 1984); these include free radicals causing oxidation, sugars causing glycation and cyanate causing carbamylation. Cyanate is derived from urea in renal failure and also from cigarette smoke. Ascorbate may also produce a form of protein glycation. Ultraviolet light is an additional factor in the production of free radicals and in protein denaturation (Taylor *et al.* 1988). It

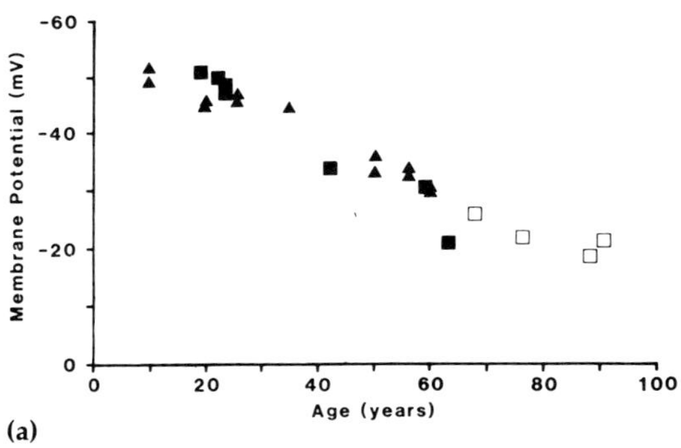

(a)

Figure 9.21(a) Human lens membrane potential measured in donor lenses (filled symbols) and nuclear cataractous lenses (open symbols) as a function of age. Data were obtained in two laboratories: ■, □ Norwich, England; ▲ Rochester, Michigan. The open symbols were obtained from lenses with pure nuclear cataracts.

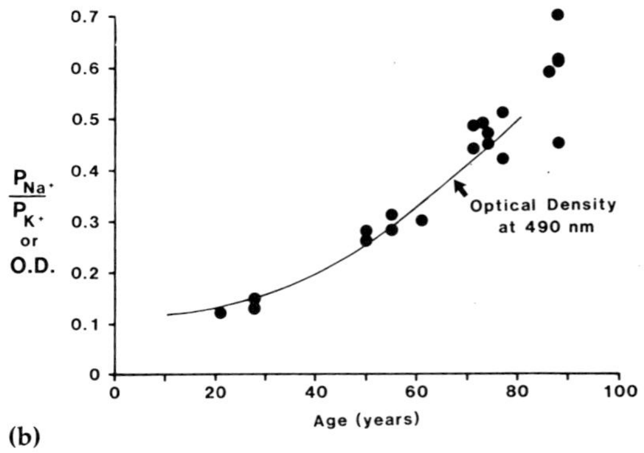

(b)

Figure 9.21(b) Relative permeability P_{Na^+}/P_{K^+} of human lenses plotted as a function of age. The solid line shows the change with age of the mean optical density of the human lens measured at 490 nm. Note that the scales for optical density and permeability ratio are the same. (From Duncan *et al.* 1989 with permission.)

is likely that the various factors act in combination (Figure 9.22).

Studies show that carbamylation or glycation of lens crystallins encourages unfolding of these protein molecules by reduction of surface positive charges. Such unfolded proteins are susceptible to aggregation in conditions of oxidative stress by the formation of disulphide bonded covalent crosslinking to form molecular aggregates. In addition, advanced glycation products are brown and fluorescent.

In disorders of sugar metabolism, such as diabetes mellitus or galactosaemia, there is an accumulation of alcohol in the lens, which, because of its relative impermeability in relation to the lens cells, results in an osmotically driven influx of water into the lens. This leads to an increase in extra- and intracellular water with disruption of the lens fibres. Clinically this is said to be responsible for a characteristic snowflake cortical cataract with subcapsular features in the juvenile diabetic (Figure 9.23), and an 'oil droplet' kind of refractive change in the case of galactosaemia (or galactokinase deficiency – see below). In either case, in the absence of treatment of the primary sugar disorder, the cataract may progress to total opacification.

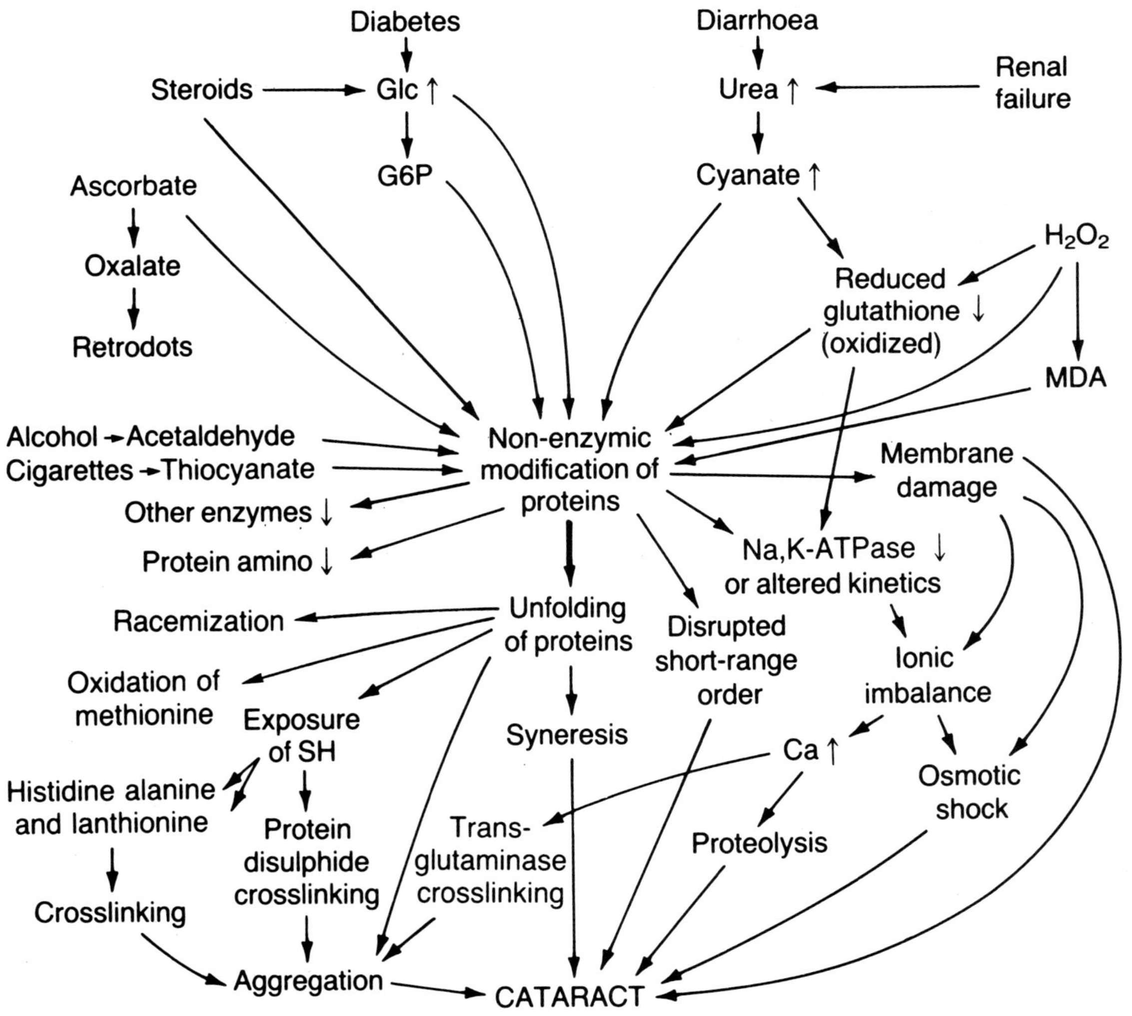

Figure 9.22 The pathways leading to lens protein degradation and cataract. (From Harding 1991 with permission.)

This osmotic mechanism, and the role of sugar alcohol, is less certain in the human situation than in the experimental rat.

Enzymes

Several calcium-activated proteolytic enzymes are present in the lens cortex and their activity may increase in cataract maturation as the calcium concentration increases (de Beradinis 1950; Shearer *et al.* 1987) with the resultant breakdown of proteins to peptides and amino acids. These diffuse through the capsule and the lens content may eventually liquify, with the exception of the senile nucleus. The enzymes associated with respiration and also glutathione reductase are depleted (Friedburg 1973).

Glutathione

This sulphydryl-containing molecule is important in lens respiration (p. 64) and is normally present in high concentrations. Its concentration declines with age and there is a marked fall in cataract levels, particularly in subcapsular cataract and in cataract maturation (Pau *et al.* 1990).

Vitamins

Ascorbic acid (vitamin C) is found in high concentration in the normal lens and declines with age and in cataract (Consul and Nagpal 1968). The fall in ascorbic acid and in gluthathione levels may be the result of oxidative stress and would itself

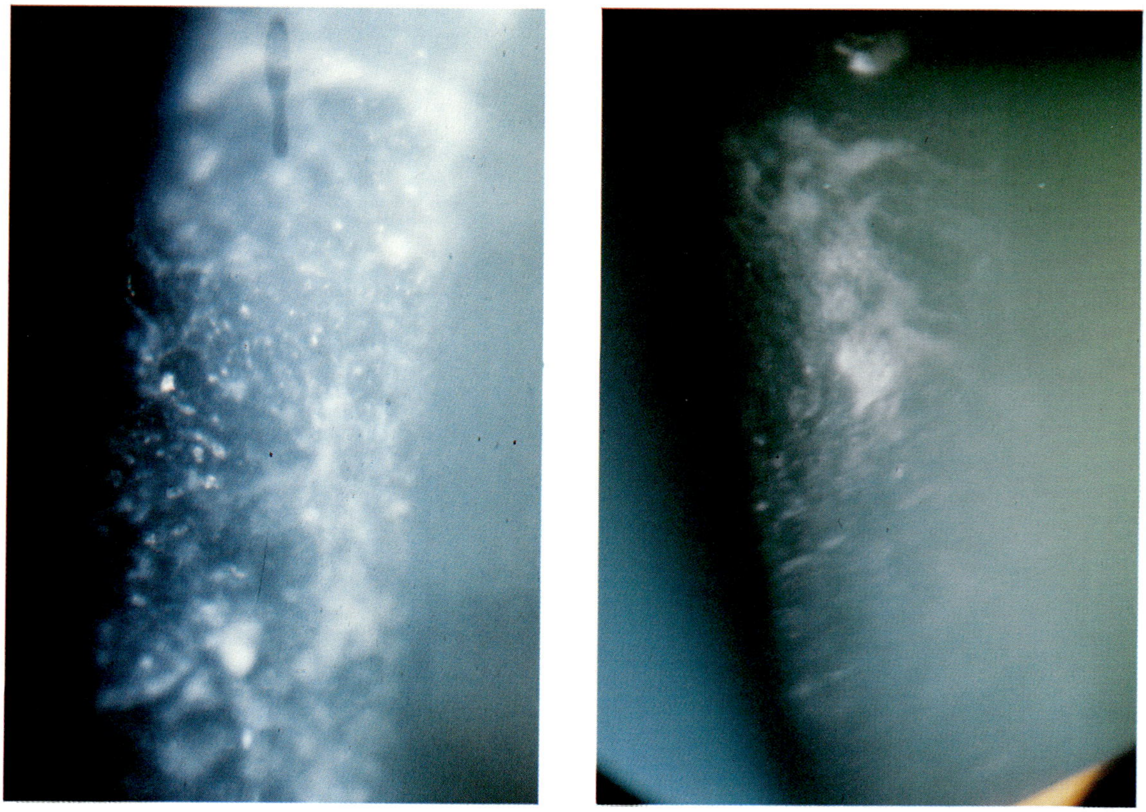

(a) (b)

Figure 9.23 Acute diabetic cataract (original magnification × 10).

render the lens susceptible to further oxidative damage. Oxidation of ascorbic acid itself could contribute oxalate as a component of retro-dot lens opacities (Bron and Brown 1987), although it appears that calcium phosphate is the major component. However, oxalate has been found in the hypermature cataract (Harding *et al.* 1983) and in the spheroliths of Morgagnian cataract (see Bron and Habgood 1976). However, lenses with retro-dot opacities do not have high oxalate levels (Lewis *et al.* 1994; Vrensen *et al.* 1994).

Degradation of lens proteins occurs by oxidation due to free radicals in the lens (Harding and Crabbe 1984). The free radicals may be neutralized by the anti-oxidant vitamins. Thus the presence of vitamins C, E and β-carotene may be important in preventing cataract.

Ions

In the normal lens, the sodium content is low and the potassium content high. In cortical cataracts the sodium content increases (van Heyningen 1972) and the potassium content falls (Mackay *et al.* 1932). The calcium content also increases. Failure of the pump mechanisms, increased membrane permeability and loss of integrity of the fibre cell walls are the likely causes.

Experimental cataract (Table 9.2)

A number of experimental models for cataract have been developed which have indicated targets for lens damage, and which may have relevance to human cataract. There is often considerable overlap in mechanism between one aetiology and another.

Basic mechanisms

Damage to certain key structures or mechanisms in the lens leads to cataract. The manner in which these targets may be damaged is introduced here and dealt with later in further detail.

Table 9.2 Experimental cataract

1. BASIC MECHANISMS OF CATARACT
   (a) Inhibition of cation pump [Nakano mouse]
   (b) Increased lens permeability [Anticholinesterases]
   (c) Osmotic swelling [sugar cataract]
   (d) Disturbed glycolysis [2. deoxyglucose]
   (e) Disturbed metabolism [2.4 DNP]
   (f) Oxidative stress and loss of protective mechanisms
2. DRUGS CAUSING LOSS OF GSH AND FREE RADICAL SCAVENGERS
   (a) Naphthalene and its derivatives
   (b) Selenium
   (c) Mercaptoundecahydrododecaborate
   (d) Iodoacetate
   (e) Methionine sulphoximine
   (f) 4-chlorophenylalanine
   (g) Diquat
3. PROTEIN DENATURATION
   DMSO
4. RADIATION CATARACT
   (a) X-radiation
       Age and Species
       Radiation damage
       Fractionation
   (b) Beta and gamma radiation
   (c) Neutrons, protons and heavy ions
   (d) Ultraviolet radiation
   (e) Infra red cataract
   (f) Electric cataract
   (g) Microwave cataract
5. POSTRANSLATIONAL MODIFICATION OF PROTEINS
   (a) Cyanate
   (b) Glycation
   (c) Other
6. PROTEOLYTIC ENZYMES AND THE LENS
7. DISTURBANCE OF LIPID METABOLISM
   (a) Inhibitors of cholesterol synthesis
       i Triparanol
       ii DEEA
       iii HMG Co A reductase inhibitors
8. DEHYDRATION CATARACT
9. COLD CATARACT
10. OTHER AGENTS
11. NUTRITIONAL CATARACT
    Malnutrition
    Vit A deficiency
    Vit B deficiency
    Amino acid and protein deficiency
12. GENETIC CATARACT
13. INFECTIVE CATARACT

Inhibition of the cation pump

In the Nakano cataract strain of mouse, a pinhead lens opacity develops at 3 weeks of life, which is associated with a sudden increase of lens sodium and water. This increases as the cataract matures. Radioactive studies (^{86}Rb and ^{22}Na) have shown defective transport of potassium inwards and of sodium extrusion in the presence of normal permeability in the early stage. At 13 days there is a 50%

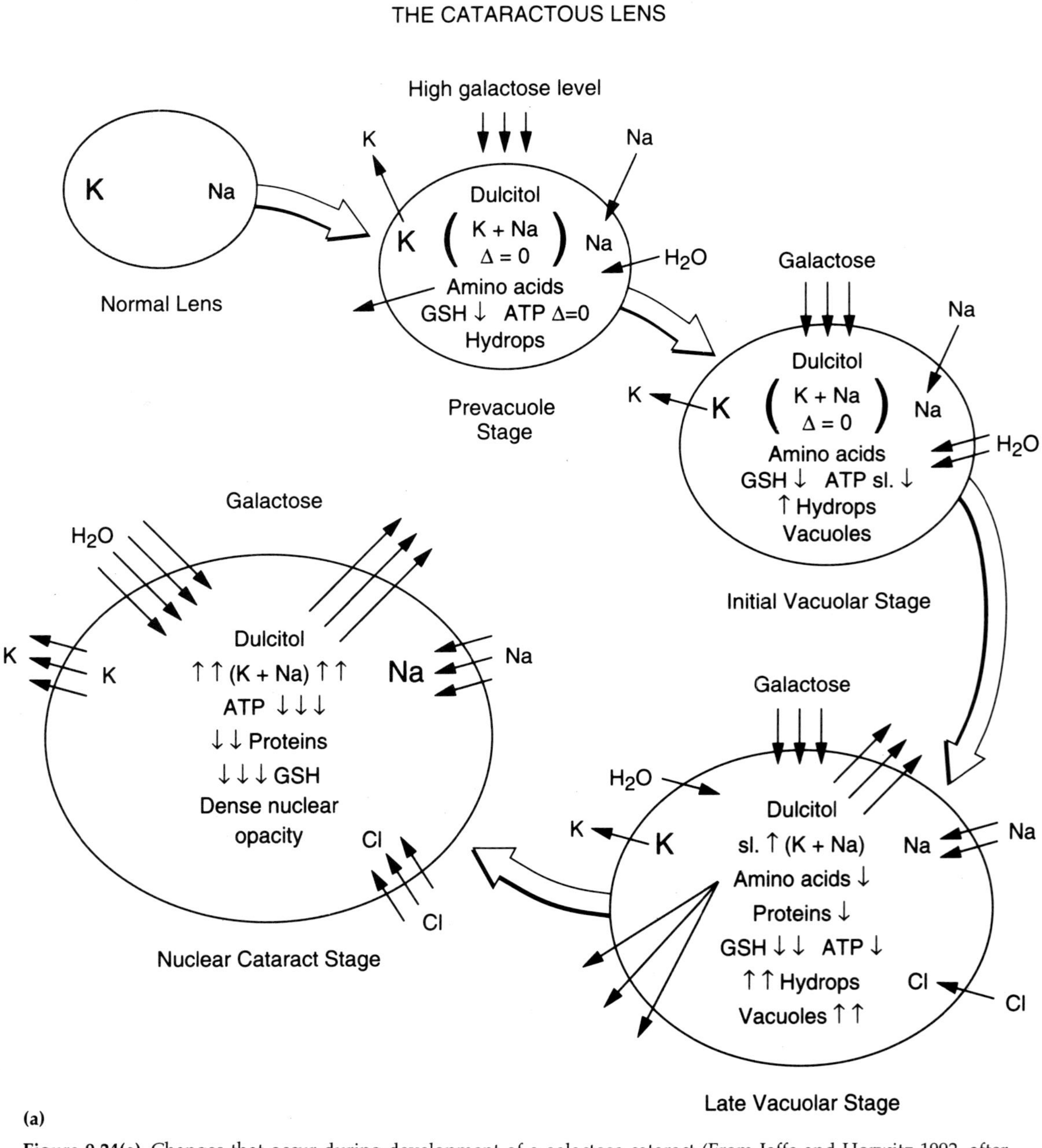

(a)

Figure 9.24(a) Changes that occur during development of a galactose cataract (From Jaffe and Horwitz 1992, after Kinoshita 1965b) inhibition of Na^+K^+ATPase. Inhibition appears to be due to the presence of a heat labile inactivator (Kinoshita 1974; Iwata and Kinoshita 1971). Ouabain in a concentration of 10^{-4} inhibits 90% of (rabbit) Na^+K^+ATPase activity, with a resulting rise in water and a loss of potassium.

Increased lens permeability

In vitro studies of anticholinesterases demacarium bromide and phospholine iodide (Michon and Kinoshita 1968) and of surface active agents (Cotlier and Apple 1973) have demonstrated an increase in lens permeability which is regarded as a possible basis of experimental cataract with these agents. Other factors may be involved with the anticholinesterases.

Osmotic swelling – sugar cataracts

A rise in aqueous sugar levels initially induces lens fibre swelling by osmotic means, and later causes a rise in lens fibre permeability resulting in disruption of the fibre.

The cataractogenic sugars, xylose, galactose and glucose entering the rat lens are converted into their respective sugar alcohols in the presence of the enzyme aldose reductase. These alcohols accumulate within the lens fibre, which is poorly permeable to them. The hypertonicity created is corrected immediately by an influx of water (Kinoshita *et al.* 1964; van Heyningen 1959a,b, 1962a,b, 1969a) (Figure 9.24).

Initially the activity of the cation pumps compensates for the increased water content of the fibre. This results in extracellular vacuole formation. Eventually, fibre membrane permeability breaks down and both water and electrolyte content of the fibre increases. At the stage of dense nuclear cataract, there is loss of free amino acids and the sugar alcohol itself, associated with disruption of the fibre (Sakuragawa *et al.* 1975).

Other early changes include a fall in glycolysis, a marked fall in glutathione, and a small fall in ATP, which could itself be important to cation pump function (Sippel 1966; van Heyningen 1963).

Disturbed glycolysis

Glucose enters the glycolytic pathway through the action of the pacemaker enzyme, hexokinase,

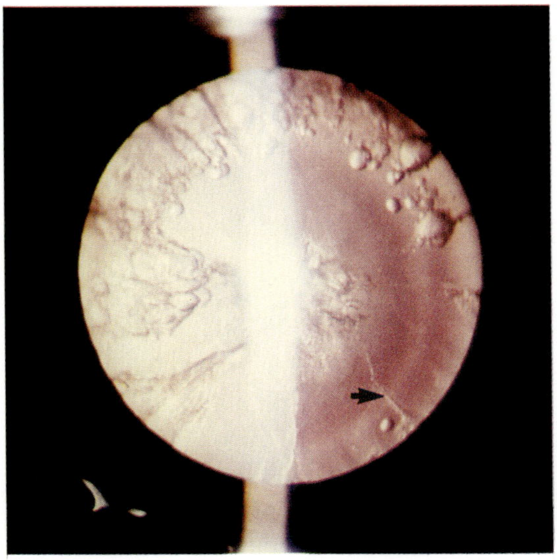

(b)

Figure 9.24(b) Red reflex image of the diabetic cataract in the BN (Brown-Norway) rat, vacuole cluster together with spokes (arrow) are typical features in the outer cortex of the lens. (Courtesy of A. Wegener.)

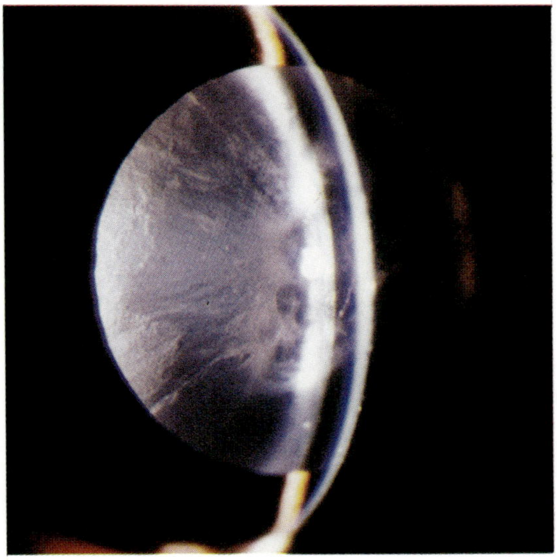

(c)

Figure 9.24(c) Optical section of the anterior eye segment of the diabetic rat, showing inhomogeneous, patchy opacities in the lens cortex. (Courtesy of A. Wegener.)

which is involved in the formation of glucose-6-phosphate. This enzyme is competitively inhibited by the glucose analogue 2-deoxyglucose. This compound is capable of inducing cataract *in vitro* in the same way as a low glucose concentration, presumably acting by reduced production of ATP, affecting the cation pump, and reduced pentose shunt activity (which provides ribose-5-phosphate for ribonucleotides and coenzymes, and NADPH coenzyme needed for fatty acid synthesis and maintenance of reduced glutathione) (Chylack 1975; van Heyningen 1977). Chylack (1977) believes that the cataract associated with neonatal hypoglycaemia is caused through such as mechanism, and that a secondary loss of hexokinase activity occurs due to the thermolability of this enzyme at body temperature in the absence of glucose.

Disturbed aerobic metabolism

2,4-dinitrophenol (DNP) uncouples oxidative phosphorylation from the respiratory chain and prevents the generation of ATP by aerobic respiration. Cataract has been produced in ducklings and chickens by feeding with DNP, but not in mature rabbits. This species difference appears to be related to the ability of DNP to enter the aqueous in different species (Gehring and Buerge 1969), and in the immature rabbit, whose blood–aqueous barrier is more permeable than the adult, cataract can also be produced by ingestion.

Since lenses may be maintained clear *in vitro* in the presence of glucose but the absence of oxygen, it is not certain that the action of DNP is due to its inhibition of aerobic metabolism, but this appears to be the most likely mechanism. It may be relevant that the initial location of the lens opacity in this condition is subepithelial while the major location of aerobic metabolism is in the epithelium.

Oxidative stress and loss of protective mechanisms

Many insults to the lens lead to a loss of free radical scavengers and decrease its protection from oxidative damage. A list of those forms of experimental cataract resulting in a fall in glutathione levels is given in Table 9.3.

There is excellent experimental evidence that oxidative stress, whether generated by radiation or by hydrogen peroxide (Figure 9.25), or by exposure to hyperbaric oxygen, will increase reactive species in the lens which cause damage to lens DNA, lipid and protein. Functionally this may impair ion pumps and membrane transport, increase membrane permeability, interfere with lens mitosis and ultimately lead to cataract formation. Such stress is associated with a fall in the level of scavengers in

Table 9.3 Experimental cataracts associated with low levels of reduced glutathione (GSH)

Diabetic	Naphthalene
Galactose	Dimethylsulphoxide
Xylose	Methionine sulphoximine
Cyanate	X-ray
Uveitis	Microwave
Traumatic	Nakano
Dinitrophenol	Philly
Mercaptoundecahydro-dodecaborate	Emory
Selenite	*ICR/1*
Steroid	Iodoacetate
4-Chlorophenylalanine	Tryptophan deficiency

From Harding (1991) with permission.

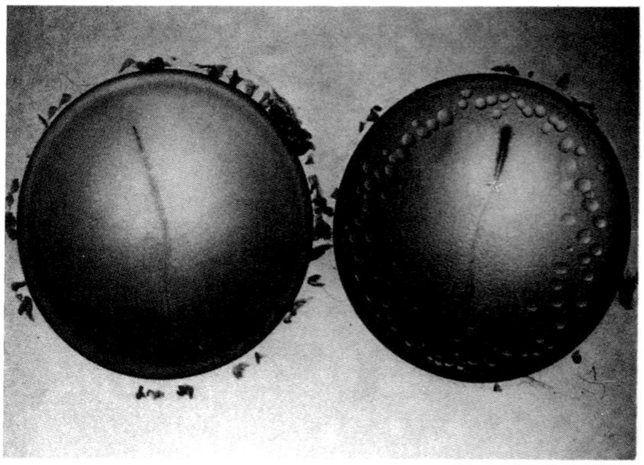

Figure 9.25 Rabbit lenses incubated for 6 hours. Left lens in control medium is clear (the oblique linear feature is the anterior suture). The right lens was pretreated for 3 hours with BCNH, a relatively specific inhibitor of glutathione reductase, which is required for glutathione synthesis. The lens was then exposed to 0.05 mM H_2O_2. Note the numerous vacuoles at the periphery of the experimental lens. (From Giblin *et al.* 1987 with permission.)

the lens. Cataract may be inhibited experimentally by a restoration or supplementation of scavengers, or the use of synthetic antioxidants in specific circumstances.

There is evidence that scavengers are diminished in human cataract and it seems likely that a deficiency of scavenger molecules, or of their regeneration, and the cumulative effect of oxidative stress plays a role in human cataract. However, the sequence of events is difficult to establish, and this role is chiefly inferential.

Zigler and Lucas (1986) have demonstrated the importance of glutathione reductase, the regenerating enzyme for reduced glutathione (GSH), in the defence of monkey lenses exposed to hydrogen peroxide or singlet oxygen. Damage is exacerbated when the enzyme is inhibited with 1,3-bis(chloroethyl)nitrosourea (BCNU). The ability of rabbit epithelial cells in culture to resist the effects of hydrogen peroxide toxicity (e.g. a lowering of lens GSH levels) is directly related to the age of the cells and inversely related to cell density. This may in turn be related to the lower levels (50%) of glucose-6-phosphate dehydrogenase and glutathione reductase in older cells, both of which are required for glutathione regeneration.

Hydrogen peroxide can induce oxidation and aggregation of total lens extracts. In the intact lens a rise of the phase reversal temperature occurs at 5–20 mmol, associated with oxidation of exposed thiols and major shifts in molecular weight distribution. There is a loss of beta H-crystallin and a dissociation to beta L-crystallin with the formation of HMW aggregates.

Exposure of rabbit lenses to long wave ultraviolet (UVA) radiation (peak 365 nm) results in a rise in aqueous hydrogen peroxide levels and lens malondialdehyde levels, and a fall in lens GSH and protein thiol levels.

In animal studies by Reddy *et al.* (1986), reduction of lens GSH by X-radiation leads to an increase in disulphide cross-linked membrane proteins. Oxidation of GSH with tertiary butyl hydroperoxide (1 mmol) leads to increased permeability of fibre and epithelial cell membranes. This is partially reversible in the fibres.

Inhibition of glutathione reductase with BCNU has a similar effect when combined with exposure to hydrogen peroxide. Binding of membrane thiols by a non-penetrating sulphydryl reagent (PCMBS) increases epithelial and fibre permeability to calcium and to sodium, and this is associated with lens opacification. This is partially reversible by GSH or cysteine (95 mmol).

A number of workers have shown inactivation of the lens pumps by UV exposure. Torriglia *et al.* (1986) have demonstrated a relationship between loss of Na^+K^+ATPase activity and the rate of swelling of the rat lens; the epithelial enzyme was more sensitive than the cortical enzyme. Pump activity is also inhibited by hydrogen peroxide generating systems (Garner *et al.* 1983, 1986a,b; Garadi *et al.* 1986). It is likely that a Na^+-binding site of the ATPase, accessible on the outside of the membrane, is affected by the hydrogen peroxide.

Garadi *et al.* (1986) have demonstrated a protective *in vitro* effect of ascorbate on Na^+K^+ATPase activity and membrane transport functions (studied using ^{86}Rb and ^{3}H choline uptake) especially when the lens was pre-dosed. Blondin *et al.* (1986) were able to show that dietary vitamin C would reduce the ability of UV exposure to induce HMW protein aggregates, and protease inactivation in guinea-pig lens homogenates.

Trevithick *et al.* (1980) and others (Ross *et al.* 1982; Charalampous and Hegsted 1950) demonstrated the prevention of sugar cataract *in vitro* by vitamin E or GSH, and also by butylated hydroxytoluene (BHT), another agent with reducing properties. These were effective without reducing the sorbitol levels in affected lenses. In further studies this group has shown, in a model system, that BHT and vitamins C and A will prevent cataract and crystallin leakage in galactosaemic rats, while vitamin E and taurine will inhibit the protein leakage alone.

Drugs causing a fall in free radical scavengers

A number of other chemicals cause oxidative stress to the lens and result in a fall in free radical scavengers, including glutathione.

Naphthalene and its derivatives

Naphthalene in high doses causes cataract in rats and rabbits through the production of 1,2-naphthaquinone, which reacts with free amino groups and the thiol groups of proteins, and reduced glutathione (Rees and Pirie 1967; Harding and Crabbe 1984) (Figure 9.26a). Reaction with ascorbate generates hydrogen peroxide in the aqueous.

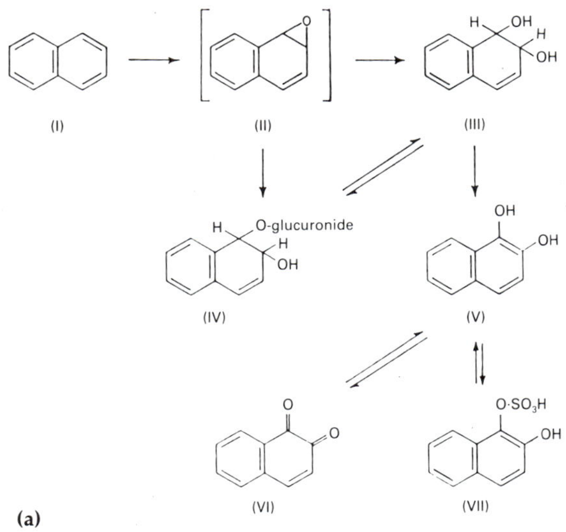

(a)

Figure 9.26(a) Metabolism of naphthalene. (From van Heyningen 1969 with permission.)

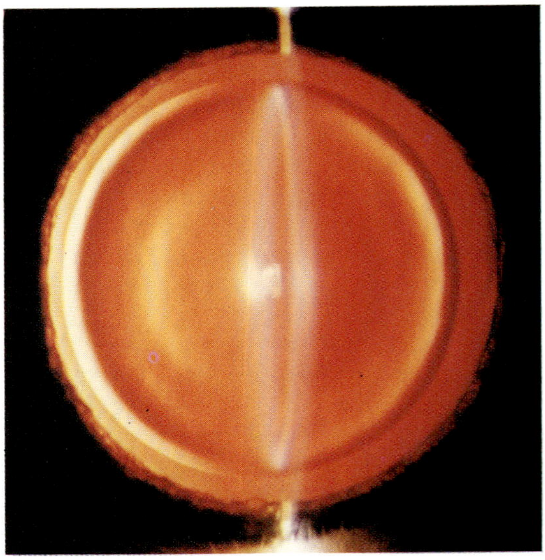

(c)

Figure 9.26(c) Red reflex image of the last stage of a naphthalene cataract in the BN rat, the 'spokes' merge into a spherical swollen zone in the lens cortex. (Courtesy of A. Wegener.)

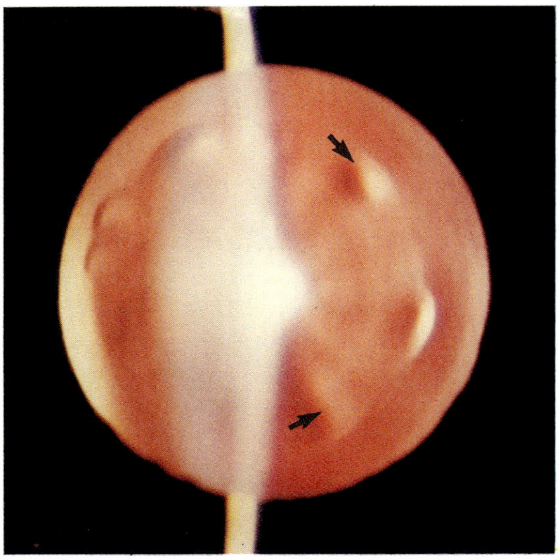

(b)

Figure 9.26(b) Red reflex image of the first stage of a naphthalene cataract in the Brown-Norway (BN) rat. Spoke-like swollen zones appear in the lens cortex (arrows). (Courtesy of A. Wegener.)

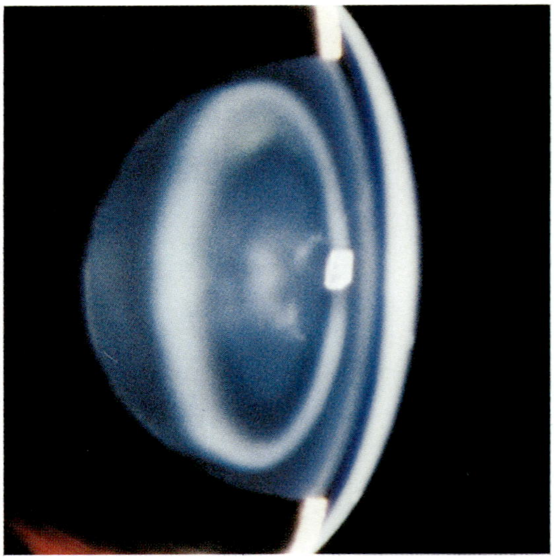

(d)

Figure 9.26(d) Optical section of the anterior eye segment of a rat, showing a zonular opacity in the cortex which is typical for the naphthalene cataract. (Courtesy of A. Wegener.)

The dehydro-ascorbate formed is recycled to ascorbate in the lens, whose levels remain high, while its glutathione levels are low (van Heyningen 1976). Kinsey and Merriam (1950) suggested that glutathione synthesis is impaired.

The cataract starts with cortical clefts and vacuoles and evolves into a swollen lens with a reduced protein content. Lens opacities have been produced in chick lenses incubated in 1,2- and 1,4-naphthoquinone, menadione and 4-amino-2-methyl-1-naphthol (Edwards *et al.* 1973).

Selenium

Injection of selenite into young rats at a critical age (10–18 days) produces a perinuclear cataract within about 20 days, which proceeds to a reversible, cortical cataract (Figure 9.27). Early changes in the lens are a sharp fall in reduced glutathione and an increase in oxidized glutathione, a fall in NADPH and an increase in NADP, and a loss of protein thiols (Shearer *et al.* 1987). There is an early decrease in mitosis, a loss of DNA, and a decrease in DNA synthesis by almost 60% (Cenedella 1987, 1989). With the development of cortical cataract there is overhydration and a decrease in dry weight (Anderson *et al.* 1988). It has been suggested that the marked rise in lens calcium which occurs in selenite cataract, probably as a secondary event, may activate proteolysis by calpain II, (David and Shearer 1986; Hightower *et al.* 1987), but leakage of crystallin polypeptides into the rat aqueous appears to be a late event (Watanabe and Shearer 1989).

Mercaptoundecahydrododecaborate

Mercaptoundecahydrododecaborate causes acute cataract in mice (Fukui *et al.* 1977), while the dimer causes swelling in incubated rabbit lenses associated with reduced GSH levels and inhibition of Na^+K^+ATPase.

Iodoacetate

Iodoacetate is a powerful inhibitor of thiol enzymes. It causes posterior cortical cataract in

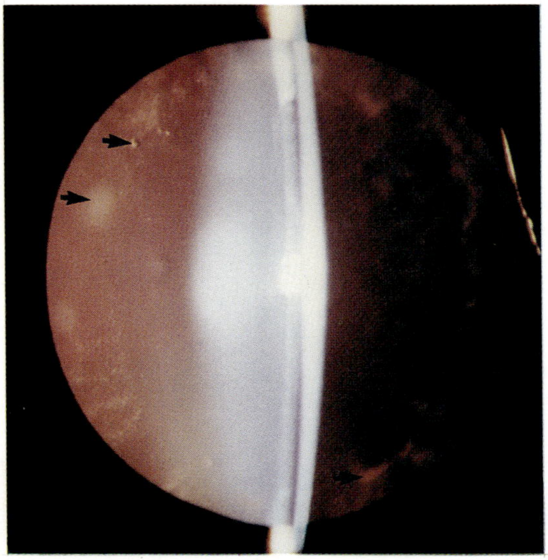

(3)

Figure 9.26(e) Red reflex image of the early stage of a naphthalene cataract in the pigmented rabbit. Areas of faint vacuoles appear in the subcapsular region close to the iris rim (arrows). (Courtesy of A. Wegener, from Hockwin *et al.* 1992.)

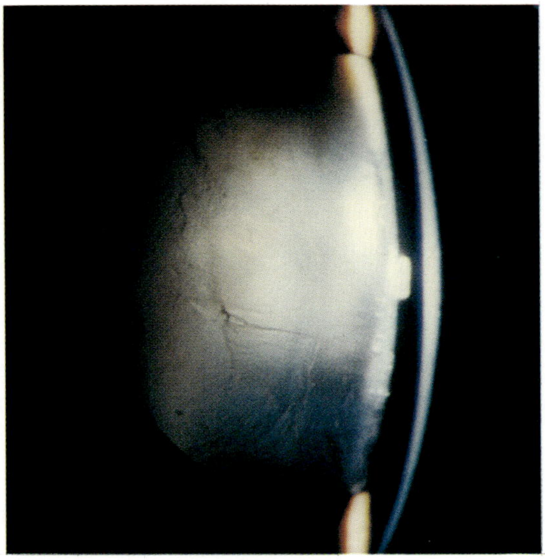

(f)

Figure 9.26(f) Mature naphthalene cataract in the pigmented rabbit with yellow discolouration of those regions of the lens close to the iris. (Courtesy of A. Wegener, from Hockwin *et al.*, 1992.).

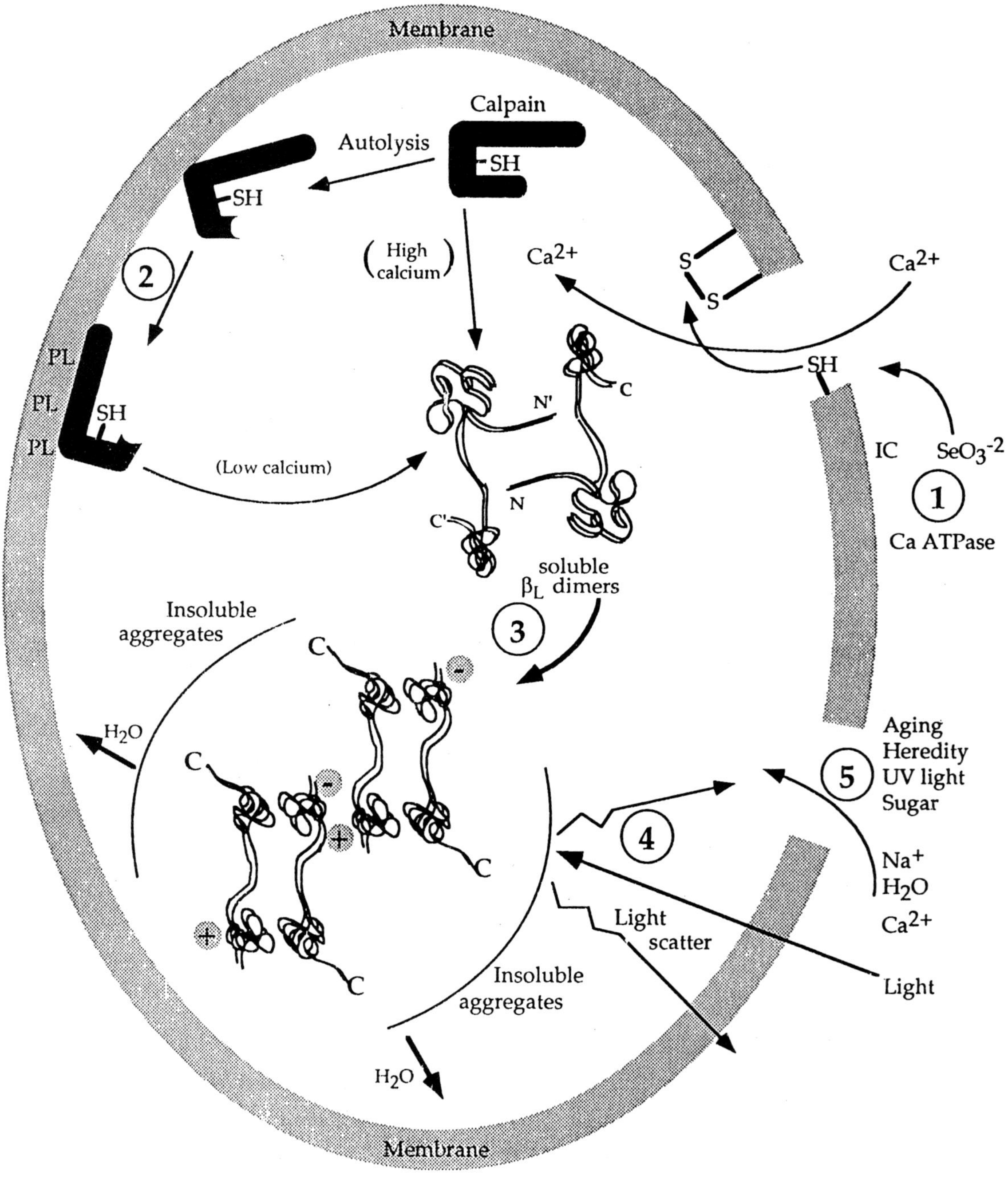

Figure 9.27 See facing page for full caption.

rabbits after intravenous administration, with lens fibre swelling and epithelial damage (Cibis and Noell 1955)

Methionine sulphoximine

Methionine sulphoximine causes cataract in the rat, which is preceded by an early fall in glutathione and a reduction in protein thiols (Bagchi 1959). It is an inhibitor of gammaglutamyl cysteine synthetase, which may explain the fall in GSH. The cataract may be prevented by dietary supplementation with methionine.

4-Chlorophenylalanine

4-Chlorophenylalanine causes subcapsular cataracts in rats, which in time progress to maturity. It is an inhibitor of tyrosine and phenylalanine hydroxylases. Free amino acids and GSH are diminished in affected lenses and little soluble protein is present.

Figure 9.27 Hypothesis for selenite cataract. Step 1: Selenium oxidizes the critical sulphydryl groups on Ca^{2+} ATPase, opens ion channels (IC) in the epithelial membrane, or inhibits synthesis of membrane transport enzymes. This allows influx of calcium from the aqueous. Step 2: High levels of calcium activate cytosolic calcium-activated protease (calpain) by causing autolysis, which exposes a buried sulphydryl group in the active site of calpain. Elevated Ca^{2+} also causes the translocation of calpain to the plasma membrane, where phospholipids (PL) lower the calcium activation requirement for calpain. The membrane may provide a localization site for hydrolysis of substrates. Large amounts of activated cytosolic calpain are also available for proteolysis. Step 3: The N-terminal extensions on soluble β-crystallin dimers are cleaved by calpain. This destabilizes the dimers leading to subunit exchange. The dimers insolubilize directly or interact to form insoluble aggregates, which are stabilized by hydrophobic intractions. Calpain hydrolysis of cytoskeletal and membrane proteins causes further leakiness and cellular disruption. Step 4: The cumulative effect is light scatter and opacity. Step 5: Other cataractogenic agents such as sugars, heredity, UV light and ageing may allow influx of calcium to activate this scheme. (From Shearer *et al.* 1992 with permission.)

Diquat

This insecticide produces posterior subcapsular cataract when fed to rats and dogs, which later spreads to involve the whole lens (Clark and Hurst 1970; Pirie and Rees 1970). Pirie and Rees (1970) suggested lens damage is due to the formation of diquat radicals. These generate superoxide, which is capable of reacting with ascorbate and GSH. Ascorbate levels fall in this form of cataract, but the GSH levels are maintained, probably because the diquat radical reduce $NADP^+$ to NADPH, and this in turn is required for GSH regeneration.

Protein denaturation

Oral administration of dimethyl sulphoxide (DMSO) in dogs and rabbits produces a curious refractive change in the lens nucleus after some months, in the absence of lens opacity (Rubin and Mattis 1966). The excised nucleus is harder than normal (Wood *et al.* 1967) and there is a marked increase of insoluble at the expense of soluble lens protein (mostly gamma crystallin) (van Heyningen and Harding 1972). It is suggested that DMSO, or its metabolic products, may react with -SH groups to encourage denaturation.

Radiation cataract

X-radiation

The first demonstration of experimental X-radiation cataract was in 1897 (Chalupecky). The clinical implications of these observations were not appreciated for some time, probably because of the delay between onset and exposure, and the variable delay in relation to dose. Subsequent animal studies established the clinical features of radiation cataract and their dependence on type of radiation, age, species and dose fractionation (see Lerman 1980).

Clinical features The clinical features are very similar in animals and in human subjects (Figure 9.28).

In the rat exposed to 440 c/kg it has been shown that, after 3 weeks, anterior cortical clefts appear and also granular dots which follow the line of the fibres (Koch *et al.* 1974). There is fibre swelling and the appearance of interfibrillar clefts (von Sallmann and Munoz 1951; Friedenwald and Rytel 1955).

This change is followed by the appearance of multiple posterior subcapsular opacities due to the posterior displacement of abnormal epithelial cells (Grzedzielski 1935; Kruckmann 1940; Cogan *et al.* 1952a; Evans *et al.* 1960; Fujinaga 1969). This is associated with a swelling of these psuedoepithelial islets to form balloon (or Wedl) cells. Clinically the posterior subcapsular cataract expands in area as a granular white opacity. With low doses, some degree of recovery occurs with the formation of clear new fibres between the opacity and the posterior capsule.

In the rabbit, in the first week following irradiation, posterior subcapsular vacuoles appear at the ends of the horizontal suture or at the equator (von Sallmann 1951). By three weeks, after irradiation with 20 Gy, all lenses show a wedge-shaped haze passing forwards from the posterior, horizontal suture, to the centre of the lens. This is associated with a nuclear haze. There is progression of the subcapsular opacities to form a complete ring and occupy the posterior subcapsular space and this may be followed by a period of rapid swelling and the formation of water clefts, nuclear and cortical opacities and ultimately the development of a mature cataract.

Histological changes precede the clinical changes by days or weeks, with epithelial degeneration

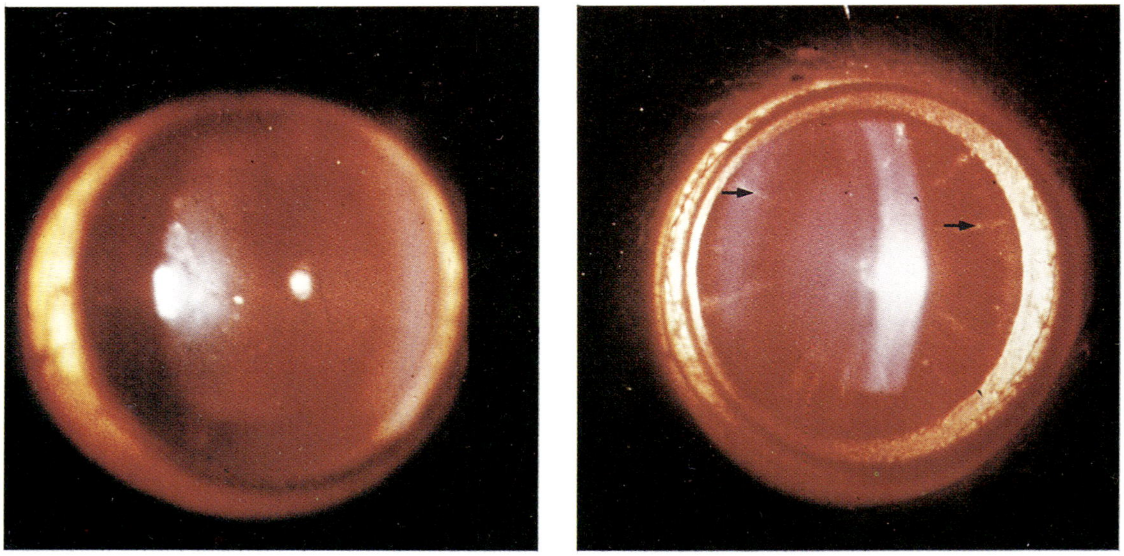

(a)

Figure 9.28(a) Late stage of X-ray cataract in the rat. Spoke cataracts (arrows) have developed in the cortex (right) together with a posterior subcapsular opacity in the sutural area (left). (Courtesy of A. Wegener, from Hockwin *et al.* 1992.)

Figure 9.28(b) Micrographs of mouse lenses, 2 weeks after X-irradiation. Lens fibres are normal in the anterior (i) and posterior (ii) subcapsular region. In the equatorial region (iii) there are small vacuoles and high density material in epithelial and meridional row cells. TEM micrographs show thickened transitional zone cells with reduced organelles (iv), small vacuoles in meridional row cells (v) and vacuoles and high density material in the low zone cells, (vi). Superficial fibres immediately behind the low zone are swollen (viii). (From Taura *et al.* 1985 with permission.)

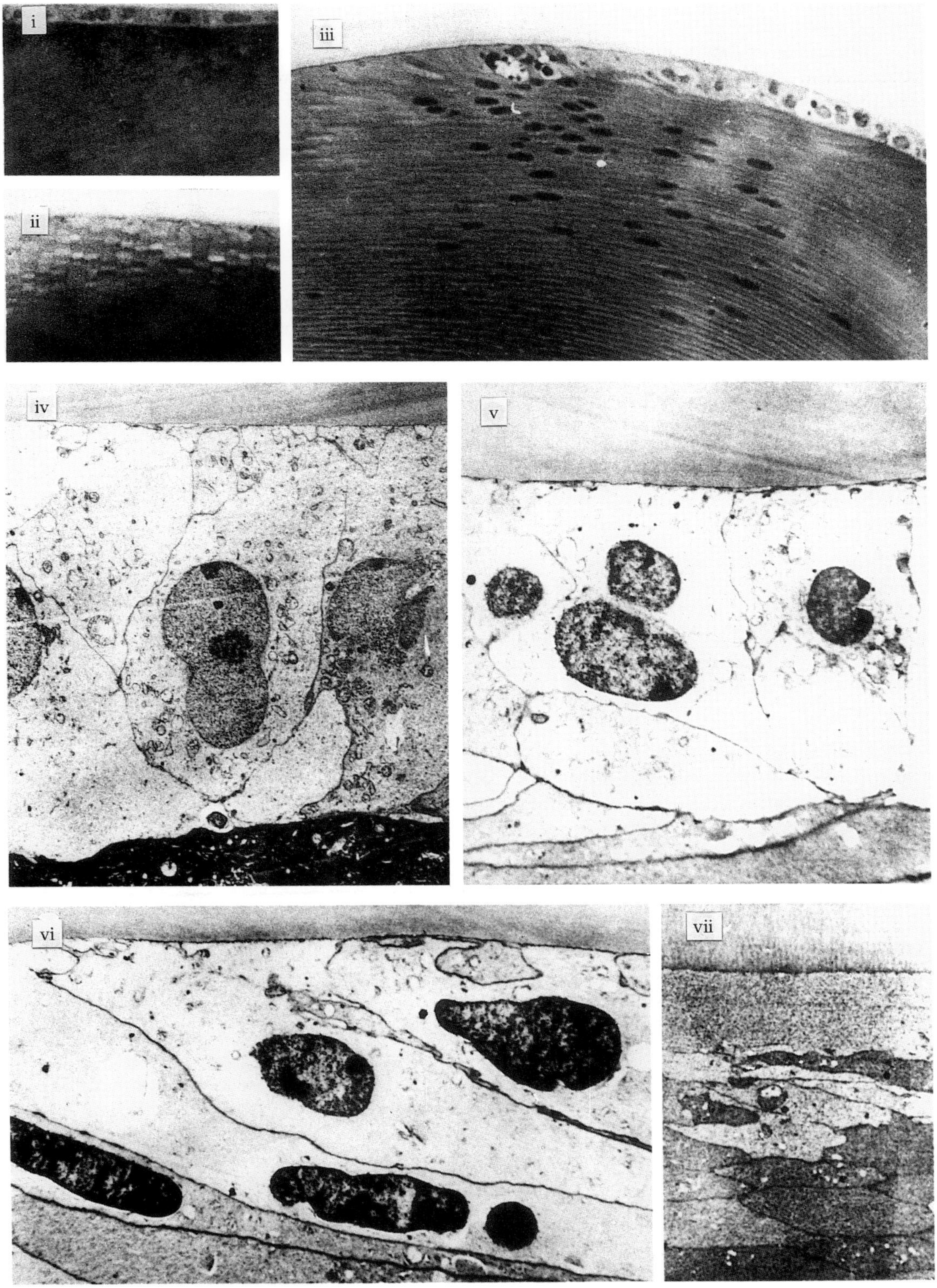

(b)

being seen within hours of exposure. The primary and major site of damage is the germinative zone of the epithelium (von Sallmann 1950a,b, 1957, 1959). Mitotic arrest occurs within 30 minutes of exposure. Nuclear fragmentation and extrusion occur with recovery after 4 days. There is broadening and irregularity of the nuclear bow. Abnormal mitoses occur and, ultimately, mitotic recovery with an increased rate of mitosis.

There are many associated biochemical and other changes. In the rat, iritis occurs in about 3 hours (Worgul *et al.* 1977). Lens ascorbate and GSH thiol levels fall (Hockwin 1962), the latter initially as a direct result of radiolysis (Hockwin 1962) and subsequently due to a breakdown in glutathione synthesis (Pirie *et al.* 1953; Lerman 1967, 1972) and inhibition of glutathione reductase (Hockwin 1962; Giblin and Reddy 1978; Daisley 1955). There is also an increase in cell membrane permeability. Enzyme changes occur, and an increase in the concentration of water insoluble at the expense of water soluble crystallins.

Effect of age Radiation damage is in general greatest in young lenses which show the highest mitosis rate (e.g. fetal and postnatal). However at low dose rates (200–400 c/kg) the young lens may be more resistant, perhaps because of better repair mechanisms (Merriam and Szechter 1973; Gajewski *et al.* 1977).

Species and radiation damage There are quantitative differences in the delay before the onset of opacity in different species. The delay is longer in the dog and monkey than in the mouse, rat, rabbit, cat and guinea-pig, possibly because of the lower epithelial mitosis rate in the former group of animals.

Radiation dosage The dose causing damage varies with the type of radiation, with greater damage being associated with a higher LET value. (The term linear energy transfer function or LET, refers to the transfer of energy to tissue by ionizing particles which traverse it. Heavy charged particles generate a much higher ion density within tissues than X- or gamma-rays of the same photon energy, resulting in a higher LET value. This influences the damaging biological effects of such radiation. The difference in biological effect of different sorts of radiation is expressed by a quality factor [Qf] for each sort. The quality factor for X- and gamma-rays is set at 1, while that for heavy charged particles and neutrons is between 10 and 20 [neutrons act by the generation of heavy charged particles within a medium]. Thus the latter sources of radiation have potentially more damaging effects than X- or gamma rays of the same energy. Because heavy charged particles have greater mass, they have however lower tissue penetrability).

Thus, whereas a cataractogenic dose for X-ray and gamma radiation is about 2 Gy, that for neutrons is 75.8 Gy (Lerman 1962; Hall 1963; Haye *et al.* 1965; Britten *et al.* 1967; Riley 1970).

Fractionation of dose Fractionation of X-ray or gamma radiation dose decreases the damage, probably because of the opportunity which it provides for repair. With neutron radiation this is not the case, perhaps because there is primary damage to both epithelium and fibres; in experimental studies fractionation does not decrease the degree of opacity or the delay (Lerman 1980).

Beta and gamma radiation

Despite the poor penetrating power of beta radiation, cataract has been produced during the treatment of pterygium (Tarr and Constable 1980). It causes cataract experimentally *in vivo* (von Sallmann *et al.* 1953), and *in vitro* causes cataract and increases cation permeability (Lambert and Kinoshita 1967).

Neutrons, protons and heavy ions

Neutron irradiation causes cataract in mice (Evans 1948) and rabbits (Hosokawa 1967), producing a posterior subcapsular cataract similar to that caused by X-irradiation (Cogan *et al.* 1952b). In mice the cataract may take over a year to develop (Di Paola *et al.* 1978).

Protons also cause cataract, similar to those produced by X-rays (Geeraets *et al.* 1971). Monkeys irradiated with heavy ions with an energy equivalent to that found in outer space have developed cortical opacities (Bonney *et al.* 1977).

Ultraviolet radiation

The cornea transmits wavelengths above 300 nm, while the lens transmits above 400 nm. Therefore the action spectrum of the lens, lying within its region of absorption, is about 300–400 nm. Exposure of mice to this waveband caused changes in lens bow nuclei at 35 weeks, and lens opacities by 50 weeks (Zigman and Vaughan 1974; Zigman *et al.* 1974) and at this intensity a corneal haze also occurred. The earliest lens change is a prominence of the anterior suture line (Pitts *et al.* 1977) (Figure 9.29). Laser radiation within the action spectrum (e.g. 325 nm and 327 nm) produced anterior subcapsular and cortical cataracts in rabbits (MacKeen *et al.* 1973; Thomas and Schepler 1980), while radiation at 325, 337, 351 and 364 nm also caused lens opacities in monkeys (Ebbers and Sears 1975; Zuclich and Connolly 1976).

Photosensitization of the lens by exposure to ultraviolet light after administration of 8-methoxypsoralen, resulted in anterior cortical cataract in guinea-pigs, in addition to other tissue damage (Cloud *et al.* 1960, 1961). Photo-sensitization probably contributes to the anterior capsular and subcapsular opacities occurring in eyes receiving chlorpromazine, or 2,6-dichloro-4-nitroaniline and exposed to sunlight (Siddall 1965; Bernstein *et al.* 1970). Johnson *et al.* (1989) working in Somalia observed a 'frosting' and plateau-like elevation of the lens capsule in the pupil, which in advanced cases was herniated forwards through the pupil. Plateau and hernial changes were strongly associated with climatic droplet degeneration, and by inference, with UV exposure in excess.

Infrared radiation

Clinical infrared cataract occurs in glass-blowers and furnacemen exposed to radiation furnaces for periods of 10 years or more (p. 205). It is generally held that lens damage is due to heat transfer from the iris (Langley *et al.* 1960), as originally proposed by Goldmann (1935). Exfoliation of the zonular lamellar of the anterior capsule is the pathognomonic feature of the disorder, although it is not always present and posterior subcapsular cataract develops as a later event.

Electric cataract

Experimental electric cataract may be caused by application of voltages as low as 14 and has features closely resembling that in humans (Long 1962).

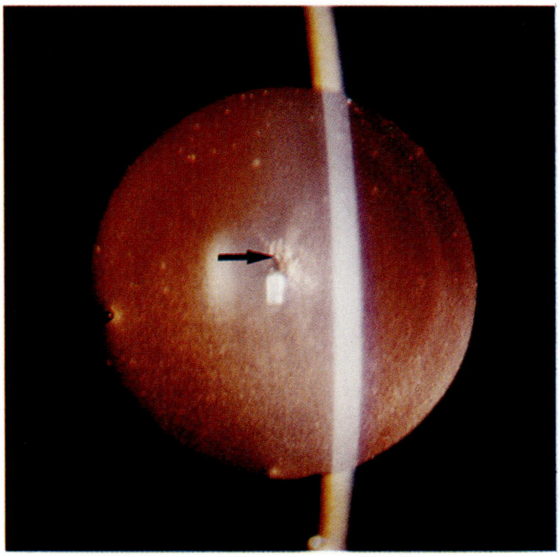

(a)

Figure 9.29(a) Anterior polar cataract due to UV-B damage to the BN rat lens (arrow). Also the cornea is slightly cloudy as a response to radiation damage. (Courtesy of A. Wegener.)

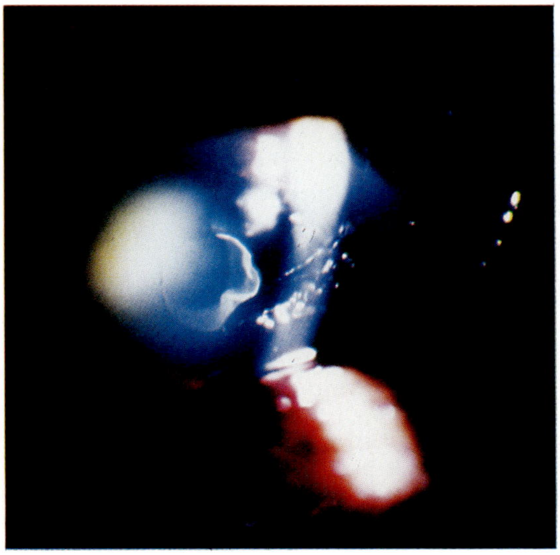

(b)

Figure 9.29(b) Herniation of lens capsule protrusion through pupil of a Somalian nomad – attributed to solar UV – exposure (From Johnson *et al.* 1989 with permission.)

Microwaves

Microwaves have a wavelength of 1–1000 nm within the electromagnetic spectrum with a frequency of 300 MHz–300 GHz. The interest in microwave cataract stems from the possibilities of exposure to domestic, commercial and military sources such as various forms of oven, and radar.

Microwaves produce posterior subcapsular and cortical cataracts in rabbits and dogs (Daily *et al.* 1950, 1951; Richardson *et al.* 1952; Carpenter *et al.* 1960). At low intensities vacuoles and membranous lamellar material have been demonstrated pathologically in the posterior opacities (Hirsch *et al.* 1977) and similar changes have been seen in biomicroscopically clear lenses (Williams *et al.* 1975).

Microwaves raise the temperature of the lens and the role of temperature in causing microwave cataract has been considered by a number of authors. A threshold temperature for the production of cataract has been suggested in the region of 45°C (Kalant 1959), but the ability to cause cataract by the cumulative effect of subthreshold doses of microwaves argues against this view (Belova and Gordon 1956); Carpenter *et al.* 1977). Pulsed microwaves of higher peak power are more effective in causing cataract in rabbits than continuous wave radiation of the same average power, which would have the same thermal effect (Carpenter 1958, 1959). This, and the inability to cause cataract by lens temperatures above the supposed thermal threshold, have supported the existence of an additional non-thermal mechanism (Kramer *et al.* 1976; Carpenter *et al.* 1977). However, hypothermia protects rabbits from cataractogenic doses of microwaves (Kramar 1975) even when exposures are subthreshold (Baillie *et al.* 1970). The biological effects of microwave radiation are reviewed comprehensively by Baransky and Czersky (1976), and by Harding and Crabbe (1984).

The cataractogenic dose varies with intensity, duration and frequency of exposure. Thus, in the rabbit, irradiation at 280 mW/cm^2 for 3 min causes no cataract (despite a vitreous temperature of 47.2°C) while irradiation at 120°C for 35 min does, even though the vitreous temperature remains below 45°C).

Carbamylation of proteins

Cyanate ions are highly reactive, and will carbamylate proteins, including the lens crystallins, to cause a change in tertiary protein structure. Treatment of patients with sickle-cell anaemia with oral sodium cyanate to inhibit the sickling of haemoglobin resulted in posterior subcapsular cataract and the treatment was withdrawn (Nicholson *et al.* 1976). Cyanate causes lens opacity in rabbit lenses *in vitro* (Kinoshita and Merola 1973) and in dogs *in vivo* (Kern *et al.* 1977). In both instances there is a fall in lens GSH.

N-methyl-*N*-nitrosourea causes anterior and posterior subcapsular cataracts in rats which do not seem to depend on its alkylating properties. Harding and Crabbe (1984) have suggested that the toxicity of this, and other urea-containing compounds, may depend on their breakdown to cyanate (Knox 1976). Urea itself is in equilibrium with ammonium cyanate in solution.

Proteolytic enzymes and the lens

A number of proteolytic enzymes are present in the normal human lens whose functions are not precisely established. These include leucine aminopeptidase (whose levels, while high in the bovine lens are low in the human lens) and certain neutral proteinases and cathepsins.

It has been suggested that such proteinases may be involved in the removal of unwanted proteins in the lens (such as crystallins and cytoskeletal proteins) which have outlived their usefulness. Normal adult lenses contain crystallin polypeptide fragments which could be derived from such digestion, but their concentration is not increased in cataract. A proteinase may determine the conversion of MP26 (the main intrinsic polypeptide of the lens, probably a channel protein in the aquaporin series), to its functionally less active form, MP21. It is thought to be concerned with water movement. Both beta and gamma crystallins have been detected in normal human aqueous and in increased concentration in cortical, but not nuclear, cataract. This suggests that there is an outward leakage of small protein fragments associated with the turnover of crystallins, with the implication that crystallin protein is lost over periods of time.

In the normal lens, proteolytic digestion might be related to central compaction, which is a normal feature of lens growth. Enzymatic loss of protein from the lens centre would permit compaction without a rise in protein density and this appears to be the case. The increased aqueous level of crystallin in cortical cataract presumably reflects the breakdown of lens fibres which occurs in this situation. (The lens capsule is a limiting factor in the diffusion of protein into the aqueous humour.) The limiting size is in the region of the protein albumin 70 kDa (Fisher 1973). It appears that lens crystallin fragments entering the aqueous humour reach the general circulation, since antibodies against crystallins have been found in the serum of normal adults and, more often so, in those with cataract.

Van Heyningen (1976) demonstrated the presence of a calcium-activated neutral proteinase whose preferred substrate is alpha crystallin (p. 65). Proteolytic digestion was accelerated by removal of LMW peptide products. Bovine lens calpain is also a neutral proteinase, and effects a limited proteolysis of crystallin A and B chains from the carboxy terminal end of the protein molecule.

Calpain II is another calcium-activated neutral proteinase which may digest cytoskeletal proteins during fibre maturation. It is normally inhibited by a native inhibitor in the cell whose activity is highest in the epithelium. Once activated, calpain II may cause extensive crystallin degradation in experimental cataracts.

The digestibility of human crystallins varies. For instance, the HMW crystallins associated with the dense nucleus of advanced nuclear cataract are poorly digestible. UVA exposure of crystallin homogenates decreases their proteolytic digestibility. Taylor *et al.* (1986) have demonstrated ubiquitin labelling of bovine and rabbit crystallins, which in the proteins of other tissues is a prerequisite to physiological proteolysis. Since ubiquitin labelling of crystallins is dramatically reduced in older lenses it would be expected that they would be relatively resistant to proteolysis.

In contrast, Wagner *et al.* (1986) have shown enhanced proteolysis of oxidized forms of lens crystallins such as are encountered in cataract, by neutral proteinase. Harding (personal communication) has found enhanced proteolysis of lens crystallins from human cataract compared to normal, implying increased conformation change. Carbamylation is one form of post-translational modification of protein. These different accounts may not be fully in conflict, since enhanced and retarded proteolysis may be encountered clinically in the same lens, as in Morgagnian cataract.

Disturbance of lipid metabolism

Inhibitors of cholesterol synthesis

Cholesterol is the main sterol present in the lens (Andrews and Leonard-Martin 1981) and the cholesterol to phospholipid ratio in the lens is the highest of any tissue in the body (Zelenka 1984). Compounds which inhibit cholesterol synthesis are known to cause cataract:

1. Triparanol blocks cholesterol synthesis at a late stage, at the enzymic reduction of 2,4-dehydrocholesterol to cholesterol. It was introduced as a hypocholesterolaemic drug in the 1950s, but was withdrawn after it was found to induce posterior subcapsular cataract (Kirby 1967).

   In the rat there is fibre swelling and breakdown with the accumulation of a sudanophilic material (von Sallman *et al.* 1963). Harris and Gruber (1969) demonstrated increase lens permeability in experimental triparanol cataract.
2. The compound (DEEA), 3-beta-(2-diethylaminoethoxy) androst-5-en-17-one HCl, like triparanol, blocks the reduction of desmosterol to cholesterol. Unlike triparanol, it causes a nuclear cataract in rats and, unexpectedly, although there is a decrease in cholesterol synthesis and reduced lens growth prior to the development of cataract, there is no accumulation of desmosterol in affected lenses (Cenedella and Bierkamper 1979; Cenedella 1983; Rintoul *et al.* 1987). Changes in the gap-junctional structure occur which may be important in cataractogenesis (Kuszak *et al.* 1988; Fleschner and Cenedella 1988).
3. Hydroxymethylglutaryl-CoA reductase is the rate limiting enzyme for cholesterol synthesis. Inhibition of enzyme leads to a fall in cholesterol, but not to an accumulation of metabolites. Hypocholesterolaemic drugs of this kind are able to cause cataract in dogs, in doses outside the clinical therapeutic range. A strong relationship exists between the plasma level of the drug and their cataractogenic potential (Gerson *et al.* 1990).

Drug-induced phospholipidosis

Lüllman *et al.* (1975) have advanced the hypothesis that certain cationic amphiphilic drugs (having both hydrophilic and hydrophobic moieties) are capable of inducing a generalized phospholipidosis, which may include the lens, by binding firmly with cell phospholipids. The complexes so formed are poorly digestible by lysosomal acid lipases, and accumulate within lysosomes as membranous lamellar and crystalloid inclusions. The amphiphilic compound chloroquine produces cataracts in rats and such lamellar inclusions are found within the opacities. This mechanism may also be relevant to the formation of lens opacities due to triparanol and phenothiazine (chlorpromazine).

Dehydration cataract

A reversible cataract may be induced in rats by keeping the lids open. A similar result is achieved by drugs which inhibit blinking. Subcutaneous injection of morphine-like compounds produces a deposit on the surface of the rodent lens within minutes of injection (Goldmann and Rabinowitz 1928; Fraunfelder and Burns 1962, 1966; Weinstock and Stewart 1961).

Cold cataract

Cooling of the lens *in vivo* (Nordmann 1954; Klass and Berns 1964) and *in vitro* gives rise to a reversible nuclear cataract due to separation of its proteins into protein-rich and protein-poor zones (phase separation) (Clark and Benedek 1980a,b). There is also a change in bound water (Lerman *et al.* 1982). In the calf lens the light-scattering moieties increase from 2000 Å to 5000 Å in size (Delaye *et al.* 1982). The ability to induce cold cataract is age-dependent, and is lost in the rat by the eighth week of life. Only gamma crystallin is cold-precipitable although its ability to precipitate may be prevented by alpha and beta crystallins. Cyanate in sub-cataract dosage raises the phase separation temperature of incubated rat lenses, and this system has been used to explore the efficacy of potential anticataract drugs based on their ability to lower the phase separation temperature (Harding 1991; Clark and Benedek 1980a). With heating, a lens becomes opaque above 65°C, due to irreversible coagulation of its proteins.

Other agents

3-(2-phenylhydrazino)-propionitrile causes cataracts in rats, with an early loss of ATP and then soluble protein before the onset of gross opacities and swelling (Dasler and Wang 1972).

3-aminotriazole causes sutural cataracts in rabbits, which spread to involve the anterior and posterior cortex (Bhuyan *et al.* 1973). It is an inhibitor of $Na^{+}K^{+}$ATPase and of catalase, and cataract formation is associated with an accumulation of hydrogen peroxide in the aqueous and vitreous (Bhuyan and Bhuyan 1977).

Bleomycin is a polypeptide antibiotic used in the treatment of certain carcinomas and lymphomas. Intraperitoneal injection causes cataract in newborn but not in older rats (Edwards *et al.* 1975), and may be due to faulty post-translational processing of lens proteins (Weill *et al.* 1980).

Myeleran is an alkylating agent used in the treatment of leukaemias and lymphomas. It produces cataracts in rats in about 8 weeks, which are initially anterior and posterior in type (Solomon *et al.* 1955). The increase in epithelial mitosis and in nuclear fragmentation resembles changes seen in X-ray cataracts (von Sallmann 1957).

Thallium acetate causes cataract in rats, occasionally bilaterally. The animals develop alopecia, gastrointestinal changes, polyneuritis and optic neuritis. There may be late uveitis and corneal neovascularization (Donski 1932; Buschke 1943).

Cobalt chloride feeding causes cataract in rabbits and rats, which is partly prevented by simultaneous feeding with cysteine.

For a more extensive account and referencing, see van Heyningen 1969a.

Nutritional cataract

Vitamin A deficiency

Experimentally, vitamin A deficiency causes epithelial keratinization in the rat lens (Pirie and Overall 1972) and lens capsular wrinkling or cataracts are said to be a feature of β-carotene deficiency in calves and bullocks (Lahiri 1938; Moore 1939). However, it is not a primary feature of xerophthalmia.

Vitamin B deficiency

Riboflavin is the B vitamin whose deficiency is most closely associated experimentally with cataract. In addition to corneal vascularization, cataract occurs in 63–94% of rats after about 60–87 days of starting a riboflavin deficient diet, with changes being most frequent in animals with the slowest growth (Day *et al.* 1931, 1934; Day and Darby 1936). However, van Heyningen (1969) was not able to duplicate these experiments.

Cataract has been reported in mice, chicks, cats guinea pigs and possibly in monkeys deficient in riboflavin (McLaren 1980).

In baby pigs, Miller *et al.* (1954) found that cataract was present at about 35 days after starting the deficient diet at the age of 72 hours. Initial opacities, just posterior to the lens equator, were due to swollen lens fibres, and there were vesicular changes in the lens epithelium. Pigs studied by Wintrobe *et al.* (1944) developed cataract in the absence of corneal vascularization.

The role of deficiency of the other B vitamins in cataract is less certain, but is discussed by McLaren (1980).

Deficiency of amino acids and protein

Tryptophan deficiency is a well-recognized cause of cataract in the rat. The mechanism is not fully understood (Curtis *et al.* 1932; Totter and Day 1942). A relationship to vitamin B metabolism is emphasized by the occurrence of corneal vascularization in both deficiency states. Acute tryptophan deficiency cataract in the rat proceeds to maturity in 3 weeks. It progresses through a feathery posterior cortical change, with accentuation of the sutures, through to a perinuclear and nuclear opacity. In the chronic form there are fine cortical dots, which do not mature over a 9-week period (Buschke 1943). In the rat model studied by van Heyningen (1976) the lens weight was reduced compared with non-deficient controls, and there was a reduction in lens protein. A singular feature was broadening of the lens bow with a granular persistence of degenerating nuclei (Figure 9.30). The opacity appeared clinically as a refractive separation of cortex and nucleus. The nucleus became cloudy, but the cataract did not mature. The growth rate of deficient animals was about 60% of that of controls.

Deficiency of all the essential amino acids, except arginine, have been associated with some degree of lens damage in the rat, especially histidine and phenylalanine (Hall *et al.* 1948). A fuller account is given by McLaren (1980).

Although there are reports of cataract in protein deficient diets, McLaren (1980) was unable to confirm this. However, he found that cataract was the most striking ocular lesion produced in pigs, occasionally progressing to maturity by 1 year (McLaren 1959). Initial changes included peri-equatorial fibre swelling and vacuolar separation, ultimately with formation of 'bladder cells'. The process spread gradually to a degeneration of all of the lens fibre cells.

Genetic cataracts (Table 9.4)

Various genetic forms of cataract have been summarized by Clayton (1985), Harding (1991), Gelat and Das (1984), and Gelatt (1991). Many cataracts have been induced experimentally by agents such as nitrosourea or X- irradiation and have assisted in the mapping of cataract associated genes.

Mouse (Figure 9.31. Table 9.5)

1. *Fraser cataract* is a dominantly inherited mouse cataract. The mutant gene is carried on chromosome 10. It is characterized by a shrivelled lens with a thickened capsule, duplicated epithelium, anterior polar cataract, and destruction of nuclear fibres (Zwaan and Williams 1969). There is no postnatal thickening of the lens. Beta and gamma crystallins are deficient in the lens, with a deficit of gamma mRNAs after the age of 40 days (Garber *et al.* 1985).
2. *Lop cataract* is a related, but more severe, form of dominant cataract which appears to be due to a mutant gene, allelic to the Fraser cataract (Muggelton-Harris and Higbee 1987).
3. *Nakano cataract*, as noted earlier (p. 106), is a recessive form of mouse cataract which starts 24 days after birth, and proceeds to a total cataract by 100 days (Iwata and Kinoshita 1971). Lens growth ceases after the age of 2 weeks and there is retarded protein synthesis (Fukui *et al.* 1976). Gap junctions in the cortex are reduced in size and number and the amount of 26 kDa polypeptide falls (Tanaka *et al.* 1980). Loss of $Na^{+}K^{+}$ ATPase activity occurs at about 7 days after birth, due to the presence of an inhibitor in the epithelium, and this may be the major factor in cataract formation (Fukui *et al.* 1978; Russell *et al.* 1977). Swelling of the posterior ends of the lens fibres also occurs at this time, contrasting with the finding in Fraser cataract in which swelling of the anterior fibre end occurs (Sakuragawa *et al.* 1975). The fully

opaque lens shows reduced levels of potassium, glutathione, ATP, ascorbate and protein thiols.

Crossbreeding of Nakano mice produces a strain with delayed cataract formation, at 60 days in females, and at 90 days in males (Matsuzawa and Wada 1988).

4. *The Philly mouse* is a recessive cataract trait which starts as an anterior subcapsular opacity, spreads to involve the sutures, and, between

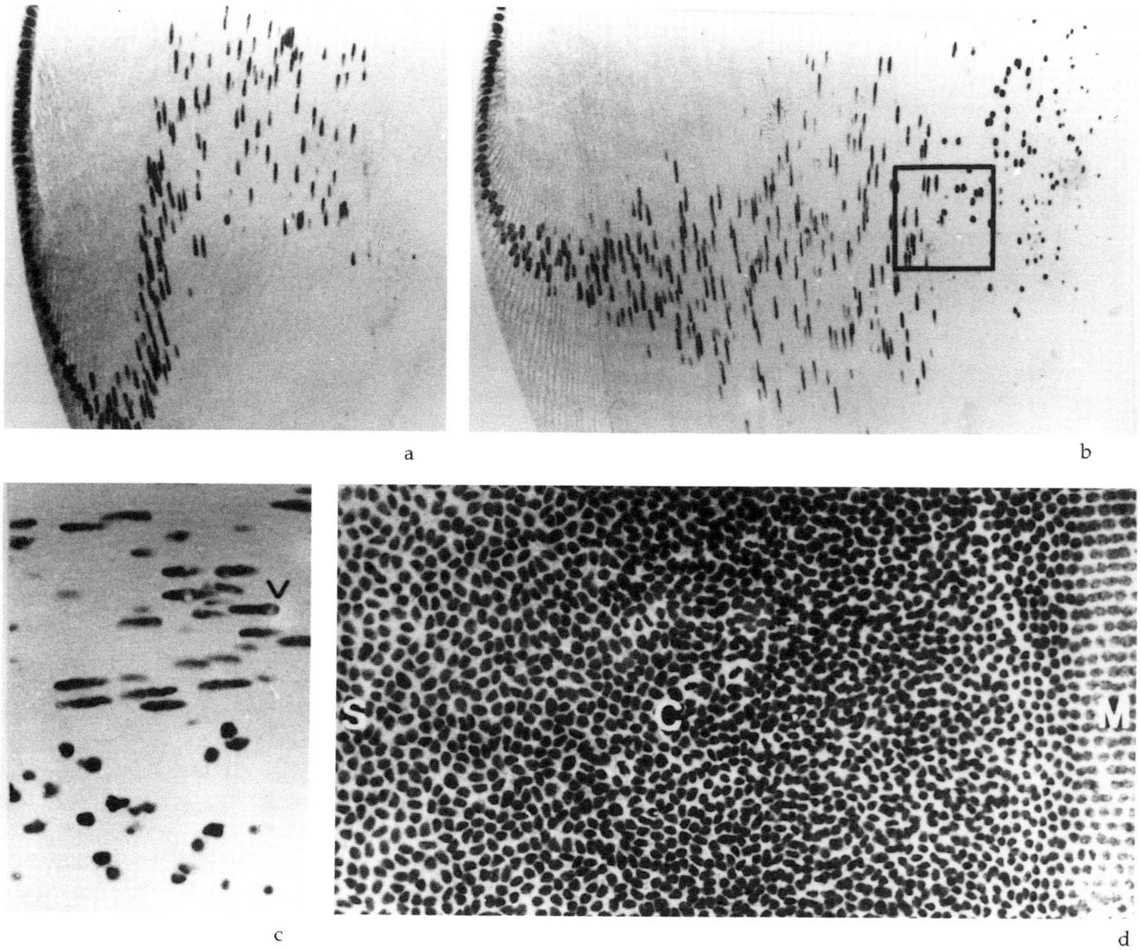

Figure 9.30 The Lens bow a) The lens bow of litter mates after four weeks on the control diet, and b) on the tryptophan deficient diet. Note the inhibition of the denucleation process leading to a broadening of the lens bow deep within the cortex. Nucleated fibres are 2–3 times more numerous than controls. Nuclei are abnormal in shape. The field included in c is outlined in b (original magnification × 150). c) Detail of the lens bow in a tryptophan deficient rat. Nuclei with prominent vacuoles (V) are adjacent to densely staining nuclei. One dense nucleus has a central clear zone (arrow). (× 480). d) Detail of the periphery of the lens epithelium of a seven-week old rat. There is a gradual transition between squamous cells (S) and cuboidal-columnar cells (C). A sharp junction between the cuboidal-columnar cells and the meridional rows (M) (× 220). (Haematoxylin). e) Detail to show the abnormal size and morphology (arrows) of fibre cells in the deeper region of the lens bow in a tryptophan deficient rat (haematoxylin and phase contrast) (From McAvoy *et al.* 1976 and 1979, with permission).

the 30th and 40th day after birth, progresses to affect the lens nucleus, when the cataract becomes visible to the naked eye (Kador *et al.* 1980a,c). Epithelial differentiation is disturbed by the seventh postnatal day, when there is posterior lens fibre swelling and subsequent degeneration and vacuolation (Uga *et al.* 1980). There is a deficiency of mRNA for a beta crystallin polypeptide, which is normally located in the bow zone, and persistence of nuclei in the lens cortex. There is an in-frame deletion in a beta-crystallin gene which probably results in an imperfectly folded beta crystallin. The beta crystallin is assumed to play a role in normal development of the lens (Carper *et al.* 1986).

5. *Elo (eye obsolescence)* is a dominant disorder in mice, in which fibre elongation is retarded and the lens is small at birth (Oda *et al.* 1980a,b). The mutation is on chromosome 1, in the

Table 9.4 Animal models with inherited cataracts

Breed	*Age of onset*	*Cataract characteristics*	*Mode of inheritance*
Mice:			
1. Fraser	3 weeks to 4 weeks	cortical	autosomal intermediate
2. Deer	2 months to 1 year	posterior; subcapsular	autosomal recessive
3. Nakano	3 weeks	nuclear	autosomal recessive
4. Philly	5 weeks to 6 weeks	anterior; subcapsular, nuclear	autosomal recessive
5. Emory	6 months to 8 months	posterior; cortical	autosomal dominant
Rats:			
1. Sprague-Dawley	congenital	anterior subcapsular; sutural	autosomal recessive
2. Wistar	senile	posterior subcapsular; supranuclear	unknown
Wistar	congenital & early postnatal	anterior polar; cortical	autosomal recessive
3. Sherman	4 months	anterior cortical; subcapsular	unknown
4. RCS	7 weeks to 8 weeks	posterior; subcapsular	associated with retinal dystrophy
Dogs:			
1. Afghan Hound	6+ months	equatorial/posterior cortex	autosomal recessive
2. American Cocker	6+ months	posterior/anterior cortex	autosomal recessive/ polygenetic
3. Beagle	congenital	posterior sutures/nuclear	autosomal recessive
4. Boston Terrier	congenital	nuclear; cortical usually progressive	dominant/incomplete penetrance
5. Chesapeake Bay Retriever	1+ years	nuclear/cortex	incomplete dominant
6. German Shepherd	8+ weeks	Posterior sutures/cortex	incomplete dominant
7. Golden Retriever	6+ months	posterior subcapsular (triangular)	incomplete dominant
8. Labrador Retriever	6+ months	posterior subcapsular (triangular)	incomplete dominant
9. Miniature Schnauzer	congenital	nuclear/posterior cortex	autosomal recessive
	6+ months	posterior cortex	autosomal recessive
10. Old English sheepdog	congenital	nuclear/cortex	autosomal recessive
11. Siberian Husky	6+ months	posterior subcapsular/ posterior sutures	autosomal recessive
12. Staffordshire Bull Terrier	6+ months	posterior sutures/cortex	autosomal recessive
13. Standard Poodle	1+ years	equatorial cortex	autosomal recessive
14. Welsh Springer Spaniel	congenital	nuclear/posterior cortex	autosomal recessive
15. West Highland, White Terrier	congenital	posterior sutures	autosomal recessive

Table 9.4 (*Continued*)

Breed	*Age of onset*	*Cataract characteristics*	*Mode of inheritance*
Sheep:			
1. Romney	1 month to 2 months	anterior; posterior cortical	autosomal dominant
Cattle:			
1. Holstein-Friesian	congenital	nuclear; cortical	autosomal recessive
2. Jersey	congenital	cortical	autosomal recessive
3. Hereford	congenital	nuclear	unknown
4. Shorthorn	congenital	nuclear; cortical	possible autosomal recessive
Other:			
1. Bobwhite quail	3 months	anterior central, or posterior cortical	possible autosomal recessive
2. Cichlid	early life	nuclear; cortical	unknown
3. Elk	2 months to 10 years	cortical	unknown
4. Degu	congenital	cortical, may be associated with diabetes mellitus	
5. Tuco-tuco	3 months	posterior; polar	hyperglycaemia
6. Timber wolf	1 week to 4 weeks	posterior subcapsular	nutritional; arginine deficiency
7. Turkey	3 months to 7 months	cortical, associated with retinal detachment	autosomal recessive
8. Rabbit	congenital	bilateral triangular nuclear and cortical axial posterior capsule and cortex	unknown
9. Cat	congenital	nonprogressive	unknown
10. Pig	variable	cortical	unknown, may be secondary to hygromycin
11. Woolly monkey	congenital	mature, cortical	unknown

middle of the third (and last) exon of the mouse gamma E crystallin gene (Griffin *et al.* 1992; Cartier *et al.* 1992). Expression of these crystallins is reduced, even though the genes themselves are not mutated (Masaki and Watanabe 1988).

6. *Nop* is a dominant cataract associated with a nuclear lens opacity. Lenses contain more oxidized glutathione and superoxide dismutase but, surprisingly, normal amounts of reduced glutathione. There are reduced amounts of several glycolytic enzymes relative to the wet weight of the lens (Graw *et al.* 1985).
7. *Scat* is a dominant mouse mutant with a sutural cataract in the cataract and vacuolated lenses in a small eye in the homozygote (Graw *et al.* 1989).
8. *The Emory cataract* develops as a dominant trait in older mice. It shows as a hazy nuclear change, which progresses in months to a total cataract (Kuck and Kuck 1983). There is a decrease in glutathione and an increase in GSSG and in protein unfolding. Lens fibre Na^+K^+ATPase decreases and there are changes in the fibre gap-junctional protein (Unakar *et al.* 1986; Takemoto *et al.* 1988).
9. *Senescent cataract.* Mice bred with features of accelerated ageing show cataract of late onset in addition to other ocular features. Cataract in one strain develops at between 12 and 18 months, while in another (SAM-R/3) it occurs from about 15 weeks. Later, the lens develops a posterior polar protrusion (Hosokawa *et al.* 1988).
10. *The Deer mouse* exhibits two forms of autosomal recessive cataract along with other ocular anomolies. Neither are congenital (Burns and Feeney 1975; Burns *et al.* 1980; Feeney-Burns *et*

al. 1980). In the early form (type I) there is abnormal closure of the fetal fissure, with hyaloid vascular abnormalities. Disorganization of the lens bow and posterior migration of abnormal fibre cells precedes the development of posterior subcapsular cataract. Nuclear opacity also occurs, as a shell or in a discrete dot pattern. Type II starts later, progresses more slowly, and lacks extensive hyaloid anomalies.

Rat (Figure 9.32)

1. A congenital, anterior subcapsular cataract, with sutural opacities, occurs in the Sprague Dawley rat as a recessive trait. It is associated with skull malformation. There is proliferation of lens epithelium and thickening of the lens capsule (Smith *et al.* 1969).
2. An autosomal recessive ocular malformation was induced in Wistar rats by X-radiation (Leonard and Maisin 1965). Changes include polar cataract, retinal folding and extensive malformation of the anterior segment, which may play a role in cataract formation (Gorthy and Abdelbaki 1974; Gorthy 1979; Gorthy 1979).
3. Inherited retinal degeneration of the RCS rat (Royal College of Surgeons) type, is associated with a posterior subcapsular cataract detectable

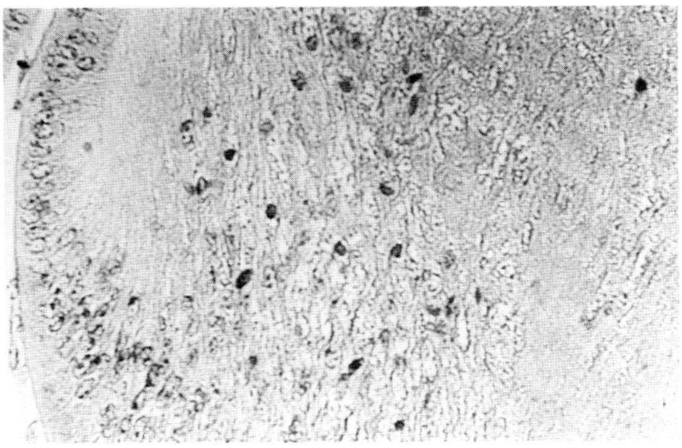

(a)

Figure 9.31(a) Fraser cataract. Older fibres are swollen and pyknotic.

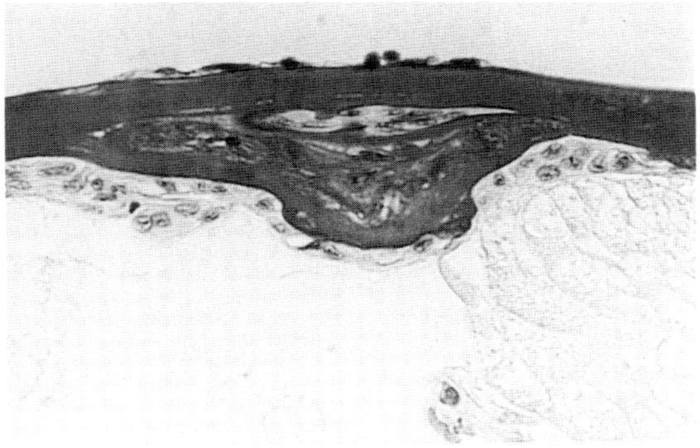

(c)

Figure 9.31(c) Epithelial plug enmeshed with thickened capsule.

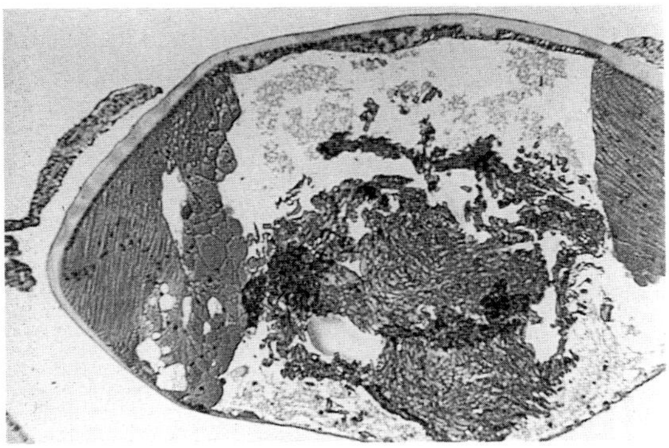

(b)

Figure 9.31(b) The nuclear area is filled with debris and surrounded by greatly swollen fibres.

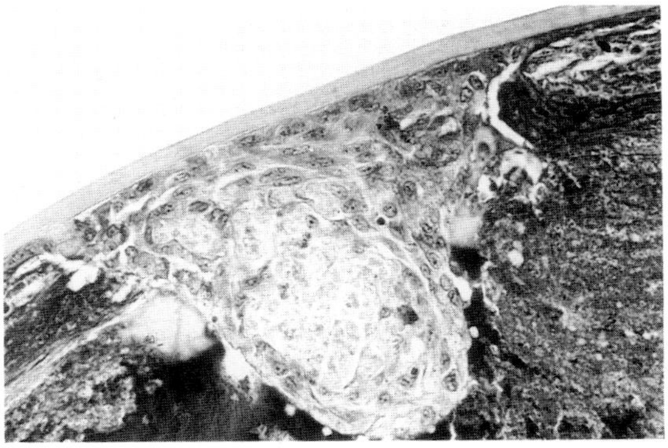

(d)

Figure 9.31(d) Subcapsular plug of epithelium. (Figures courtesy of J. Zwaan.)

Table 9.5 Inherited mouse cataract

Description	*Symbol*		*Comment*	*INH**	*Ref*
	Current	*Past*			
1. Fidget	fi		Pleiotropic effects: small eye or anophthalmia. Lens small vacuolate or absent. Lens-corneal fusion. Absent semicircular canals	r Chr 2	g
2. Eye, ear	ie	Ie	Anophthalmia or small eye	Chr X	af
3. Microphthalmia	mi	Mic	Asymmetrical cataract; lens and corneal vascularization; microphthalmos	Chr 6	b
4. Iris dysplasia	Ids		Irregular unreactive pupils; cataract fused to cornea	D	b
5. Iris anomaly cataract	Lac		Oval or slit-like pupils, colobomata and cataract	D	b
6. Ocular retardation	or		Cessation of lens growth, vacuolated lens fibres		a, w
7. Small-eye	Sey		Manifestations vary, heterozygote may show ant. polar cataract, or lens may be represented by thickened capsule or a shrunken eye at the back of the orbit. Mutation in the PAX 3 gene. Allelic with Sey^{dey}. Homozygous lethal	Chr 2 D	x
8. Dickie's small eye	Sey^{dey}	Dey	Small eye; cataract. Lens-iris-corneal adhesion Allelic with Sey. Mutation in PAX 3 gene	Chr 2	j
9. Anophthalmia	ey 1;	ey 2	Anophthalmia or microphthalmus	r	h
10. Aphakia	ak		Lens vesicle fails to separate. No primary fibres; small eye	r	
11. Nuclear cataract	Nuc		embryonic and posterior sutural	D	b
12. Blind	Bld		Eyelids open at birth. Corneal damage	Chr 15	ag
13. Gorthy's anterior polar cataract			Retinal dysplasia; small eye; forward displacement of cataract		k
14. Eye blebs	eb		Small body size and skeletal defects. Microphthalmus; anophthalmus. Cataract	Chr 10	e
15. Senescence-accelerated	SAM		Persistent hyaloid remnant. Posterior polar cataract		y
16. Anterior polar cataract	Apoc		Concentric ant. polar opacities; pupillary remnants	D	b
17. Anterior capsular cataract	Acc		Irregular dustlike capsular opacity; pupillary ant. embryonal opacity; remnant embryonal opacity	D	b
18. Dysgenetic lens	dyl		Dysgenic lens with small eye, corneal opacity; iris adhesion, cataract	r	l
19. Cataract-Fraser	Cat^{Fr}		Affection of primary and secondary lens fibres, with capsular thickening and epithelial hyperplasia	Chr 10 D	m
20.	Cat^{wp}		Allelic with Cat^{Fr}	Chr 10 D	ak
21. Nuclear + zonular	$Cat\text{-}2^{no}$	Nop	Heterozygote: nuclear opacity, Homozygote: Same. Loss of a single γ-crystallin protein	Chr 1	n

Table 9.5 *(Continued)*

Description	*Symbol*		*Comment*	*INH**	*Ref*
	Current	*Past*			
22.	Cat-2ro	Rop	Heterozygote: Radial opacity Homozygote: homogeneous opacity	Chr 1	e
23. Nuclear + zonular	Cat-2^{nz}	Nzc	Heterozygote: nuclear and zonular opacity. Homozygote: nuclear opacity	D	p
24. Total cataract with microphthalmia	Cat-2^{t}	R324	Heterozygote: total opacity; iris/lens dysplasia Microphthalmia. Homozygote: same altered pattern of crystallins. Increased ATPase activity	Chr 1	f
25.	Cat-2^{ns}	Scat	Heterozygote: nuclear and anterior suture opacity. Homozygote: same	Chr 1	q
26. Vacuolated lens + microphthalmia	Cat-3^{vl}	Vlm	Heterozygote: extensive vacuoles; microphthalmia. Homozygote: same	D	b; p
27. Vacuolated lens with axial opacity	Cat-3^{vao}	R-341	Heterozygote: vacuoles and axial opacity Homozygote: same	D	b, f
28. Ant. pyramidal cataract	Cat-4^{a}	A pyc	Heterozygote: ant. polar cataract; pup. remnant. Homozygote: closed eyes; microphthalmia		b; c; r
29. Anisocoria with polar	Cat-4^{b}	Anc	Heterozygote: Ant. polar cataract in 20% Anisocoria; pupillary remnant Homozygote: lethal	D	b
30. Polar cataract; small eyes	Cat-4^{c}	R7 PCS2	Heterozygote: Ant. polar cataract; corneal opacity dysplasia; microphthalmia Homozygote: lethal	D	f
31.	Cat-4^{d}		Heterozygote: Ant. polar cataract; Homozygote: lethal	D	f
32.	Cle	H-9	Heterozygote: closed eyes, lens, iris dysplasia microphthalmos Homozygote: same	D	d
33. Total cataract with microphthalmia	Tcm	X-11	Heterozygote: total cataract, dysplasia of lens and iris. Homozygote: same	D	d
34. Iris anomaly with cataract	Iac		Microphthalmos; corectopia; coloboma	D	b
35. Iris dysplasia with cataract	Idc		Microphthalmia; dysplasia of iris	D	b
36. Anterior lenticonus with microphthalmia	Alm		Ant. polar opacity and lenticonus; opaque cornea; pupillary remnants; microphthalmia	D	b
37. Polar cataract and small eyes	Pcs-1		Microphthalmos; dysplasia; corneal opacity	D	p; s
38. Anterior sutural cataract	Asc-1		Sutural opacity; pupillary membrane	D	f
39. Anterior sutural cataract	Asc-2		Sutural opacity; pupillary membrane	D	f
40. Anterior polar opacity	Hfi	538	Heterozygote: hydropic fibres Homozygote: total opacity	D	d
41. Embryonic + nuclear cataract	Enc		Embryonic and nuclear cataract	D	n; s

Table 9.5 (*Continued*)

Description	*Symbol*		*Comment*	*INH**	*Ref*
	Current	*Past*			
42. Coralliform cataract	Coc	R-322	Heterozygote: coralliform flecks Homozygote: same	D	f
43. Bare-patches	Bpa		Skin defects, skeletal defects and lens opacities	Chr X	ah
44. X-linked cataract	X cat		Homozygotes: total opacity Heterozygotes: variable	Chr X	t
45. Lens opacities – 4	Lop–4		Clusters of reflectant specks in nuclear or perinuclear region	Chr 2	ai
46. Eye lens obsolescence	Elo		γ crystallin mRNA reduced in mutant eyes; mutant maps close to γ gene cluster. Primary fibres degenerate. Associated microphthalmus	Chr 1	u
47. Cataract and small eye	Cts		semidominant defect of secondary lens fibres	D	v
48. Paget's mouse			Persistent hyaloid artery; posterior polar lens change		z
49. Nakano mouse	nct		Onset of pinpoint central lens opacity; presence of Na^+K^+ATPase inhibitor	r	aa
50. Philly mouse			Anterior subcapsular and sutural cataract; deficient β crystallin mRNA. In-frame deletion of βB2-crystallin gene	r	ab, al
51. Emory mouse	Em		Onset in older mice. Nuclear haze progresses to total cataract	D	ac
52. Deer Mouse			Hyaloid vascular anomalies and posterior subcapsular cataract in type I; later onset with less vascular change in type II	r	ae
53. Total opacity – 2	Cat-5		Total lens opacity	Chr 10	aj
54. Opacity	Op	ENV-410	Heterozygote: opacity due to poor secondary fibre junctions Homozygote: total opacity	Chr 16	aj
55. Nuclear-posterior	Npp	ENV-712	Heterozygote: nuclear-posterior polar opacity Homozygote: Total opacity	Chr 5	aj
56. Nuclear opacity	Cat-2^{no2}	ENV-3018	Nuclear opacity	Chr 1	aj
57.	Cat-2^{tol}	ENV-369	Heterozygotes and homozygotes: total opacity with lens vacuoles	Chr 1	aj

* Inheritance pattern or affected chromosome, if known; r = recessive trait; D = dominant trait; x = X-linked

at 7–8 weeks and visible to the naked eye at 9–15 months (Bourne *et al.* 1938). It has been suggested that lipid peroxidation products, released into the vitreous from the degenerating retina, are responsible for an increase in lens permeability (Zigler and Hess 1985). In RCS rats fed with a diet supplemented with sunflower kernels, visible cataract failed to develop (Hess *et al.* 1981).

Table 9.5 *(Continued)*

Key	*General References*
a	Clayton
b	Kratochvilova 1981
c	Kratochvilova and Favor 1988
d	Kratochvilova and Favor 1992
e	Green 1981, 1989; Graw *et al.* 1984; Graw *et al.* 1990
f	Graw *et al.* 1986
	Selected references
g	Truslove 1956; Konyukhov and Vakhrusheva 1969
h	Chase and Chase 1941; Silver and Hughes 1974; Harch *et al.* 1978
i	Varnum and Stevens 1968
j	Theilier *et al.* 1978
k	Gorthy 1981
l	Sanyal and Hawkins 1979
m	Zwaan and Williams 1969; Duke Elder 1969; Raffety 1965; Srinavasan and Harding 1965, Muggelton-Harris *et al.* 1987
n	Graw *et al.* 1984
o	Kratochvilova *et al.* 1988
p	Kratochvilova and Ehling 1979b
q	Graw *et al.* 1989
r	Petiers 1987
s	Ehlmy *et al.* 1982
t	Favor and Pretsch 1990
u	Oda *et al.* 1 1980; Quinlan *et al.* 1987; Cartier *et al.* 1992
v	Ikeda *et al.* 1981
w	Truslove 1962
x	Clayton 1979
y	Takeda 1991
z	Paget and Baumgartner-Gamauf 1953
aa	Kador *et al.* 1980
ab	Carper *et al.* 1986
ac	Takemoto *et al.* 1988
ad	Garber *et al.* 1985
ae	Feeney-Burns 1980
af	Hunsicker, P. 1974 *Mouse News Lett.* 50: 51–52
ag	Teicher, L. S., E. W. Caspari, 1978, *J. Hered.* 69: 86–90
ah	Happle, R., Phillips, R. J. S., Roesseur, A. and Junemann, G. 1983, *Human Genet.* 63: 21–27
ai	West, J. D., and Fisher, G. 1986, *Mutation Res.* 164, 127–136
aj	Everett, C. A. *et al.* 1994, *Genomics* (in press)
ak	Lyon *et al.* 1981
al	Chambers and Russell 1991
am	Hogan *et al.* 1987

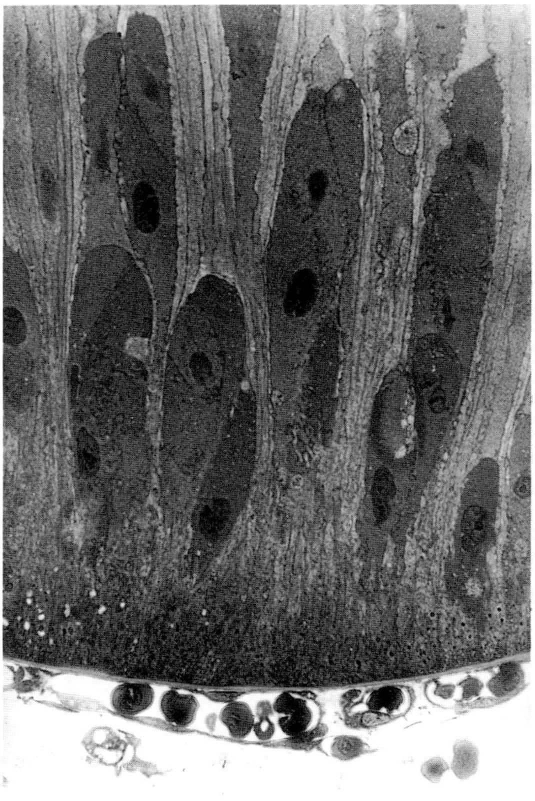

Figure 9.32(a)

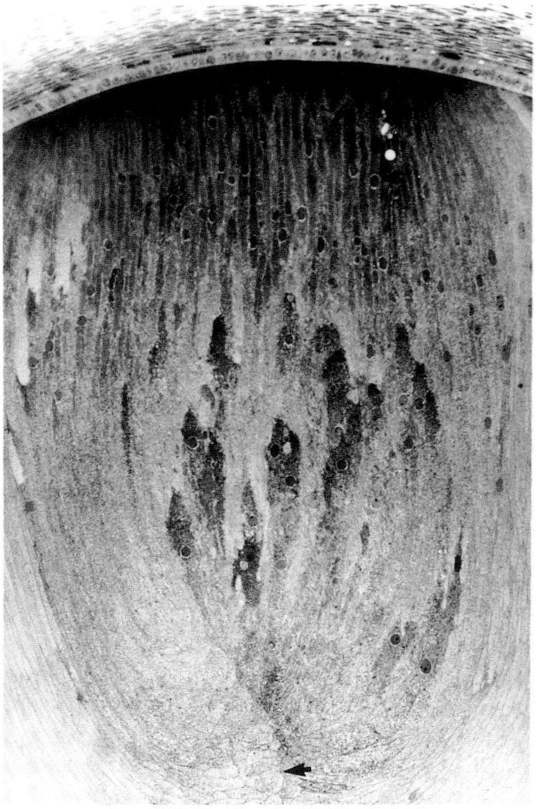

Figure 9.32(b)

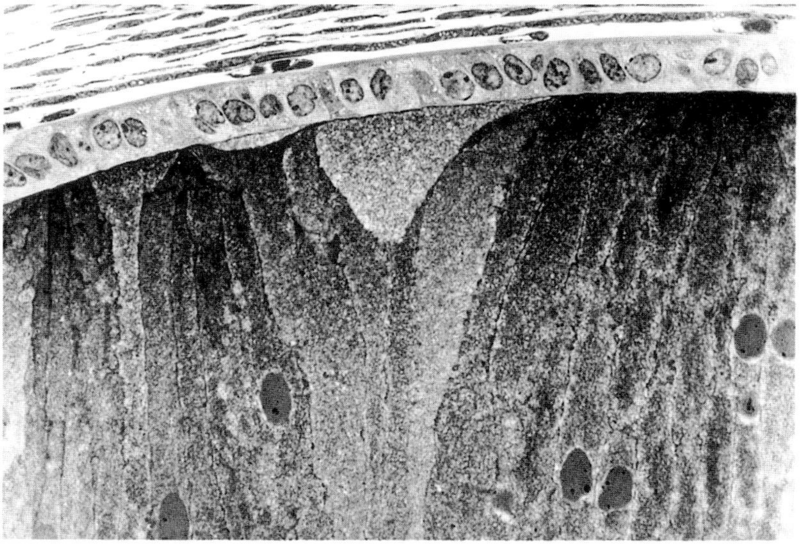

Figure 9.32(c)

Dog

About 65 breeds of purebred dog are disposed to cataract, and in 14 of these the inheritance is documented. The initial opacity is often confined to a particular region of the lens. Thus it is posterior, cortical and triangular in the golden retriever, and equatorial in the afghan hound, siberian husky (Figure 9.33) and standard poodle (Gelatt 1991).

In the miniature snauzer, congenital nuclear and posterior cortical cataract is associated with microphthalmos (Figure 9.33b). The cataract begins in fetal life. It matures, often with early stages of lenticonus, lentiglobus and capsule rupture, to hypermaturity by 2–4 years (Gelatt *et al.* 1983a,b).

Sheep

Focal, anterior and posterior cortical cataracts appear in the lenses of New Zealand Romney sheep at 1–2 months of age. They are inherited as an autosomal dominant trait, and reach maturity

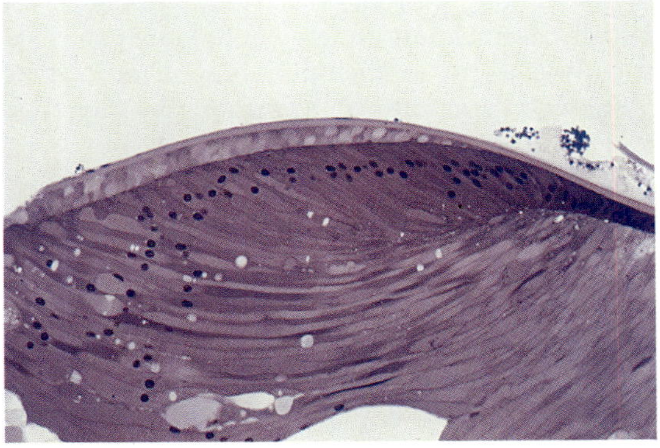

(bi)

Figure 9.33(bi) Neonatal cataract in the miniature snauzer. Bow nuclei pattern and mid-cortical region showing vacuolated areas, some of which contain liquefied material (arrow) (magnification × 240). (From Monaco *et al.* 1984 with permission.)

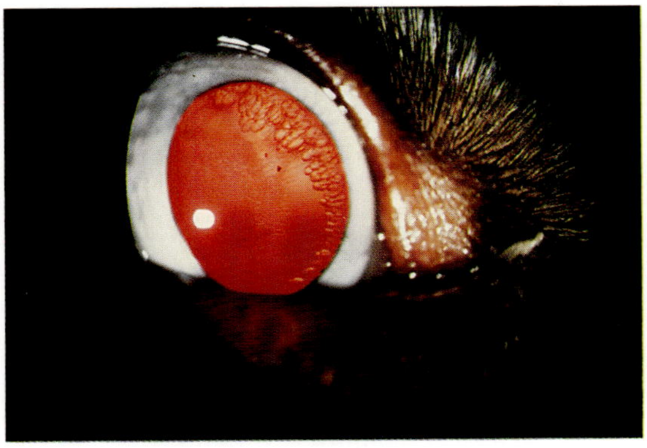

(a)

Figure 9.33(a) Slit-lamp photograph of an equatorial cataract in the Siberian husky dog. The vacuoles in both anterior and posterior cortices of the equator are clearly evident in this wide angle-slit beam (magnification × 10). (From Gelatt and Das 1984 with permission.)

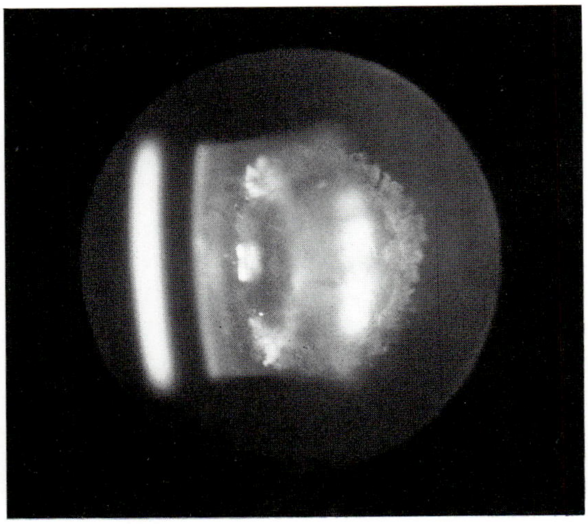

(bii)

Figure 9.33(bii) Miniature snauzer: as viewed by slit-lamp biomicroscopy. The posterior aspect (arrows) of the lens is malformed (lenticonus). (From Gelatt 1991 with permission.)

Figure 9.32(a) Abnormal elongation of primary fibre cells at the posterior pole of the rat lens at day 15 post conception (p.c.), mutant *cat*, magnification × 720.
Figure 9.32(b) At day 18 p.c. *(cat)*, malformed 1° fibre cells are visible in the nuclear area. No anterior suture system has been formed, although the posterior suture is already discernable (arrow). Numerous rounded cell nuclei indicate the inability of primary and secondary fibre cells to mature. Magnification × 180.
Figure 9.32(c) Disoriented fibre cells at the anterior lens pole, instead of converging they diverge away from the pole. Magnification × 720. (Courtesy of A. Wegener.)

by 10–11 months (Brooks *et al.* 1982). Lens fibres are initially normal, but undergo subsequent swelling and lysis. The epithelium shows vacuolation, hyperplasia and, ultimately, metaplastic migration under the posterior capsule (Brooks 1983).

Guinea-pig

There is a congenital guinea-pig cataract, associated with a genomic splice-site mutation in the zeta crystallin gene (Rodriguez *et al.* 1992).

Infective cataract

Various virus-induced congenital cataracts occur in animals, caused either by direct viral invasion or secondary to virus-induced inflammation or retinal degeneration or dysplasia.

1. *Herpes simplex virus type I* induces cataract in mice after corneal inoculation, in association with intraocular inflammation. Virus has been demonstrated within lens fibres and occasionally epithelium (Pfeiffer *et al.* 1983; Mitchell *et al.* 1992).
2. The *canine herpesvirus* crosses the placenta to cause various ocular anomalies, including retinal dysplasia and cataract. Also, experimental infection in newborn pups induces a panuveitis associated with cataract.
3. In *Marek's disease,* herpesvirus-induced lymphoma in chickens, cataracts occur secondarily to the intraocular inflammation (Smith *et al.* 1974).
4. Intracerebral injection of *St Louis encephalitis* subviral particles in 4-day-old rats produces cataract in 86% of the animals. Cataracts are initially posterior subcapsular and, if they develop early, are accompanied by microphthalmia, microcornea and microphakia. Virus is present within the eye (Hanna *et al.* 1968).
5. In the cataract which occurs in *induced lymphocytic choriomenengitis* in newborn rats, virus is not found in the lens. Cataract has been attributed to the extensive retinal damage (Monjan *et al.* 1972).
6. *Avian encephalomyelitis* (picornavirus/enterovirus) affects chickens between the ages of 1 and 21 days. Mortality in this neurological disorder may exceed 50%. A posterior subcapsular cataract is often seen in association with anterior uveitis, and virus is present in the lens (Bridges and Flowers 1958; Gentry *et al.* 1968).
7. Intraocular injection of *feline leukaemia virus* (oncorna) into fetal and newborn kittens induces tumour, retinal dysplasia and cataract, the latter occurring with intraocular inflammation (Albert *et al.* 1977).
8. The *Enders strain of the mumps virus* injected into chick blastoderm, prior to capsule formation, causes cataract following entry of virus into the lens fibre (Williamson *et al.* 1957). Newcastle disease and influenza virus A can also cause cataract in chick embryos.
9. *Bovine viral (togavirus) diarrhoea–mucosal disease* causes congenital cerebellar hypoplasia and ocular malformations, including microphthalmos, optic neuritis, retinal atrophy and cataract. The cataract is cortical and occurs in the absence of retinitis or uveitis. The lens may be misshapen (Bistner *et al.* 1970).
10. Injection of *rubella virus* into pregnant albino rats induces a congenital syndrome in the newborn which parallels the human disease. Cataract is due to viral invasion and destruction of lens epithelium and fibres (Cotlier *et al.* 1968).

10

Forms of human cataract

Cataracts of a given cause may contain many different morphological elements; for instance 'senile cataract' may exhibit cortical, subcapsular and nuclear features. It is helpful to classify the various forms which cataract may take before considering their aetiology (Figure 10.1).

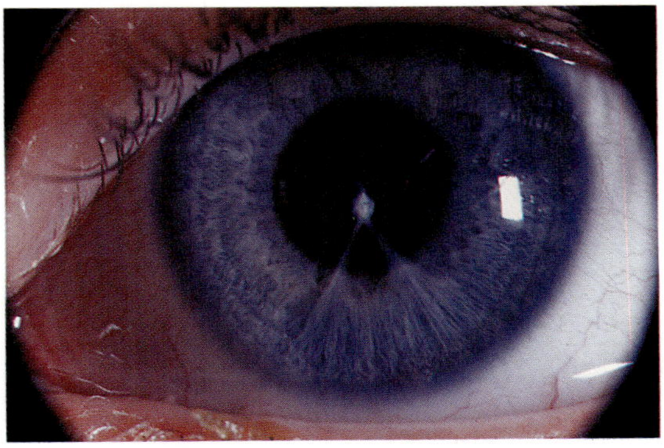

Figure 10.2 Anterior polar capsular opacity associated with a pupil membrane remnant, with strands passing from the iris collarette to the opacity, which is typical of this condition.

Capsular abnormalities

Capsular opacities

Capsular opacities are either congenital or acquired.

Congenital capsular opacities

The common congenital opacity is situated at the anterior pole of the lens (Figures 10.2, 10.3).

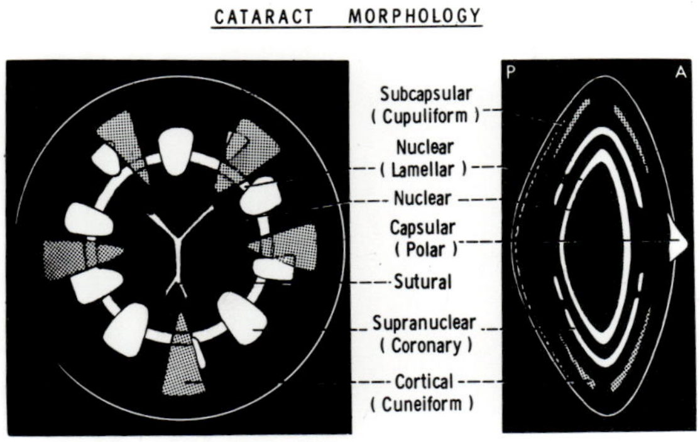

Figure 10.1 Classification of cataract.

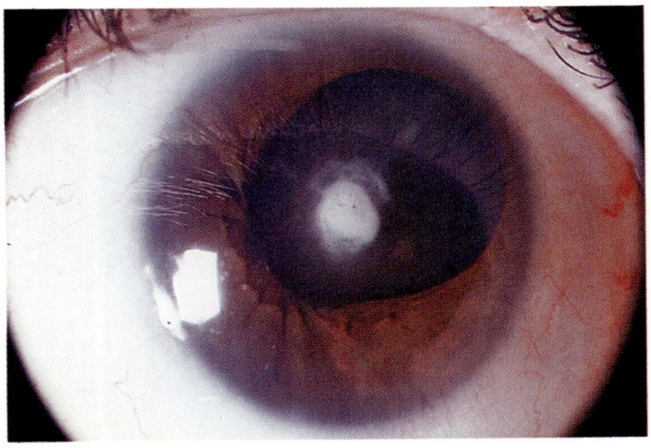

Figure 10.3 An anterior polar capsular opacity with a disc-shaped subjacent anterior cortical cataract associated with partial aniridia.

Inheritance is dominant or the changes may be sporadic. The opacity forms a plaque, or occasionally projects forwards from the lens as a cone (as part of an anterior polar pyramidal cataract) (Figure 10.4) (Brown and Lewis 1972). Histology has shown these plaques to be of hyaline material. The congenital anterior capsular opacity is often joined to a persistent pupillary membrane and occasionally associated with a corneal opacity. A corneal opacity and maldevelopment of the anterior chamber angle occur in Peter's anomaly (Kivlin *et al.* 1986).

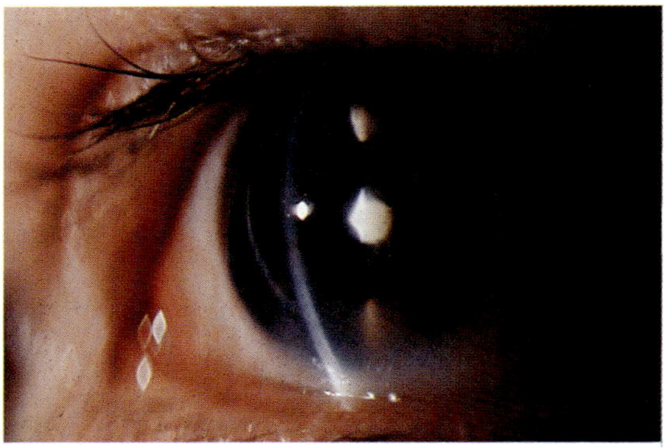

Figure 10.4 A rare and striking anterior polar pyramidal cataract which projects as a cone into the anterior chamber.

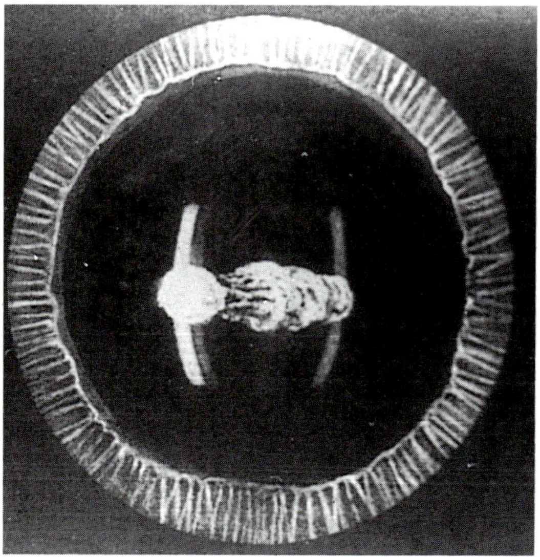

Figure 10.5 Drawing of reduplication cataract.

An opacity in the subjacent lens fibres is common and it must be assumed that the subjacent epithelium is affected. It appears that the capsular defect, lying at the anterior pole of the lens, interferes with the sutural interdigitation of the anterior tips of each new generation of lens fibres. They fail to meet at the anterior pole, and, in their place, an irregular stack of opacities gradually builds up like a stack of plates (anterior and posterior polar cataract) (Figure 10.3). If there is a break in the column of opacity, this is a reduplication cataract (Figure 10.5). Vision is affected if successive plates increase in diameter.

Congenital capsular opacities may also occur posteriorly and in association with persistent hyaloid artery remnants. The Mittendorf dot, which is tiny, is the common example. It is sited about 1.5 mm nasal to the posterior pole. The opacity may be more gross than this. Subjacent cataract may

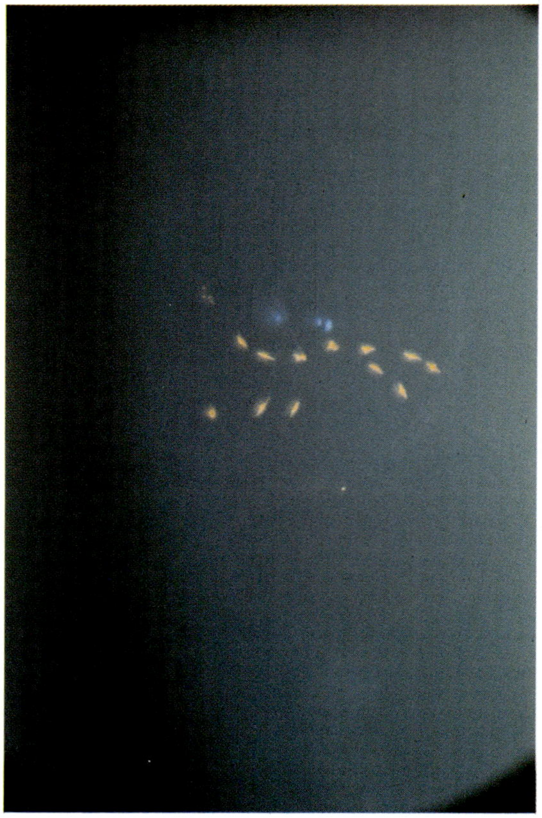

Figure 10.6 Epicapsular stars (magnification × 10).

occur and the condition needs to be distinguished from cataract related to posterior lenticonus.

Pupillary membrane remnants in the form of epicapsular stars (Figure 10.6) are fairly common and not usually associated with a capsular opacity.

Acquired capsular opacities

Vogt (1921, 1931) described occasional dot-like features in the anterior lens capsule seen in the periphery of the adult lens. In specular reflection they are convex forwards or may be doughnut shaped. They do not affect vision. Other acquired capsular opacities are usually the result of inflammation or of trauma. Thus they are seen following iritis, or keratitis, particularly when there are posterior synechiae which are associated with anterior capsular opacities. Posterior capsular opacities may develop in the presence of mature cataract and these are found at the time of an extracapsular cataract extraction when they become distinguishable from the fibre element of a posterior subcapsular cataract.

A penetrating eye injury may cause a capsular rupture. A small penetration of the anterior capsule is often healed by the action of the epithelium, which proliferates, some cells undergoing a metaplastic change to resemble fibroblasts. A capsular opacity is formed (Figure 10.7), but, if the perforation of the capsule is at all large, it does not heal and the lens is unable to cope with the water influx, presumably because of the coexistent breach in the epithelium. The condition then passes rapidly to the development of a mature cataract.

The capsule may also be opaque in association with anterior or posterior lenticonus.

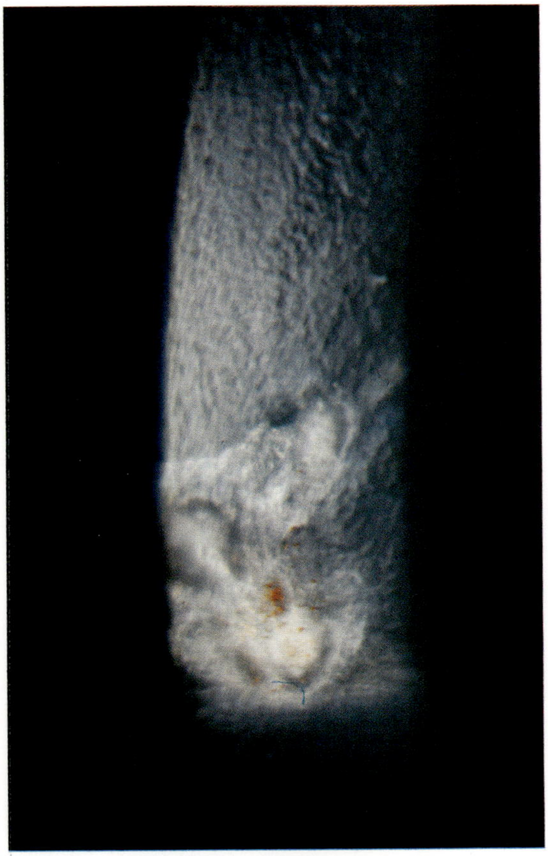

Figure 10.7 Traumatic capsular opacity following capsular penetration (magnification × 10).

Capsular pigmentation and other cellular deposition

Jaeger (1983) has described a green coloration of the peripheral anterior capsule as a dominantly inherited disorder without visual effect (Figure 10.8). Three sisters and one brother were affected. Changes were less in the brother. There was increased light scattering from the capsule in slit-image photographs. No disorder of copper metabolism was found and the capsular change in

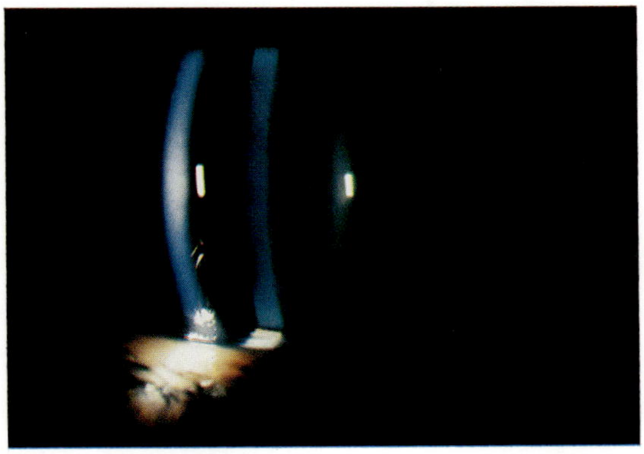

Figure 10.8 Green capsular abnormality of a member of the family described by Jaeger in 1983. (Courtesy of W. Jaeger.)

Wilson's disease (p. 199) differs in that it is central, and a yellowish-brown colour.

Radial pigmented lines at the periphery of the older lens have been described as retro-iridial lines (Sturrock and Tripathi 1976). These represent forwardly migrated zonular fibres which have taken up uveal pigment.

Flecks of pigment on the anterior capsule are common following iritis and often represent the site of previous posterior synechiae. Other cellular deposits, together with fibrin, are also found on the anterior capsule in association with iritis.

A fine pigment deposition is often present in the pigment dispersion syndrome, occurring on both capsular surfaces and in the trabecular meshwork. On the posterior capsule the pigment forms a ring at the site of a vitreo-lenticular adhesion.

A ring of pigment, known as the Vossius ring, and corresponding in diameter to the pupil, occurs occasionally as a result of blunt trauma. It is due to deposition of pigment from the iris epithelium imprinted at the pupil margin.

Products of abnormal metabolism may deposit as fine white granules and these have been reported in Fabry's disease (Franceschetti 1976).

Drugs and metals may precipitate in the capsule, commonly producing a fine dusting, as is seen with chlorpromazine and gold (p. 197). The deposit takes on the star shape of the lens sutures because of deposition occurring also in the superficial lens cortex. Mercury produces a fine grey sheen in the capsule (Figure 10.9).

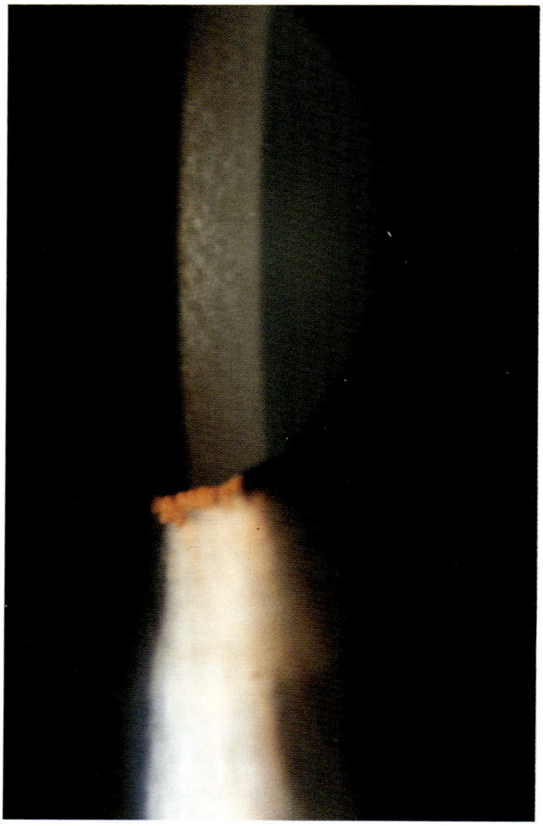

Figure 10.9 Mercuria lentis (magnification × 10).

Capsular pits

This is a rare condition in which a collection of bleb-like defects are seen nearly centrally in the anterior lens capsule (Harris *et al* 1992) (Figure 10.10). They are best observed by indirect retro-illumination when they repeat the distribution of light and shade in the background (Figure 10.11), known as the unreversed effect (Brown 1971). They are also seen by specular illumination which suggests that they may be due to dimples in the surface. Their significance is not yet known (Figure 7.6).

Exfoliation and pseudoexfoliation

Exfoliation

True exfoliation, in which an anterior lamella of the capsule peels forward into the pupil, is an

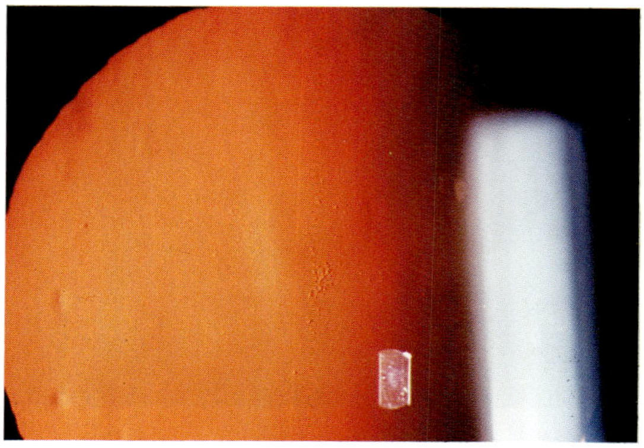

Figure 10.10 Capsular bleb disorder.

extremely rare disorder today and is limited to small numbers of idiopathic cases (Cashwell *et al.* 1989) (Figure 10.12). It used to be reported in glass blowers and furnace workers and was considered to be due to the heating of the lens by infrared radiation absorbed by the iris pigment. However, it is now known that infrared radiation may also damage the lens directly. A somewhat similar condition with herniation of an anterior layer of the capsule into the pupil has recently been reported in desert dwellers (Johnson *et al.* 1988).

Pseudoexfoliation

Pseudoexfoliation syndrome (PXS) is a systemic fibrillopathy affecting a wide range of tissues, which in the eye involves the lens, zonule, ciliary body, iris and drainage angle. It gives rise to a secondary open angle glaucoma and zonular laxity. Details have been summarized by Streeten and Dark (1994).

Prevalence Generally, females are affected more frequently than males (2.3:1) (Hiller *et al.* 1982) although the finding was reversed in Australian aboriginals (Taylor *et al.* 1977). Prevalence has been said to be highest in Scandinavia, but variation is so great from region to region, that this is still in debate. In northern Finland, Lapland, Iceland and parts of (former) Russia the prevalence is 10–13% in persons of 50–69 years, and 21–35% in those over 70 years of age. Similar figures apply to the Navajo Indians (Faulkner, 1971), Australian aboriginals (Taylor *et al.* 1977), and in Saudi Arabia (Summanem and Tonjum 1988). In a study of geriatric homes in Birmingham, England, Bonn and Bergen, Aasved (1969) found 3% in the seventh decade, rising to 11% in the tenth decade. The disease occurs in 2–7% of persons over 60 years in most of Europe and in parts of the US, and is virtually absent in the Inuit peoples (Forsius, 1988).

PXS is rare before the age of sixty, but has been recorded in the fourth decade (Horven and Hutchinson; Tarkkanen 1962), and even in the second decade in a patient who had suffered a penetrating injury in childhood (Sugar 1976). The prevalence of PXS rises with age.

The condition is unilateral at diagnosis in 48–76% (Aasved 1971; Klemetti 1988; Tarkkanen 1962), and 13–15% of these become bilateral by 10

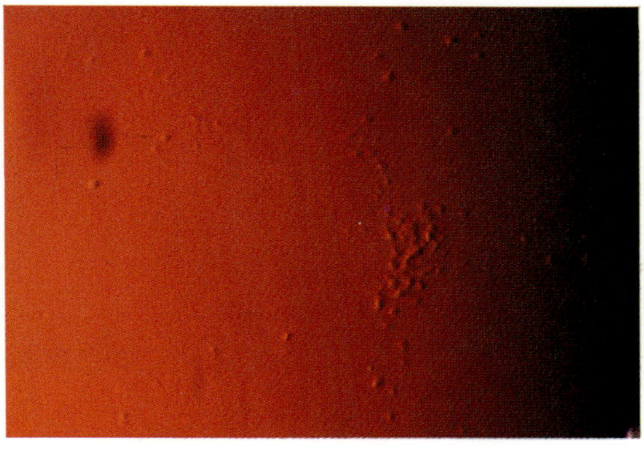

Figure 10.11 Capsular bleb disorder (magnification × 8).

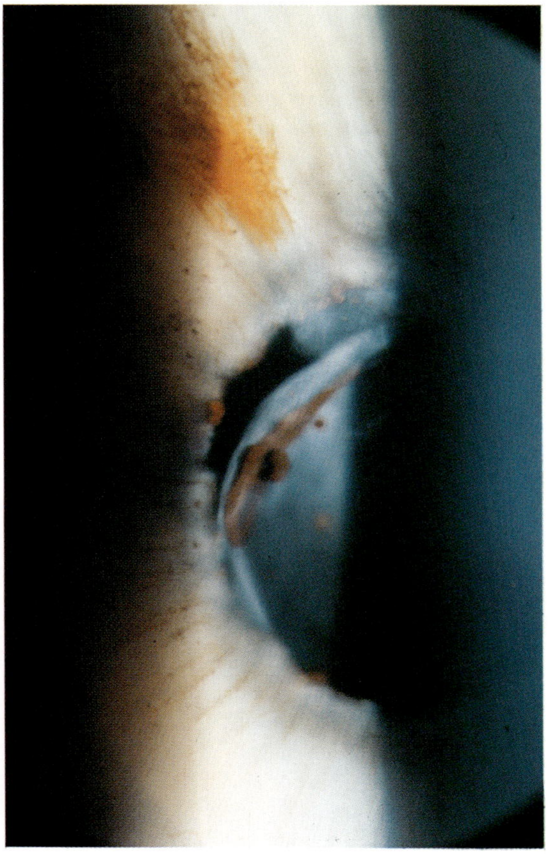

Figure 10.12 True exfoliation of the lens (magnification × 10).

years (Knorr *et al.* 1981; Roth and Epstein 1980; Yanoff 1988). Unilateral cases are typically younger than bilateral by about 2–6 years, suggesting that it is an earlier stage of the disease. Indeed, in apparently unilateral cases, deposits may be detected on the zonules and ciliary processes in 77% of fellow eyes by gonioscopy (Mizuno and Muroi 1979) and typical changes may be preceded by a greyish layer on the anterior capsule (Dark and Streeten 1990) which may show radial striations (Bartholomew 1971), holes, or an association with extensive iris pigmentary loss (Tetsumoto *et al.* 1992).

Features In pseudoexfoliation of the lens there is a fine deposit on the anterior lens capsule resembling a coating of icing sugar which is most evident in the mid periphery. It is therefore best seen after pupil dilatation (Figure 10.13). The deposit has a bull's eye arrangement, with a central disc of fine material with a well-defined margin and a peripheral ring of more granular material. A clear ring is found between the two. The disc is present in 80–90% of patients (Horven 1937; Tarkkanen 1962). The margins of the central peripheral zones may become raised, and curl away from each other. The granular zone may form in the presence of a traumatic coloboma (Tarkkanen 1962), but may be absent opposite a surgical coloboma (Sunde 1956).

The intervening clear ring is attributable to contact between the lens capsule and pupil margin, whose movements maintain a clear capsular surface. A radial pattern is common and may well relate the iris movement (Figure 10.14). Small particles of material on the pupil margin are a useful clue to the presence of PXS on the lens (Figure 10.15).

The material may deposit on the zonule and on the ciliary processes, and this may be associated with zonular weakening, although the mechanism is not known. PXS material may also be seen on the anterior hyaloid after cataract extraction and rarely, on the back of the cornea. Corneal endothelial density may be reduced, in association with polymegathism and pleomorphism (Knorr 1991).

Flakes of PXS material are seen occasionally on the trabecular meshwork and a heavily pigmented trabeculum is a frequent finding, often associated with an undulating pigment line and dense pigmentation of the posterior meshwork which is more frequent in this condition (64%), than in primary open angle glaucoma (POAG) (9%) (Layden and Schaffer 1974). As in the pigment dispersion syndrome, which may coexist, lines of pigment may be seen in the drainage angle anterior to Schwalbe's line (Layden *et al.* 1990; Sampaolesi *et al.* 1988). Pigment deposited along the trabecular meshwork is probably derived from the iris pigment epithelium by the abrasive action of the capsular deposits. The iris may show loss of pigment from the pupillary ruff, transillumination of the peripupillary and pripheral iris and release of pigment into the aqueous on mydriasis (Prince and Ritch 1986; Repo *et al.* 1990). These features are sometimes the only clinical indication of PXS in some patients diagnosed by conjunctival biopsy (Tetsumato *et al.* 1992).

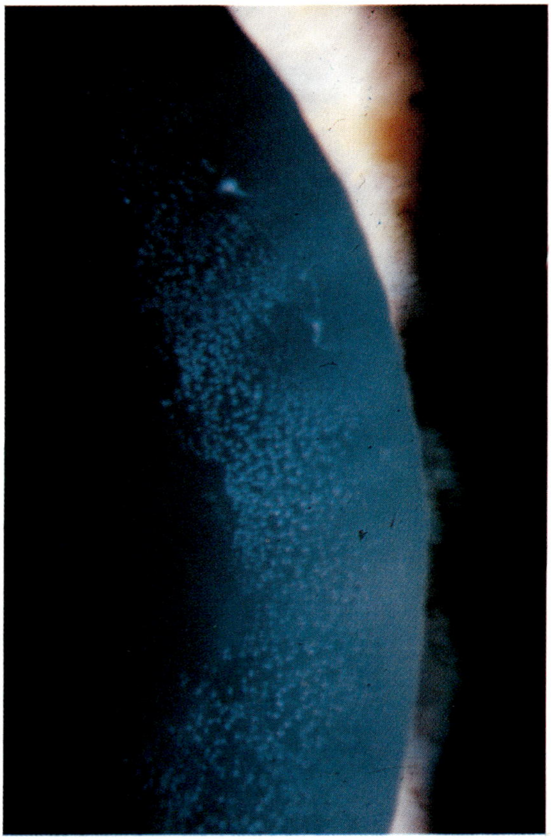

Figure 10.13 Pseudoexfoliation of the lens. The ring of particles is seen after pupil dilatation (magnification × 10).

Iris angiography in PXS demonstrates hypoperfusion, leakage and a fine focal neovascularization which is not usually visible on biomicroscopy alone (Brookes and Gilles 1987; Vannas 1969).

PXS material is found at other ocular sites and in extraocular tissues. It was shown to be present in the limbus and lid conjunctiva by Ringvold (1972, 1973) and in unaffected fellow eyes by Speakman and Ghosh (1976). It has been demonstrated in the orbit, the lid and buttock skin and in various viscera (Streeten *et al.* 1990; Schlötzer-Schrehardt 1991, 1992a), so that the disorder may be truly regarded as a systemic condition.

Structure By light microscopy the deposit appears to be granular in the mid-periphery of the lens but confluent on the zonule, iris and anterior hyaloid face. There is a deep fibrogranular layer in the pre-equatorial zone of the lens, into which vertically oriented fibres insert, arising from the underlying lens epithelial cells (Bertelson and Seland 1972; Ashton *et al.* 1965).

Ultrastructural studies show the central capsular disc to be fibrillar, while the granular zone is made up of stump-like aggregates. Deposits are made up of two types of fibre: type A fibres are thin, 15–20 nm wide and up to 1 um long, and frequently with a cross-banding (20–25 or 40–50 nm) which may exceed the fibre width. Type B fibres are shorter (45 nm), more elctron dense, and have less definite banding. Fibres have a filamentary structure and are bound in places, at the 50 nm cross-band to fine (3–7 nm) fibrils, or to scattered, banded (8–10 nm) fibrils with a tubular cross-

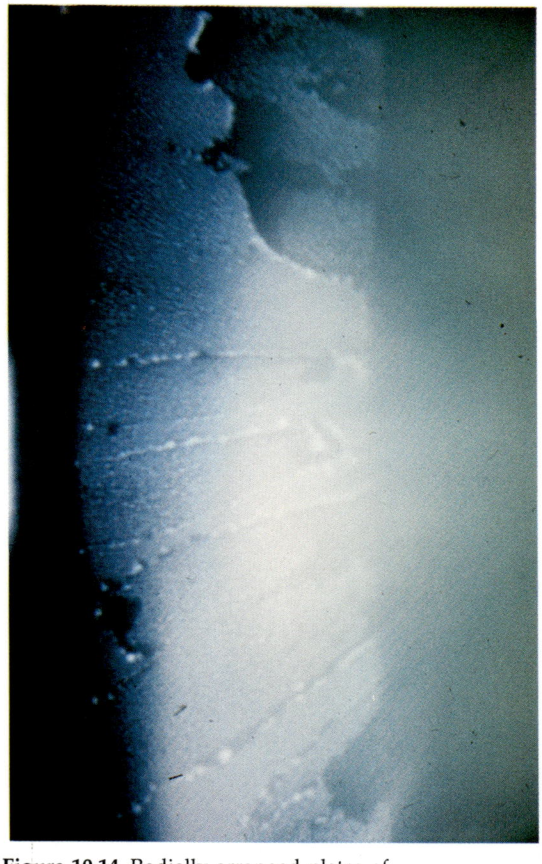

Figure 10.14 Radially arranged plates of pseudoexfoliative material.

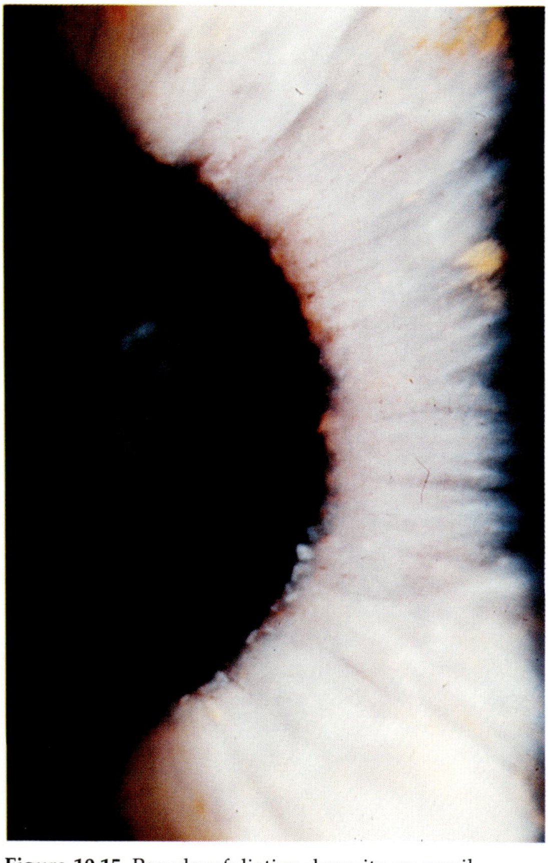

Figure 10.15 Pseudoexfoliative deposits on pupil margin (magnification × 10).

section (Streeten and Dark 1994). The central capsular deposit contains a mixture of PXS fibres and fibrils some of which attach to the capsule, and including fibrillin, the major component of the zonule (Sakai *et al.* 1986). The precapsular film, noted earlier, which may be a precursor of the PXS disc, contains fibrillin and laminin (Dark and Streeten 1990; Tetsumoto *et al.* 1992), but is also found on 20–50% of lenses undergoing cataract extraction.

The fine branching fibrils of the deep fibrogranular zone insert into pits in the underlying epithelial cells. The deposit contains fibrillin, and although the zonules are themselves intact, PXS fibres percolate freely between them. Full details of the ultrastructural features of PXS material at other sites in the eye and elsewhere is given by Streeten and Dark (1994).

Composition Various carbohydrates and proteins have been demonstrated within PXS material. Both heparan sulphate and chondroitin sulphate proteoglycan have been demonstrated (Harnisch *et al.* 1981; Schlötzer-Schrehardt *et al.* 1992b) and also hyaluronan (Fitzsimmons *et al.* 1992). The carbohydrate associated with the PXS material contains both O-linked sialomucin-type and N-linked oligosaccharide chains. (Hietanen and Tarkannen 1989; Streeten *et al.* 1986). Protein components include nidogen/entactin, fibronectin, amyloid P, fibrillin, alpha elastin, vitronectin and possibly laminin. Other components which have been identified are shown in Table 10.1.

Origins The source of the PXS material is uncertain. One view is that it derives from the abnormal synthesis of basement membrane components (Konstas *et al.* 1990). Focal interruption of the basement membrane is found at many of the sites where PXS material is located both within and outside of the eye. Another view is that the condition arises as an abnormality of the elastic system particularly affecting the microfibrils (Streeten *et al.* 1987), or that the condition is due to disordered regulation of extracellular matrix synthesis (Li *et al.* 1988; Schlötzer-Schrehardt 1992a,b; Streeten *et al.* 1992). Viral, immune and genetic factors have also been considered.

Clinical significance of PXS Open angle glaucoma is more common in PXS than in the normal population. This is presumed to be due to the deposition of material in the trabecular meshwork, although the precise relationship between the deposit and the glaucoma is not known. The frequency of glaucoma ranges from 0% in the Framingham study (Hiller *et al.* 1982) to over 60% in various other reports in Europe, Asia and South America. (Overall, a frequency of 20–40% is representative.) PXS glaucoma accounts for 5–20% of open angle glaucoma in most European countries, but from 50–93% in parts of Scandinavia. The risk of developing raised intraocular pressure is moderate: 5% at 5 years and 15% at 10 years (Henry *et al.* 1987). Trabeculectomy in PXS is more effective than in POAG, while laser trabeculoplasty is initially more effective but not so after one year, (Hetherington 1988).

There is a higher incidence of narrow angle glaucoma in PXS, perhaps reflecting laxity of the zonule (Layden and Schaffer 1974; Franks *et al.* 1990).

Lens subluxation has been recorded and zonular dialysis during extracapsular cataract extraction may occur (Skuta 1987). Subluxation or dislocation (usually inferiorly) can cause pupil-block glaucoma. In Giffords long-term series (1957) spontaneous dislocation occurred in about 5%. Zonular rupture occurs near the ciliary attachment where the zonules are said to be focally thin. In extracapsular cataract extraction (ECCE), zonular dialysis can cause dislocation, implant decentration, or

Table 10.1 Immunoidentity of pseudexfoliative deposits

Basement membrane related material	***Positive***	***Negative***
Collagen IV		MC
Laminin	PC; MC	
Nidogen/entactin	PC	
Heparan sulphate	PC; MC	
Elastic tissue related		
Fibrillin	MC	
Zonular peptides	PC	
MAGP	PC	
α-elastin, aortic	PC; MC	
Amyloid P protein	PC	
Vitronectin	PC; MC	
Other matrix components		
Fibronectin	MC	
Amyloid A protein	PC	

From Streeten and Dark (1994). PC = polyclonal antibody; MC = monoclonal vitreous loss, which is increased up to 10-fold, and may necessitate sulcus fixation (Raitta and Setala 1986; Naumann *et al.* 1986; Tarkkanen 1986; Guzek *et al.* 1987; Picnalosa *et al.* 1989).

Adhesion between lens periphery and iris occurs in PXS, which may explain poor mydriasis and capsular rupture during intracapsular cataract extraction (ICCE) or zonular dialysis during ECCE.

Non-opaque lens defects

The non-opaque lens defects occur in association with cataract and probably represent an aspect of the cataract forming process, although their precise role has yet to be evaluated. These defects are: fibre folds (lamellar separation), water clefts and vacuoles.

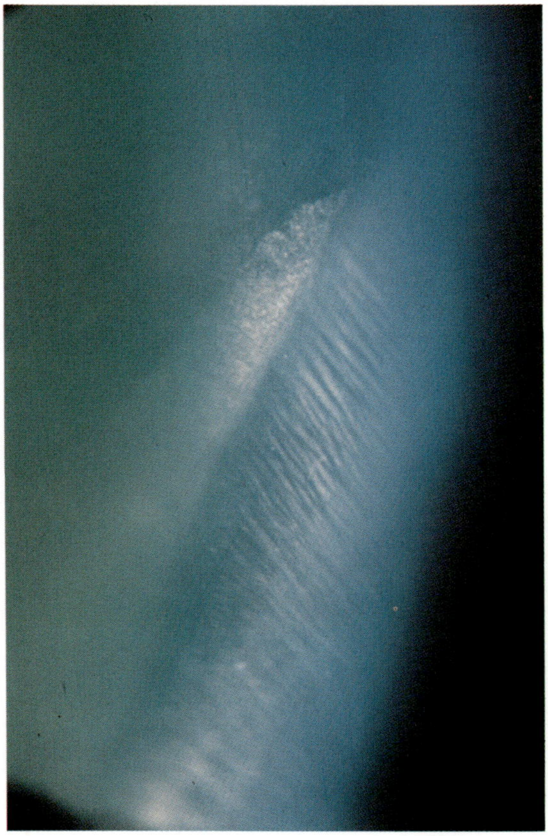

Figure 10.16 Fibre folds interrupted by a spoke cataract (magnification × 10).

Fibre folds (lamellar separation)

Fibre folds (Brown *et al.* 1989) are a common concomitant of senile cataract, but are occasionally seen in the absence of evident cataract. The folds (Figures 10.16, 10.17), which are seen best with focal illumination, consist of approximately parallel white lines, which occasionally branch and rejoin. Their direction is roughly parallel to the lens equator and they are most commonly found in the lower half of the lens superficial cortex, where they are more evident anteriorly than posteriorly. The extent of a group of folds may be limited by a spoke cataract (Figure 10.16), a water cleft, or by a lens suture. The lines may continue beyond the lens suture with a change in direction, forming a fishbone pattern (Figure 10.18). It can be seen that they extend in depth into the lens (Figure 10.19), and are therefore a three-dimensional structure of layers of fibres folded in the same place. Their appearance gave rise to the previous name of lamellar separation, but electron microscopy has shown that they are due to corrugations in the fibres (Figures 10.20, 10.21). Electron microscopy also showed (Figure 10.22) that there is an associated break in the pre-equatorial part of the affected fibres which appears to explain their undulating contour, resulting from a release of

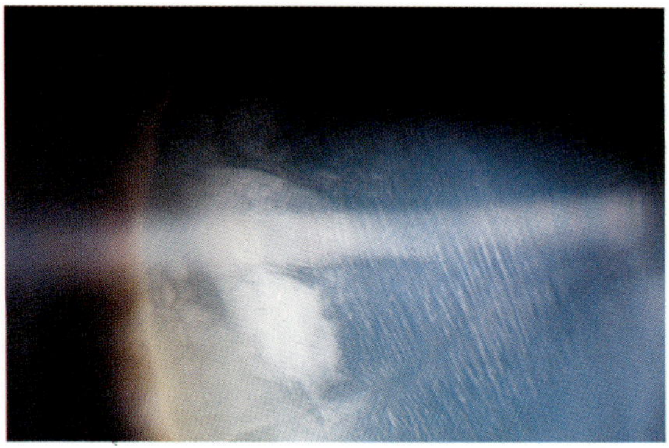

Figure 10.17 Fibre folds are seen as parallel ridges. (Courtesy of A. Shun-Shin.)

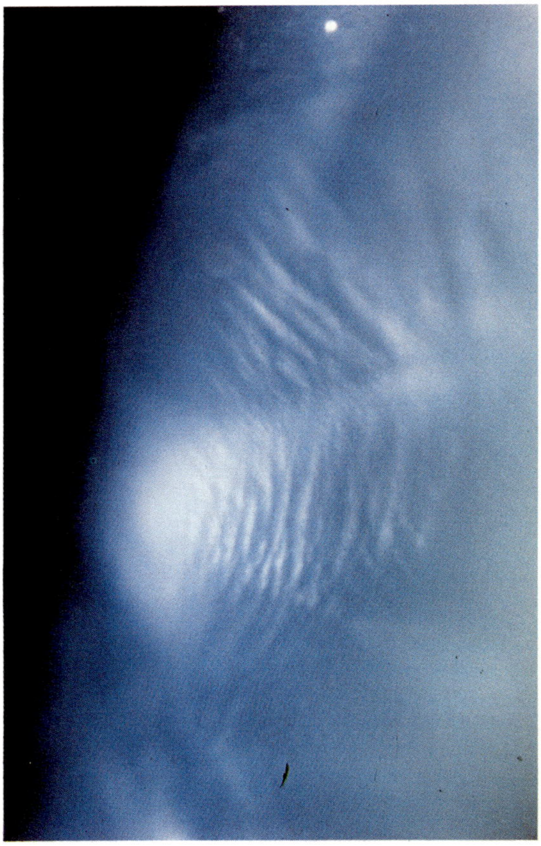

Figure 10.18 Change in direction of a fibre fold when interrupted by a suture, creating a fishbone pattern.

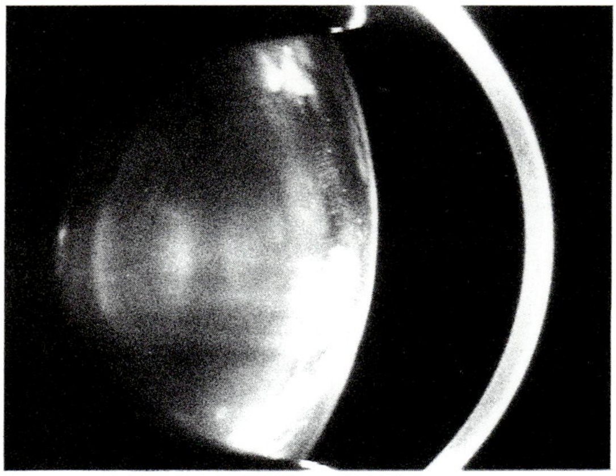

Figure 10.19 Fibre folds extending in depth into the anterior cortex in a lens with spoke cataract.

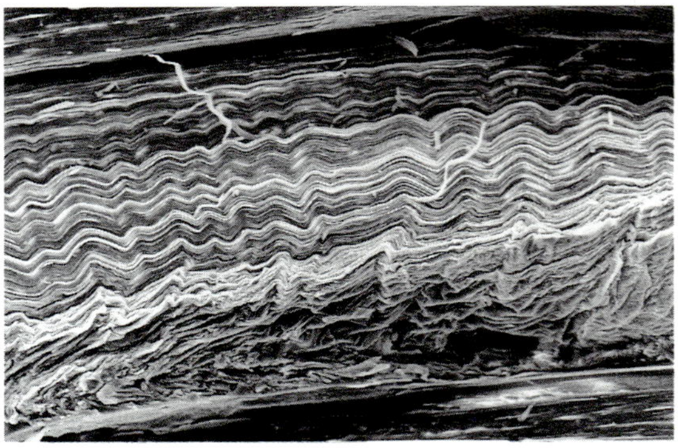

Figure 10.20 Fibre folds. SEM. (From Brown *et al.* 1989 with permission.)

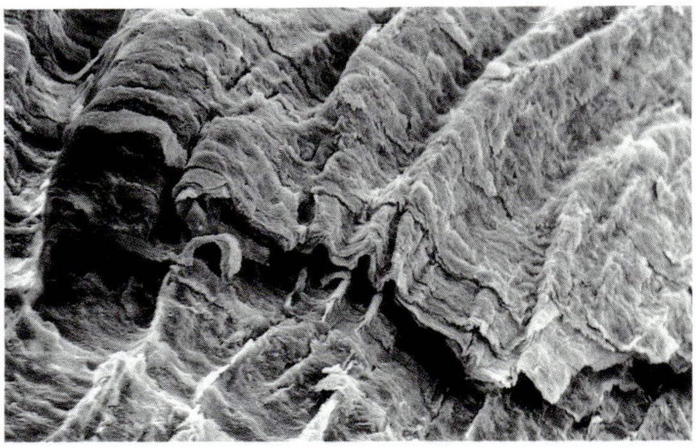

Figure 10.21 Fibre folds at higher magnification. Their three-dimensional nature is appreciated. SEM. (From Brown *et al.* 1989 with permission.)

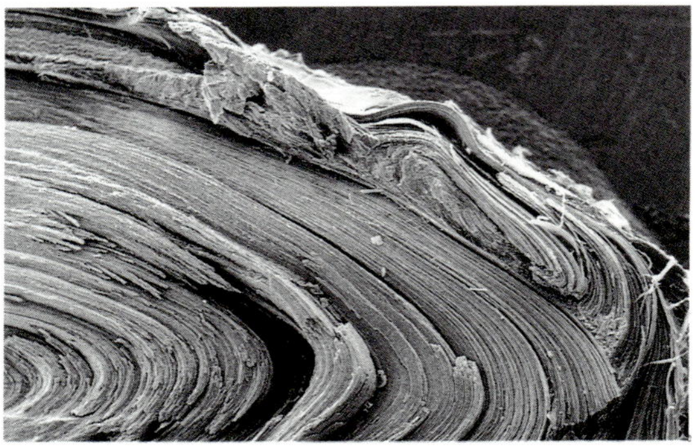

Figure 10.22 Fibre breaks. Fibre folds are seen in the top left of the picture and breaks are seen in these same fibres at the right of the picture. SEM. (From Brown *et al.* 1989 with permission.)

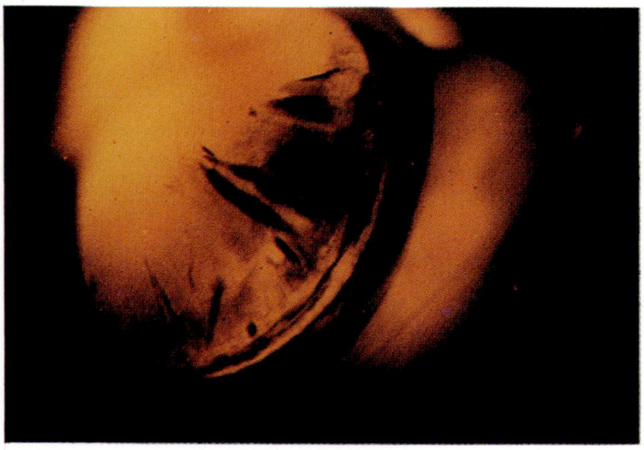

Figure 10.23 Circular shades as described by Obazawa are seen when the eye is turned down. Spoke cataract is also present.

tension along the length of the fibre. The line of breakage gives rise to a crescent-shaped defect which appears to correspond to the features described by Obazawa *et al.* (1983) as circular shades (Figure 10.23). These can be found by examining the periphery of any lens affected by fibre folds.

Water clefts

Water clefts are a common feature of the ageing lens and may precede the development of cataract (Figures 10.24–10.26). They consist of radial wedge-like clefts in the lens cortex and are more evident anteriorly than posteriorly. The clefts arise in C2 as a wedge-shaped split running in the line of the suture and greatly broadening it. They may first be

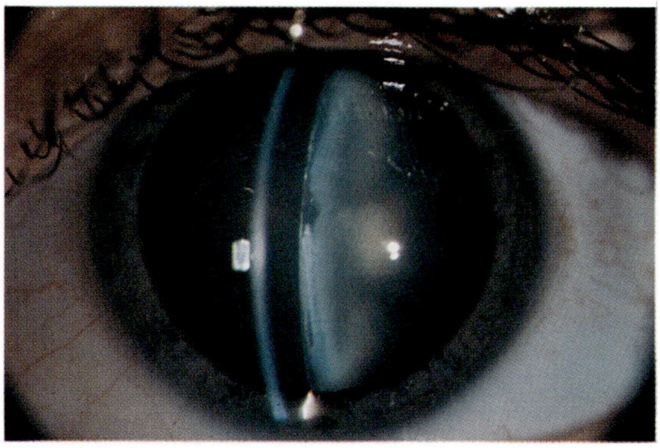

Figure 10.24 An anterior cortical water cleft affecting the axial region of the suture system.

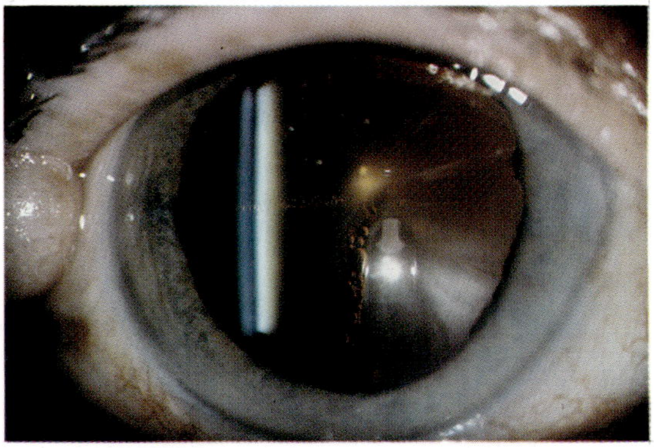

Figure 10.25 Water cleft with contained globules.

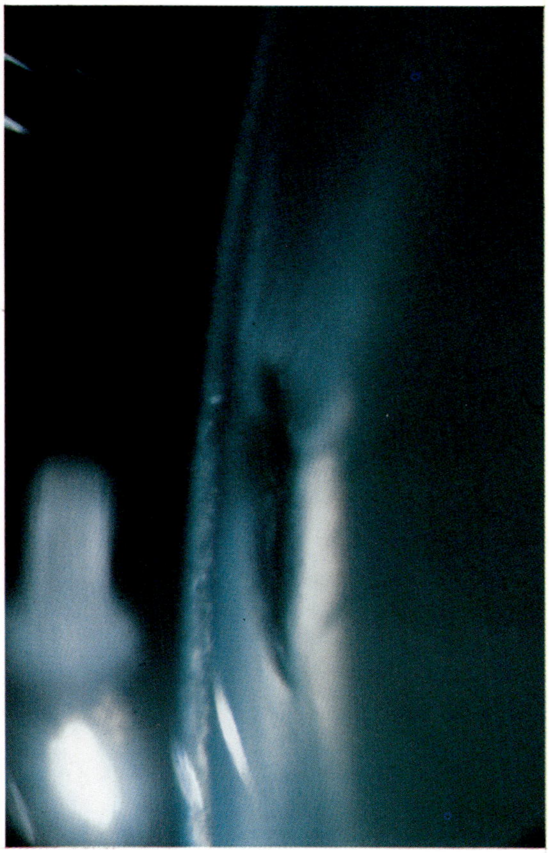

Figure 10.26 Water cleft in the anterior cortex (magnification × 10).

noted as a tiny, optically empty blip within an otherwise normal suture, but are more obviously seen as an expansion occupying a limited anteroposterior segment of a suture, being of variable cross-section. They commonly extend to the central confluence of the adult suture but their radial extension does not reach the equator, presumably reflecting the peripheral limit of the suture arrangement. Along their anteroposterior length they may show insinuations in the plane of the fibre shells, which imply an extension of the water cleft between consecutive layers of lens fibres. An interesting feature of the water cleft is its initial exclusion from the most superficial cortical zone, C1, which suggests that there is some physical obstruction to its expansion forwards from C2 across C1β. Ultimately, this barrier is negotiated, and the water cleft breaks through into C1. A similar barrier appears to restrict the extension of water clefts into the deep cortex (C3 and C4) (Figure 10.24). Water clefts occasionally result from trauma (p. 201).

The visibility of water clefts depends on the condition of their walls and of their contents. The walls and contents may be clear (simple water clefts), or may be lined by opaque fibres and/or contain opaque globules, like strings of pearls. These are complex water clefts, which are visible on retro-illumination and form one variety of spoke cataract. Electron microscopic examination shows globules both lining the walls and free in the cavity (Figures 10.27, 10.28). Spongy material is also often present.

All water clefts are visible by focal illumination as a clear space with no light-scattering properties (Figure 10.26), which distinguishes the water cleft from adjacent normal lens fibres. The picture of the complete, simple water cleft is built up by the examiner scanning the lens with the slit-beam. Water clefts without opaque elements are not visible by retro-illumination at the slit-lamp, which implies that the refractive index of their contents is very similar to that of the surrounding lens fibres. Water clefts are visible as 'spokes' with the retinoscope. This is because the retinoscopic examination is at 1 metre and is therefore sensitive to very small changes in angle produced by small differences in refractive index. The posterior wall of the cleft can be demonstrated as a bright strip by specular illumination, again implying a refractive interface.

The relationship between water clefts and true spokes is not fully established. Complex water clefts may become sufficiently opaque to resemble spokes, but their axis is at an angle to the fibre direction since they run, with variable obliquity, along the sutures into which the fibres insert. Water clefts may be found at the tips of a spoke, at the point of which the fibres involved in the spoke opacity insert into the suture.

The origin of the water cleft is at present obscure. It may arise either by separation between adjacent lens fibres with a localized expansion of the

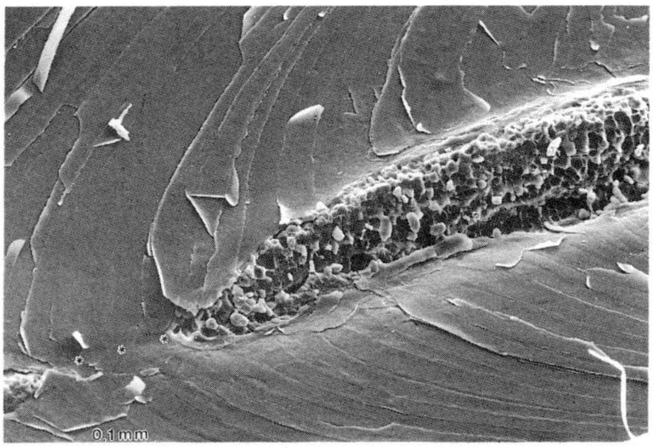

Figure 10.27 Water cleft. The cleft is seen as a separation along the suture line and has a globular content. The suture line is marked by asterisks. SEM. (From Shun-Shin *et al.* 1991b with permission.)

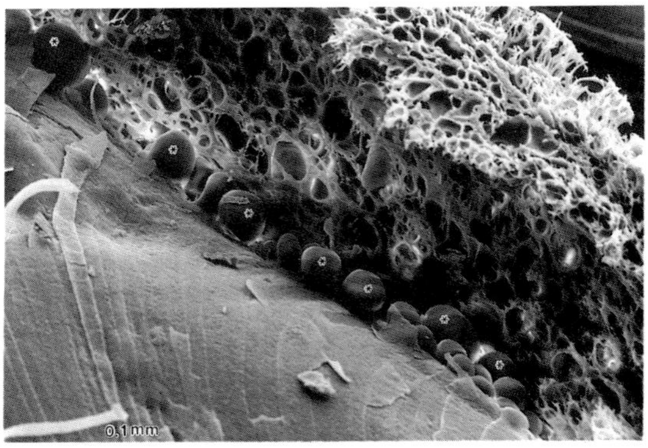

Figure 10.28 Water cleft containing globules (asterisks) emerging from the tips of distrubed fibres and spongy material. SEM. (From Shun-Shin *et al.* 1991b with permission.)

extracellular space, or by the absorption of lens fibres. Scanning microscopy of water clefts in the region of the suture shows swelling of the fibre interdigitations, free vacuoles, and sprouting of vacuoles from the walls of the water cleft (Shun-Shin *et al.* 1991). There is no overall increase in the volume of lenses with water clefts.

Water clefts have a minor effect on vision and can be responsible for monocular diplopia (p. 220).

Lens vacuoles

These are approximately spherical cystoid spaces in the superficial lens cortex (usually in C2, at the C2/C1 interface). They are well seen by indirect retro-illumination (Figures 10.29, 10.30) (Brown 1971), when they exhibit the unreversed light effect indicating that they contain fluid of low refractive index. They are visible by specular illumination which produces a bright reflection from the anterior and posterior surfaces. They vary in size from the smallest discernible at about 10 μ up to 1.3 mm in diameter.

Vacuoles are a common finding in lenses over the age of 45 years and their incidence increases with age. Vacuoles are a somewhat transient phenomenon and any recorded vacuole may be seen to disappear after a period of months. Their effect on vision is at most minimal. They have been noted to occur following trauma (p. 201), but their relationship to cataract development has not been studied. Transient lens vacuoles have been induced in normal adults by limited topical steroid administration (Burde and Becker 1970).

Transient vacuoles have been reported in premature neonates, when they have been observed after 1 week of life and persist for a further 2 weeks. The vacuoles are superficially situated near to the anterior and posterior lens poles, usually at the junction of the first and second cortical zones. Electron microscopy shows intracellular spaces within the fibres (Yanoff *et al.* 1973).

Vacuolar changes are a component of subcapsular cataract and should in this instance be regarded, for the purposes of quantification and grading, as a component of the cataract and not separately as vacuoles (p. 79).

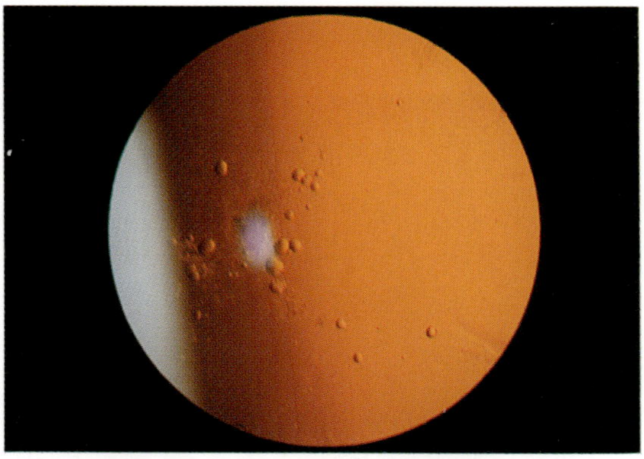

Figure 10.29 Lens vacuoles. The unreversed effect is seen by marginal retro-illumination with the vacuoles appearing bright on the same side as the brightness of the background illumination. (Courtesy of A. Shun-Shin).

Figure 10.30 Lens vacuole. Indirect retro-illumination (magnification × 10).

Table 10.2 Morphological cataract groups

Fibre-based cataracts		*Non-fibre-based cataracts*
Sutural	*Non-sutural*	
Developmental	Lamellar	Subscapsular
Concussional	Congenital nuclear	Glaucoma fleck
Myotonic	Adult spoke	Coronary
Storage disorders	Adult nuclear	Focal-dot
Material deposits		Retro-dot
		Christmas tree

Morphological groups

Cataracts are separated on morphological grounds into two major groups (Bron and Brown 1986) (Table 10.1):

1. *Fibre-based cataracts,* in which the form of the cataract (Figure 10.31) is determined by the arrangement of the lens fibres (Figure 10.32). The fibre-based cataracts are further subdivided into sutural and nonsutural, according to their relationship to the sutural system of the lens.
2. *Non-fibre-based cataract,* in which the form of the cataract is unrelated to their organization.

Fibre-based cataracts

Sutural fibre-based cataracts

Developmental sutural cataract This is the cataract commonly named 'sutural cataract'; it is usually congenital in origin and familial (Figures 10.33, 10.34). An X-linked inheritance occurs in which the males (Figure 10.35) have a significant cataract and the females a minor opacity (Figure 10.36). The opacity follows the line of the anterior or posterior Y sutures and is therefore in the fetal nucleus, where it is to be seen later in the adult. In an uncommon form the opacity remains subcapsular (Figure 10.37). This opacity is usually

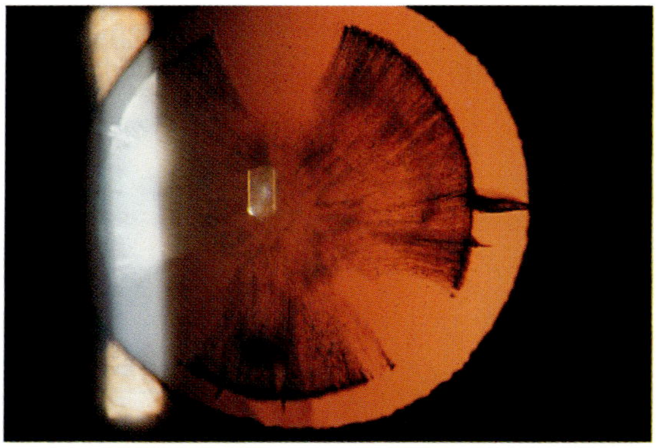

Figure 10.31 The form of this lamellar cataract shows that it is based on the anatomical arrangement of the fibres.

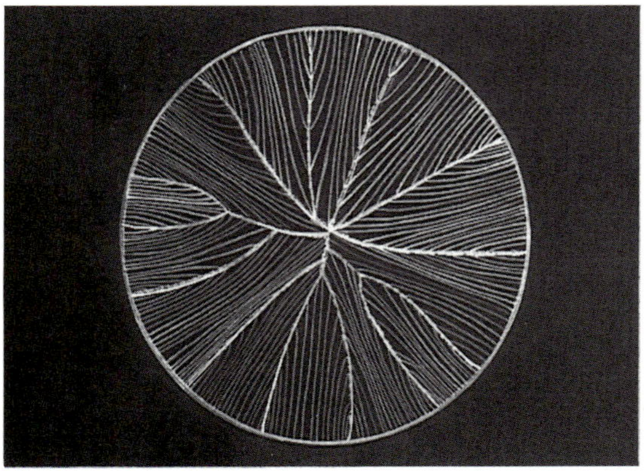

Figure 10.32 The arrangement of the cortical lens fibres and sutures.

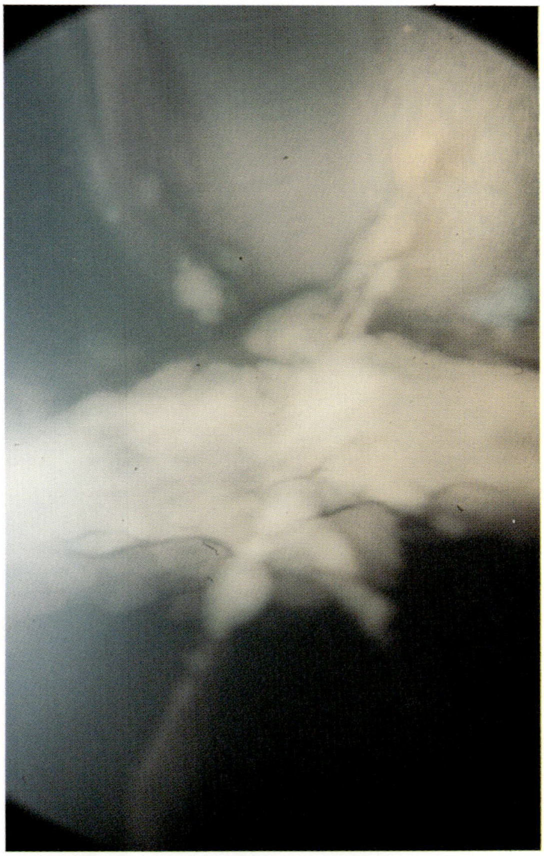

Figure 10.33 Posterior sutural X-linked cataract in male child (magnification × 10).

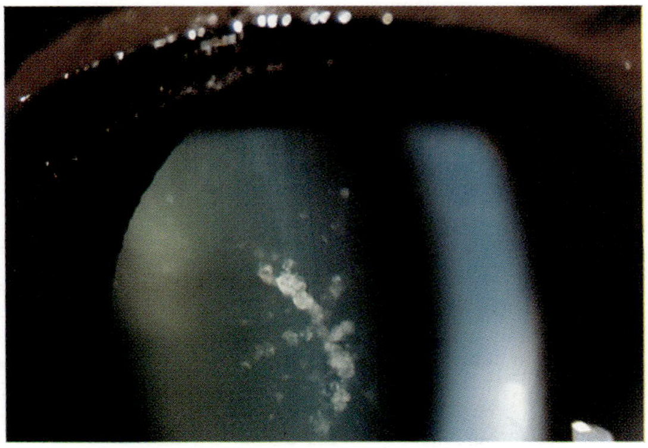

Figure 10.34 An anterior sutural cataract depicting the anterior Y suture. (Courtesy of A. Shun-Shin.)

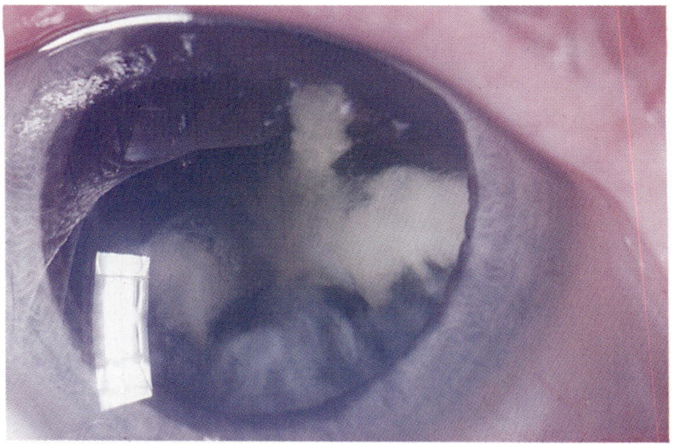

Figure 10.35 A dense anterior sutural cataract in a male child in a family with X-linked sutural cataract.

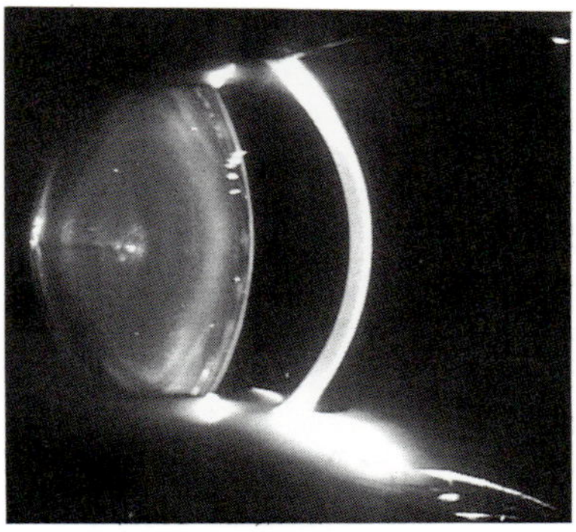

Figure 10.36 Punctate cortical opacities along the Y sutures in a female carrier of X-linked sutural cataract.

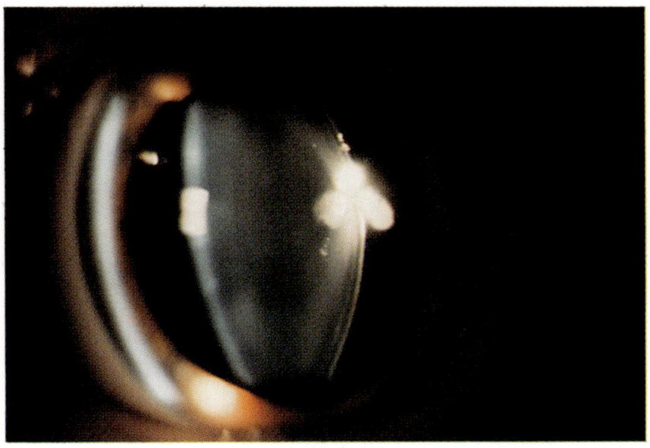

Figure 10.37 A sutural cataract at the posterior pole.

limited to the Y suture and does not follow the branches of the postnatal sutures. It occurs during lens development and is not progressive. Vision is usually unaffected, but, in the X-linked form, male children have a significant cataract, which spreads beyond the suture.

Concussional cataract The typical concussional cataract is the result of blunt trauma to the lens. Initially it affects the subcapsular fibres, commonly both anteriorly and posteriorly. It is not always easy to observe initially, but loss of the subcapsular clear zone is the easily identifiable clue to its presence. The visibly affected fibre tips are initially oedematous (Figure 10.38) and then become more obviously opaque. This gives rise to the expression 'delayed traumatic cataract', but it is really only the identification that is delayed. The opacity extends for a limited distance along the fibre end on either side of the suture so that a herring-bone appearance is produced.

A possible cause of the typical flower shape is rupture of the superficial lens cortex at the suture lines, allowing fluid to enter the tips of the fibres and to spread for a variable distance up the fibre, so determining the size of the flower. It is assumed that the fibres anneal peripherally to the oedematous zone so that the remaining fibres retain their clarity. In minimal cases the result is a delineation of the lens suture alone. In some severely traumatized cases, actual separation, forming a Y-shaped water cleft, is seen at the suture lines. These cases continue to deteriorate, whereas the typical concussional cataract remains of constant size and appears to sink away from the capsule as the lens grows (Figure 10.39). This allows the dating of a traumatic cataract whose time of origin is unknown (Brown 1976).

The cataract is not always flower-shaped and may follow the fibre pattern in a peripheral segment of the lens (Figure 10.40), particularly if the trauma is peripheral (Figure 10.41).

Another form of concussional cataract occasionally seen is the anterior subcapsular punctate opacity, which resembles the glaucoma fleck. It probably has the same cause and is due to necrosis of groups of lens epithelial cells.

Dystrophia myotonica Patients with this condition, which is inherited as an autosomal dominant

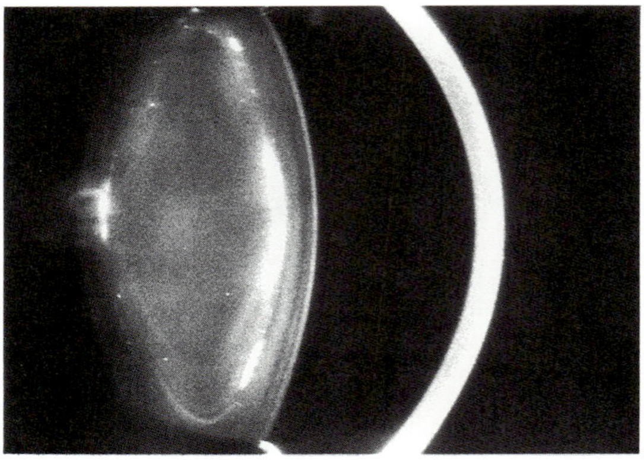

Figure 10.39 A traumatic cataract in a 28-year old subject that had occurred 14 years previously.

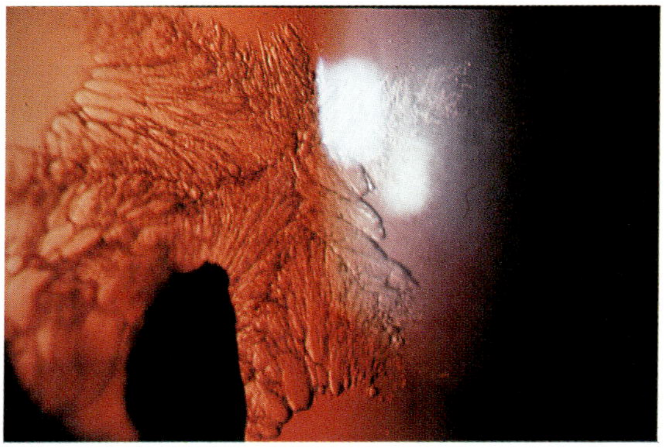

Figure 10.38 A newly formed traumatic cataract due to penetration of the lens by a foreign body. The affected lens fibres are oedematous.

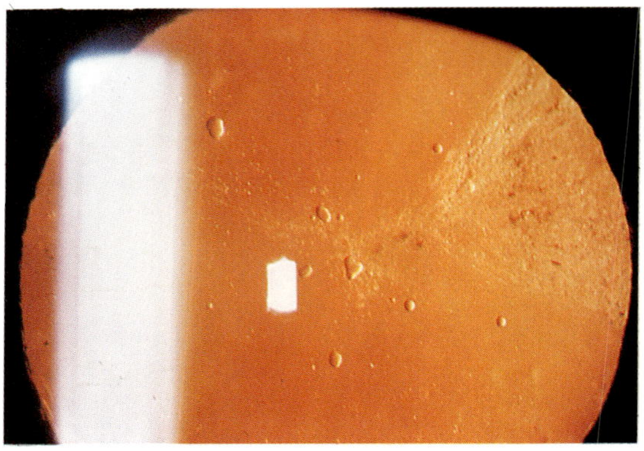

Figure 10.40 A cortical segmental traumatic cataract with associated vacuoles.

trait, gradually develop a posterior cortical stellate cataract (Figure 10.42, 10.43) based on the posterior fibre system. It has the appearance of a fine orange granular material. It is preceded by fine polychromatic granules in the posterior subcapsular region. The penetrance in terms of cataract formation is complete. Ocular hypotony is an associated feature. Electron microscopy (Eshagian *et al.* 1978) shows whorls of intracellular plasma membranes and increased intercellular spaces. (A fuller description is given on p. 180).

Storage disorders In Fabry's disease, a glycolipid storage disorder, the posterior sutures become visible, probably because of the accumulation of abnormal glycolipid (ceramide trihexoside) within the fibre membranes and because of the high density of the membranes within the sutural zones (e.g. at the posterior lens suture). Initially this defines the posterior inverted Y suture, and subsequently the secondary branches of the Y suture (Franceschetti 1976).

In mannosidosis, a posterior spoke opacity occurs which is based on the posterior sutures (Murphree *et al.* 1976a,b). A similar explanation may be offered to that suggested for Fabry's disease, in this case reflecting the accumulation of mannose-containing glycolipids within the fibre membranes.

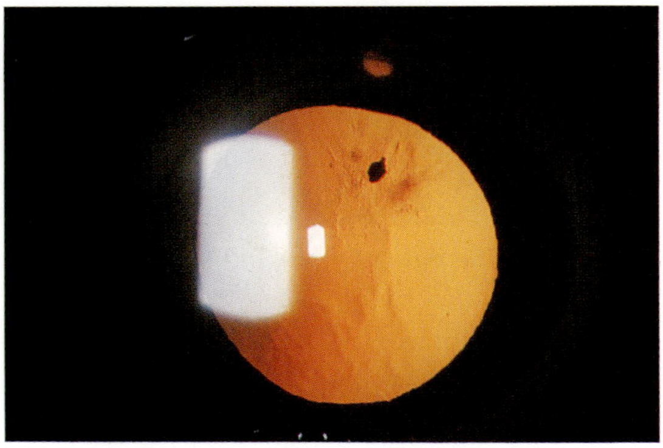

Figure 10.41 A segmental traumatic cataract following a surgical iridectomy.

Deposition of material in the lens Various metals and drugs may be deposited in the lens and may be strikingly visible. The source of these materials, when known, is either from local application, or from raised systemic levels. It is not always possible to differentiate the various deposits on appearance alone and a melanin pigment deposition can also occur.

The deposition is in the superficial cortex, and consists of fine granules. Commonly the capsule has a coloured metallic sheen. The cortical granules are often arranged at the anterior pole, in a star-shaped pattern, reflecting their proximity to the lens fibres at the confluence of the sutures.

Copper (chalcosis) (Figure 10.44) Copper deposits occur in the lens as a result of raised serum copper levels (Wilson's disease), or from the application of eye drops containing copper sulphate. The capsule takes on a copper-coloured sheen and fine multi-coloured granules form in the lens, sometimes creating a radiating figure (sunflower cataract).

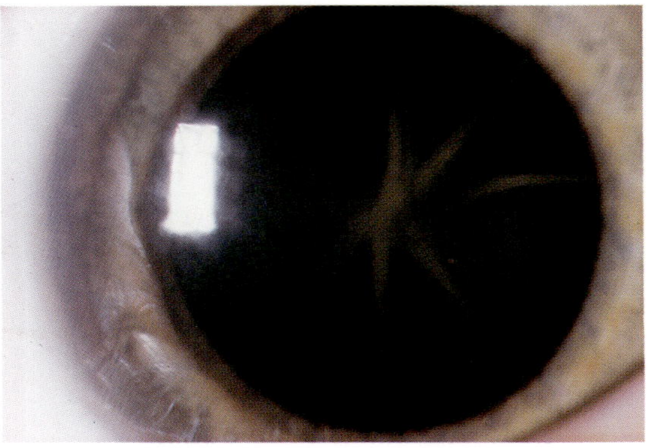

Figure 10.42 The typical stellate myotonic cataract.

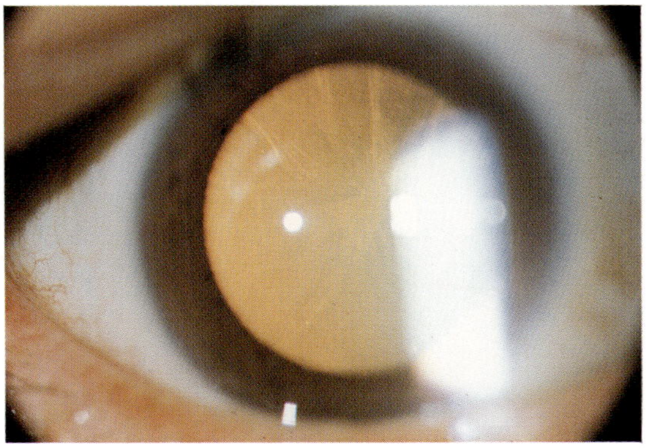

Figure 10.43 Myotonic cataract (retro-illumination).

Gold Gold deposits in the capsule and superficial lens appear as fine golden granules, which may form a star shape. It occurs as a result of long-term systemic administration.

Silver (argyrosis) Bluish granules form in the pupillary area of the capsule and anterior cortex (Cowan 1961).

Iron (siderosis) Iron produces a brown rust colour of the capsule and the lens (Figure 10.45), and iris heterochromia (Figure 10.46). It is more invasive than the other metals and is toxic to the lens fibres. The lens becomes coloured throughout and loses transparency due to cataract.

Drugs Various drugs (or their metabolites) have been reported to cause precipitates in the lens. This

Figure 10.44 Chalcosis of the lens (magnification × 10).

Figure 10.45 Siderosis of the lens (magnification × 10).

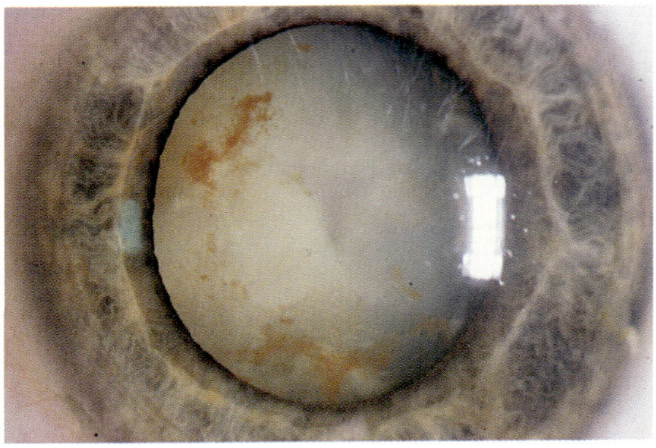

Figure 10.46 Siderotic cataract.

occurs most frequently with the long-term use of chlorpromazine which produces a typical, golden star-shaped opacity in relation to the anterior capsule (Mathalone 1967) (Figure 10.47). Opacities have also been reported with chloroquine.

Pigment granules Anterior axial pigment stippling of the lens suture (Vogt 1931) is due to the deposition of very fine brown granules. It is a common occurrence in the older lens. With fine beam focal illumination, the granules can be seen to be light brown in colour and to extend in depth from the capsule, where they appear to occupy the epithelium to the full depth of the cortex in some cases (Cowan 1961). The brown coloration usually makes it possible to differentiate this precipitation from that of metals and drugs.

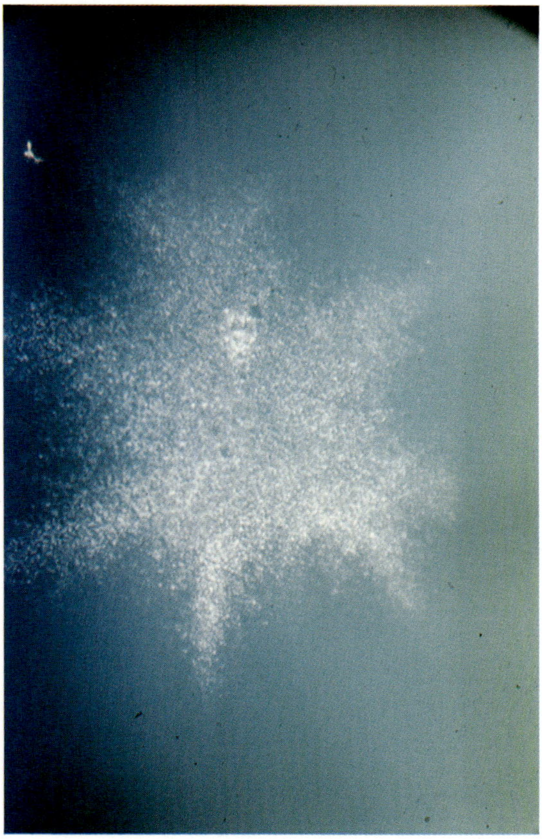

Figure 10.47 The characteristic star-shaped opacities of largactil toxicity (magnification × 10).

Non-sutural fibre-based cataract

Lamellar cataract A lamellar cataract (Figures 9.2, 10.48) is one that affects a particular lamella of the lens both anteriorly and posteriorly. At its onset it is initially subcapsular and it is due to an insult affecting the young lens fibres for a limited period and causing a shell-like opacity. Its diameter at the time of formation depends on the diameter of the lens at that time, which at birth is about 6.5 mm. It occurs *in utero* as a result of rubella, or as a hereditary form with either dominant or recessive inheritance. Whatever influence is responsible for formation of the original shell in the hereditary form, it appears to continue to a lesser degree after that event, so that subsequent lamellae are partially affected in the form of 'riders' – narrow radial opacities which lie in the suture lines. Possibly these are equivalent to radial opacities laid down in the suture lines in relation to water clefts in the adult lens (Figures 9.23, 10.49). The affected lamella has a very fine punctate white granular appearance. Sometimes the lamella is incomplete so that a wedge of perfectly transparent fibres is inserted into the shell of opacity (Figure 10.31).

Metabolic insults after birth, including diabetes (Figure 12.10), galactosaemia and hypocalcaemia, can cause lamellar opacities, which proceed no further if the condition is treated in time. Juvenile diabetic cataract is a rare, acute cataract, which forms a subcapsular snowstorm of opacities in uncontrolled young diabetics. It should be distinguished from cataract in the diabetic adult,

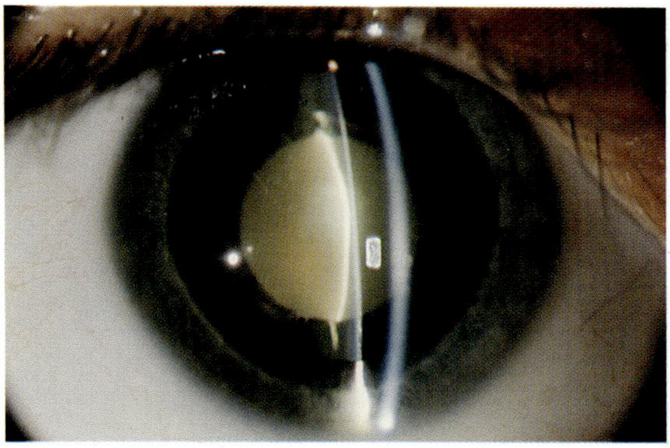

Figure 10.48 A lamellar cataract with riders and a centre affected by cataract.

whose morphology resembles that of age-related cataract in the non-diabetic (p. 178). After treatment, the cataract is seen to sink into the lens with time and the diameter of the affected lamella becomes smaller (Brown *et al.* 1988). Thus these opacities can come to have a lesser effect on vision with time.

Congenital nuclear cataract These cataracts are commonly lamellar, as described above. Alternatively the entirety of the nucleus is affected as a total congenital cataract (Figure 10.49), or the cataract is limited to the embryonic nucleus forming a small nearly spherical opacity (Figure 9.8) consisting of fine white granules (cataracta centralis pulverulenta). These bilateral opacities are complete by 6 weeks of gestation. A dominant inheritance is well known, as in the Coppock cataract. Rubella is the commonest cause of the total congenital cataract.

Senile spoke cataract (cuneiform cataract) This is the commonest form of senile cataract (Figures 9.5, 10.50–10.52). The opacities are usually situated in cortical layer C2 (see Figure 10.19) and begin peripherally. They are often wedge-shaped, but may take different forms, according to the organization of the fibres in different zones. The natural history is for a slow spread centripetally along the course of the fibres, and also a spread to adjacent lens fibres, so that the spokes tend to increase both in width and in length. Spokes are more prevalent in the lower part of the lens, which is the region most affected by solar radiation; this may be contributory. Water clefts and fibre folds are associated features.

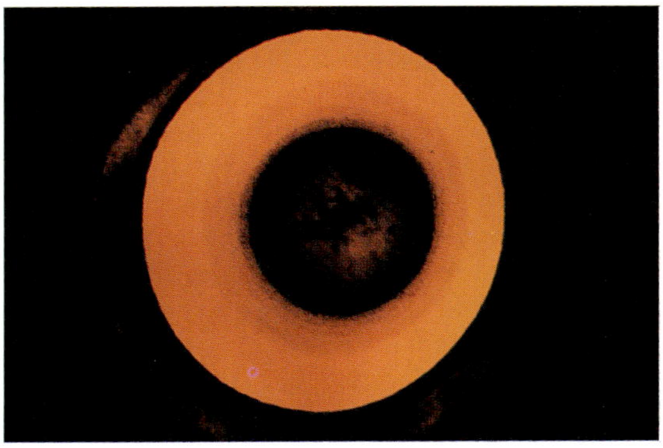

Figure 10.49 A dense congenital lamellar cataract affecting the nucleus with a fine outer affected lamella.

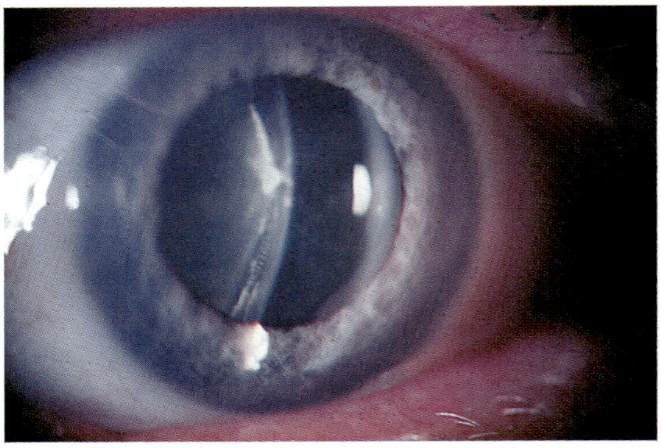

Figure 10.51 Cortical spoke cataract.

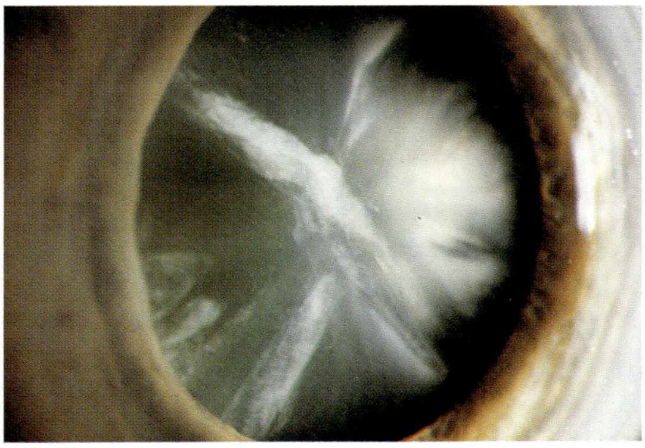

Figure 10.50 Senile cortical spoke cataract.

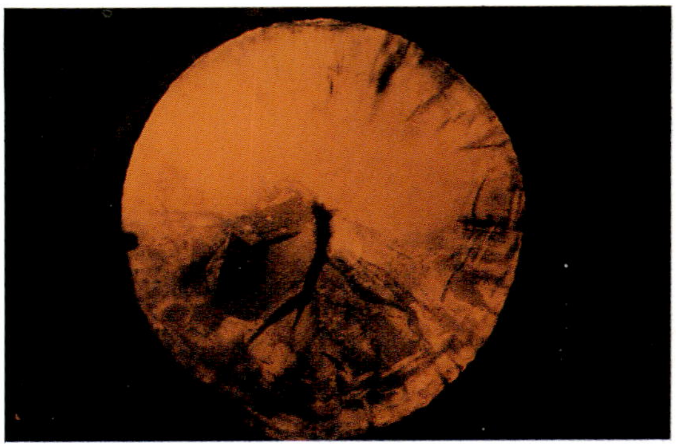

Figure 10.52 A less usual appearance of a senile cortical spoke cataract with a more elaborate appearance.

Senile nuclear cataract The changes in nuclear light scatter and colour which represent nuclear cataract involve that envelope of fibres which defines the lens nucleus; this therefore entitles nuclear cataract to be termed fibre-based. The changes within the nucleus are diffuse. There are two distinct components to the senile nuclear cataract, which are commonly seen together in the same lens but occasionally separately. These components are nuclear white scatter (Figure 9.14) and nuclear brunescence (Figure 9.15). The old term 'nuclear sclerosis' is not very useful since it describes the mechanical, rather than the optical, properties of the ageing nucleus. Increased fluorescence is associated (Lerman *et al.* 1989).

Nuclear white scatter The normal ageing nucleus undergoes a gradual increase in light scattering with age. When this exceeds the normal for the age then it is properly described as cataract. White scatter may become gross (Figure 9.14). The degree of white scatter can be graded at the slit-lamp by reference to standard neutral density chips (Sparrow *et al.* 1986).

Nuclear brunescence In nuclear brunescence, brown pigments (chromophores) accumulate within the fibres of the nucleus to give it a colour which varies from amber through brown to virtually black ('cataracta nigra') (Figure 10.53). The degree of brunescence can be graded at the slit-lamp by reference to a standard colour chart (Sparrow *et al.* 1988). Densitometry of slit-images of lenses with brunescence always shows increased scatter. This may be due to scatter by the brunescent chromophores themselves, to the coexistence of non-pigmented light-scattering aggregates, or to both of these features. In both nuclear white scatter and brunescence there is a myopic shift which implies an increased nuclear refractive index. Nuclear white scatter appears limited to the nucleus, whereas, in advanced brunescence, the effect spreads beyond the nucleus.

Non-fibre based cataracts

Subcapsular cataract

Posterior subcapsular cataract is the least common of the three major senile cataract types and, when it occurs alone, it tends to occur at a younger age. There may be a positive family history. It also occurs in response to eye disease, radiation and drugs, specifically corticosteroids.

The subcapsular site of posterior subcapsular cataract is determined with focal illumination (Figure 9.14) and the detailed structure is seen best with retro-illumination (Figures 10.54, 10.55). It forms a granular or lace-like material with vacuolar elements immediately beneath the capsule posteriorly. This material is in a state of flux and can be seen to undergo changes when photographs are made at intervals as short as 4 weeks (Shun-Shin *et al.* 1989). The posterior subcapsular cataract tends to be disposed around the posterior pole of the lens ('cupuliform' or cup shaped), but the earliest sign

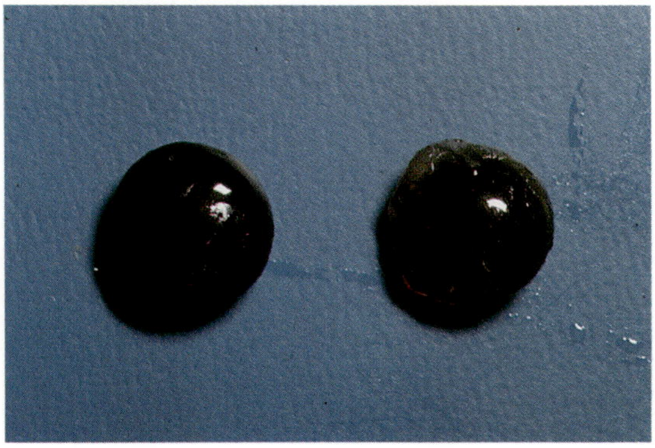

Figure 10.53 Cataracta nigra. Two nuclei removed on extraction.

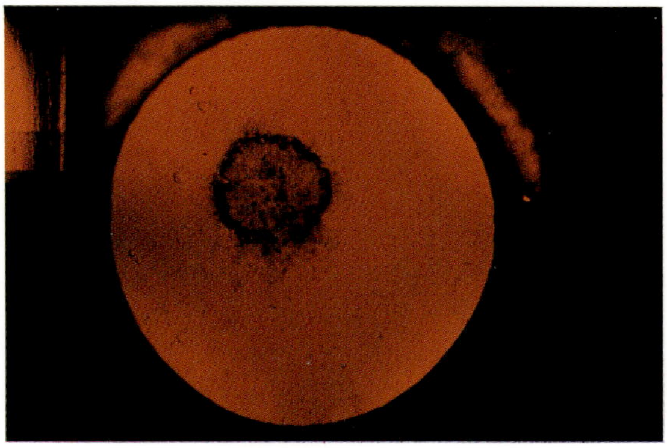

Figure 10.54 A typical compact posterior subcapsular cataract of granular material.

of a posterior subcapsular cataract is fine granules, often in radial lines in the lens periphery. Alternatively, specular illumination may show polychromatic lustre (Figure 9.11) preceding visible opacities. This change is characteristic of complicated cataract.

The granules move centripetally to form the cataract at the posterior pole. Thus these cataracts do not represent opacification of previously clear lens fibres, but abnormal material, which is probably generated by faulty mitosis and fibre differentiation in the germinal epithelium. This process is clearly established in radiation cataract and may be common for other types of posterior subcapsular cataract. The histology shows migrant epithelial cells and bladder cells, which may account for the clinically observed vacuolar components (Eshagian and Streeten 1980).

Anterior subcapsular cataracts are less common and less easily recognized at the slit-lamp, but a frequent finding in the presence of posterior subcapsular cataract is loss of the anterior subcapsular clear zone (C1α) of the lens, probably reflecting a relative deficiency of differentiating fibres and a lack of normal, anteriorly migrating fibre tips (Figure 9.23). The histology of the most anterior lens fibres shows them to have become cataractous (Figure 9.16). Thus this cataract is truly present anteriorly and posteriorly.

Anterior subcapsular cataracts occurring alone have been shown to consist of proliferation of the epithelium with degeneration of the subjacent lens fibres.

Posterior subcapsular cataract is situated axially, where it has the most destructive effect on vision. It is probably the axial position rather than the relationship to the nodal point of the eye that is the more significant in this cataract's effect on vision. It also tends to deteriorate faster than other cataract types.

Glaucoma flecks

These opacities can be seen immediately following an acute attack of glaucoma. They consist of small round or oval forms, sometimes budded like yeast cells. The overall picture has been likened to 'spilt

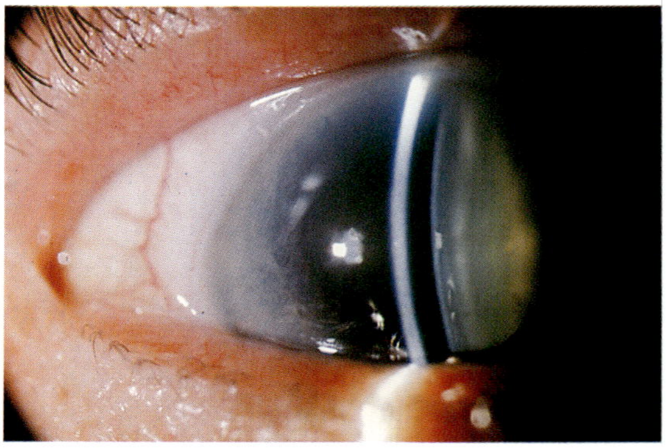

Figure 10.56 Glaucoma flecks.

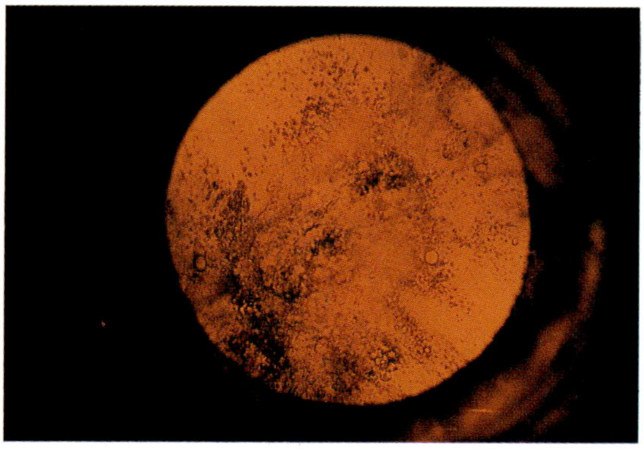

Figure 10.55 A diffuse posterior subcapsular cataract with lacy and vacuolar components.

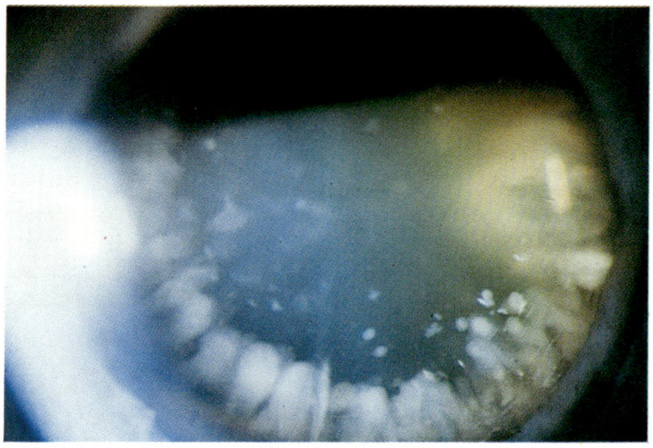

Figure 10.57 Coronary cataract. (Courtesy of Shun-Shin)

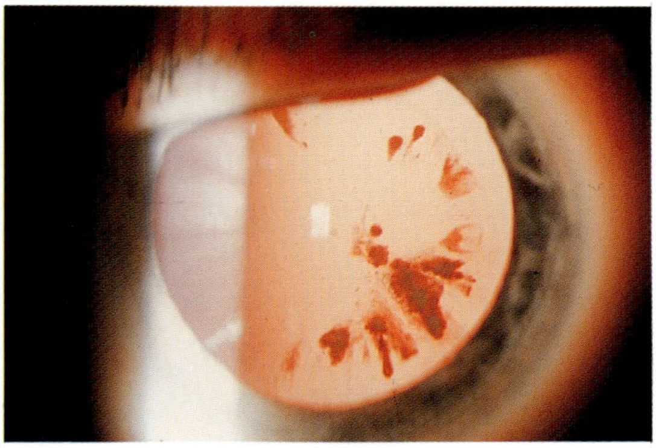

Figure 10.58 Coronary cataract (retro-illumination).

milk' at the anterior surface of the lens. Initially, they are immediately subjacent to the capsule (Figures 9.12, 10.56), where they are considered to represent islands of epithelial necrosis (Winstanley 1961). With time they then pass to a deeper level in the lens, as new fibres are formed superficial to them (Brown and Tripathi 1974).

Coronary (supranuclear) cataract

These opacities occur in the deep cortex (C3) (Figure 9.9), where they form a corona around the nucleus (Figures 10.57, 10.58), from which their name is derived. These opacities may be classed as developmental, since they form during the otherwise normal growth of the lens. Apart from the greater depth at which these opacities are sited, they are also distinguished from spoke cataract by their rounded form (Figure 10.59). Focal dot opacities are commonly associated and may have the appearance of being seeded from the corona. The occurrence of coronary opacities is occasionally familial, but other causes have not been identified. There is no significant effect on vision, unless the associated focal dot opacities are very numerous.

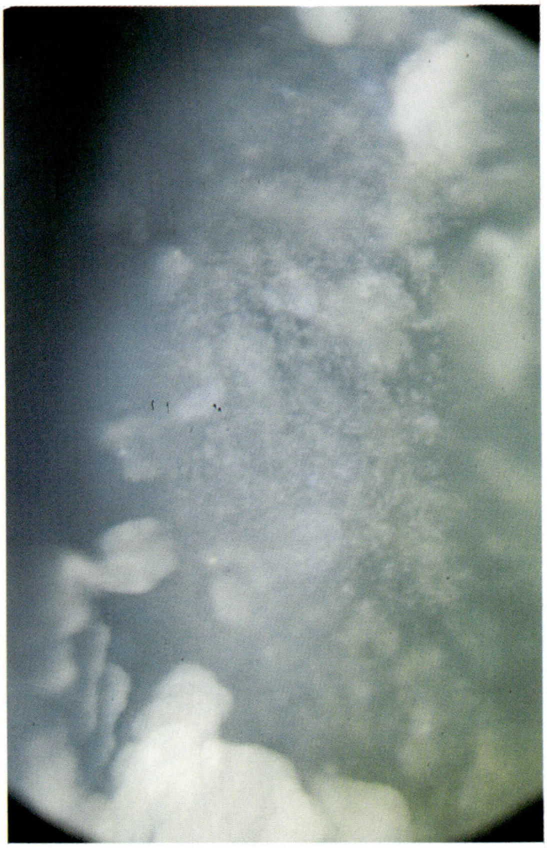

Figure 10.59 Coronary and focal dot opacities (magnification × 10).

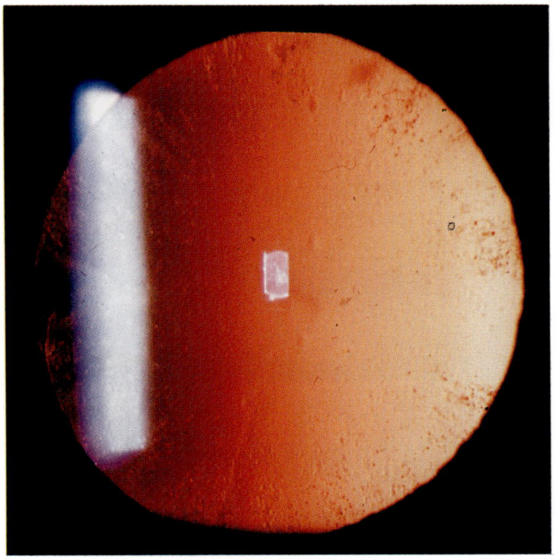

Figure 10.60 Focal dots in a female carrier of Lowe's syndrome (retro-illumination).

Focal dot opacities (punctate, or blue dot opacities)

These are common in the peripheral cortex and are to be found in some numbers in most lenses (Figure 10.60). They are seen best by focal illumination and the light that they reflect is often coloured and may be blue (Figures 10.61, 10.62). The clinical significance appears to be limited to the identification of the female carrier state in Lowe's syndrome (Figure 10.63). The effect on vision is insignificant, except when the axial cortex is involved; in these

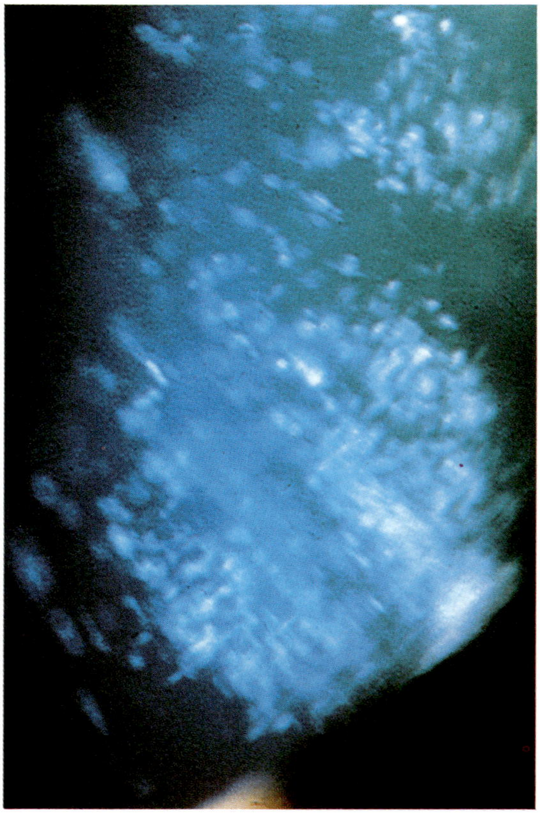

Figure 10.62 Blue focal dots in a female carrier of Lowe's syndrome (magnification × 10).

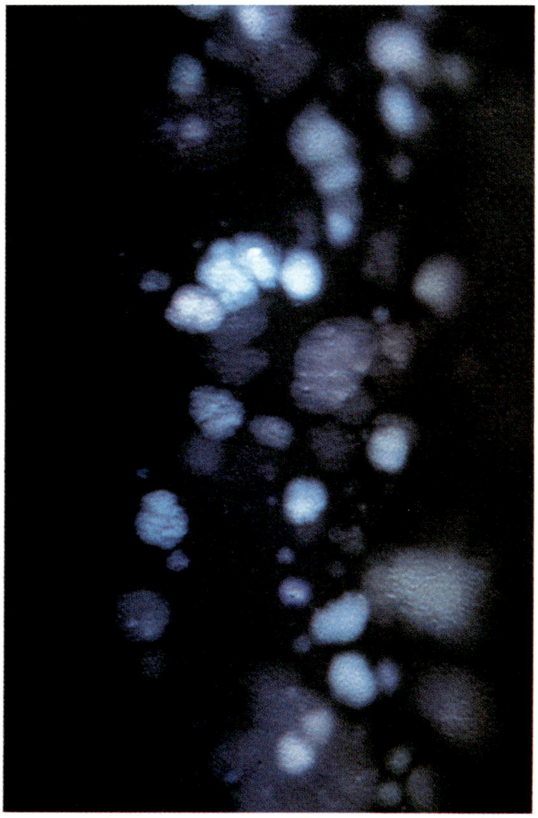

Figure 10.61 Multicoloured focal dots (magnification × 10).

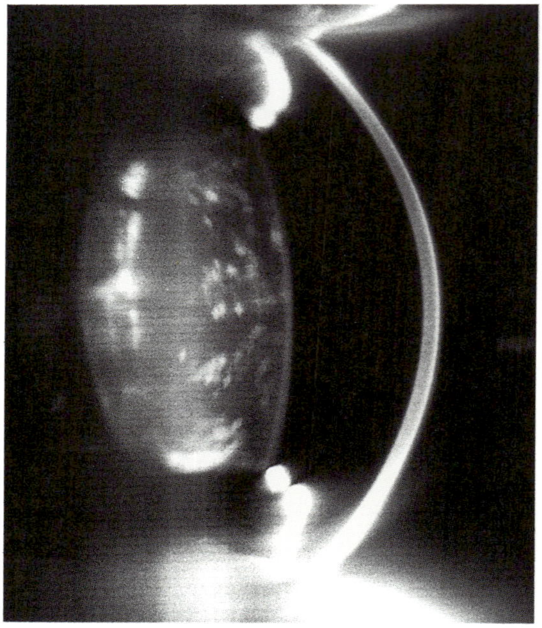

Figure 10.63 Focal dot cortical opacities in a female carrier of Lowe's syndrome (off axis image).

cases vision may gradually deteriorate over the years as the opacities accumulate (see developmental cataract p. 171).

The rare and peculiar floriform and coralliform cataracts begin as punctate opacities, but do not remain static (Figures 10.64, 10.65). They expand into the zones anterior to their point of origin as these layers develop. The forward coralliform growths are tubular.

Retro-dot opacities

These opacities (Figure 10.66) are common in the ageing lens, where they are situated in the perinuclear cortex (C3 and C4) and in the superficial nucleus (Bron and Brown 1987). They vary in number from one or two, to hundreds. They are found in the lenses of adult eyes, in particular in relation to nuclear and other forms of cataract. They consist of smooth contoured discoid structures of between 80 μm and 500 μm diameter, which are best seen by retro-illumination. They then demonstrate reversal of illumination, indicating that they are of high refractive index. By specular illumination (Figure 7.7) they show as elevations in the deep cortex, at the level of the relief pattern in this region. By focal illumination, they appear as small empty clefts (Figure 10.67) and birefringence is demonstrable in polarized light (Figure 10.68). It was previously considered

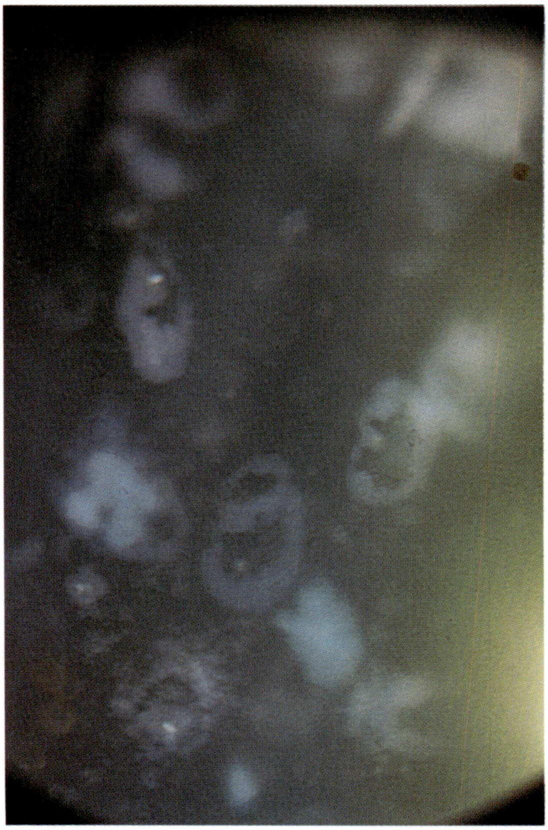

Figure 10.65 Coralliform cataract (magnification × 10).

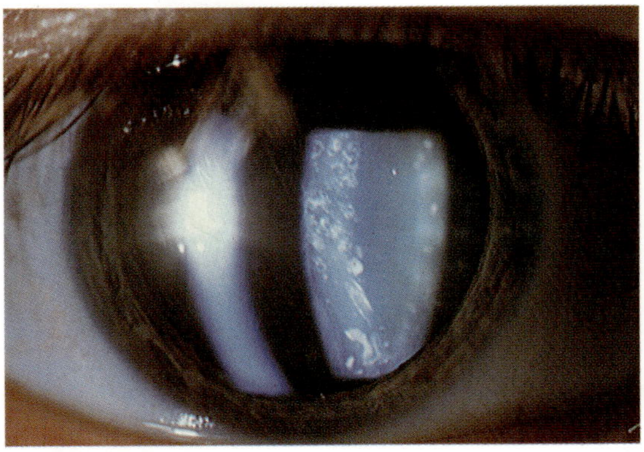

Figure 10.64 The curious coralliform cataract.

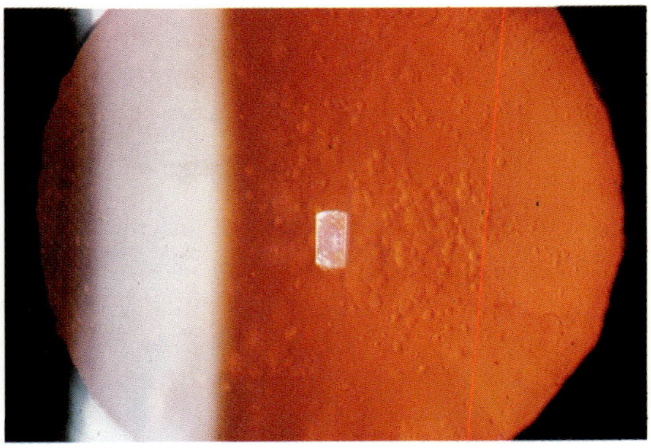

Figure 10.66 Retro-dots by retro-illumination.

that they were composed of calcium oxalate because of their resemblance to the nuclear inclusions in Morgagnian cataract (spheroliths) (Figures 10.69, 10.70) (Bron and Habgood 1976; Bron and Brown 1987). This would have been of great interest since oxalate is the final oxidation product of ascorbate, and ascorbate is abundant in the human aqueous and lens. However, studies by Vrensen *et al.* (1994) show their major component to be calcium phosphate, with oxalate a possible minor constituent (Figure 10.71). The effect on

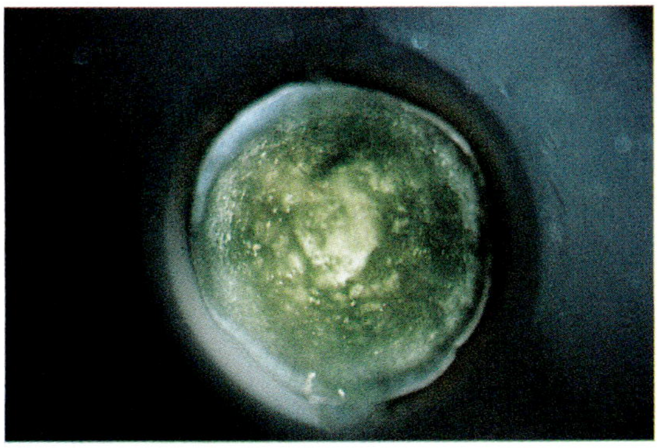

Figure 10.68 Birefringence of retro-dots by polarized light *in vitro*.

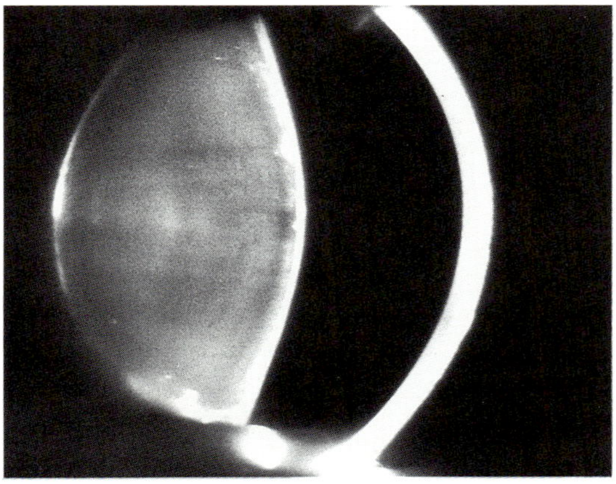

(a)

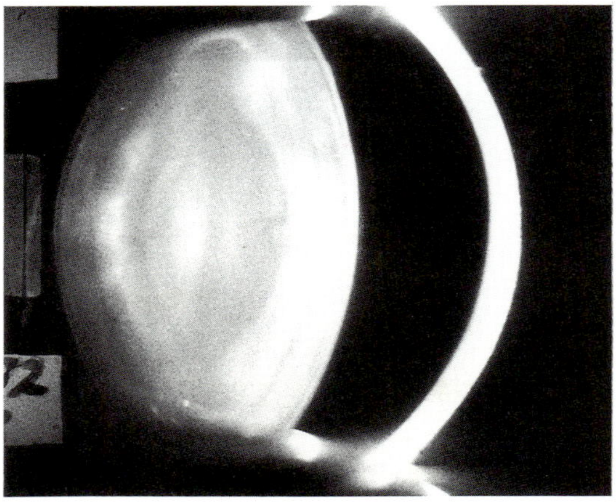

(b)

Figure 10.67(a) The affected left lens shows an abnormally small lens size for age (71), a posterior subcapsular cataract and loss of the anterior subcapsular clear zone. The small dark clefts are due to retro-dots. **(b)** The fellow right lens is normal.

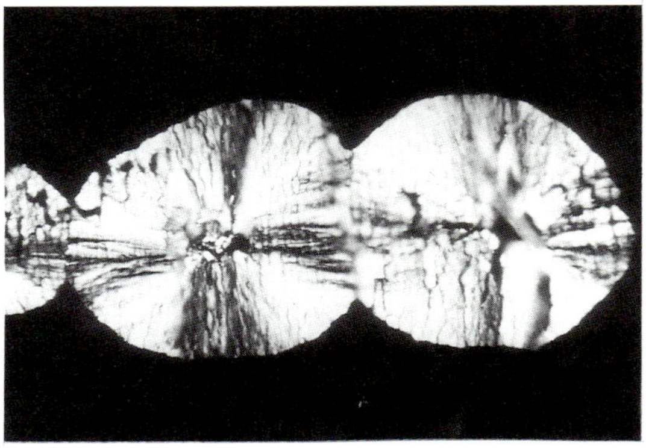

Figure 10.69 Birefringence of a spherolith cut in cross-section and viewed in polarized light, showing the typical Maltese cross pattern.

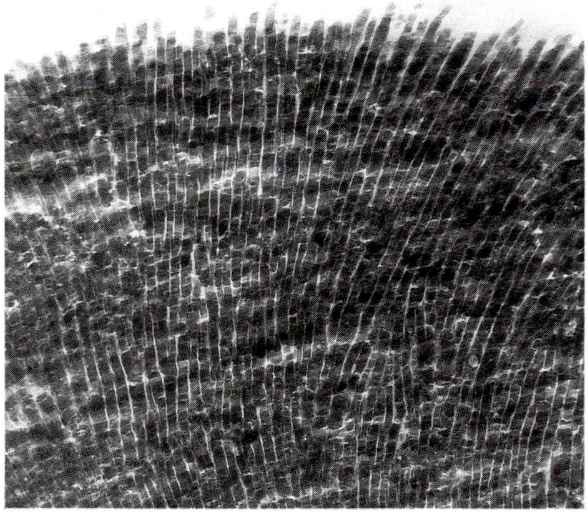

Figure 10.70 TEM of a spherolith from a Morgagnian cataract nucleus, demonstrating a typical cluster of electron-dense rods of the crystal. (From Habgood and Bron 1976 with permission.)

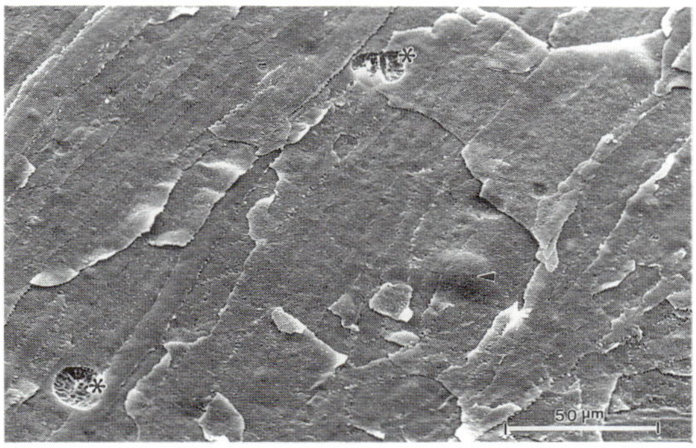

(a)

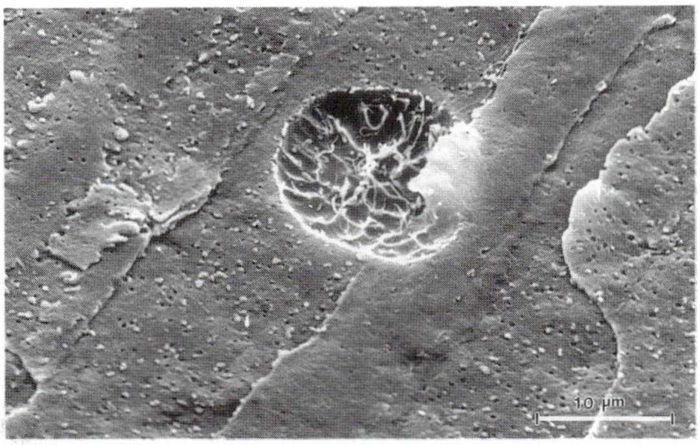

(b)

Figure 10.71(a) The craters left by two retro-dots (asterisks) that have lost their contents. A retro-dot (arrow) is still covered by overlying fibres that are relatively normal. **(b)** The interior of a retro-dot contains membranous elements. X-ray microanalysis showed chiefly calcium phosphate and possibly some oxalate. SEM. (Courtesy of Vrensen and Willekens)

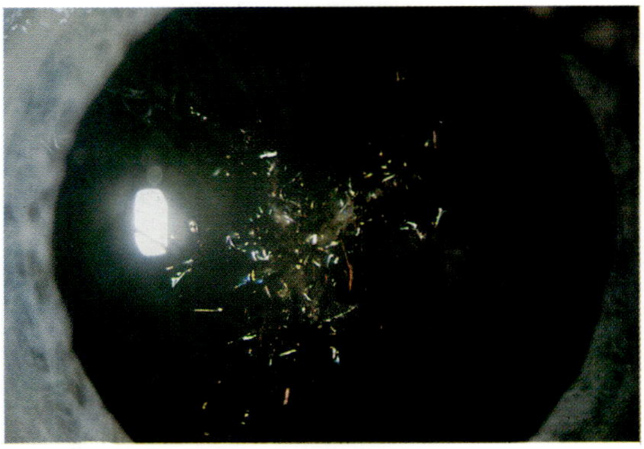

Figure 10.72 Christmas tree cataract (Courtesy of Shun-Shin).

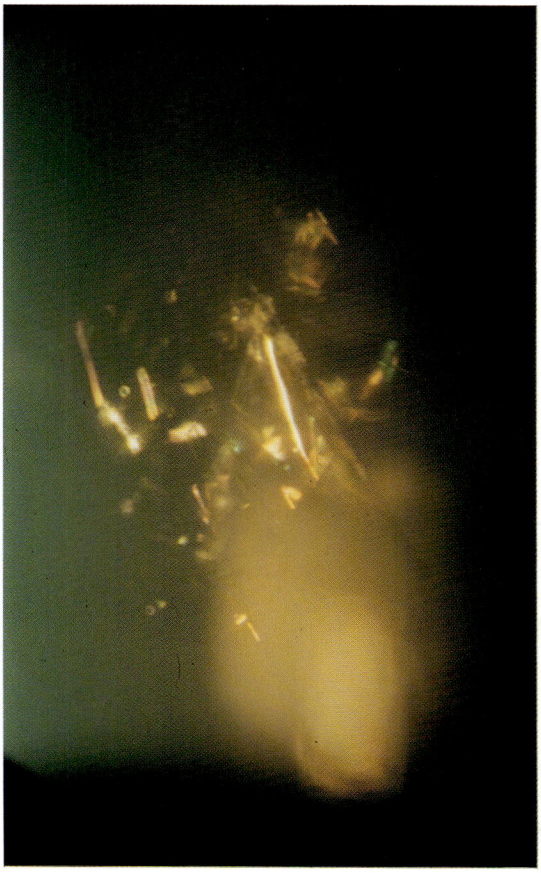

(a)

Figure 10.73(a) The crystal-like structures in Christmas tree cataract (magnification × 10).

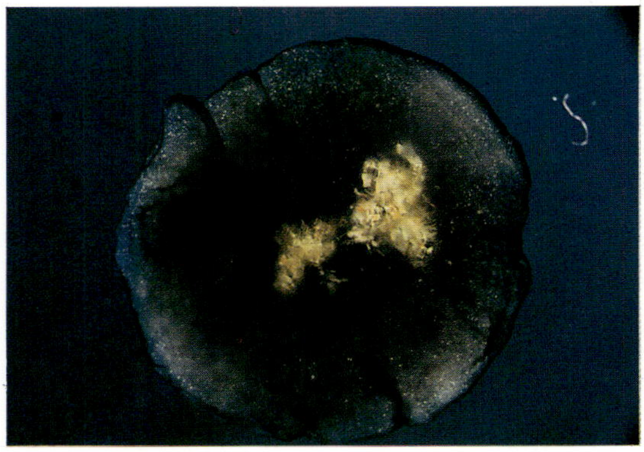

(b)

Figure 10.73(b) Christmas tree cataract in extracted nucleus showing birefringence in crossed polarized light.

vision is minor, but may become moderate if these opacities are profuse or when they are associated with nuclear cataract, when their effect on vision is amplified. Both retro-dots and nuclear scatter increase in frequency with age and a significant association has been shown between them (Shun-Shin *et al.* 1992).

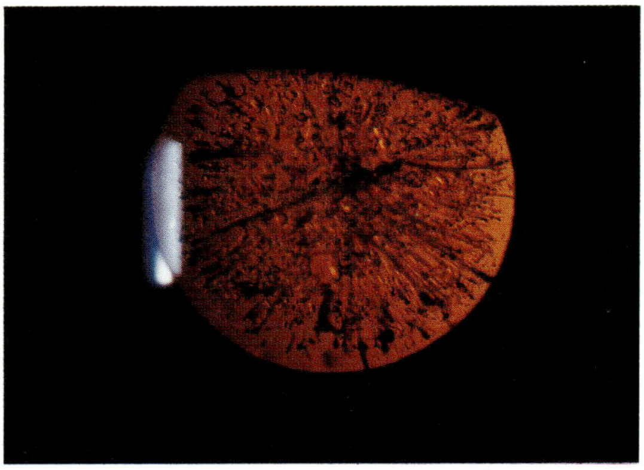

Figure 10.74 Crystalline cataract occurring in the syndrome of 'uncombable hair'. (Courtesy of P.T.V.M. de Jong.)

Christmas tree cataract

This striking and uncommon form of senile cataract presents the appearance of highly reflective crystalline deposits in the deep cortex and nucleus of the lens. The polychromatic, needle-like structures are remarkable in that they pass cleanly through the growth rings in which they lie, without interfering with the transparency of the intervening lens substance (Figures 10.72, 10.73). It appears that such polychromatic structures are not actually crystalline (Hayes and Fisher 1984), but are made up of multilamellar membranes that reflect light. The multicoloured effects are then explained by destructive interference. An SEM study by Shun-Shin *et al.* (1992b, 1993) showed irregular, plate-like structures bordered by membrane. Repeating structures were shown on TEM with a spacing of 5 nm. X-ray microanalysis and Raman spectroscopy showed crystals with a high sulphur content, and with pronounced S-S, CS-SC and CS vibrations, which could be cystine. Examination in crossed polarized light shows that the christmas tree structure is birefringent (Figure 10.73b), which is characteristic of a crystalline structure.

An unusual form of crystalline cataract, associated with uncombable hair, is shown in Figure 10.74 (de Jong *et al.* 1990). Analysis of the crystals showed them to contain carbon, oxygen, nitrogen and sulphur, suggesting cystine.

11

Aetiological classification of cataract: infantile, inherited and systemic causes

Transparency of the lens may be reduced by many events. Cataract aetiology is considered here on the basis of individual causes, but there is good experimental evidence to suggest that multiple factors may act together, in what is termed co-cataractogenesis (Hockwin and Wegener 1987). It will be seen that there is necessarily some overlap between groups.

In some cases a particular cause predisposes to a specific morphological type of cataract and in others there is a disposition to cataract of the common senile types: cortical, nuclear and subcapsular.

Infantile cataract (Table 11.1)

Infantile cataract embraces both congenital and early postnatal cataracts and may be familial or non-familial. They are of particular importance as a cause of amblyopia and squint and, if bilateral, of nystagmus and blindness. Francois (1963) reported that 10–38% of childhood blindness was due to cataract. Other figures are given in Table 11.2. About 0.4% of newborns have some form of cataract; not all are associated with poor vision. Visual loss (and the development of amblyopia) are dependent on the size and location of the cataract, and particularly on density (Merin and Crawford 1971a).

The causes of congenital cataract have been variously reported as: rubella (19%); systemic disease (21%); genetic (8%) and local ocular disease (6%). Prematurity and perinatal problems are also important. Central nervous system impairment is the most common association with cataract (23%) (Merin and Crawford 1971a; Merin 1986). Currently, aetiology is determined in about 25–33% of cases (François 1963; Verrey 1957). Of the inherited forms, the dominant are most common and the recessive least. Recessively inherited congenital cataract was reported in various pedigrees by Saebo (1949); the proband of one family had Usher's syndrome. Recessive inheritance was found to be relatively frequent in Cyprus (Merin *et al.* 1972), and in Japan (Nakajima 1964). Shokeir and Lowry (1985) found nine instances in four sibships of an inbred Lehrerleut Hutterite community. Ogata *et al.* (1979) found an association between the 'i' phenotype and congenital cataract. Macdonald *et al.* (1983) reported a brother and sister (the offspring of half-sisters) with cataracts and an I positive/i negative phenotype. Yamaguchi *et al.* (1972) suggested linkage between congenital cataract and the I-blood group locus. In X-linked families the female carriers may show a minor defect (Figure 10.36). Thus, in the pedigree of Fraccaro *et al.* (1967), males showed nuclear cataract while carrier females showed sutural changes. Crews and Bundey (1982) have also suggested that this could occur in a dominant pedigree where the cataract was more fully expressed in the male.

There are several different types of infantile cataract and many variations (Cordes 1961). The more common forms are given here.

Table 11.1 Causes of cataract: inherited and sporadic causes*

Description	*Comment*	*McKusick No. D, r, XL*
Anterior polar	May be dominant, recessive or X-linked inheritance. Also translocation t (2;14) (p25,p24)	115650
Capsular flakes	–	–
Circular capsular	–	–
Reduplication	–	–
Spear-shaped, frosted	–	115700
Coralliform	Crystalline, coralliform	115800
Floriform	–	115900
Lamellar	+/– finger malformation	116800
Coronary	–	D
Central pulverulent	Maps to chromosome 2 (Coppock)	123660
Zonular pulverulent	Maps to chromosome 1	116200
Total nuclear	Central pulverulent discoid	212700 116400
Nuclear	–	212600
Nuclear diffuse	–	116300
Congenital cerulean	–	115660
Congenital anterior	–	–
Embryonal	–	–
Congenital sutural	–	D
Mittendorf dot	–	–
Posterior polar	+/– choroideraemia myopia	116600
Disciform	–	–
Membranous	–	116100
Morgagnian	–	D
Total	–	116400
Congenital	'i' phenotype; also Lehrerleut people	212500
X-linked	Severe in males, sutural in females, – early sutural in hemizygotes	302200
Pseudo-X-linked	Simulating XL, cataract marked in males, mild in females	–
Cataract with other ocular disease:		
Retinitis pigmentosa	Pigmentary retinopathy, night blindness	180100 268000 312600
Usher syndrome	Deafness, RP, mild and severe forms – 7 genotypes	276900
Cockayne syndrome	Dwarfism, deafness, premature aging, mental retardation, pigmentary retinopathy, cataract. Three types	216400 216410 216411
Bardet-Biedl syndrome	(see CNS section)	209900
Microcornea	–	116150
Gyrate atrophy	With hyperornithaemia	258870
Microcornea/microphthalmos	(see CNS section)	156850
Microphthalmos	–	302300
Aniridia	With glaucoma, corneal pannus, foveal hypoplasia, +/– cataract	106200

Table 11.1 (*Continued*)

Inherited and sporadic causes:	***Inherited infantile cataract***	***McKusick No. D, r, XL***
Cataract with other ocular disease (*Continued*):		
Prenatal infection	a. Viruses – rubella, rubeola, varicella, variola, zoster poliomyelitis, infectious mononucleosis, CMV	–
	b. Bacteria-syphilis	–
	c. Protozoa-toxoplasma	–
	d. Helminthiasis-distoma	–
Glaucoma	–	–
Uveitis	–	–
Retinal disease	Retinal detachment and its surgery; high myopia	–
Ocular tumour	–	–
Ischaemia	Various associations cited: megalocornea, keratoconus, sclerocornea, anterior cleavage syndrome, aniridia, heterochromia iridis, persistent pupillary membrane, coloboma	–
Chromosomal disorders:		
Trisomy 13	Microcephaly, cleft palate, cardiac defect, polydactyly; haemangioma, CNS malformation, vitreoretinal dysplasia	–
Trisomy 18	Mental retardation, characteristic facies, cardiac defect, ptosis, microphthalmos	–
Trisomy 21	Mental retardation, characteristic facies, Mongoloid lid slant, Brushfield spots, cataract	–
Monosomy	Turner's syndrome: XO. Ovarian dysgenesis, webbed neck, coarctation of aorta, epicanthus, squint, lacrimal abnormality and occasional cataract	–
Deletions:		
Wolf-Hirschorn syndrome	Mental defect, microcephaly, 'Greek helmet' facies, cleft lip, coloboma. (4pc)	194190
Cri du chat syndrome	Mental retardation, slow growth, cat-like cry, rare catarat. ($5p^-$)	–
Rings	Chromosome 13q 18q;p	–
	Chromosomes 13, 18, 21	–
Syndromes, metabolic and systemic disorders. Disorders of carbohydrate metabolism:		
Galactosaemia	gal. uridyl transferase deficiency	230400
	galactokinase deficiency	230200
	gal. 4. epimerase deficiency	–
Gluc. 6. P deficiency	–	230350
Diabetes mellitus	–	125850
Hypoglycaemia	Therapeutic, or perinatal difficulty	222100
Disorders of lipid metabolism:		
Fabry disease	Burning pain, vascular dermatosis, renal failure, hypertension; cornea verticillata, vessel tortuosity cataract	301500
Cerebrotendinous xanthomatosis	Defective bile acid synthesis leads to cholestanol and cholesterol deposits in tissues. Mental defect, tendinous xanthomata, xanthelasma, neural defect cataract	213700

Table 11.1 (*Continued*)

Inherited and sporadic causes:	*Inherited infantile cataract*	*McKusick No. D, r, XL*
Disorders of glycoprotein metabolism:		
Mannosidosis	alpha type	248500
	beta type	248510
Disorders of metal ions		
Hypocalcaemia	Hypoparathyroidism	–
	Pseudohypoparathyroidism	–
	Pseudopseudohypoparathyroidism	103580
Hypercupremia	Wilson's disease: liver failure, dysarthria, incoordination; Kayser–Fleischer ring, sunflower cataract	203330
Lowe syndrome	Mental retardation defective renal tubular function cataract, glaucoma. Lens dots in carriers.	300800
Alport syndrome	Haemorrhagic nephropathy, renal failure, sensorineural deafness, lenticonus, cataract, flecked retina	277900 309000 104200
Muscoloskeletal disorders:		
Muscular Disorders–		
Dystrophia myotonica	Myotonia, wasting, CNS abnormality, premature baldness, testicular atrophy; cardiomyopathy, blepharitis, cataract, hypertension. 19q 13.3	160900
Mitochond. myopathy	Face, pharynx, limb	–
Mitochond. cardiomyopathy	Lactic acidosis on exercise	–
Skeletal disorders–		
Apert syndrome	Acrocephalosyndactly; occasional cataract	101200
CAMAK syndrome	Cataract, Microcephaly, Arthrogryposis Kyphosis; cerebral/cellular calcification	212540
Chondrodysplasia	Skeletal dysplasia, flat facies, punctate skeletal calcification	118650
Ellis van Creveld syndrome	Chondroectodermal dysplasia, dwarfism, short distal limbs, polydactyly, nail dystrophy, partial cleft lip, cardiac and dental abnormality, occ. cataract	225500
Engelman disease	Progressive diaphyseal dysplasia, leg pain and weakness, occ. cataract	131300
Lanzier disease	–	–
Mandibulofacial syndromes:		
Crouzon	Acrocephaly, beak nose, maxillary hypoplasia, prognathism, exophthalmos, occasional cataract	123500
Hallerman-Streiff	Bird's head dyscephaly, dwarfism, skin atrophy, dental abnormality, microphthalmos, and cataract	234100
Treacher Collins	Oblique lid fissures, lower lid colobomata, hypoplastic zygomata, dysplastic ears, micrognathia; occasional cataract	154500
Pierre Robin syndrome	Microphthalmos, micrognathia glossoptosis; occasional cataract	261800
Marshall syndrome	Similarities to Stickler syndrome	154780
Meckel-Gruber syndrome	–	249000
ODD syndrome	Oculodentaldigital dysplasia: thin nose, alar hypoplasia, narrow nostrils, campodactlyly of 4th and 5th fingers, enamel hypoplasia, microcornea, iris anomalies, glaucoma, congenital cataract	164200

Table 11.1 *(Continued)*

Inherited and sporadic causes:	***Inherited infantile cataract***	***McKusick No. D, r, XL***
Muscoloskeletal disorders *(Continued)*:		
Mandibulofacial syndromes *(Continued)*:		
Osteogenesis imperfecta	Brittle bones, blue sclerotics, otosclerosis dentogenesis imperfecta; varies with type	166600 25970 1/2/3
Osteogen impf. congen.	Lethal: microcephaly, cataract	259410
Oxycephaly	Exophthalmos, optic atrophy, infantile zonular cataract	D
Rubenstein-Tabyi syndrome	Facial dysmorphism, broad thumbs and toes, mental retardation, ocular signs, occ. cataract	268600
Stickler syndrome	High myopia/large globes, vitreo retinal disorder; arthropathy of wrists, hips, knees, ankles with epiphysical X-ray changes	108300
Disorders of the central nervous system:		
Bardet-Biedl syndrome	Mental retardation, obesity, hypogonadism, polydactyly, retinitis pigmentosa, squint	209900
Marinesco-Sjögren	Mental retardation, spinocerebellar ataxia, congenital cataract	248800
Martsolf syndrome	Mental retardation, dwarfism, minor cephalic and digital abnormalities and cataract	212720
Myoclonus-cerebellar dyssynergy	Early onset (under 10 years), of tremor and myoclonus; pre-senile cataract described	–
Norrie syndrome	Mental retardation and progressive blindness due to retinal dysplasia (pseudoglioma) and cataract with onset in the first year	310600
Smith-Lemli-Opitz	Mental retardation, microcephaly, high forehead, anteverted nostrils, polydactyly syndactyly, cataract	270400
Cataract ataxia deafness retardation	Polyneuropathy, short stature	212710
Other	Oligophrenia, keratoconus, cataract, vitreous ectopia, optic atrophy and cataract	–
Dermatological disorders:		
Anhydrotic Ectodermal	Microphthalmos, PHPV and occasional cataract in congenital form	–
Dysplasia		
Atopy	Atopic dermatitis, asthma, hay fever, shield cataract, keratoconus	–
Goltz syndrome	Dermal atrophy and linear pigmentation, fat herniation, dermal/mucous membrane papillomata, poly/compo/syndactyly, bone striation and mental retardation, dental hypoplasia; coloboma of iris/choroid, microphthalmos, ectopia lentis. Lethal in the male	305600
Ichthyosis	Thick skin and nails, anhydrosis, increased cataract risk, hypertrophic icthyosis at birth, on scalp, ears, neck, abdomen, flexures; deep corneal dots, rare cortical and nuclear lens opacities	–
Congenital ichthyosis	–	212400
Incontinentia pigmenti	Pigmented grey dermal patches and streaks, hypo/anhydrosis, alopecia in females, dental anomalies; congenital cataract, persistent hyperplastic vitreous, squint, nystagmus	308300

Table 11.1 (*Continued*)

Inherited and sporadic causes:	*Inherited infantile cataract*	*McKusick No. D, r, XL*
Dermatological disorders (*Continued*):		
Rothmund syndrome	Poikiloderma atrophicans vasculare, telangiectasia, brownish skin. Also saddle nose, bony defect, hypogonadism, and disturbed hair growth. Cataracts are congenital or acquired in the 3rd to 5th year of life	268400
Schäffer syndrome	Palmarplantar keratosis, hyperhydrosis, patchy alopecia, thick nails, hypogonadism, congenital cataract	–
Siemen syndrome	Hypoplasia or atrophy of the skin, congenital cataract	–
Werner syndrome	Short stature, stocky trunk, beak nose prematurely aging facies, premature arteriosclerosis, scleroderma-like skin, subcutaneous calcification, cataract	277700
Other syndromes:		
Progeria	Variegated translocation in fibroblasts. Premature ageing and death in the first years of life. Cataract	176670
Zellwegger syndrome	Cerebrohepatorenal syndrome. Developmental abnormalities of skull, face, eyes, ears. Abnormal chondral calcification (e.g. patella). Polycystic kidneys, biliary dysgenesis. Minor lens opacities. Absent peroxisomes	214100 214110
Cataract, aberrant frenula	Aberrant frenula and growth retardation	115645
Endocrine disorders:		
Diabetes mellitus	–	138190 125850 222100
Hypothyroidism	–	–
Infective causes:		
Rubella	–	–
Nutritional:		
Malnutrition	–	–
Anorexia nervosa	–	–
Toxic causes:		
Drug-induced:		
Corticosteroids	–	–
Anticholinesterases	Nitrogen, mustard, TEM, methyl amino	–
Phenothiazines	Stryl quinoline, trenimon, mimosine	–
Radiomimetic drugs	Busulphan, allopurinol, antimalarials chloroquine	–
Chemical induced:	Dinitrophenol, dinitrocresol, trinitrotoluene, naphthalene	–
	Paradichlorobenzene heptachlor, tetracaine	–
Metal ions		
Copper	Systemic Wilson's disease, topical copper sulphate	–
	IOFB	–
Iron	–	–
Gold	–	–
Silver	topical: e.g. thiomersal	–
Mercury	–	–

Table 11.1 (*Continued*)

Inherited and sporadic causes:	***Inherited infantile cataract***	***McKusick No. D, r, XL***
Physical factors:		
Dehydration	–	–
Trauma	Concussion, penetrating injury	–
Electric shock	Concussion, penetrating injury	–
Radiation	X-ray, gamma rays, beta rays	–
Ionizing	Heavy charged particles, neutrons infra red, ultraviolet, microwave	–
Non-ionizing	–	–

* Designation here as inherited does not exclude the possibility of non-genetic causes.
Note: In the McKusick nomenclature the initial number 1 implies a dominant trait, 2 = recessive and 3 = X-linked.

Anterior polar cataracts

Anterior and polar cataract

This is a sharply circumscribed opacity of the anterior capsule which may be the size of a pin-head or of the pupil (Figures 10.2, 10.3, 10.4). There may be associated radiating lines or an anterior or posterior conical projection, with or without cortical involvement. Fine strands may pass between the opacity and the cornea. Vision is invariably affected.

Postulated mechanisms include imperfect separation of the lens from surface ectoderm at the 5th week of intrauterine life, epithelial damage with the formation of a mass at the anterior pole, or incomplete resorption of the vascular tunic of the lens. When there is a posterior projection, this maintains contact with the surface of the fetal nucleus so that an extended cylinder is formed which spans the cortex in adult life. The deepest location of the cylinder in the lens indicates the time of onset of the causative insult.

Anterior polar cataracts are usually dominantly inherited (Merin 1986). Moross *et al.* (1984) reported a family in whom dominant cataract occurred in four members of three generations, associated with a balanced translocation (t(2i14) (p25;q24)).

The cataract may take one of three forms:

1 Associated with other zonular lens opacities, mainly lamellar (Wolfsohm-Jette 1933).
2 Associated with microphthalmos (Harman 1910a, b).

Table 11.2 Congenital cataract in some recent blindness surveys

Survey reference	***Country***	***Conclusions***
Potter, 1991	Central African Republic	13.5% of blindness
Goggin and O'Keefe, 1991	Ireland	4.6% of blindness
Department of Health, 1991	United Kingdom	15.8% partial sight; 4.2% blindness
Stoll *et al.*, 1992	France	2.3/10 000 live births
Hansen *et al.*, 1992	Scandinavia	6/100 000 population
Moriarty, 1988	Jamaica	39% of blindness
Robinson, 1987	British Columbia	18.8% of blindness

3 Associated with a hyperplastic pupillary membrane covering the pupil, and in three of four families described, attached to the lens. (Pagenstecher 1925; Waardenburg 1949; Cassady and Light 1957; Merin *et al.* 1971).

Capsular flakes

These are dense, white, multiple oval or round opacities up to 1 mm in diameter, which are often associated with deeper lens changes, superficial pigment threads and epicapsular stars.

Circular capsular cataract

Circular capsular, or subcapsular, cataract (Figures 10.2, 10.3) is made up of white, bluish white or brownish opacities arranged in a radial or circular pattern (e.g. 1–2 mm wide). Pupillary remnants may be attached, and vision is variably affected. Anterior chamber malformations may coexist (Kivlin 1986).

Reduplication cataract

There is a localized opacity of the anterior capsule, separated from a similar cortical opacity by a layer of deep cortex (Figure 10.3). It has been suggested that it is due to focal intrauterine or, rarely, postnatal damage to the anterior capsule and subjacent cortex with the subsequent interposition of normal lens fibres between the damaged capsule and cortical fibres. It appears that the capsule defect has a variable adverse effect on lens fibre formation, so that the ends of the fibres inserting beneath it are sometimes opaque and sometimes clear. Thus the subjacent lens opacity gradually builds up like a stack of plates. Successive plates, which may be attached together by a narrow pillar, may increase in diameter.

Fusiform cataract

The opacity extends into the cortex as a rod shape, which occasionally passes through the nucleus to the posterior capsule (Figure 10.5).

Spear cataract

Spear cataract is a polymorphic cataract which presents branching needle-like clusters of opacity, up to 1 mm in length. The needles may be polychromatic, are often axial, and do not respect the fibre arrangement. Variations include a central compacted mass with concentric outer clusters and branching nuclear clusters with neighbouring petalloid opacities. Needles are found in both nucleus and cortex. The cataract may be dominantly inherited (Vogt 1921). Vision may be almost normal (Gifford and Puntenney 1937).

Crystalline cataract

A crystalline cataract with snowball-shaped clumps of crystals and a dominant inheritance is shown in Figure 11.1.

Coralliform cataract (Figure 10.65)

This is an unusual form of cataract which may be inherited as an autosomal dominant and possibly as a recessive. It consists of rounded and oblong opacities grouped towards the centre of the lens and resembling a piece of coral. The opacities may extend from anterior to posterior capsule (Nettleship 1909; Gunn 1895; Jordan 1955).

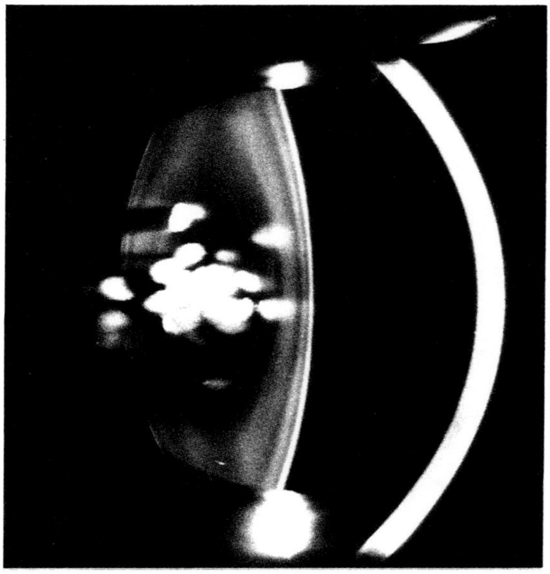

Figure 11.1 Familial snowball nuclear cataract.

Floriform cataract

This is a rare congenital form of cataract which may be inherited as a dominant (Doggart 1957). Opacities are 0.25–0.75 mm wide, ring-shaped, bluish or white, and sometimes diaphanous. They are commonly in the axial part of the lens, often in the region of the fetal sutures and their arrangement gives the appearance of a flower. They may be associated with the development of lens opacities in later life.

Lamellar cataract (Figures 9.2, 9.4, 11.2)

Lamellar cataract is one of the most frequent infantile forms. It may be inherited as a dominant trait (McKusick 1988) or it may have a metabolic or inflammatory cause. Hypocalcaemia or galactosaemia are important infantile causes. In the family of Harman (1910a), malformation of the fingers was associated. Lamellar cataract appears as a round grey shell of opacity surrounding a clear nucleus. It is nearly always bilaterally symmetrical. With time, and the laying down of normal fibres outside the shell, a clear zone of cortex appears outside it which increases throughout life. The opacity represents a shell of several generations of secondary lens fibres which have become opacified in response to a specific insult when these fibres were at their most metabolically active stage (i.e. at or shortly after their formation). This may occur *in utero* or postnatally. Neonatal hypocalcaemia was once a common cause of lamellar cataract and was due to maternal calcium and vitamin D deficiency. Restoration of calcium balance in such instances would lead to the formation of clear new fibres outside the lamellar shell.

The lamellar opacity may be formed of sheets which emphasize the fibre pattern, or of fine punctate opacities, sometimes involving the fetal sutures, the embryonic nucleus, or concentric lamellar zones. Sometimes clear, pie-shaped sectors are present (Figure 10.31) which indicate that fibres occupying this zone are of normal transparency and function. The location of the lamellar opacity implies the laying down of fibres which opacify at a particular point during lens development. The common occurrence of 'riders' (radial cataractous extensions into overlying cortex) implies that abnormality of fibre formation persists beyond this time (Figure 10.48).

Lamellar cataract varies between 2–8 mm in diameter with its shell between 0.5–0.7 in thickness. With time, because of the compaction of the central parts of the lens, there is a reduction of the diameter and sagittal width of the opacity (Brown *et al.* 1988), and an increase in density which may lead to a further loss of vision. The diameter of a lamellar cataract is determined by its time of onset since it affects the newest fibres formed at this time. Thus prenatal lamellar cataracts are smaller than postnatal cataracts. When it is small the effect on vision may be limited, and there may be insufficient image degradation to reduce acuity or to induce amblyopia, squint or nystagmus. Children with lamellar cataract must be kept under surveillance and may be assisted visually by mydriatics.

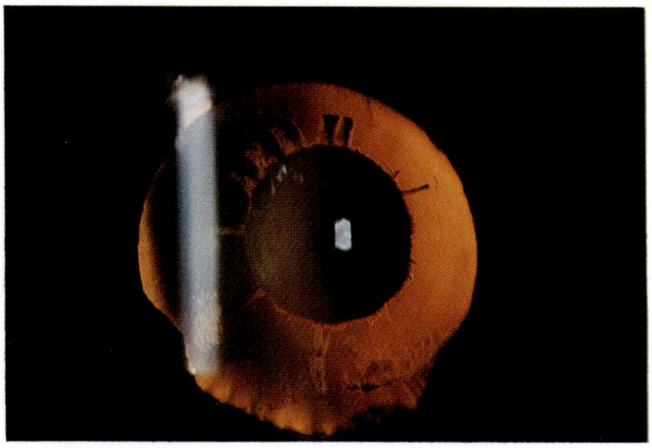

Figure 11.2 The riders of a lamellar cataract are well shown in this retro-illumination picture.

Congenital cataracts confined to the embryonic or fetal nucleus

Central pulverulent cataract (Figures 9.8, 11.3)

This cataract, described by Nettleship and Ogilvie (1906) is dominantly inherited, non-progresive and limited to the embryonic or early fetal nucleus. It was named 'Coppock', after the family in whom it was first described. It has also been called 'Doyne's discoid cataract', after Robert Doyne, who observed the first patients. The opacity consists of fine white powdery dots which form a small grey spheroidal or biconvex opacity within the lens nucleus, retaining the shape of the embryonic or early fetal lens. The centre of the cataract is more or less clear. Vogt (1921, 1922, 1931) used the term 'cataracta pulverulenta centralis' to describe what is probably the same condition (Gifford 1924) but noted both inner and outer ring opacities. Within a pedigree the cataract is bilateral and symmetrical and of similar density although in some instances the opacity may be quite faint. The opacity measures 1–4 mm in width. Gifford (1924, 1927) described equatorial diameters of 2 mm in one patient and 3 mm in another, Rados (1947) cited diameters of 2–4 mm, and a diameter of 4 mm was mentioned in the paper by Nettleship and Ogilvie. Vogt (1921) measured a central component of 0.72 mm and a peripheral one of 1.04 mm in one patient, compared to 0.8 and 2.2 mm in another. Because of their small size these cataracts generally have little or no effect on vision. These descriptions suggest that there may be considerable phenotypic variation in this form of cataract which may reflect genotypic variation. Recessive pedigrees of Coppock cataract have been reported by Rados (1947) and by Robinson (1975).

Linkage analysis of a pedigree of a Coppock-like cataract suggested that the cause of the cataract is a mutation in a crystallin gene mapping to the human gamma crystallin gene cluster on chromosome 2 (2q) (Lubsen *et al.* 1987). The lod score for this association was 7.58 maximum at theta = 0. The nucleus of the lens is relatively rich in gamma crystallins which are only expressed in and around the prenatal period. It was inferred from this study that the cataract was due to a disturbance of the tertiary structure of a mutated gamma crystallin, resulting in an alteration of the short-range order of

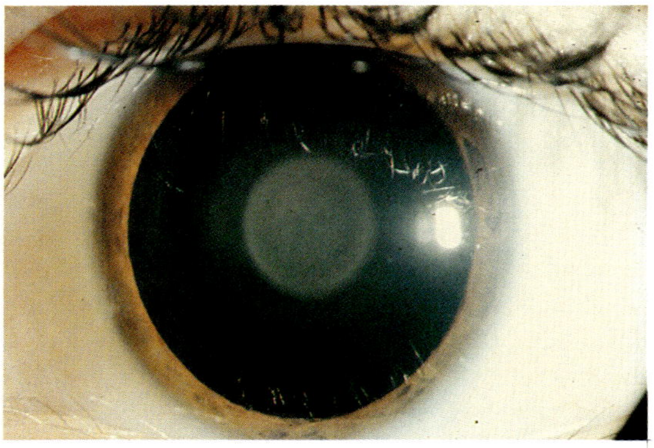

Figure 11.3 Cataracta centralis pulverulenta.

the crystallins of the prenatal lens and a loss of transparency. A further study by this group has narrowed the gamma gene defect to an upstream mutation in the promoter region of the gamma E gene, leading to over-expression of gamma E crystallin (Brackenhoff *et al.* 1994). It should be noted that the gamma E gene is designated a pseudogene on the basis of an in-frame stop codon and it had been assumed that gamma E was not normally expressed in the lens. However, Brackenhof *et al.* (1994) have demonstrated that the gene is transcriptionally active to a minor degree in the normal human lens and is therefore not completely inactive functionally. As noted in Chapter 6, the gamma crystallins are folded into four *Greek Key* motifs, organized in 2 domains. The protein strands are intercalated so that the 4th strand of the *Greek Key* of the first motif derives from the second motif, and vice versa. The gamma E protein lacks the fourth chain required to complete the motif structure and is unlikely to fold correctly. It is assumed that in Coppock cataract activation of the gamma E promoter greatly increases the amount of gamma E in the lens. This improperly folded, single motif gamma crytallin then disturbs the organization of the fibre crystallins during fetal life and leads to the nuclear opacity found in the postnatal lens.

Lubsen *et al.* (1987) have commented that the 'embryonic' manifestation of the Coppock cataract is in keeping with the developmental timing of gamma crystallin synthesis in the calf and rat (Slingsby and Miller 1983; Siezen *et al.* 1986; van Leen *et al.* 1987). However, in the human lens the situation is different. Thomson and Augustyn (1985) reported that gamma crystallin synthesis proceeded throughout prenatal life and ceased thereafter, while Bours (1980) has reported that gamma crystallin synthesis continues to the age of 5–6 years. Gamma crystallin genes are said to be activated simultaneously, although the initial expression of human gamma crystallin is delayed compared to the rat (Brackenhof *et al.* 1990). This might explain the clear centre of the Coppock cataract (Adams 1942) although it might also be determined by the relative concentrations of the crystallins in the central fibres. The outer dimensions of the Coppock cataract must be determined by the period over which the faulty gamma fragment is expressed. Down-regulation of the gamma crystallin genes occurs differentially in development, with the gamma D gene being the last to be active. The period of expression of the mutated gamma E gene is not known, but the size of the Coppock cataract indicates that there is not sufficient of the improperly folded, gamma E protein in the fibres to cause opacity in late fetal life. This is either because the protein is no longer expressed, because its concentration is too low to interfere with the supramolecular organization of the crystallins as a whole, or because the organization of the crystallins is conserved by the chaperone function of alpha crystallin (Horwitz 1992). Variations in these events both within and between family members could explain phenotypic variations in cataract morphology, including differences in size and density and the shells of opacity which may be seen from time to time.

In 1963, Renwick and Lawler described linkage of another dominant cataract type to the Duffy blood group locus (Fy) which maps to chromosome 1 (Donahue *et al.* 1968). The cataract, about 4 mm in equatorial diameter, was said to consist of innumerable powdery opacities, such as those depicted as a zonular, pulverulent cataract in Waardenburg, Francesschetti and Klein (1961: Figure 689a) except that riders were present in only one patient (patient IV 32). Many of the cataracts showed numerous irregular fluffy opacities such as those depicted by Vogt (1931: Figure 969). The cataracts were bilateral and bounded by a smooth envelope consisting of a thin layer of particularly fine opacities. Outside this the lens was clear in about five out of six eyes. In the remaining eyes this outer zone had one or more shells or parts of shells also consisting of these powdery opacities.

No such linkage was found in a morphologically identical kindred by Hammerstein and Scholt (1974), but Coneally *et al.* (1978) found linkage to markers on chromosome 1 in one of several families with this form of cataract, although in this case the opacities involved the fetal nucleus and were associated with incomplete cortical 'riders' such as those described in the pedigree of Nettleship (1909).

Congenital punctate cerulean cataract

There are small bluish dots scattered throughout the lens, with clear lens between them (Figures 10.61 and 10.62, plate X). Opacities are found in the fetal lens and pass into the superficial cortex. The condition is bilateral, non-progressive in the sense that the density of the dots does not increase, and has little effect on vision.

Congenital anterior embryonal cataract

This is a stationary form of cataract with chalk white or iridescent dot opacities lying at or close to the anterior embryonal suture. Opacities are sometimes surrounded by a halo. They are not always bilateral.

Congenital sutural (stellate) cataract (Figures 10.35, 10.36)

This is a dominant form of cataract affecting one, especially the posterior, or both fetal sutures. It is stationary and usually bilateral. The opacity is made up of fine white or bluish dots, sometimes with a feathery configuration, or may be a dense chalky band which may take on many shapes. It may sometimes interfere with vision.

Posterior lens changes

Mittendorf's dot is a white condensation on the posterior pole of the lens capsule, slightly inferonasal to its geometric centre. It is without lens fibre involvement. It may be up to 1 mm in diameter, is attached to a freely floating thread in the vitreous gel, and represents the anterior part of the hyaloid artery remnant. It is often unilateral and is non-progressive.

Posterior polar cataract

There are various forms:

1. A dense, saucer-shaped opacity may cover the posterior pole of the lens and involve the underlying lens fibres. It is thought by some to represent a remnant of the vascular sheath of the lens, as a mild form of persistent primary hyperplastic vitreous. The visual effect may be marked.
2. Posterior polar cataracts may occur as opacities affecting the capsule and underlying lens fibres; they vary in size from under 1 mm to large saucer-shaped opacities. Larger opacities may affect vision. They may be associated with other lens opacities. Dominant inheritance is described by Nettleship (1909, 1912) and Tulloh (1955) and their occurrence in association with dwarfism, choroideraemia and myopia reported by Valk and Binkhorst (1956). Linkage has been

described to the haptoglobin locus on chromosome 16 (Marner type of cataract and autosomal dominant, posterior polar cataract).

3. Posterior lenticonus (Figure 11.4) is a rare, often unilateral, anomaly with a conoid protrusion of the posterior lens substance. The nucleus is not always involved in the deformation, in which case a postnatal basis is suggested. The altered lens shape produces a poorly correctable, high myopia. Eighty per cent of such cases are complicated by posterior lens opacities and a hyaloid artery remnant is often present. In the absence of a lens opacity there is an 'oil droplet' appearance against the red reflex. The condition is usually unilateral.

Other forms of infantile cataract

Congenital disciform (annular) cataract

In this cataract the axial part of the lens is thinned to a central membranous sheet while the remainder is of normal size, thickness and clarity. The lens takes on a doughnut shape. The central depression never exceeds the diameter of the embryonic nucleus, and for this reason Mann (1956) has suggested that the embryonic nucleus fails to develop. (The condition must be distinguished from a residual opacity following lens absorption, Soemmering's ring.) The cataract may be inherited as a dominant trait.

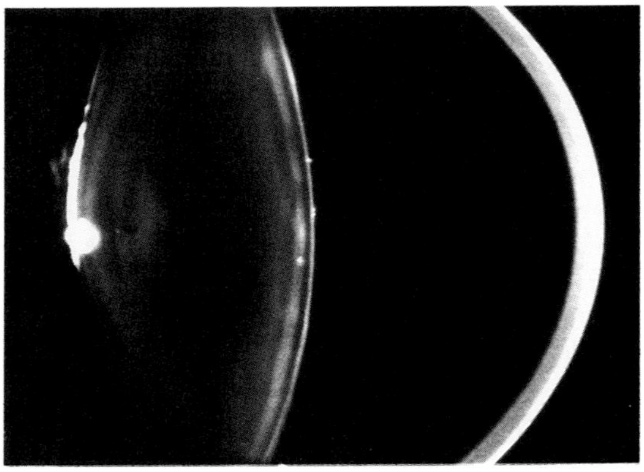

Figure 11.4 Posterior lenticonus with posterior cortical cataract formation.

Total cataract

The lens is totally white at birth, or becomes so shortly afterwards. The lens may be shrunken in size. The condition may be bilateral, or be associated with another form of cataract in the other eye. It may progress to form a Morgagnian or membranous cataract. Dominant inheritance of total nuclear cataract is reported by Brown (1924) and Parrow (1955). Reese *et al.* (1987) reported cataract in a father and son with a translocation 4(3;4) (p26.2; pl5), suggesting a gene change at or near the breakpoints, 3p26.2 or 4p15. In the child, the opacities were not noted at birth, but progressed to maturity between 7–9 weeks.

In another family, linkage with the haptoglobin gene was suggested (Richards *et al.* 1984; Maumenee 1979). A dominant, non-progressive cataract, limited to the fetal nucleus, is described by Vogt (1931). Recessive pedigrees of total nuclear cataract have also been reported by Wagner (1940), Bane (1944) and Saebo (1949).

It will be recognized that there is some possibility of confusion and misclassification with the terminology in use here. For instance, a total cataract at birth will be described as a nuclear cataract in later life if the cortex grows normally postnatally. It is therefore not always clear that distinct entities are described.

Membranous cataract

In this condition, the whole of the lens substance is absorbed, leaving a thin grey-white or chalky-white capsular membrane. Occasionally posterior capsule rupture may occur. The condition may be preceded by a Morgagnian cataract. Dominant inheritance is described (Gruber 1945).

Morgagnian cataract

The condition is rare in childhood and resembles the condition seen in the adult. The cortex liquefies, and is either absorbed, or provides a milky fluid in which the 'nucleus' floats. It may be the outcome of a total cataract and may proceed to membranous cataract.

Coronary cataracts

Developmental opacities include coronary cataracts (Figures 10.57, 10.58, 10.59, Plate VII) which may occur in a lens already affected by congenital cataract, or in a previously clear lens (Figure 10.58). They are said to be inherited as a dominant trait, but the family history may be lacking because the condition does not usually affect vision. However, it must be remembered that coronary cataract is very common, occurring in about 25% of adults (Gjessing 1920), so that the impression of inheritance may be spurious. Onset is at or around puberty. The opacities are found in the periphery of the superficial cortex (C2), where they form a crown-like circle which gives the cataract its name. The opacities are chiefly whitish and club-shaped and flattened in the plane of the lens surface. They are accompanied by lines, discs and rings within the same zone. It is not uncommon for coronary cataract to be associated with cerulean dot opacities in the lens nucleus (Berliner 1949). Vogt (1921) suggested that coronary cataract was commonly associated with cortical spots as a hereditary combination.

Although coronary cataracts may appear to be stationary, most of them progress over long periods of time, increasing in number and density. Vision is usually spared but may be affected when opacities are more axial.

Persistent hyperplastic primary vitreous

In this condition there is an imperfect development of the secondary vitreous, with persistence and hyperplasia of the primary vitreous. There is unilateral (90%) microphthalmos with prominent iris vessels, shallow anterior chamber, and elongated, dentate ciliary processes which are dragged centrally (Reese 1955; Kazuhiko *et al.* 1986; Karr and Scott 1986). The lens is clear initially but intralenticular haemorrhage may occur. Cataract usually occurs, with time, and the anterior chamber may become shallow if the lens is swollen.

Hereditary cataract

Many of the cataract types cited above are inherited, but not all inherited cataracts present in infancy. Some present in later life.

A proportion of inherited cataracts are associated with wider systemic syndromes such as dystrophia myotonica, while others, for instance certain sugar cataracts, are inherited in the sense that they are secondary to a metabolic disturbance which occurs as an inherited disorder. These are dealt with later in this chapter. A list of inherited cataracts is presented in Table 9.5 (see also Table 11.3).

Chromosomal disorders

Chromosomal disorders occur in about 1 in 160 newborn infants (Thompson and Thompson 1980) and account for about 10% of congenital malformations (Wilson and Frazer 1977). They take various forms. Aneuploidy is a deviation from the normal chromosome number (Figure 11.5) and includes the trisomies (e.g. trisomy 21 – Down's syndrome) and monosomies (e.g. 45, X, Turner's syndrome). Structural aberrations include the translocations (i.e. the transfer of one part of a chromosome to another) and the deletions (i.e. the loss of a portion of a chromosome, either terminally or interstitially, between 2 breaks). Loss of both ends of a chromosome allows a ring chromosome to form. Trisomy 21 is the most common of the autosomal trisomies with a frequency of 1:800 births (Thompson and Thompson 1980); the incidence rises to 1 in 32 with a maternal age above 44 years (Hook 1982). Trisomy 18 is the next most common (1:8000 births). The frequency of Turner's syndrome is about 1:10000. (Gieser *et al.* 1986)

Trisomy 13

Trisomy 13 is associated with major malformations including holoprosencephaly, facial clefting, congenital heart defect and polydactyly. The gross ocular defects include microphthalmos, coloboma, retinal dysplasia and persistent hyperplastic primary vitreous. Cataract and, rarely, aphakia occur. Death occurs in the first months of life.

Trisomy 18

In trisomy 18 (Edwards' syndrome) there is facial dysmorphism with low set ears and slanting lid fissures, epicanthus, ptosis and thickened lids. The frontal region is narrowed. Systemic features include cardiomyopathy, skeletal muscle hypoplasia, short sternum, flexion contracture of the fingers and 'rocker bottom' feet. Eye signs include microphthalmos, corneal clouding, coloboma, cataract, glaucoma and retinal dysplasia. Aphakia is also reported (Gieser *et al.* 1986). The karyotype is shown in Figure 11.6.

Trisomy 21

More than 90% of people with Down's syndrome have a trisomy 21, due to non-disjunction. About 5% have a translocation of the long arm of the chromosome, usually with a break at the centromere (Robertsonian type). Based on those cases of Down's syndrome cause by reciprocal translocations, it appears that trisomy of only the distal one-third of the long arm of chromosome 21 is all that is needed for the complete phenotype. Systemic findings are of mental retardation, short stature, cardiac defects, muscle hypotonia, gonadal dysplasia, dry skin and characteristic dermatoglyphs and transverse palmar creases. Ocular findings include epicanthus and a mongoloid lid slant, blepharitis, iris hypoplasia and Brushfield's spots. Keratoconus is associated (Figure 11.6).

Cataract occurs in 60–85% of those affected, usually becoming manifest after puberty, but occurring in a few before the age of 8 years (Eissler and Longenecker 1962) or even congenitally (Merin and Crawford 1971a, Alden 1978; Jaeger 1980).

Lowe (1949b) has described the opacities as follows:

1. *Arcuate opacities*. These arch around the early layers of the fetal nucleus and are the earliest type of cataract seen.
2. *Sutural or stellate cataract*. Although these occur in the line of the Y sutures, they are seldom seen at an early age, and usually manifest in the teens or later. This is a reminder that, although the lens grows throughout life, location is not always an indicator of time of occurrence. Fetal nuclear opacities are present in a small proportion at birth (Alda 1973).
3. *Flake opacities* are formed in the cortex in early life (Ginsberg *et al.* 1977). These are often subcapsular, but a proportion may represent excrescences of the lens capsule, such as are seen in Lowe's syndrome.
4. *Lamellar and posterior polar cataract* are observed uncommonly.

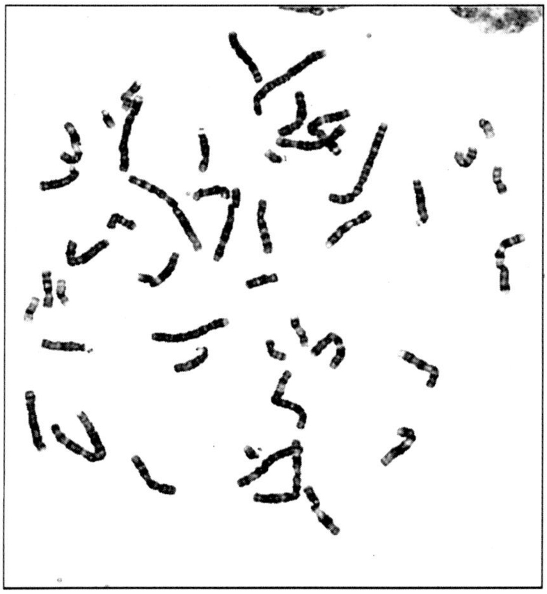

Figure 11.5 A normal female metaphase spread. (Courtesy of M. Fitchett.)

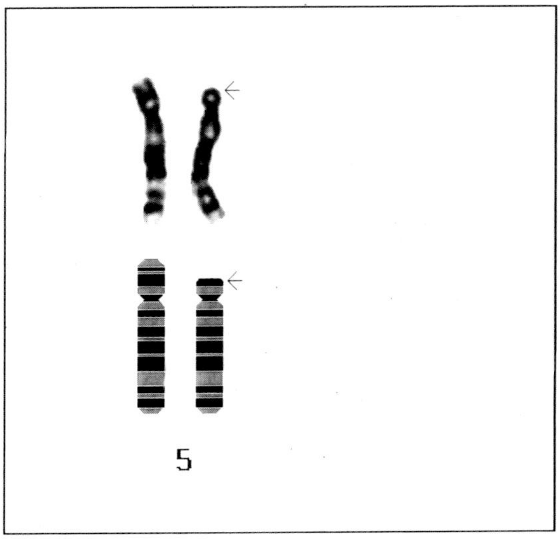

Figure 11.6 Trisomy 18. (Courtesy of M. Fitchett.)

Other chromosome abnormalities

Cataract is reported with deletions of the short arm of chromosome 4 (Wolf–Hirschorn syndrome) and chromosome 5 (Figure 11.7) (Cri du chat syndrome) (Farell *et al.* 1988), of the long arm of chromosome 13, and of either the short or the long arm of chromosome 18. It is also found with ring chromosomes 13, 18 and 21 (Gieser *et al.* 1986). Reese *et al.* (1987) described autosomal dominant cataract with a reciprocal translocation involving chromosomes 3 and 4 (t[3;4] [p26.2; pl5]). It is also described with a balanced translocation between chromosomes 2 and 14, and with a familial translocation (t[2;16][p22.3; p. 13.3]) in balanced and unbalanced forms, where it is associated with a syndrome of autosomal dominant cataract and microphthalmia.

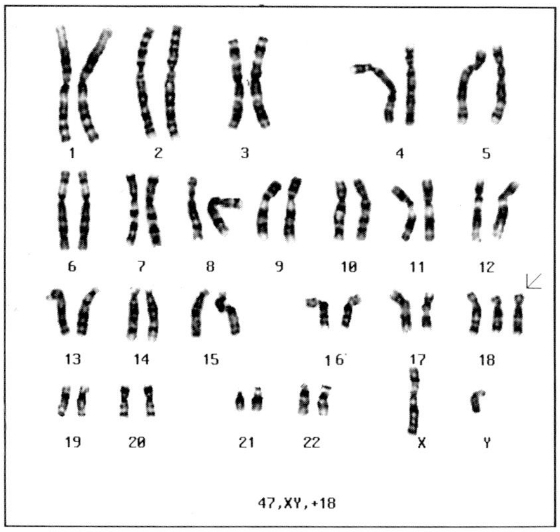

Figure 11.7 Partial karyotype and ideogram showing a deletion of the short arm of chromosome 5 at band p14 [del(5) (p14)]. (Courtesy of M. Fitchett.)

Cataract in systemic disease and syndromes

Cataract is encountered with a variety of systemic diseases and syndromes. Some of these are discussed below.

Disorders of sugar metabolism

The conversion of galactose to glucose in the tissues involves three enzymes. An absence of any one of these may cause cataract as part of an autosomal recessive disorder. The cause of cataract is an accumulation of galactitol (the sugar alcohol of galactose) within the lens and a subsequent osmotic disruption of the lens fibres (Figure 11.8).

Galactosaemia results from a deficiency of the enzyme galactose-1-phosphate uridyl transferase. Galactosaemia and galactosuria in infancy are associated with failure to thrive, hepatosplenomegaly, mental retardation and cataract. Untreated, the condition leads to death in early infancy (Fanconi 1933).

The earliest lens change is an oil droplet effect seen on retinoscopy, due to a refractive change in the nucleus. Anterior and posterior subcapsular opacities develop within a few days or months of birth, and progress through a nuclear cataract to maturity (Figure 11.9) (Nordmann 1966). The progression of early cataract may be prevented by withholding galactose from the diet.

CHO		CH_2OH		CH_2OH
HCOH	→	HCOH	→	CO
HOCH	aldose reductase	HOCH	polyol dehydrogenase	HOCH
D-Glucose	⇌	Sorbitol	⇌	D-Fructose
D-Galactose	⇌	Dulcitol (Galactitol)		
D-Xylose	⇌	Xylitol	⇌	D-Xylulose
L-Arabinose	⇌	L-Arabitol		

Figure 11.8 Sorbitol pathway. Configuration of the first three carbon atoms of the sugars and polyols. (Adapted from van Heyningen 1962a.)

Galactokinase deficiency is associated with galactosaemia and cataract in the absence of systemic manifestations (Beutler *et al.* 1973). The cataract may present in infancy (Benson *et al.* 1976) but was first reported in childhood (Gitzelmann 1967). This was also the case in one series with a low mean red cell galactokinase level (Beutler *et al.* 1973). Congenital cataract has been described in the offspring of heterozygous mothers with low levels of galactokinase activity during pregnancy which suggests that dietary restriction during pregnancy might prevent these cataracts (Harley 1974; Winder *et al.* 1982). However, later studies did not confirm greater risk in heterozygotes (Winder *et al.* 1985). Prchal *et al.* (1978) associated heterozygosity for galactokinase or uridyl transferase deficiency with presenile cataracts.

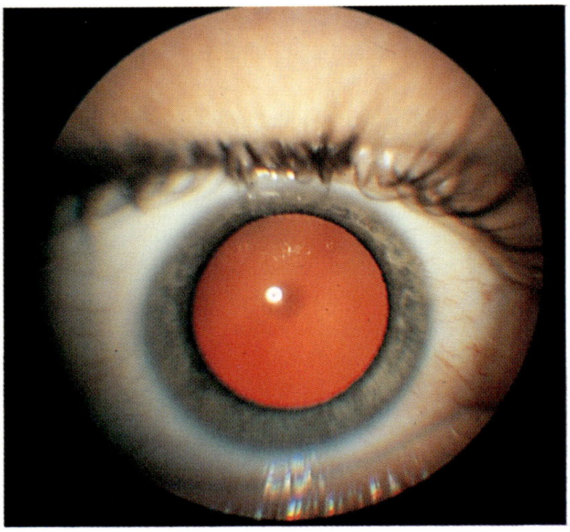

(a)

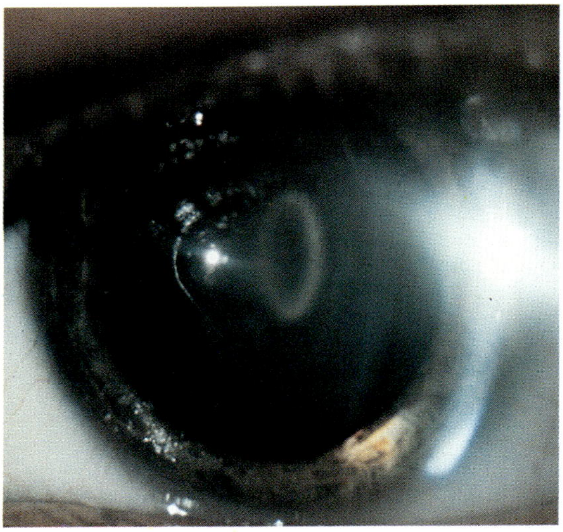

(b)

Figure 11.9 Galactose cataract. (Courtesy of W. Wilson.)

Reduced levels of galactokinase were found in patients with presenile cataract by Skalka and Prchal (1980) (30%), and by Stambolian (1988) (8%), but not by Stevens *et al.* (1989). For uridyl transferase, the figures were 13% (Skalka and Prchal 1980) and 7% (Stevens *et al.* 1989). The role of such abnormalities in presenile cataract appears unresolved.

Galactose-4-epimerase deficiency has been reported to cause both mild and severe forms of galactosaemia (Gitzelmann 1972; Henderson *et al.* 1983).

A high prevalence of lactose absorbers has been reported in adults with senile and presenile cataract in a population in which lactose malabsorption is the norm (Rimaldi *et al.* 1984). Lactase activity is high in the gut of young mammals and commonly declines in the adult human. When lactase persists in the gut, lactose continues to be absorbed and is converted to galactose, which may explain the excess prevalence of cataract in lactose absorbers.

Glucose-6-phosphate dehydrogenase is an enzyme involved in the pentose shunt pathway. There is a large number of enzyme variants. A deficiency may be associated with haemolytic anaemia. Orzalezi *et al.* (1981) reported a red cell deficiency in 30% of patients with cataracts compared with 10% of those without, while Costagliola *et al.* (1988) encountered a deficiency only in diabetic patients with cataract. The latter suggested that the deficiency was not genetic, but was due to inhibition by oxidized glutathione.

Diabetes mellitus

Diabetes causes physical, refractive and cataractous changes in the lens.

The age-related increase in light scattering and fluorescence is greater in diabetics than non-diabetics. An increase in fluorescence has been shown by several workers (Helve and Nieminen 1976; Zeimer and Noth 1984; Sparrow 1992).

The increase in autofluorescence is more pronounced in type 1 and type 2 diabetics, and in the former there is a strong duration-dependent annual increase of about 50% more than that due to age.

Nuclear light scatter is also dependent on diabetes duration and is similarly associated with fluorescence (Sparrow *et al.* 1992). Diabetic retinopathy has been strongly associated with increased autofluorescence, especially in those with shorter duration of disease. With each 1% increase in HbA1c, there is said to be an 11% increase in autofluorescence, suggesting a relationship with diabetic control (Sparrow 1988; van Wirdum 1989).

The fluorescent material has similar fluorescent characteristics to the reaction products of glucose or ascorbate with the lens crystallins (Bensch *et al.* 1985). The blue-green autofluorescence (excitation around 420–430 nm, emission around 520 nm) shows a strong association with duration of disease in early onset diabetes, and a correlation with nuclear brunescence independent of age or diabetic duration, which is not shown by non-diabetics. The association between fluorescence and duration is less strong in late onset diabetes (Sparrow *et al.* 1992).

The clear lenses of diabetics are larger for age than lenses of non-diabetics (Figure 3.10), have a widened subcapsular clear zone (C1α) and a widened zone of disjunction (C1β) (Brown and Hungerford 1982). This is a sufficiently reliable sign to make possible the diagnosis of diabetes at the slit-lamp. The adult diabetic lens is about 15 years older than its non-diabetic counterpart. It has not been determined whether this is due to an accelerated growth rate, hypertrophy of the lens fibres, or to an increase in extracellular water.

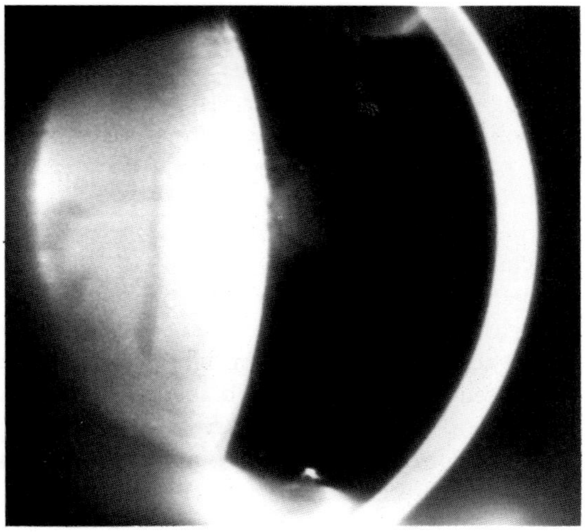

Figure 11.10 An acute diabetic cataract in a child with uncontrolled diabetes. The snow-storm effect extends throughout the cortex.

Refractive changes may be a presenting feature of hyperglycaemia or associated with therapeutic reduction in blood glucose levels. Changes occur in youth and into the eighth decade. This contrasts with the occurrence of juvenile diabetic cataract which is confined to the early decades of life. Visual symptoms occur in about 34% of diabetics at onset, most of which are of refractive origin. Refractive changes occur in another 47% (Granstrom 1933).

Symptoms may evolve over a few hours in untreated hyperglycaemia and resolve over 20 weeks or more on treatment. Eva *et al.* (1982) have emphasized the occurrence of hypermetropia with hyperglycaemia, although myopia was stressed in the earlier literature (Bellows 1944b). Both may occur. A hypermetropic shift has also been reported in response to both insulin and oral hypoglycaemics, which Duke-Elder (1925) suggested might be preceded by a myopic change.

No adequate explanation has been advanced to explain the refractive changes in diabetics. It is assumed to involve changes in refractive index, a result of a relative movement of water into or out of the lens, due to changes in membrane permeability, ion pumps or osmotic events. However, this awaits clarification.

Juvenile diabetic cataract True diabetic cataract, with a characteristic morphology, is seen in uncontrolled young diabetics with onset of disease before the age of 30 years. Rarely, it occurs in infants (Figures 9.23, 11.10). It is now relatively uncommon (Vinding and Nielson 1984). It is assumed to be an osmotic cataract due to the accumulation of sorbitol within the lens, as occurs in experimental diabetes in the rat. The failure of this kind of cataract to occur in older age groups may reflect factors which limit the ability of the older lens to swell, or perhaps limit the production of sorbitol, but it contrasts with the wide age span over which refractive changes occur. Sorbitol is produced by the reduction of glucose in the presence of the enzyme aldose reductase. Its activity is much higher in the murine than the human lens but as noted elsewhere, its role in sorbitol production awaits clarification (p. 74) (Figure 11.11).

The onset of cataract may be preceded by myopia. The cataract forms quickly with dense white anterior and posterior subcapsular opacities in the cortex ('snowflake' cataract). There are also fine needle-shaped polychromatic cortical opacities and subcapsular vacuoles. The opacities may be arrested by treatment in which case they form a lamellar cataract, or may mature to a total cataract within weeks or months (Caird *et al.* 1969).

Cataract in diabetic adults A number of studies suggest that cataract has a higher prevalence in diabetics, is diabetes duration dependent, with a greater risk for women, and has a more rapid progression to surgery (Harding 1988). The morphology of such cataracts cannot be distinguished from that of senile cataract in non-diabetics, but the increased risk applies to cortical and subcapsular cataract rather than to nuclear cataract (Leske *et al.* 1991), which is surprising in view of the presumed role of glycation in nuclear cataract.

Ederer *et al.* (1981) found an excess risk of cataract in diabetics in two population studies. The relative risk for cataract in the 50–64 years age group was increased, at 4.02 (Framingham study) and 2.97 (HANES study) with a decreased risk in the older age groups, possibly reflecting a higher mortality in diabetics with cataracts. In a case control study, van Heyningen and Harding (1986) found an increased risk for cataract extraction in the age group 50–79 years, with a threefold greater risk for women. Hiller *et al.* (1983) showed an association between diabetes duration and cataract, so that in this respect duration is as critical for cataract as it is for other diabetic complications such as retinopathy (Davis *et al.* 1979).

The mechanism for the excess of cataracts in diabetic adults is not known; there is no evidence for an osmotic mechanism. Although sorbitol levels may be increased in the cataractous lenses of diabetics, the amounts found would not cause osmotic damage.

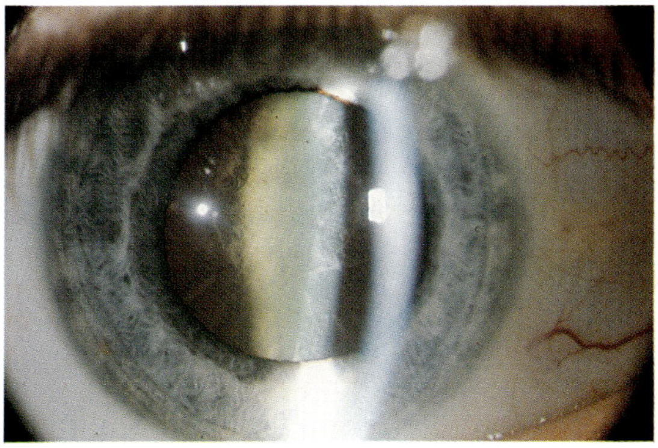

Figure 11.11 Acute diabetic cataract in a child with anterior subcapsular opacities.

It has been suggested that diabetes may render the lens more susceptible to oxidative stress. An increased flux through the polyol pathway could lower the levels of reduced NADPH available for the regeneration of reduced glutathione (GSH). This has an important protective role against oxidative stress and free radical damage.

Another potential mechanism for cataract formation in diabetes is by post-translational modification of lens proteins. Glycation of the lens crystallins is thought to result in the formation of high molecular weight aggregates which scatter an increased amount of light or form brown chromophores which absorb excess light. Similarly, carbamylation of crystallins could be responsible for the formation of crystallin aggregates. It is envisaged too that increased cyanate levels could arise from raised blood urea levels in some diabetics. Such post-translational changes might also affect ion channels and membrane functions. Whatever the actual mechanisms, it is likely that they converge in those responsible for senile cataract.

Hypoglycaemia

Infantile cataract occurs with various forms of hypoglycaemia (idiopathic, ketotic or neonatal) (Brooks 1975). The majority are in males and are associated with prematurity, low birth weight and complicated pregnancy. The cataracts are usually lamellar, which suggests that they may have been subcapsular, but not observed at onset. Subcapsular opacities have been recorded. They are often bilateral, but not necessarily of simultaneous onset. They may be congenital, or appear later in life, when treatment of the hypoglycaemia and therefore of the cataract may be feasible (Merin and Crawford 1971b).

Reversible cataracts have been reported in diabetic hypoglycaemia, whose onset coincided with the institution of diet or insulin therapy. These opacities cleared after treatment, within hours, days or weeks after onset (Brown and Burman 1973; Jackson 1955; Alt 1906). They are assumed to be due to the relative or absolute hypoglycaemia during therapy (Vinding and Nielsen 1984).

Glucose is the major energy source of the lens and it is not surprising that a deficiency can lead to cataract; however, Chylack and Cheng (1978) have also demonstrated that hexokinase, a rate-limiting enzyme for entry of glucose into the glycolytic pathway (Figure 6.14), is destabilized in the presence of hypoglycaemia.

Disorders of lipid metabolism

Fabry's cataract

Fabry's disease is an X-linked lysosomal storage disorder in which cataract of mild degree is found. The condition maps to Xq 21.33–q22.

A deficiency of the enzyme alpha-galactosidase results in the tissue accumulation of a glycolipid, ceramide trihexoside. Affected males suffer from episodic fever and burning pains, hypertension, renal disease and a characteristic skin rash.

A typical spoke-like cataract is found not only in the affected male, but also in a proportion of female carriers (Spaeth and Frost 1965) (Figure 11.12). Also, unusual wedge-shaped opacities, anterior sutural opacities and subcapsular opacities are described (Franceschetti 1976). It is likely that opacities result from the incorporation of the abnormal glycolipid into lens membranes and the effect of this on the structural and light-scattering properties of the fibres.

Cerebrotendinous xanthomatosis (CTX)

CTX is a rare autosomal recessive disorder characterized by dementia, spinal paresis, cerebellar ataxia, and tuberous and tendon xanthomata. Early atherosclerosis occurs, and cataract in over 70%. The basic defect is a deficiency of a 26-hydroxylase involved in bile acid synthesis, in particular of cholic and desoxycholic acids. The resulting deficiency of these acids reduces feedback inhibition of the rate-limiting enzymes for cholesterol synthesis (HMG-CoA reductase) and the increased synthesis of bile acid intermediates leads to overproduction of cholesterol and cholestanol and their deposition in the tissues (Björkhem and Skrede 1989).

Cataracts are of early onset and may require extraction in the first few decades of life.

Disorders of glycoprotein metabolism

Mannosidosis is an autosomal recessive disorder due to a deficiency of acid alpha mannosidase A and B. Mannose-rich glyoproteins and other compounds accumulate in tissues and body fluids producing a severe Hurler-like syndrome (type I) and a milder form (type II).

Lens opacities occur in both forms and appear in infancy or early childhood. They may be posterior (arranged in a wheel or broad spokes) in type I, or scattered dot-like opacities affecting the entire lens in type II. An anterior plaque-like opacity has been recorded (Letson and Desnick 1978) (Figure 11.13).

Other metabolic causes

In addition to those conditions mentioned, the lens is sensitive to many other metabolic disturbances, including: homocystinuria, Hurler's disease, Lesch–Nyhan syndrome, Miller's syndrome, Fanconi's syndrome, chronic renal failure (Berlyne 1972), hypophosphatasia and phenylketonuria.

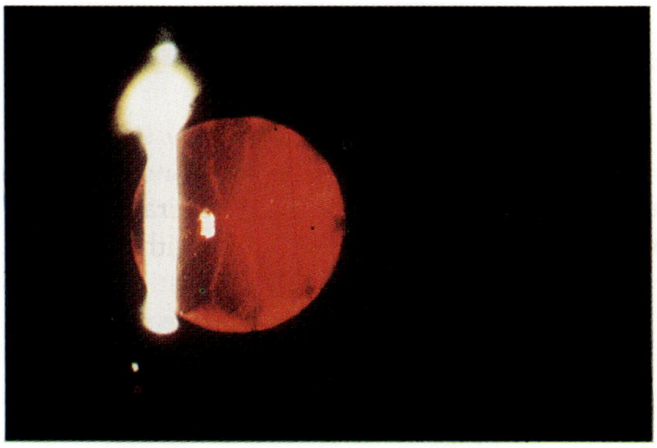

Figure 11.12 Cataract in Fabry disease. (Courtesy of M. Luxenberg.)

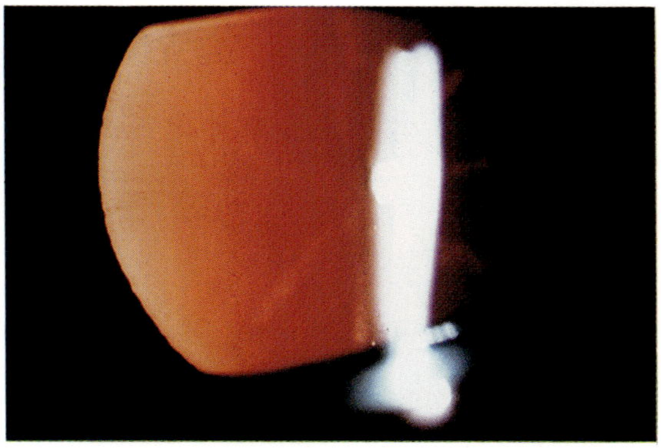

Figure 11.13 Cataract in mannosidosis.

Renal disorders

Lowe's oculocerebrorenal syndrome

This severe X-linked disorder causes mental retardation, renal tubular acidosis and hyperammonaemia, aminoaciduria and renal rickets (Abassi *et al.* 1968). Affected boys show frontal bossing, chubby cheeks and hypotonia in infancy. Blindness occurs from congenital glaucoma and congenital cataract, and corneal keloids are also present (Figure 11.14).

Cataract is usually total, and is difficult to assess clinically because of a resistant miosis. This is due to hypoplasia of the dilator pupillae. Histological study shows the lens to be small and discoid, with poor demarcation of cortex and nucleus, suggesting a defect early in lens embryogenesis (Curtin *et al.* 1967). There is epithelial metaplasia and the capsule shows variable thinning, or thickening with capsular excrescences. The posterior capsule may be adherent to vitreous. There is incomplete cleavage of the anterior segment and the retina extends more anteriorly than usual (Tripathi *et al.* 1986).

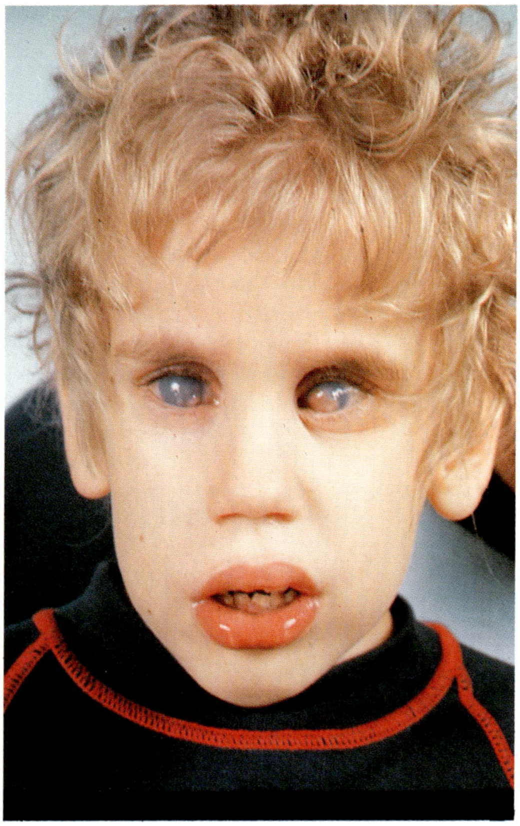

Figure 11.14 Corneal keloid in Lowe's syndrome. (Courtesy of E. Cotlier.)

An excess of focal cortical dot opacities has been reported in carrier females (Figures 10.60, 10.62) (Gardener and Brown 1976; Delleman *et al.* 1977). Lowe's syndrome maps to Xq25–q26.1.

Alport's syndrome

Hereditary haemorrhagic nephropathy with sensorineural deafness is a phenotypically variable disorder which may be inherited as a dominant, recessive or X-linked trait. There is a generalized defect of basement membranes. Ocular features may include microspherophakia and anterior or posterior lenticonus (Figures 8.5, 11.4). Congenital cataract or a postnatal cortical cataract is not infrequent. Allport's syndrome is clinically heterogeneous. There is variation in the onset of deafness and in the severity of renal disease. There are six forms of dominant Allport syndrome as well as X-linked (mapping to Xq 22.3) and possibly recessive forms (McKusick 1992).

Other renal disorders

Crome *et al.* (1963) have described congenital cataract in association with renal tubular necrosis in two sisters.

Musculoskeletal disorders

Dystrophia myotonica

This condition is a dominant disorder in which muscle wasting and tonic relaxation of skeletal muscle are associated with premature baldness, gonadal atrophy and cardiac defects. Intellectual deterioration also occurs. Cataract is a prominent feature and may be the first or only evidence of the disease in a family. Other ocular changes include blepharitis, low intraocular pressure and mild pigmentary retinopathy. Increasing severity and earlier onset of the disease may be encountered in successive generations (anticipation). Myotonic dystrophy is caused by mutational expansion of an unstable [CTG] DNA repeat, mapping to chromosome 19q13.3 and located in part of the

3'terminal exon of a gene encoding a protein kinase. Antibody studies suggest that the protein is localized at sites of neuromuscular and neurotendinous junctions (van der Ven *et al.* 1994).

Cataracts may develop as early as 10 years of age, but in most patients they appear after the age of 20, mature slowly and do not interfere with vision before the age of 40. They occur in 90% of patients (Simon 1962). The degree of cataract does not necessarily correlate with the severity of systemic manifestations (Duke-Elder 1969). There are several stages in their evolution (Bellows 1944a; Gifford *et al.* 1929; Farber 1949):

1. Biomicroscopy shows a dust-like carpet of polychromatic dots and flakes, usually red and green, which are located in the superficial cortex (C2), and avoid both the first clear zone (C1) and the nucleus. They are thus not quite so subcapsular as suggested in many texts. Changes are most marked posteriorly. There is an increase in light-scattering from the superficial cortex (C2) so that demarcation from the subjacent perinuclear cortex becomes less distinct.

   Ultrastructural studies suggest that the multicoloured dots are due to the presence of multilamellar bodies derived from fibre membranes and acting as interference gratings (Dark and Streeten 1977). The lens opacities, when encountered from the 3rd to 5th decades, are highly suggestive of dystrophia myotonica, but resemble changes seen in other diseases (e.g. diabetes and hypocalcaemia).
2. With maturation, the changes become diffuse and may be detected with the naked eye. A stellate opacity appears at the posterior pole in relation to the fibres, which is characteristic (Figures 10.42, 10.43).
3. After many years with little visual impairment, the cataract may advance to complete opacification, necessitating cataract extraction.

Chondrodysplasia Punctata

This is a condition of punctate cartilaginous calcifaction in association with skeletal dysplasia of variable degree. Conradi–Hunermann syndrome shows predominantly epiphyseal calcification, skin changes and a relatively good prognosis. It is inherited as a dominant. Spranger *et al.* (1971) considered that cataract occurred in 17% of this form while Happle (1981) suggested that it was absent. The autosomal recessive form shows stippled calcifaction of hyaline cartilage, dwarfing, proximal limb shortening and skin changes in about 27% of those affected. Cataracts occur in about two-thirds of these patients and are bilateral (Happle 1981). The condition is lethal in the first year of life.

There are also two X-linked forms of this disease, of which the recessive is the milder. The X-linked dominant form is thought to be lethal in hemizygous males; affected females show a variable degree of skeletal change and a patchy atrophic skin change which has been attributed to lyonization of the X-chromosome (Happle *et al.* 1977). Cataract too may be unilateral and of variable degree and occurs in about two thirds (Happle 1981).

Although the eye may be normal except for cataract, it may also exhibit heterochromia iridis, optic atrophy or optic hypoplasia. Histology shows normal primary lens fibres but abnormal epithelial cells, which divide but do not differentiate. It is suggested that the cataract develops at about the fifth gestational month when the lens becomes avascular (Ryan 1970).

Mandibulofacial syndromes

The features of Francois' dyscephalic syndrome (Hallerman–Streiff) include dwarfism, 'bird's head' dyscephaly (beaked nose, deep fronto-nasal angle and mandibular hypoplasia), dental anomalies, skin atrophy and hypotrichosis (Figure 11.15). Ocular signs include microphthalmos and cataract, and less common anomalies including retinal drüsen and angioid streaks. Cataract occurs in 81–90% of cases; they are always bilateral and complete (Francois 1982). The lens substance is commonly liquefied, so that a milky fluid is released at surgery. Occasionally the lens is totally absorbed. This was described in conjunction with aniridia, by Yamamoto *et al.* (1988).

Although many cases of dyscephalic syndrome are sporadic, there are sufficient reports of familial occurrence to suggest a genetic basis. The normal sex incidence and high frequency of parental consanguinity (7%) suggest a recessive disorder. Some reports of affected cases in more than one generation have also suggested dominant inheritance (Koliopoulos and Palimeris 1975), but in one family in which a father and daughter were affected, the grandparents were consanguinous, so this could be an instance of pseudodominance.

Congenital cataract is occasionally encountered in Treacher–Collins syndrome and Pierre–Robin syndrome.

In Stickler syndrome, presenile cataract may occur, in conjunction with vitreo-retinal degeneration, myopia, retinal vascular and pigmentary changes and detachment. Cataract may be of a cortical variety, thought to be congenital and stationary, or a rapidly maturing nuclear sclerosis presenting in the fourth decade (Weingeist *et al.* 1982). However, in the original pedigree of Wagner (1938), characteristic fluffy, dot-like lens opacities which were present in the cortex by the first decade (often forming a striped or stellate pattern) progressed to nuclear opacity and surgery by the age of 35 or 40 years.

Musculoskeletal changes occur in 60% of patients with kyphoscoliosis, marfanoid body habitus or joint hypermobility. Facial abnormalities include maxillary, nasal and mandibular hypoplasia with characteristic facial flattening. Features of Pierre–Robin or Treacher–Collins syndromes may be present. The condition is inherited as a dominant, with variable penetrance and expressivity. In some families Stickler syndrome has been shown to be caused by a mutation in the gene for type II collagen, which is a component of both vitreous and cartilage.

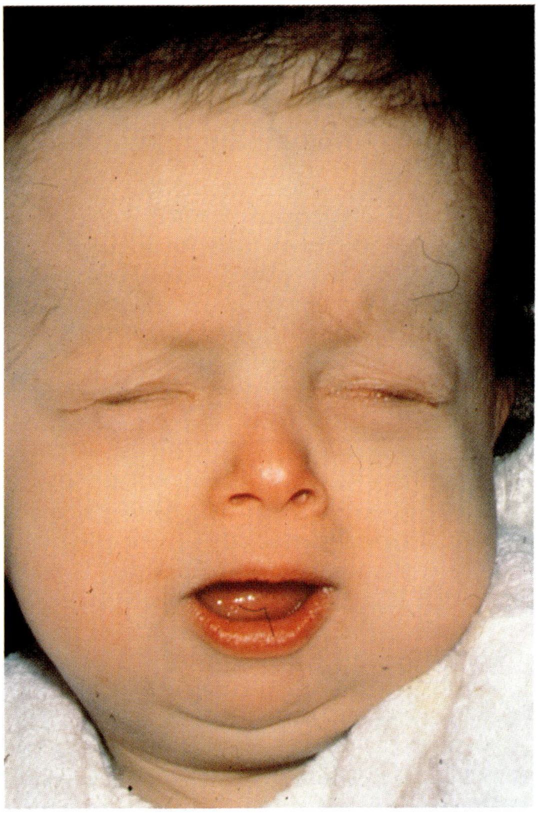

Figure 11.15 Young girl with Hallerman–Streiff syndrome, with bilateral microphthalmos and cataract (Courtesy of D. Taylor.)

Apical malformations

Congenital cataract is reported in a number of cases with apical malformations, especially polydactyly (Francois 1963). In Rubinstein–Taybi's syndrome it occurs occasionally (Roy *et al.* 1968).

Other associations

Zonular or cortical cataracts have been reported in some patients with osteogenesis imperfecta (Wenda 1949) and bilateral congenital cataract in an infant with arthrogryposis multiplex. Cataract, microcephaly, arthrogryposis and kyphosis (CAMAK syndrome) are described as a recessive association. There is a bird-like face and extensive calcification of the cerebrum and cerebellum (Lowry *et al.* 1971; Beyer *et al.* 1956). Zonular cataract has been reported in association with status dysraphicus involving the maxilla (Fonseca 1938) and also congenital cataract with Duane's anomaly.

Pepin *et al.* (1980) reported early onset cataract in a grandmother, mother and son, with mitochondrial myopathy documented in the first two. The grandmother had severe progressive ophthalmoplegia with facial, pharyngeal and limb involvement, the mother had milder signs (cataract extractions were performed at the age of 40 and 32 years respectively). The son was healthy, but had bilateral cataract surgery at the age of 3 years.

Congenital cataract is described as a recessive disorder with mitochondrial myopathy of skeletal and cardiac muscle (Sengers *et al.* 1975; Cruysberg *et al.* 1986).

Dermatogenic cataract

Cataract is associated with a number of skin disorders, many of them inherited. The association is not unexpected since the lens is of ectodermal origin.

Icthyosis

Children with congenital autosomal recessive icthyosis show hypertrophic nails and may be covered with a thick layer of keratin at birth. Sweat glands are atrophic and this may cause neonatal hyperthermia. There is an increased risk of cataract.

Rare cuneiform and nuclear lens opacities are found in X-linked icthyosis (Jay *et al.* 1968).

In congenital anhydrotic ectodermal dysplasia, microphthalmos, cataract and persistent hyperplastic primary vitreous are occasionally described (Merin 1986).

Rothmund–Thomson syndrome

Rothmund–Thomson syndrome is an autosomal recessive disorder characterized by poikiloderma, hypogonadism and cataract. A piebald skin change alternating with sclerosis and telangiectasia appears in the first year of life and hairs and nails may be atrophic (Thomson 1936). Cataracts develop between the second and fifth year of life in about 50% of affected individuals. They are bilateral and rapidly progressive (Warkany 1971).

Werner syndrome

Werner syndrome is an autosomal recessive disorder in which premature ageing occurs in the second decade of life with greying and sparseness of hair, arteriosclerosis, diabetes and hypogonadism. There is a scleroderma-like thickening of the skin, especially of the limbs. Juvenile cataracts are common in this disease (Figure 11.16) (Boyd and Grant 1959; Francois 1963). Death occurs at about the age of 40 years.

Schäffer syndrome

In dyskeratosis palmaris et plantaris, congenital cataract may occur in addition to mental deficiency, dwarfism and hypogonadism (Schäffer 1925).

Incontinentia pigmenti (Block–Sulzberger syndrome)

This is a hereditary disorder affecting eyes, skin, teeth, hair and nails, and skeletal, cardiac and central nervous systems. Inheritance appears to be by an X-linked dominant mode, which is lethal in males. Blister-like skin lesions appear at or shortly after birth, are succeeded by warty outgrowths, and, ultimately, by whorled or feathery pigmented lesions at the level of the dermis. These fade slowly over the years (McKusick 1988).

Ocular changes occur in 35% of patients (Carney 1976), causing blindness (8%) or visual disability (10%) due to cataract, uveitis, chorioretinitis, pseudoglioma, or optic atrophy. Retinal non-perfusion appears to be an early stage leading to retinal pseudoglioma (Watzke *et al.* 1976; Brown 1988; Goldberg and Custis 1992). Early, bilateral changes may lead to squint and nystagmus. Association with other skin disease is reported.

Cockayne syndrome

Cockayne syndrome is a condition of dwarfism, a precociously senile appearance, deafness, marble epiphyses, and visual loss due to pigmentary retinal degeneration, optic atrophy and cataract. There are disproportionately long limbs, with large hands and feet, and joint contractures. A congenital form exists (Lowry 1982). Cells are hypersensitive to UV exposure and show impaired DNA and RNA repair (Mayne 1979; Lehmann 1985).

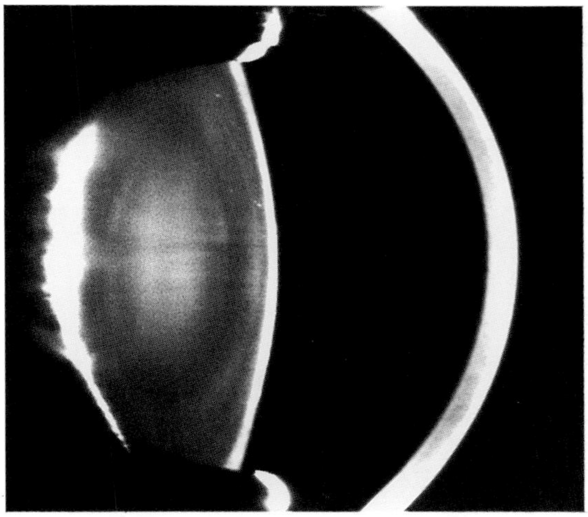

Figure 11.16 The lens in Werner syndrome, which is abnormally small for the subjects age and affected by posterior subcapsular cataract with loss of the anterior subcapsular clear zone (C1α).

Goltz syndrome

Goltz syndrome is an X-linked dominant disorder with lethality in males. There is skin atrophy with linear pigmentation, fat herniation, and multiple papillomata of the skin and mucous membranes. Digital anomalies are common (McKusick 1988). Congenital cataract has been described and Warburg (1970) has observed microphthalmos, bilateral iris coloboma and ectopia lentis in this disorder.

Atopy

Atopic dermatitis is a hereditary disorder, precipitated by a variety of environmental, psychological and infective factors and associated with immunodeficiency. Atopic eczema may present at or around birth and affect the cheeks, extensor limb surfaces and nappy area; in adults the flexures, face, hands, feet or entire body may be affected.

Cataracts occur in about 10% of adults with severe atopic dermatitis (Brunsting *et al.* 1955); they are usually bilateral (70%). Onset occurs between the ages of 15 and 30 years. Other ocular associations with atopy include keratoconjunctivitis, keratoconus and retinal detachment, which may occur in 10% of patients.

The typical form of cataract is the so-called 'shield cataract' which develops as a dense anterior subcapsular plaque with radiating cortical outriders, which wrinkle the anterior capsule as it thickens (Vogt 1921). The 'shield' opacity appears to be due to a localized proliferation of lens epithelium, causing degenerative changes in the underlying cortex (Vail 1966) (Figure 11.17).

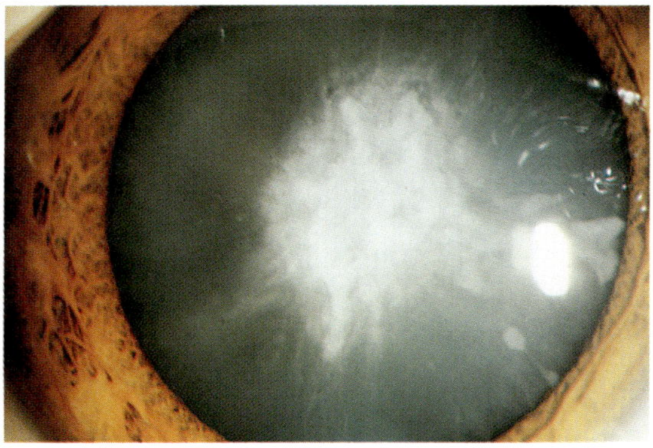

Figure 11.17 Atopy: shield cataract.

A second form involves a posterior subcapsular opacity resembling a complicated cataract, which sends out extensions which involve the anterior cortex (Beetham 1940). Both forms of cataract may progress rapidly until the entire lens is opaque. They are not associated with ocular inflammation.

The mechanism of cataract in this condition and its relation to atopy are not known. Recognition of atopy as the cause of cataract may be complicated by the patient having been exposed to corticosteroids, or the presence of psoriasis, congenital dyskeratosis, anhydrotic ectodermal dysplasia or acrodermatitis enteropathica (Cameron 1986).

Association with central nervous system disorders

Neurofibromatosis type II

Neurofibromatosis type II (NFII) (Figure 11.18) is characterized by dominantly inherited, usually bilateral, acoustic neuromata, associated with numerous intracranial and intraspinal tumours (NIH consensus report 1987). Ocular associations include retinal hamartomata (Good *et al.* 1991), epiretinal membranes, rarely Lisch nodules, and

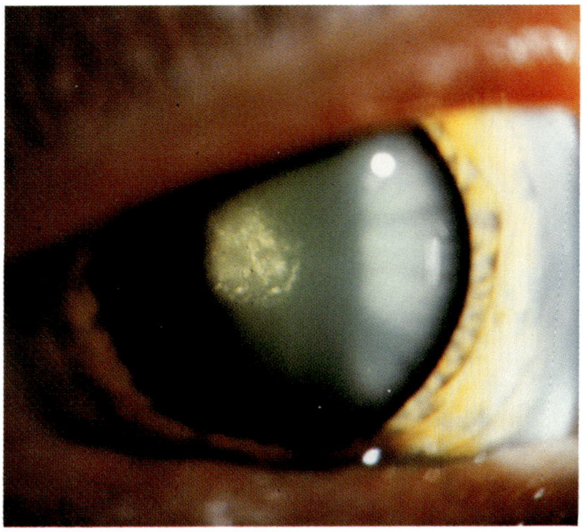

Figure 11.18 Subcapsular cataract in neurofibromatosis type II. (Courtesy of I.H. Maumenee.)

cataract detectable in the second or third decade. The cataracts are posterior subcapsular or posterior cortical, but may include peripheral wedge-shaped cortical opacities (Kaiser-Kupfer *et al.* 1989; Kaye *et al.* 1992). The gene for NFII has been mapped to the middle of the long arm of chromosome 22 (Seizinger *et al.* 1986; Rouleau *et al.* 1987), which is in the region of one of the genes controlling the expression of βB_2 crystallin (Hogg *et al.* 1987).

Törsten–Sjögren syndrome

This is an autosomal recessive disorder in which congenital cataract is found in association with mental defect (Sjögren 1950, 1970). This association is also found on a non-genetic basis.

Marinesco–Sjögren syndrome

In this autosomal recessive disorder congenital cataract is associated with mental retardation and spinocerebellar ataxia.

Crome syndrome

Crome *et al.* (1963) described two female infants with congenital cataracts, epilepsy, small stature, mental retardation, and death at 4 and 8 months respectively. Post-mortem showed encephalopathy and renal tubular necrosis. Renal change is not described in the Marinesco–Sjögren syndrome to which similarities exist.

Myoclonic cerebellar dys-synergy

Ramsay Hunt (1921–22) described progressive myoclonic cerebellar dys-synergy as a dominant disorder with progressive tremor and myoclonus of early onset (about 7 years), due to a lesion of the dentate nucleus and the superior cerebellar peduncle. Franceschetti *et al.* (1954) described bilateral presenile cataract in affected and unaffected family members.

Smith–Lemli–Opitz syndrome

Smith–Lemli–Opitz syndrome is an autosomal recessive disorder in which mental retardation occurs with microcephaly and a typical facies with a high forehead and anteverted nostrils. Syndactyly and polydactyly occur. Cataract occurs in 15% of cases (Kretzer *et al.* 1981).

Zellweger syndrome

Zellweger syndrome (or hepatocerebrorenal syndrome) is an autosomal recessive disorder characterized by dysmorphic features, neurological abnormalities, renal cysts and hepatosplenomegaly (Schutgens *et al.* 1986; Zellweger 1987). Affected infants have psychomotor retardation, hypotonia and seizures. Ocular features include corneal clouding, retinal degeneration and cataracts (Figure 11.19) (Stanescu and Draloands 1972; Hittner *et al.* 1981; Garner *et al.* 1982; Cohen *et al.* 1983). The retina shows extensive photoreceptor damage, with loss of ganglion cells and nerve fibre layer gliosis. There is an accumulation of long chain fatty acids throughout the ocular tissues due to an inherited peroxisomal disorder. Affected infants usually die in the first year of life.

Other associations

Congenital cataract, keratoconus, ectopia of the vitreous and optic atrophy, have been associated with oligophrenia (Pfändler 1950), marked microphthalmos and disorganization of the globe (Whitnall and Norman 1940; Andersen and Warburg 1961).

Cataract, microphthalmos and nystagmus were reported by Harman (1910a,b), with nine persons affected in five generations, and this was associated with extreme miosis in the pedigree of Zeiter (1963). Temtamy and Shalash (1974) suggested a recessive inheritance on the basis of an affected brother and sister with first cousin parents.

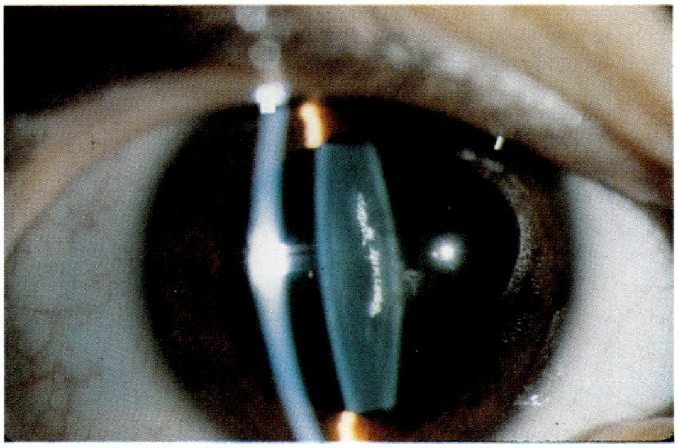

Figure 11.19 Zellweger syndrome. (Courtesy of D. Taylor.)

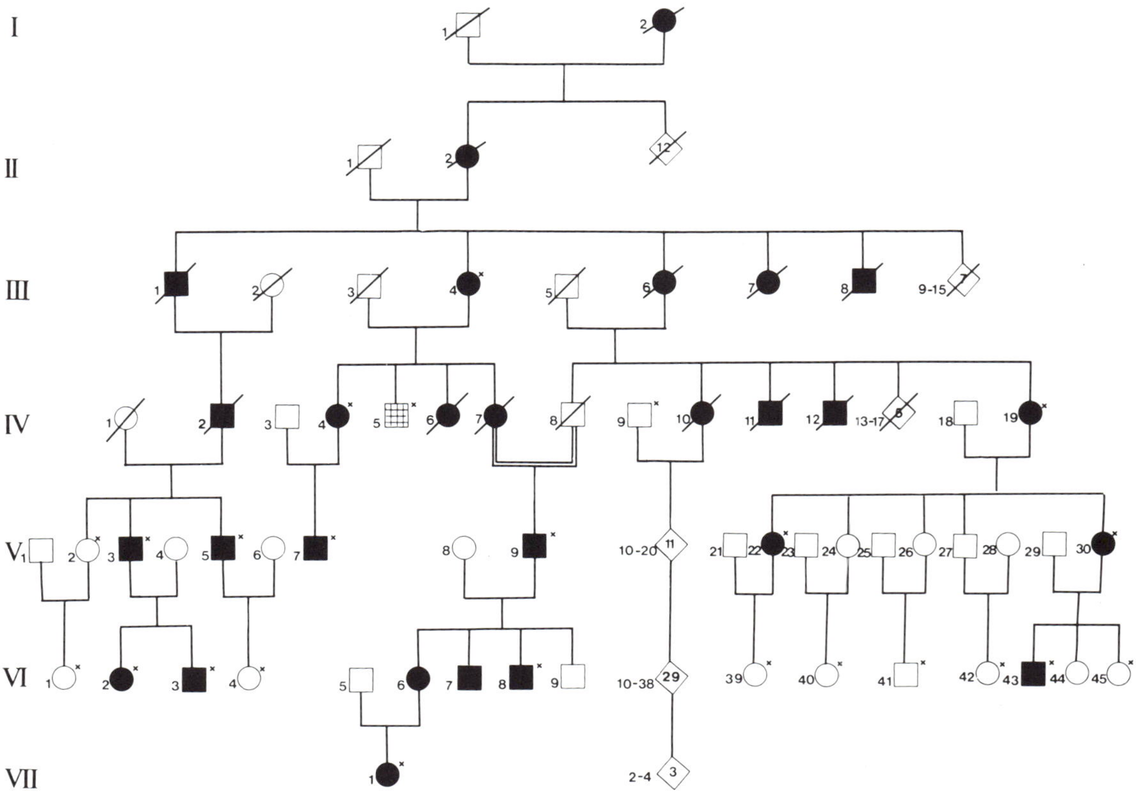

(a)

Figure 11.20(a) Dominant pedigree of microcornea and cataract (only part of the full pedigree is shown).

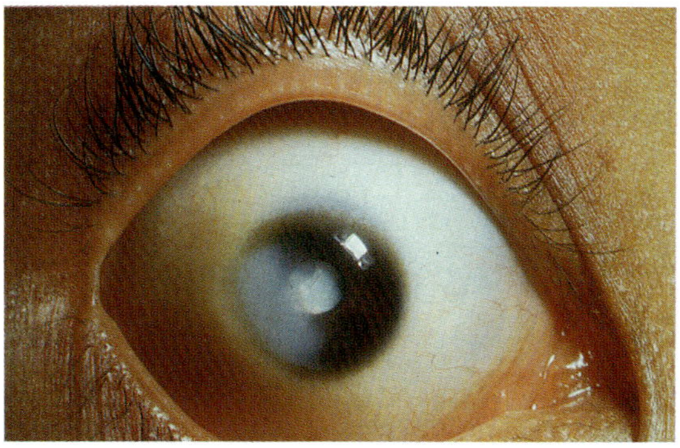

(b)

Figure 11.20(b) Posterior polar cataract (patient VI 25).

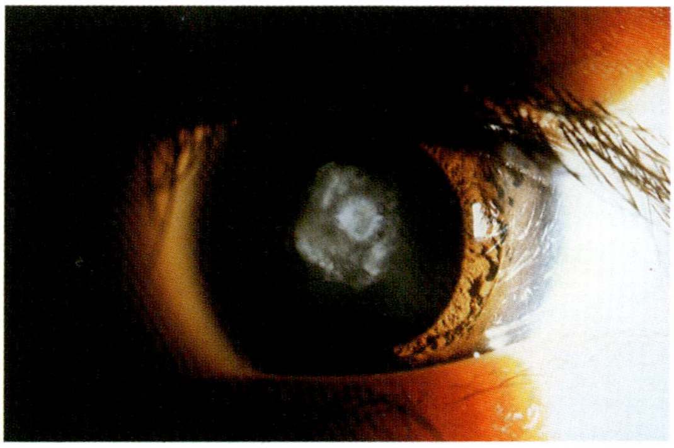

(c)

Figure 11.20(c) Microcornea, corneal opacity and mature cataract (patient VI 30). (Figures from Salmon *et al.* 1988 with permission.)

Infantile or adult onset cataracts occur in association with multiple telangiectia, some with early cardiac disease and aortic stenosis, and known as Nieden's syndrome (Nieden 1887; Terrien and Prelat 1959; Petersen 1954).

Salmon *et al.* (1988) described a family with dominantly inherited cataract with microcornea (Figure 11.20a). The cataract was posterior polar, but lamellar and cortical changes were also seen (Figure 11.20b). Affected patients had sufficient cataract to cause navigational vision by the age of six years but onset and degree were not sufficient to cause amblyopia. Eighteen affected members were described, over seven generations. All corneal diameters were below 11 mm, with the lowest being 9 mm. Six patients showed evidence of mesodermal dysgenesis, with a variable degree of sclerization of the cornea, cornea plana, corneal opacity, anterior synechiae and in one case Peters' anomaly (Figure 11.20c). Microphthalmos was not present. Cataract extraction usually restored visual acuity. The authors proposed that the disorder was due to a defective migration of neural crest cells during development, as in Peters' anomaly (Bahm *et al.* 1984). Microcornea with cataract has been described by other authors (Friedman and Wright 1952; Polomeno and Cummings 1979; Mollica *et al.* 1985; Green and Johnson 1986). In the family of Polomeno and Cummings, coloboma of the iris was associated with zonular cataract, while Mollica *et al.* (1985) described myopia in the presence of normal axial length.

Waardenberg *et al.* (1961) described a family with X-linked inheritance of congenital cataract and microcornea. Slight microphthalmia occurred in an X-linked inheritance also reported by Capella *et al.* (1963). While Witkop-Oostenrijk (1956) described a family with a probable X-linked dominant mechanism, McKusick (1992 – No. 302300) notes that this entity resembles that described by Walsh and Wegman (1937) which may be associated with microcornea (Krill *et al.* 1969).

Walsh and Wegman (1937) described a congenital X-linked nuclear cataract with severe visual impairment in affected males in the tri-racial 'We Sorts' group in southern Maryland. Heterozygous females had posterior sutural cataracts with only slight reduction in vision. Fraccaro *et al.* (1967), performing linkage studies on a similar family, found an Xg locus within measurable distance. Krill *et al.* (1969) described an X-linked pedigree in which sutural cataract is an early manifestation in hemizygous males. Goldberg and Hardy (1971) described X-linked cataracts in two sons whose mother had a sutural cataract. A posterior sutural cataract in a female carrier of X-linked congenital cataract is shown in Figure 11.21.

Crews and Bundey (1982) described a family in which the pedigree could be interpreted as an autosomal dominant inheritance with greater severity in the males. The transmitter female had small dense cataracts in each eye and was asymptomatic. X-linked cataract also occurs in the Nance Horan (Figure 11.22) and Leng syndromes.

Horan and Billson (1974) described two brothers with X-linked sutural cataract, whose two sisters and a mother with normal vision, showed punctate opacities around the Y sutures. The brothers had 'Hutchinsonian' incisors in the absence of syphilis. Nance *et al.* (1974) described a family in which affected males, and also carrier females, had dental anomalies such as supernumerary central incisors in affected males, and screwdriver incisors in heterozygotes. Affected males also showed anteverted pinnae and short metacarpals. Maumenee (1988) has suggested that this disorder, also reported by van Dorp and Delleman (1979) and Bixler *et al.* (1984) is the same as that described by Waardenberg *et al.* (1961). Nance-Horan syndrome maps to X p 21.1–22.2, close to the gene for hypophosphataemic rickets. The mouse X-linked cataract (X-cat) maps to a region of presumptive homology with Nance-Horan syndrome and is likely to be the murine equivalent. (Stambolian *et al.* 1990).

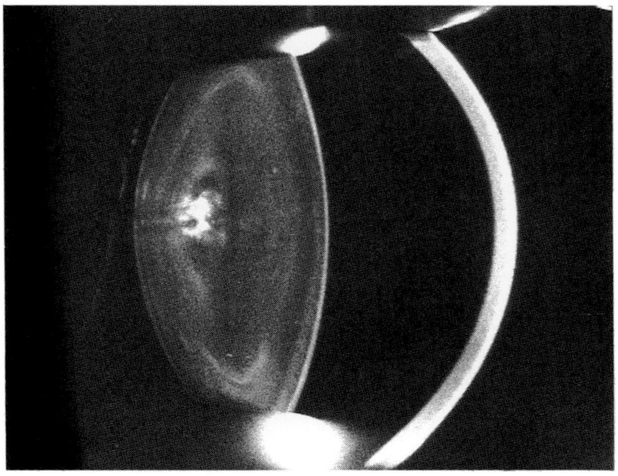

Figure 11.21 Posterior sutural cataract in a female carrier of X-linked congenital cataract.

Norrie disease (Figure 11.23) is an X-linked recessive disorder responsible for congenital or infantile blindness and associated with mental retardation in about 25% of patients, and a cochlear deafness in about 30% (Norrie 1927; Anderson and Warburg 1961; Warburg 1961, 1963). Deafness may begin in infancy or be delayed until adult life (Parving and Warburg 1977). Ocular findings include vitreoretinal dysplasia, resulting in retinal folds, retinal detachment, vitreous haemorrhage, and the formation of a white retrolental mass. Ultimately there is also cataract formation. Carrier females show no abnormality. There is a strong linkage between Norrie disease and the DXS7 locus of the X-chromosome. More recently the gene has been mapped to X p 11.4 (Diergaarde *et al.* 1989) and to Xq 11.3 (Sims *et al.* 1992). The gene may be identical to that for familial exudative vitreoretinopathy) Li *et al.* 1992).

Endocrine disorders

Cataracts have been reported in various forms of hypothyroidism (e.g. myxoedema, cretinism and even post-thyroidectomy in the absence of hypoparathyroidism) (Brooks 1975; Mahto 1972). The reported opacities resemble those of hypocalcaemia and consist of flakes, blue dots or iridescent crystals in the superficial cortex, with little effect on vision. A cause and effect relationship has not been clearly established.

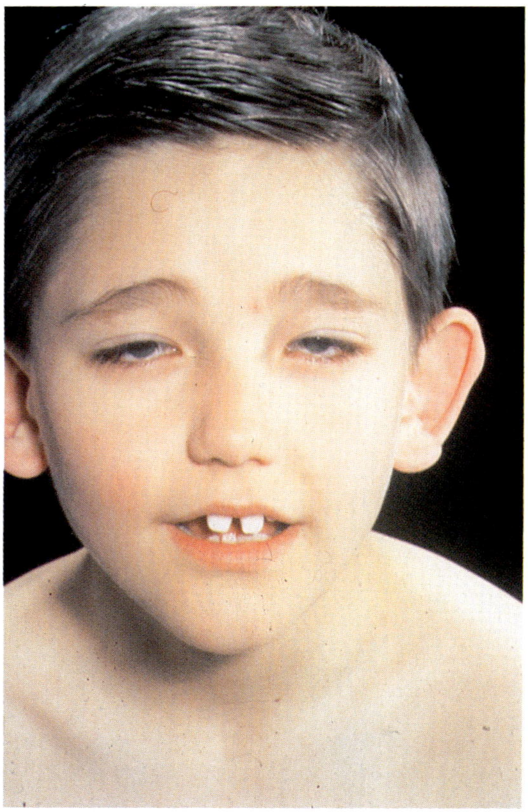

(a)

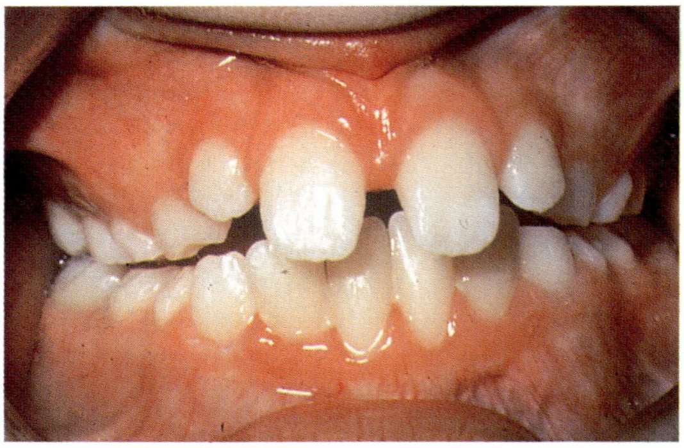

(b)

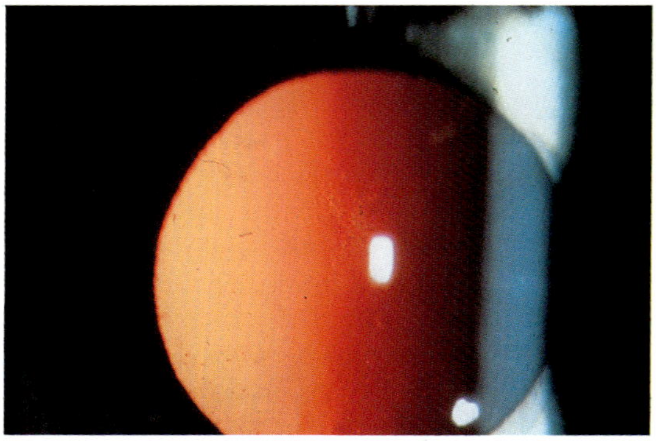

(c)

Figure 11.22(a) Boy with Nance-Horan syndrome; **(b)** showing abnormal incisor and other teeth; **(c)** minor opacities are present in his mother's lenses. (Courtesy of D. Taylor.)

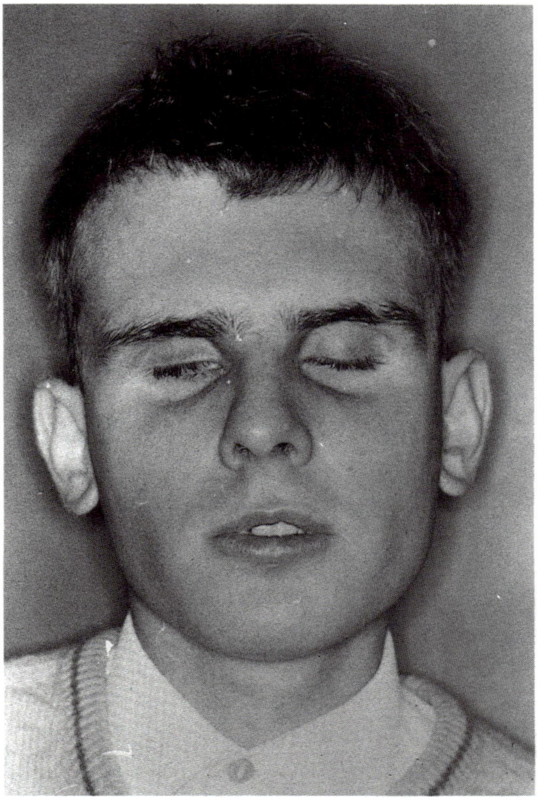

(a)

Figure 11.23(a) Patient with Norrie disease. Note bilateral enophthalmos. (Courtesy of M. Warburg.)

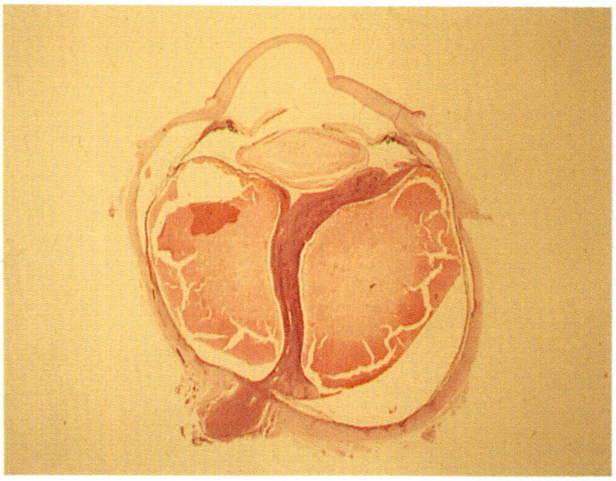

(bi)

Figure 11.23(bi) Low power view of detached and dysplastic retina in Norrie disease. (Courtesy of O. Jensen and M. Warburg.)

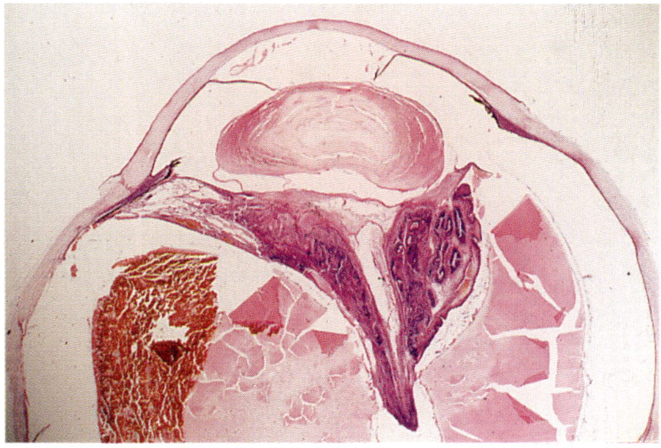

(bii)

Figure 11.23(bii) High power view (Courtesy of O. Jensen and M. Warburg.)

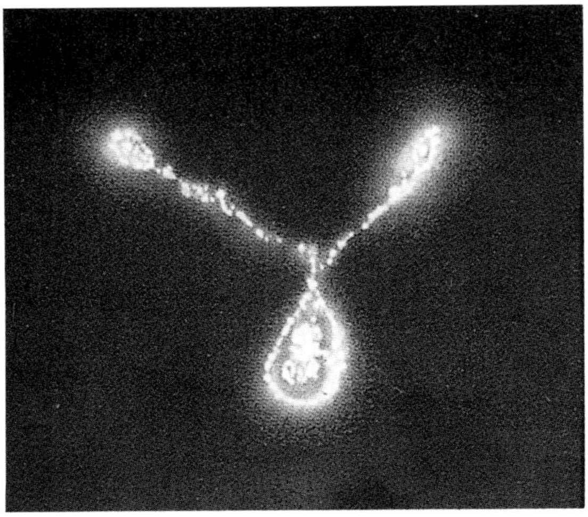

I A form of anterior embryonal sutural cataract.

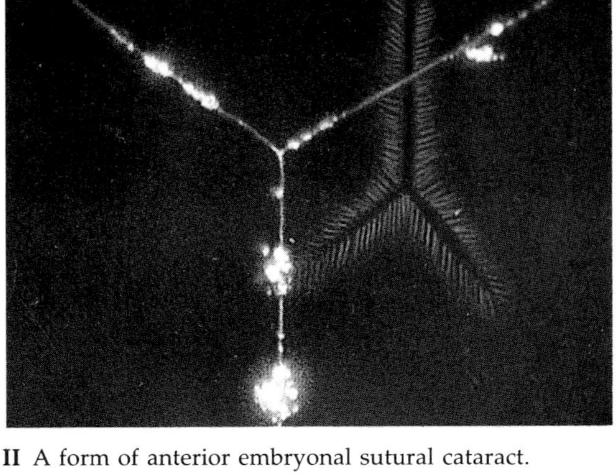

II A form of anterior embryonal sutural cataract.

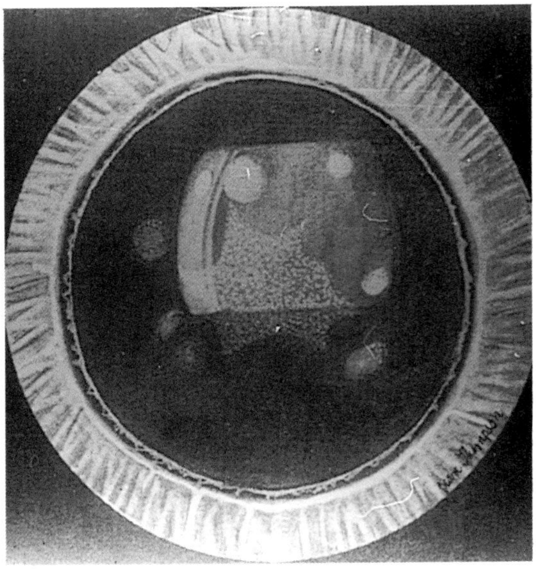

III Capsular flakes.

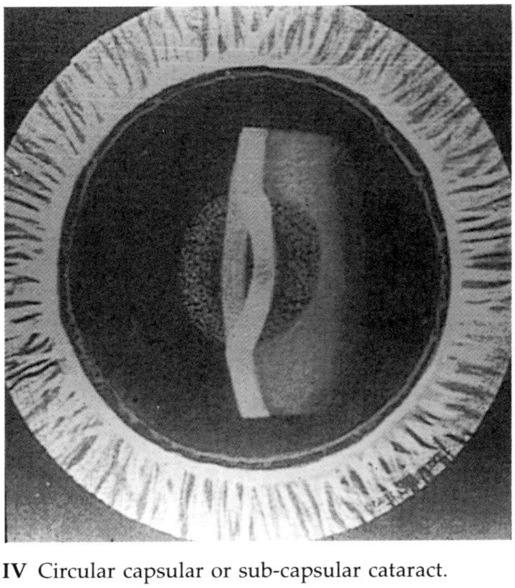

IV Circular capsular or sub-capsular cataract.

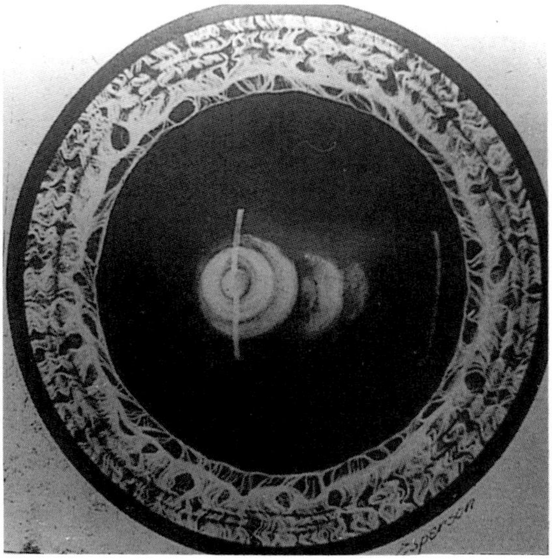

V Axial fusiform cataract in 27-year-old male in which only the anterior half of the fusiform spindle is present. This extended into the embryonal nucleus.

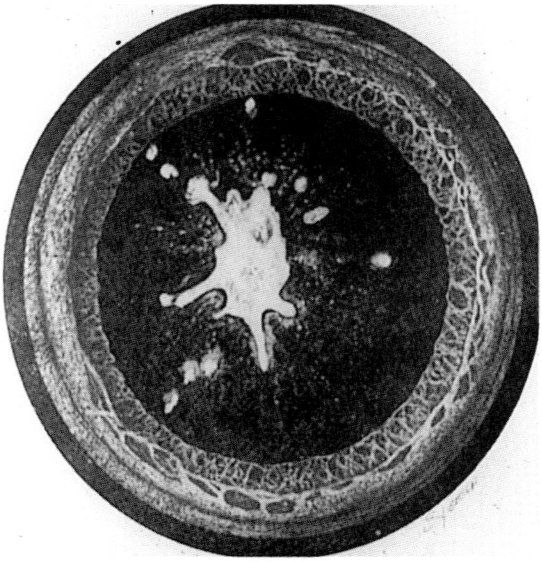

VI Cataract associated with atopic dermatitis.

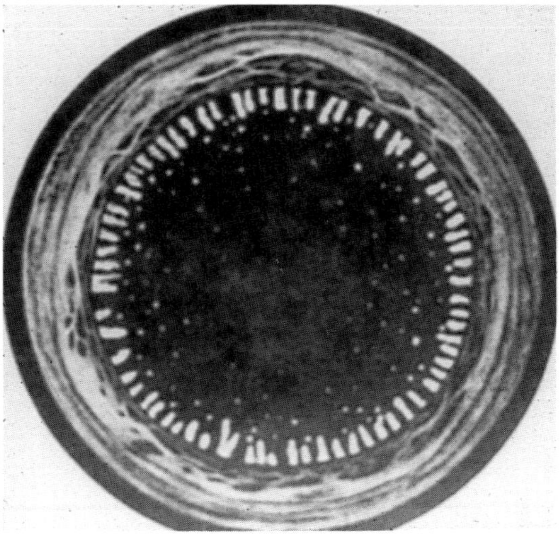

VII Coronary cataract.

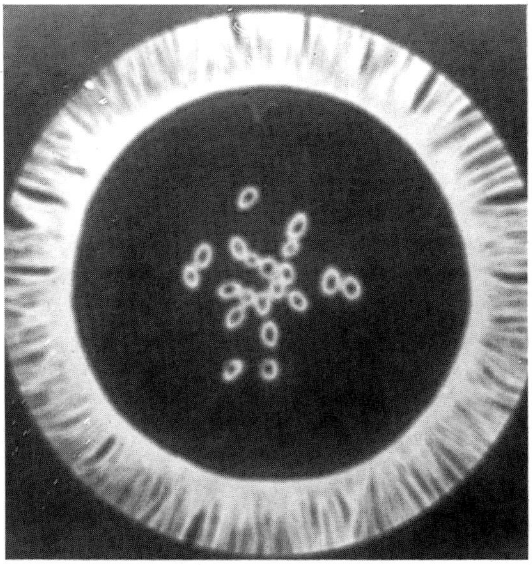

VIII Floriform cataract.

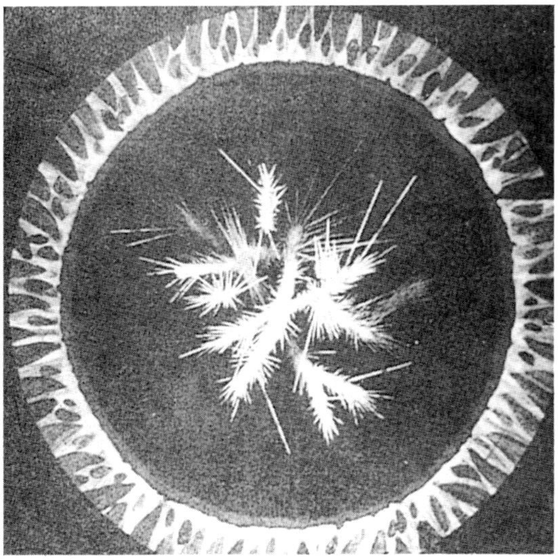

IX Spear cataract in the right lens of a 6-year-old girl.

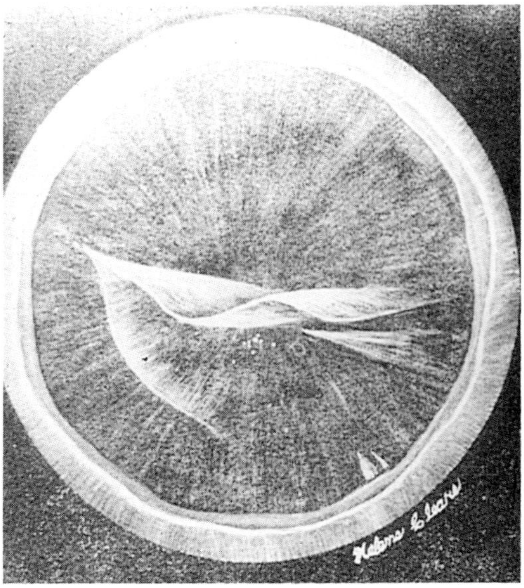

XI 'Glass-blowers cataract': note exfoliation of the lens capsule. A disc-shaped flaky opacity is present in the posterior cortex.

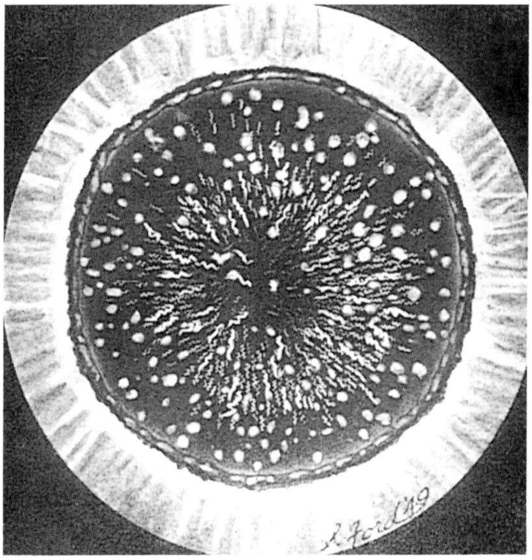

X Spirochaete-like opacities associated with cerulean cataract.

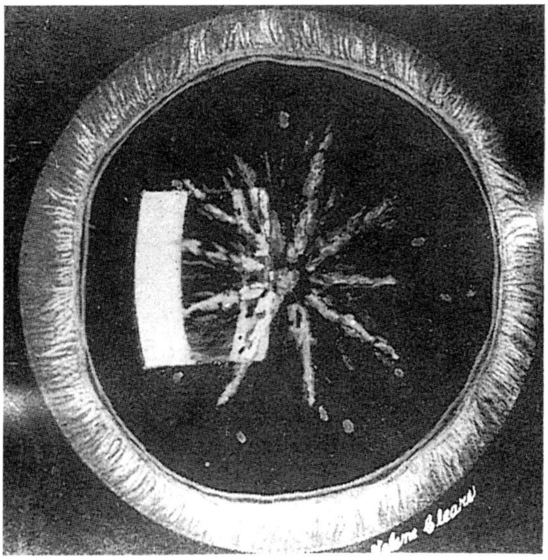

XII Stellate cataract present in Down's syndrome.

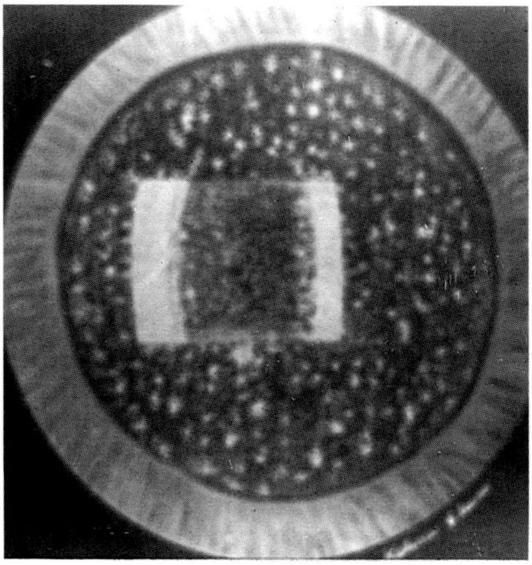

XIII Snowflake opacities present in the cortex in a juvenile diabetic cataract.

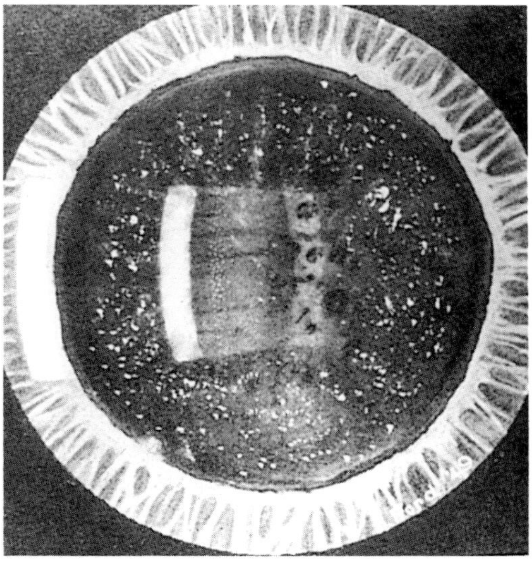

XIV Tetanic cataract present in a 38-year-old woman.

12

Aetiological classification of cataract: ocular, toxic, nutritional and physical factors, and senile cataract

Local ocular disease

Glaucoma

There appears to be little, if any, relationship between chronic simple glaucoma and cataract (Watson *et al.* 1990), but the relationship to miotic treatment has been noted (p. 196). There is an increased incidence of cataract following glaucoma drainage surgery and cataract, which tends to be anterior subcapsular, has been seen to occur as a complication of the persistently shallow anterior chamber following drainage surgery (Kanski and McAllister 1989) and related to hypotony. A localized anterior cortical cataract may follow peripheral iridectomy and is probably due to direct lens trauma (Figure 10.41).

Nuclear cataract may be seen as a sequel to angle closure glaucoma and occurs frequently in absolute glaucoma (glaucoma flecks are described on p. 153).

Uveitis

Intraocular inflammation commonly results in subcapsular cataract, but may also cause cortical and nuclear cataract. The posterior subcapsular cataract may be preceded by polychromatic lustre (Figure 9.11) when the posterior capsule is examined by specular illumination.

The posterior cortical and subcapsular cataract is typical of chronic uveitis, but it may be difficult to decide whether this is due to the disease or to corticosteroid treatment (p. 195). It is commonly seen in Fuchs' heterochromic cyclitis as an early sign prior to treatment.

Lens changes, consisting of loss of the anterior subcapsular clear zone, may be seen in acute uveitis and this change is usually followed by recovery on treatment. However, it proceeds to anterior subcapsular cataract when the uveitis is resistant to treatment as may be seen to occur in herpes zoster. Curiously, the cataract is quite commonly segmental and this may reflect the segmental involvement of the iris (Figure 12.1). The epithelium may be affected with glaucoma fleck-like opacities (Figure 9.13). In juvenile rheumatoid arthritis (ANA positive) and in intermediate uveitis (chronic cyclitis) there is a particular risk of cataract. Later, nuclear scattering and brunescence may occur.

Retinitis pigmentosa

Cataract is associated with the inherited retinal degenerations. Pruett (1983) found a frequency of 46% in retinitis pigmentosa (RP), of which 98% were posterior subcapsular. Heckenlively (1988) reports posterior subcapsular cataract in 41%, with opacities ≥ mm in diameter in 27% of patients, and of a lesser degree in the remainder. It is reported in 40–49% of eyes in patients with autosomal dominant, recessive and X-linked RP (Heckenlively 1988) (Figure 12.2).

Onset of cataract is to some extent related to the age at presentation of the disorder; it is therefore earlier in recessive and X-linked forms. In Leber's congenital amaurosis, onset is between the ages of one and ten years, with an increasing frequency with age. Posterior subcapsular cataract is said to occur in 18% of patients, and cortical cataract in 68%. Cataract is frequent in Usher's syndrome but its occurrence is not consistent (Figure 12.3). Although anterior subcapsular cataract and nuclear cataract are cited to occur in simplex retinitis pigmentosa (isolated cases without family history) (Heckenlively 1988), it is not clear that these are specific features. The former is a frequent accompaniment of posterior subcapsular cataract of any cause. Although the cataract in retinitis pigmentosa has been often described as subcapsular, the adjacent cortex is commonly seen to be affected for some depth, suggesting development over several years. Cataract extraction is worthwhile in RP, despite the presence of the retinal degeneration; vision improved to 20/50 in the series of Heckenlively (1988).

Pathologically the epithelial cells show degenerative changes, including mitochondrial swelling, and there is posterior migration of epithelial cells to form aberrant lens fibres. The posterior capsule may be duplicated (Eshagian *et al.* 1980; Fagerholm and Phillipson 1985).

The mechanism for cataract in retinitis pigmentosa has not been established. Many forms of retinitis pigmentosa result from a mutation in the gene for the photopigment, rhodopsin (e.g. there are dominant forms of RP which map to chromosomes 3, 7p, 7q, 8pter, 19q13.4, and an X-linked form of RP2 mapping to Xp11.3-p11.2, as well as dominant RP due to an RDS peripherism mutation). This knowledge makes it very unlikely that the cataract is due to a direct gene effect on the lens itself. It is more likely that lens damage results from toxic products released by the degenerating retina (e.g. malondialdehyde or lysophospholipid) or from the absence of a factor synthesized by the retina, such as $_{\beta}$FGF, which is important to normal lens growth.

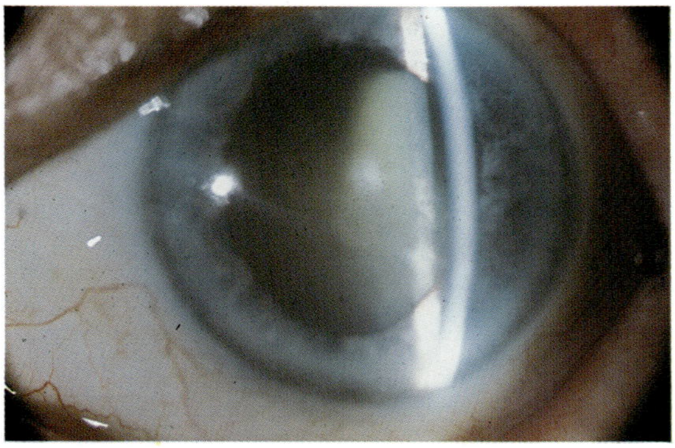

(a)

Figure 12.1(a) Segmental cataract in herpes zoster.

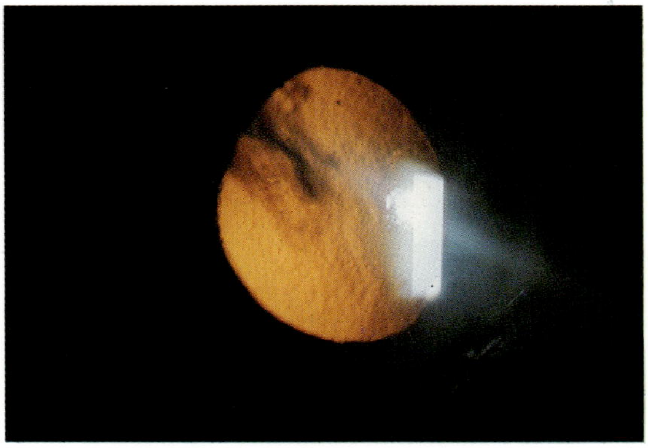

(b)

Figure 12.1(b) Segmental cataract in herpes zoster (retro-illumination).

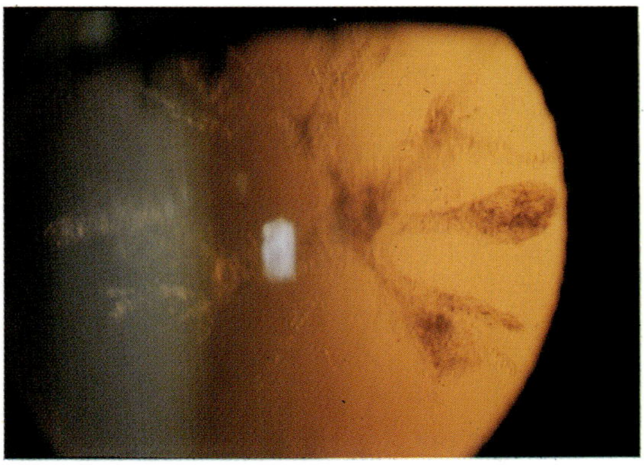

Figure 12.2 The posterior cortical complicated cataract in retinal degenerative disease.

Hyperornithinaemia with gyrate atrophy

Hyperornithinaemia with gyrate atrophy of the choroid and retina is an autosomal recessive disorder presenting in childhood with night blindness, peripheral field loss and myopia. Peripheral patches of chorioretinal atrophy develop, whose confluence and scalloped borders give the condition its name (Takki and Simell 1976; Kaiser-Kupfer *et al.* 1985, Berson *et al.* 1978, Weleber and Kennaway 1988). Subcapsular cataract develops in early adult life and includes a feathery opacification of the posterior sutures which can be traced from the capsular surface into the depths of the superficial cortex (Figure 12.4). Cataract surgery may be required in middle age. Reasonable visual acuity may be maintained until about the age of 50 years, when it is reduced by cataract or macular changes. Slight structural changes have been recorded in

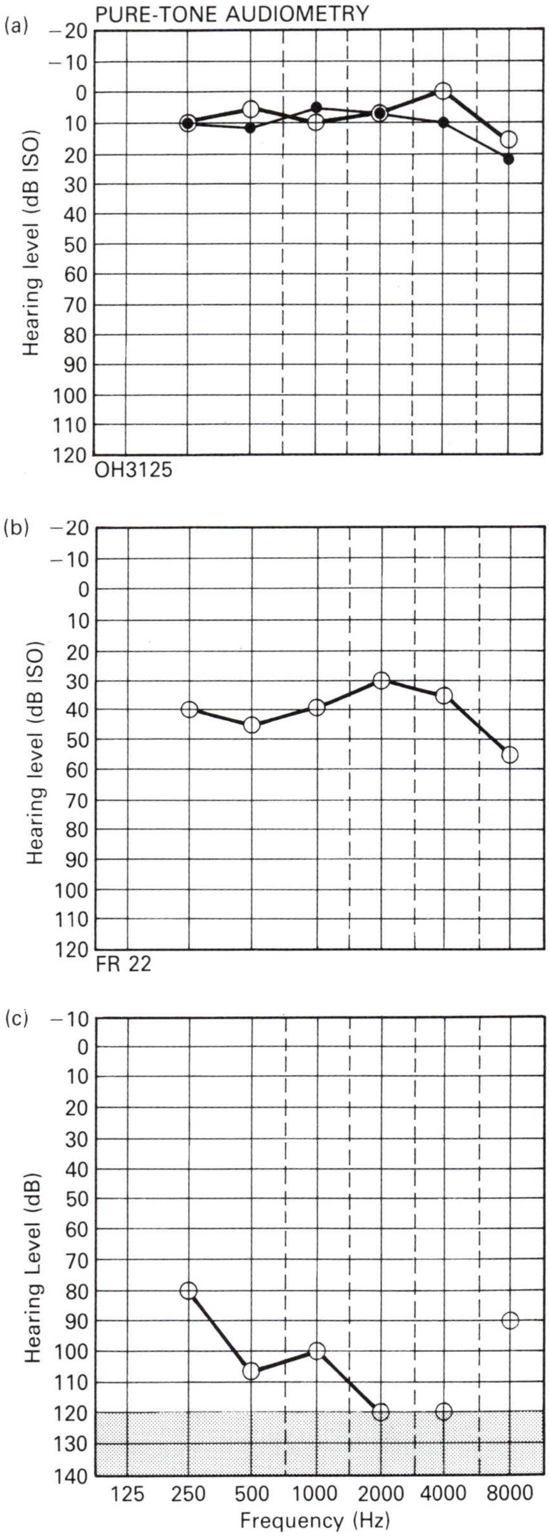

Figure 12.3(a) A normal audiogram, showing a normal auditory threshold on the right and left. (Courtesy of A. Freeland.)
Figure 12.3(b) Intermediate level of neurosensory loss in a patient with Usher's syndrome Type II (b and c, courtesy of the Usher Society.)
Figure 12.3(c) Severe neurosensory loss in Usher's syndrome Type I.

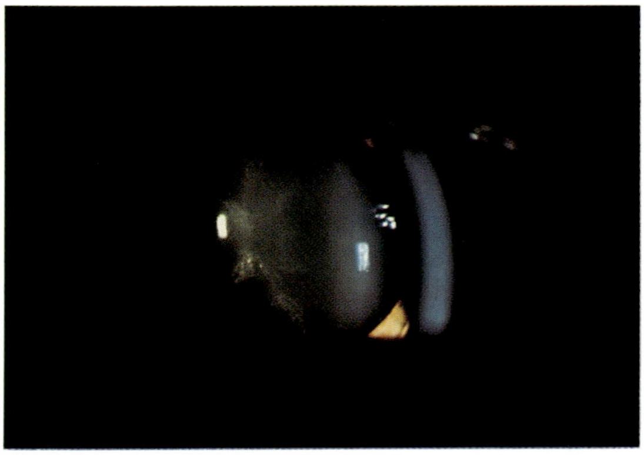

Figure 12.4 Lens opacity in hyperornithinaemia with gyrate atrophy (HOGA).

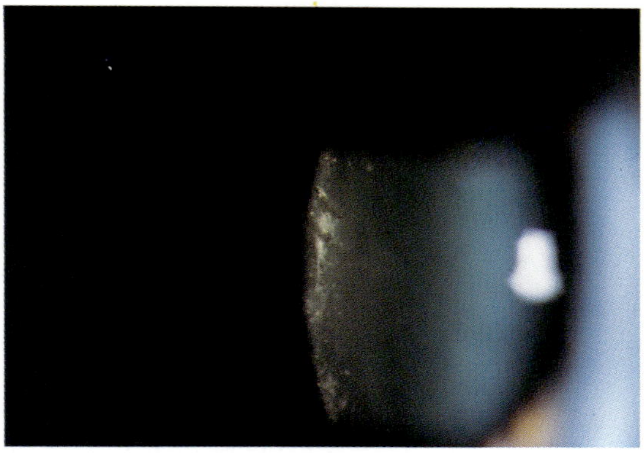

(a)

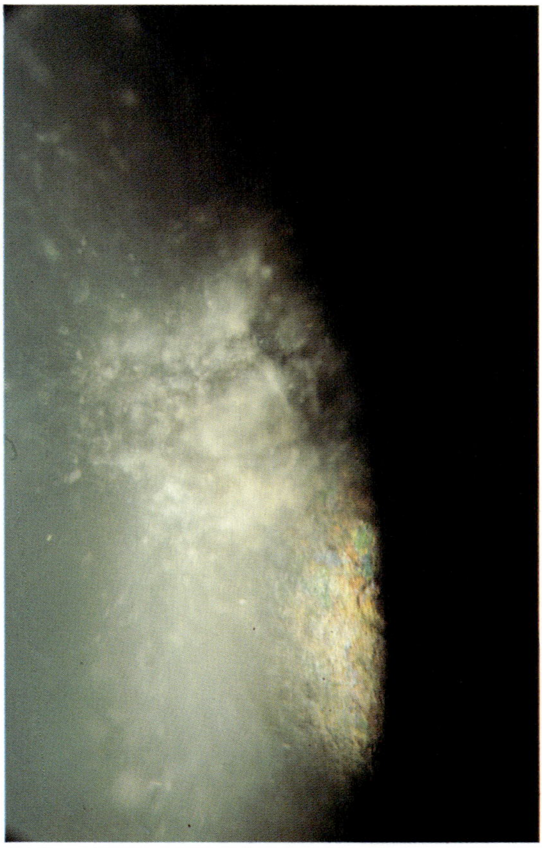

(b)

Figure 12.5(a,b) Complications of myopia.

muscle and hair, and mild mental retardation may occur (Kaiser-Kupfer 1981).

The disease is due to a mutation or deletion of the gene for the enzyme ornithine aminotransferase which is carried on chromosome 10q26 (Inana *et al.* 1988).

Myopia (Figure 12.5)

A posterior cortical, subcapsular and nuclear cataract is also seen in degenerative myopia. The posterior cortical cataract is granular and affects the axial region.

An association between cataract and non-degenerative myopia has been suggested by the finding of myopia presenting with cataract (Weale 1980; Perkins 1984). However, much of the apparent myopia is induced by nuclear cataract itself, and it appears that moderate degrees of simple myopia do not predispose to cataract (Brown and Hill 1987).

Retinal detachment and retinal surgery

Cataract, usually posterior subcapsular, follows retinal detachment and surgery for this condition (Yoshioka *et al.* 1965). It occurs frequently following vitrectomy (de Bustro 1988) and particularly with silicone oil injection (Figure 12.6) (Foulds 1987) and

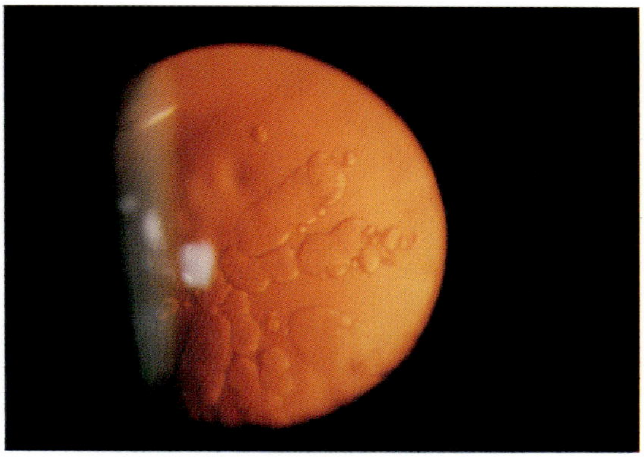

Figure 12.6 Cataract associated with periretinal vitreous retraction (Courtesy of J. Scott.)

with gas injections (see below). Scott (1979, 1982, 1990) has reviewed the relationship between massive vitreous retraction (MVR) and cataract (Figure 12.7). Watzke (1967) found cataract in many MVR patients, usually after unsuccessful surgery, and Dufour (1968) also associated cataract with persistent detachment, although one case had cataract prior to surgery. Okun (1967) reported an incidence of 51% in 300 patients reviewed at 5 years after surgery, while Leaver *et al.* (1979) found cataract over a 10-year period in 71% of patients treated with silicone oil.

Although posterior subcapsular cataract may occur with MVR, the characteristic form is anterior subcapsular, developing independently of surgery or the use of silicone oil, over a period of 9–12 months. Uveitis is unlikely to be a contributing factor since such eyes are free of uveitis in about 90% of cases (Scott 1979).

Histologically, the anterior subcapsular change is due to metaplasia of the lens epithelium central to the germinative zone. The laying down of an organized collagenous membrane may result in technical difficulties at cataract surgery. At the slit-lamp the earliest sign is wrinkling and thickening of the lens capsule. This is followed by cortical swelling and opacity, attributed to a failure of epithelial pumps (Scott 1979) (Figure 12.7).

Vitrectomy with gas tamponade

A transient posterior subcapsular cataract appears within 24 hours of surgery for retinal hole, vitreous haemorrhage or membrane peeling involving vitrectomy and gas (e.g. SF6) tamponade. A similar event follows the use of silicone oil. The cataract has a feathered appearance and consists of a branching subcapsular sheet corresponding to the posterior suture system and the fibre tips which insert into it (Figure 4.12). These features are made visible on retroillumination by relative differences in intra- and extracellular refractive index which appears to reflect a fluid overload. Superimposed on the feathered pattern are a series of flattened vacuoles aligned in the axis of the sutures and the fibres, which give the cataract a distinctive appearance. The subcapsular cataract is transient, gradually fading away over about 2 weeks. In a smaller proportion of patients the subcapsular cataract is followed by the development of a nuclear cataract, either increased scattering or brunescence. It appears to be an accelerated form of age-related nuclear cataract. The mechanism of these cataracts is not established. A possibility concerning the nuclear cataract is that it is due to a transient loss of the protective influence of the cortex at the time of posterior subcapsular cataract formation (Hsuan *et al.* 1994).

Anterior subcapsular cataract may also be encountered as a congenital disorder associated with remnants of the tunica vasculosa lentis, with anterior polar cataract (Hendkind and Prose 1967), with severe intraocular disease (Lamb 1937), and following direct lens trauma.

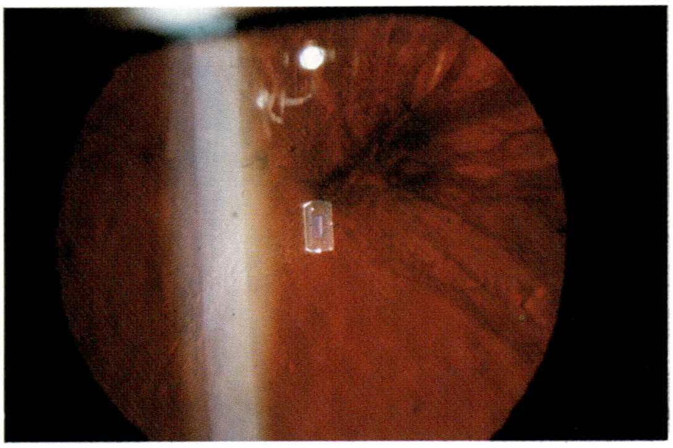

Figure 12.7 The amorphous nature of anterior subcapsular cataract. In this case the cataract is due to neutron radiation.

Tumours

Cataract occurs in association with intraocular tumours. Ciliary body tumours (Figure 12.8) may be associated with cataract in the form of cortical lamellar cataract in the affected quadrant. The contour of the lens may also be distorted by the tumour.

Ischaemia

Anterior segment ischaemia is commonly a local effect and follows encircling surgery for retinal detachment, or it may be part of a generalized cranial ischaemia, as in carotid stenosis and pulseless disease. Cataract may be subcapsular or nuclear and progress is rapid.

Complicated cataract

Cataract consequent to eye disease is traditionally described as complicated cataract. The lens is totally dependent on the health of the eye for its metabolism and so is inevitably affected when the eye cannot supply oxygen and nutrients, or when toxic substances are produced. As noted above, complicated cataract occurs in association with glaucoma, inflammation, retinal disease, tumour, ischaemia and also infection. Complicated cataracts are commonly subcapsular.

Infective cataract

A number of infective conditions, including herpes zoster (Figures 9.13, 12.1), are indirectly responsible for causing cataract by first causing uveitis. The intact capsule represents a barrier to bacteria, but organisms occasionally do gain access to the lens substance and cause abscess and cataract. Cataract is well known to occur in the neonate following maternal rubella infection and has been reported in the neonate in syphilis, cytomegalovirus disease and in herpes simplex (also see section on experimental cataract (p. 131)).

Toxic causes of cataract

Many drugs and chemicals are known to cause cataract, sometimes of a characteristic appearance. For other substances a relationship has been inferred on epidemiological grounds.

Drug induced

Corticosteroids

The cataract of glucocorticoid toxicity was first described by Black *et al.* (1960) in patients on long term systemic therapy for rheumatoid arthritis. It is now recognized to be unassociated with the systemic diagnosis, and may occur in any condition receiving long term therapy, such as asthma, systemic lupus erythematosus, nephrotic syndrome and renal transplantation. It is characteristically a posterior subcapsular cataract (Figures 10.54, 10.55, 12.9).

Posterior subcapsular cataract is said to occur in about 21% of patients on corticosteroid therapy for rheumatoid arthritis, compared with 0.2% of young adults or 0.6% of adults in their fifth or sixth decade and not receiving steroids (Spaeth and von Sallmann 1966). Early studies suggested that steroid cataract was dose-related, with an 11% incidence with treatment in a moderate dosage range and 78% in a high dosage range, when treated for between 1 and 4 years, and 57% and 83% with treatment for more than 4 years (Black *et al.* 1960). Subsequently there have been conflicting reports about a dose-response relationship, perhaps reflecting the difficulties of defining the details of dosage, scheduling and duration. In general it is unusual for posterior subcapsular cataract to be induced in

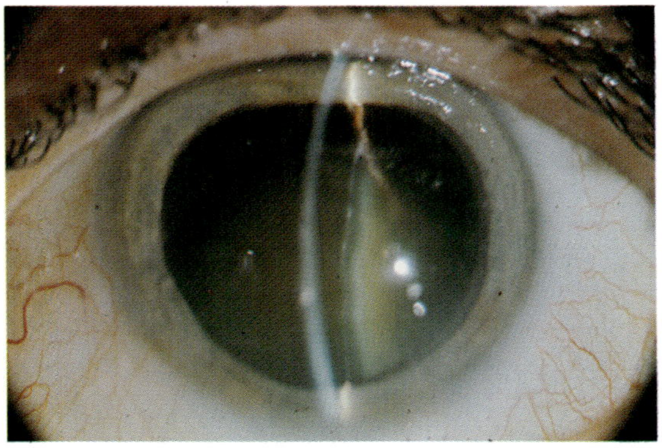

Figure 12.8 A ciliary body tumour distorting the lens and causing cataract.

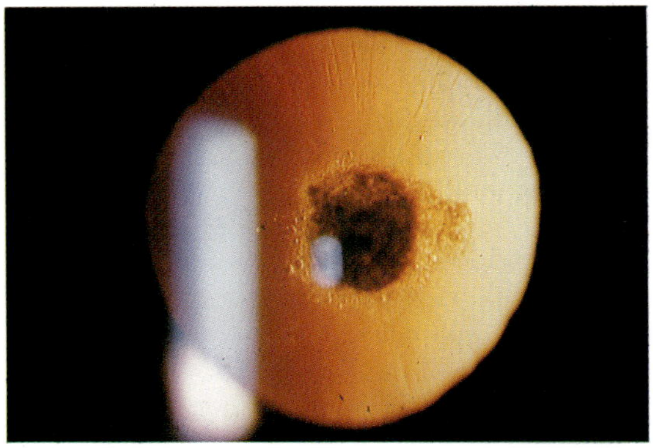

Figure 12.9 Posterior subcapsular cataract.

adults within 1 year of treatment. A dose of prednisone of 10 mg/day or less is regarded as a safe maintenance dose for at least 1 year (Giles *et al.* 1962; Crews 1963; Spaeth and von Sallmann 1966).

Children are said to be more susceptible to corticosteroid cataract than adults, with development of posterior subcapsular cataract at lower doses and within a shorter time. Some have shown changes within 6 months of starting treatment (Dikshit and Avasthi 1965; Loredo *et al.* 1972). Although, as has been stated, the relationship between dosage and incidence of posterior subcapsular cataract is unclear, the possibility that the difference in behaviour in children relates simply to body weight dosage must be considered.

Posterior subcapsular cataract can also occur with topical corticosteroid use, particularly in the presence of an epithelial corneal defect. Valerio (1963) reported cataract in a 25-year-old man treated topically for 6 months. It is also recognized as a complication in chronic treatment of corneal grafts with topical steroid therapy. Burde and Becker (1970) recorded the reversible occurrence of cortical vacuoles in two young volunteers treated topically. Reversal over a period of 10 months was reported by Streiff in posterior subcapsular cataracts in a young man treated with topical steroids for allergic conjunctivitis. Minor fluctuations in size and density of posterior subcapsular cataracts of various causes have been recorded over short periods of time (Shun-Shin *et al.* 1989).

Steroid-induced cataract has a characteristic morphology which may suggest its aetiology. The earliest change is a polychromatic lustre in the posterior capsule. In time an axial (sometimes eccentric), discoid posterior subcapsular opacity of 2–3 mm in diameter appears within the subcapsular clear zone, which gradually increases in size. This process may take many years. The borders are usually sharp but are sometimes surrounded by a grey haze. Vacuoles may be present at a distance from the main mass. The opacity is made up of opaque particles, separated by vacuoles of various sizes, appearing together as a conglomerate mass within which red, green and blue reflections occur.

Steroid cataract may resemble other forms of posterior subcapsular cataract, such as that due to ionizing radiation, uveitis and high myopia, as well as age-related and complicated cataract. In these disorders a narrowing of the anterior clear zone is universal when the opacity is of significant size, and may infrequently be accompanied by an anterior subcapsular cataract, usually of lesser density.

Usually, for instance in age-related or radiation posterior subcapsular cataract, the lens is reduced in size because of a failure of new fibre formation and differentiation. Recently it has been observed in the steroid cataracts of renal transplant patients that axial lens thickness is increased, even in the presence of posterior subcapsular cataract, which would normally be associated with reduced thickness. It is noted that the posterior cortical opacity becomes separated from the posterior capsule by a distance related to the time from transplantation. In the study of Shun-Shin *et al.* (1990) it was concluded that the cataractogenic insult occurred chiefly in the peritransplant period and that the formation of the posterior subcapsular opacity was followed by the growth and differentiation of new cortical lens fibres which interposed between lens capsule and cataract. In this way the posterior cortical clear zone is restored as normal growth resumes; the anterior clear zone was not reduced in these patients. If corticosteroid treatment is withdrawn, the opacity becomes more compact and separate from the lens surface.

It has been suggested that the pathogenetic mechanism of posterior subcapsular cataract involves the posterior migration of equatorial epithelial cells followed by the formation of abnormal fibres in the posterior subcapsular region (Eshagian and Streeten 1980). Although this has been observed with steroid cataracts, it is less easy to accept as a generalization for the early central discoid opacity where the peripheral posterior capsule may appear biomicroscopically clear.

Anticholinesterases and other miotic drugs

Anticholinesterases were used extensively in the past in the management of chronic open angle glaucoma. The ability, particularly of the irreversible anticholinesterases (such as diethyl-*p*-nitrophenol phosphate (Mintacol) and di-isopropyl-fluorophosphate (DFP) to cause cataract was first suspected in 1954, by Kreibig, who reported its development in a patient receiving treatment with DFP over a period of several weeks. These observations have been confirmed by several retrospective (Axelsson and Holmberg 1966; De Roetth 1966; Shaffer and Hetherington 1966; Tarkkanen and

Karjalainen 1966; Axelsson 1969a) and prospective studies (Morton *et al.* 1969). The cataract affects the anterior subcapsular zone of the lens, starting with minute vacuoles, which later aggregate into larger configurations associated with mossy patches and streaks. The effect on vision is severe, because the pupil is intensely miosed by such drugs.

The incidence of cataract due to phospholine iodide, in strengths ranging from 0.06–0.25%, was cited to be between 33% and 62% by Patterson (1971). The effect, which is dose related and accelerated by increasing age, may be static or progressive after stopping therapy (Drance 1969; Axelsson 1969b).

Harrison (1960) reported complete reversal of a DFP-induced cataract in a child, which had developed after three months of treatment.

Mechanism No convincing model of anticholinesterase cataract exists, but biochemical changes have been produced *in vitro*.

De Roetth (1966) demonstrated reduced cholinesterase activity in response to such drugs, and Laties (1969) showed localization to the anterior lens surface. Michon and Kinoshita (1968) demonstrated a depression of oxidative metabolism in the lens, differing in degree with different miotics. They also demonstrated an increased permeability of the lens and altered sodium and potassium content, albeit at high drug levels. It has been suggested that cholinesterase is involved in ion transport in the lens.

Phenothiazines

In the high doses required for psychotropic action the dimethylamine, chlorpromazine causes pigmentation of the skin, conjunctiva, cornea and lens. A daily dose of 300 mg/day up to a total dose of least 500 g appears to be the minimum to produce ocular effects. The incidence of skin and conjunctival pigmentation (about 0.1–1%) occurs at a high dose level (e.g. a minimum of 800 mg/day for 20–24 months. Corneal and lens changes are more frequent and occur at a lower dose (e.g. 20–35% of patients receiving over 500 mg/day for 3 years).

The lens changes precede the corneal changes and consist of fine brownish-white punctate axial opacities (Figure 10.47). These develop into a large stellate opacity related to the suture and finally into an anterior polar cataract (Mathalone 1967; Bernstein 1983).

Chlorpromazine is a photosensitizing agent. Absorption of energy by the drug leads to the formation of highly reactive free radicals which could be responsible for lens damage. Lullmann *et al.* (1975) have suggested that chlorpromazine may cause cell damage by combining with phosholipid and forming an insoluble, intra-lysosomal lipid complex, a kind of drug-induced lipidosis.

Radiomimetic drugs

Cataract has been reported experimentally with a number of antimitotic drugs after systemic administration, including nitrogen mustard, triethylene melamine (von Sallmann 1965; von Sallmann and Grimes 1966), 4-(*p*-dimethylamino-styryl) quinoline (Christenberry *et al.* 1963), 2,3,5, tris (ethyleniminο)-benzoquinone (trenimon) and mimosine (β-(3-hydroxy-4-pyridone) α-amino propionic acid (von Sallmann *et al.* 1959; Tittarelli *et al.* 1961).

Clinically, busulphan may cause a posterior subcapsular cataract (Hamming *et al.* 1976). Since radiomimetic agents may be used in combination with systemic steroids for the purposes of immunosuppression in bone marrow and renal transplant patients, it is possible that such cataracts may have a synergistic basis (see above).

Allopurinol

This drug is in common use for the treatment of gout. An association with cataract has been reported in some, but not all, studies. Liu *et al.* (1988) described an anterior subcapsular cataract.

Antimalarials

A white, flake-like posterior subcapsular lens opacity is said to occur in 20–40% of patients receiving chloroquine, but not hydroxychloroquine (Bernstein 1983). Yellowish anterior subcapsular dots have been reported in patients using amiodarone (Flach *et al.* 1983). Both these changes may be examples of toxic lipidosis (Lullman *et al.* 1975, and see above).

Chemical

Several locally or systemically administered substances can produce cataract. These include the local effects of chemicals as in chemical corneal burns and the systemic effects as in poisoning (see van Heyningen 1969, for a fuller account).

Toxic chemicals applied to the cornea produce anterior punctate lens opacities similar to glaucoma flecks and have been attributed to secondary ocular pressure rise (Houle and Grant 1973) (Figure 9.12); these are probably due to epithelial necrosis. On the rare occasions when an insect sting discharges venom into the anterior chamber, it causes a cataract that passes into maturity in days (Chen and Richardson 1986).

Other chemicals and toxins which have been implicated include: ergot, aromatic nitro compounds such as dinitrophenol, dinitro-*o*-cresol and trinitrotoluene (Teir and Grenquist-Nordén 1990), substituted hydrocarbons such as naphthalene and paradichlorobenzene, heptachlor and tetracaine.

Cigarette smoking has been identified as a risk factor for nuclear cataract (Flaye *et al.* 1989) and it has been suggested that this is due to carbamylation, or thiocarbamylation, of lens proteins by the cyanide present in smoke (Harding 1991; Harding and van Heyningen 1989). The cataract is of the nuclear type (West *et al.* 1989) which is to be expected with an agent affecting proteins (p. 96). Alcohol consumption in moderate quantities is also a risk factor for cataract (Harding 1988). Hyperbaric oxygen has been shown to cause a myopic shift and nuclear opacity, with nuclear vacuoles (Palmquist *et al.* 1984).

Some drugs may have a protective effect against the development of cataract, as suggested by the negative risk in case control studies for certain non-steroidal anti-inflammatory agents such as aspirin and ibuprofen, and analgesics such as paracetamol (Harding 1988).

Bedazac lysine, a non-steroidal anti-inflammatory has been shown to reduce the rate of development of nuclear scatter (Shun-Shin *et al.* 1994).

Metal ions

Metals tend to deposit as granules in the capsule and anterior cortex in the pupillary area of the lens, which may be due to the effect of light as in the photographic process.

Calcium

Hypocalcaemia Hypocalcaemia occurs in association with hypoparathyroidism, pseudohypoparathyroidism, rickets and hypocalcaemia of infancy. Lens opacities may occur in as many as 50% of post-parathyroidectomy patients with hypoparathyroidism (Ireland *et al.* 1968).

In the infant or child the cataract is generally lamellar. Rarely, the embryonal or fetal nucleus is involved. In the adult, hypocalcaemia produces anterior or posterior punctate subcapsular opacities which are sometimes blue in colour. With treatment of the hypocalcaemia a residual lamellar cataract is formed (Figure 12.10). Otherwise there is progression to a total cataract (Bellows 1944a; Haft 1953).

Pseudohypoparathyroidism All forms of this disorder have in common a resistance to parathyroid hormone. Patients are hypocalcaemic and hypophosphataemic despite high plasma parathyroid hormone levels. In pseudohypoparathyroidism type 1a (Albright osteodystrophy) there is resistance to multiple hormones, and patients have characteristic physical abnormalities such as short stature, obesity, round face and shortened metacarpals. Hypocalcaemia is responsible for tetany, enamel hypoplasia, basal ganglia calcification and cataracts. The genetic defect involves the lack of a G protein which couples the parathormone receptor to the synthesis of cAMP.

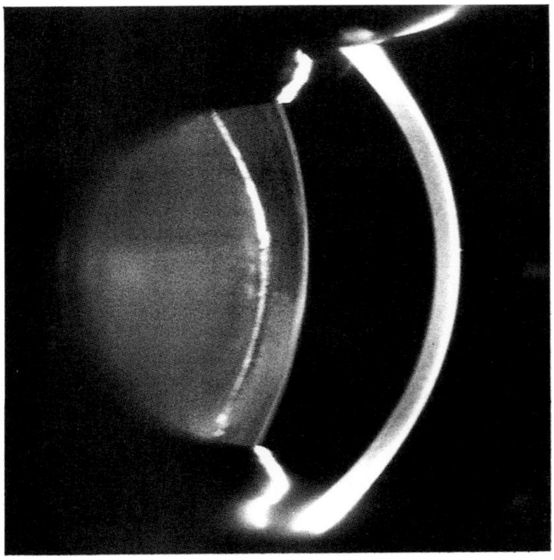

Figure 12.10 A lamellar opacity in an adult aged 58 years resulting from hypocalcaemia occurring 25 years previously.

Copper

Chalcosis of the lens (Figure 12.11) Copper may be deposited in the lens as a result of the use of copper sulphate-containing eye drops, copper ingestion, the presence of an intraocular copper-containing foreign body, or as part of Wilson's disease (hepatolenticular degeneration). The latter is an autosomal recessive disorder in which there is defective transfer of copper to the copper-carrying enzyme ceruloplasmin and reduced biliary excretion of copper. The levels of free copper in the serum are raised. Severe liver damage and other visceral features occur, in addition to involuntary movements due to involvement of the extrapyramidal system. A brown corneal ring at the level of Descemet's membrane is pathognomonic of the condition, as is the typical, sunflower cataract, which occurs in under 10% of cases.

Sunflower cataract is a disc-shaped polychromatic opacity present in the pupil zone anteriorly and extending petal-like spokes towards the periphery. Minute rainbow-coloured shimmering dots give a velvety appearance to the anterior surface of the lens. Posterior changes are less marked, and in the form of a greenish shagreen. The cataract has little effect on vision and is not visible against the red reflex (Hanna 1975). There is a deposition of metallic copper in the lens capsule (Tso *et al.* 1975). Sunflower cataract may be completely reversed during treatment of Wilson's disease with penicillamine (Walshe 1976).

Iron (Siderosis) (Figures 10.45, 10.46, 12.12, 12.13)

Cataract due to ferrous ions occurs in siderosis following the retention of an intraocular iron-containing foreign body. Iron deposits in the lens epithelium and fibres cause a brown discoloration, and iris heterochromia occurs. The ferrous ions are toxic and a flower-shaped cortical cataract occurs. This differs from the copper cataract in that there is actual lens fibre opacity in siderosis. The cataract may be sufficient to cause visual loss, although it is the associated retinal damage which is responsible for blindness.

Haemosiderosis lentis is due to iron staining resulting from intraocular haemorrhage.

Other metals

Mercury salts have been used as a preservative in eye drops and mercury is deposited in the capsule as a fine sheen after long-term use of such drops (Figure 10.9).

Gold is deposited in the lens as fine golden granules in the capsule and epithelium (Figure 12.14). This occurs after long term therapeutic use of gold. Corneal and conjunctival deposits are also a feature of gold toxicity.

Silver toxicity (argyrosis) is characterized by deposits throughout the tissues of the eye. In the lens it deposits as bluish granules in the pupillary area of the capsule and the anterior cortex (Cowan 1961).

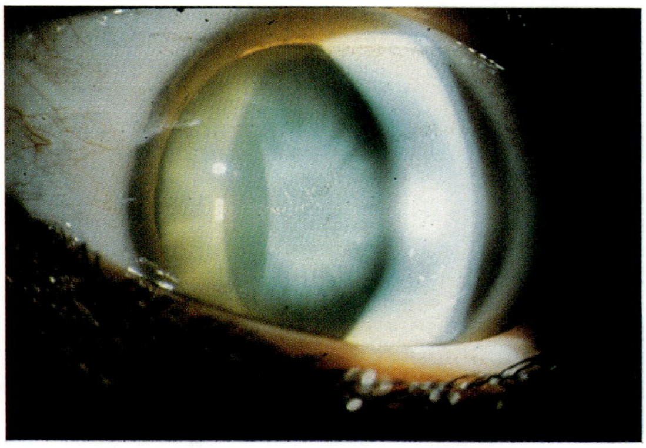

Figure 12.11 Cataract in a patient with Wilson disease. (Courtesy of J.M. Walshe.)

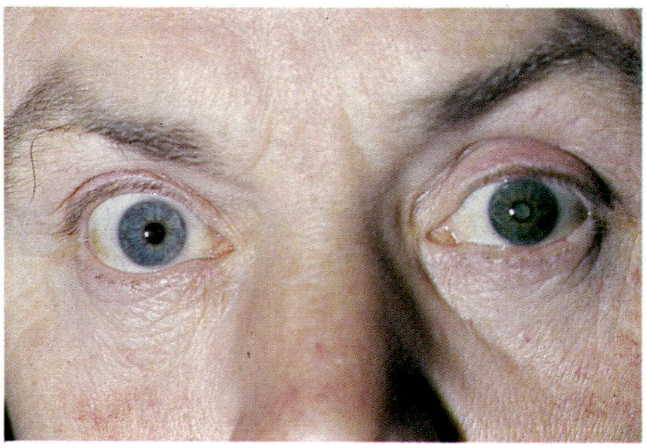

Figure 12.12 Iris heterochromia due to siderosis.

Cataract may occur occasionally on exposure to thallium. It has been reported in the deep anterior and posterior cortex (Kubesova 1949)

Nutritional factors

Epidemiological studies suggest that nutrition plays a role in the development of cataract. In areas of good nutrition, cataract is more common in those of low socio-economic status, low stature and low educational achievement (Khan *et al.* 1977). The antioxidant status of persons with cataract has been shown to be reduced compared with persons without cataract (Jacques *et al.* 1988). In other studies a vegetarian diet has been implicated (Das *et al.* 1990).

Lens proteins are denatured by chemical attack including oxidation by free radicals in the lens (Harding and Crabbe 1984). These free radicals are neutralized by the antioxidant vitamins. Lack of these vitamins may explain cataract in persons of poor nutrition.

A cataract which may pass rapidly to maturity is occasionally seen in anorexia nervosa (Miller 1958) (see Figure 13.3).

Physical factors

Dehydration

Cataract has been shown to occur in association with chronic diarrhoea in epidemiological studies

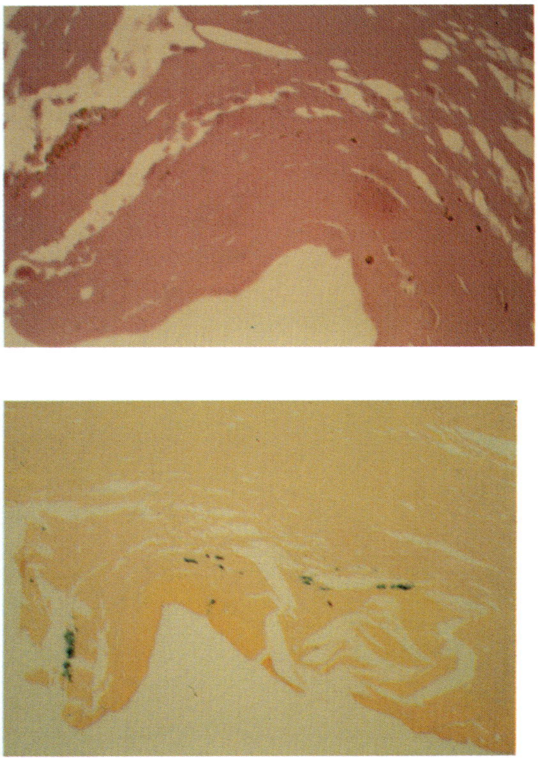

(b)

Figure 12.13 Siderosis of lens. **(a)** H & E (magnification ×100). **(b)** Perl's reaction for iron (magnification ×40.) (Courtesy of A. Garner.)

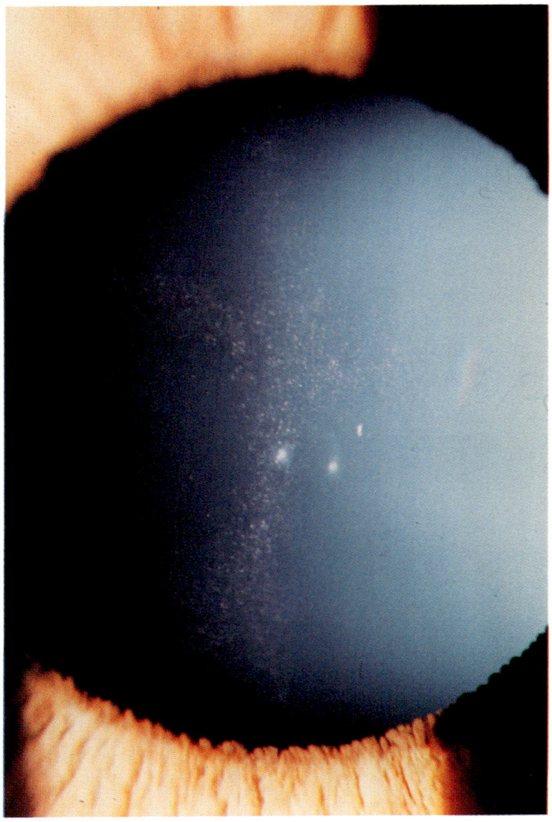

Figure 12.14 Anterior capsular and subcapsular gold deposits in a patient treated with gold injections.

(Harding 1989) and in acrodermatitis enteropathica, in which diarrhoea and zinc loss occurs (Cameron and McClain 1986). The use of purgatives may be a factor in causing cataract in anorexia nervosa.

Hyperbaric oxygen

Hyperbaric oxygen has been shown to cause a myopic shift and nuclear opacity with nuclear vacuoles (Palmquist *et al.* 1986) (Figure 12.15).

Trauma

The lens may receive physical damage from concussion of the eye, by penetration of the eye and lens with a sharp object, or by a high velocity foreign body. Electric shock is a further cause of physical damage.

The transparency of the lens may be affected by physical energy in a number of ways. The classical flower-shaped cataract is pathognomonic of trauma, but this is only one of the ways in which the lens may react.

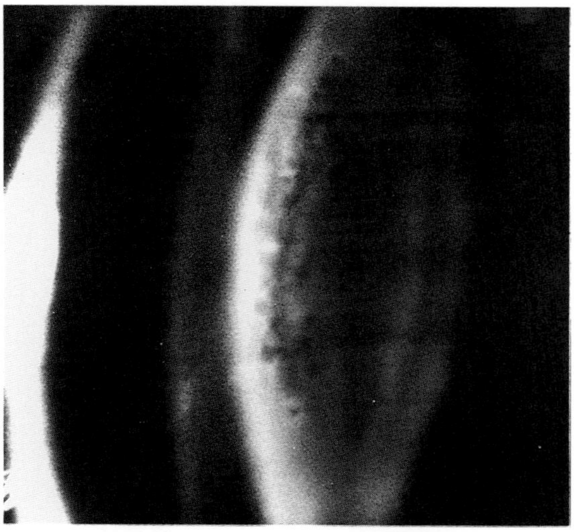

Figure 12.15 Lens of a 67-year-old female patient with hyperbaric oxygen cataract. Note the shadow of decreased turbidity behind the vacuoles. (From Palmquist *et al.* 1984, with permission.)

Concussional injury

The effect depends on whether the capsule is ruptured. Blunt injury commonly produces cataract without capsule rupture. The most readily injured fibres are in the subcapsular region, both anteriorly and posteriorly. If the lens is examined within a few days of an injury sufficient to cause cataract, the affected fibres show a thickened oedematous appearance but remain relatively transparent. The anterior subcapsular clear zone (C1α) is lost. The appearance is best identified by retro-illumination (Figure 10.38) and may otherwise be missed. Vacuoles may be seen to have formed in the adjacent lens (Figure 10.40). Following the oedematous phase the fibres lose their swelling and whiten and the characteristic flower shape or a lacy pattern becomes apparent (Figures 9.6, 9.7). It is probably this characteristic that has led to the description of the so-called delayed traumatic cataract, in which the cataract is first identified months after the injury. A Vossius ring may rarely be present (p. 135).

The flower shape forms by the spread of oedema from the fibre tips, where the fibres meet at the suture. This is probably due to rupture of the processes that link one fibre tip to the next, which permits extracellular water to enter the fibre. Occasionally the rupture is obvious, producing a Y-shaped water cleft in place of the suture. The oedema tracks along the affected fibre for a limited distance to form the characteristic flower shape. A peripheral wedge-shaped cataract may alternatively occur (Figures 10.40, 10.41).

Alternative forms of traumatic cataract are an amorphous anterior subcapsular opacity, which may be off-axis, and a punctate subcapsular opacity resembling the glaucoma fleck (Figures 9.12) and probably having the same histological basis.

Blunt trauma, insufficient to cause a definite cataract, can cause loss of the anterior subcapsular clear zone (C1α), which is seen to re-form gradually over a period of many months. In the absence of lens growth, when new fibres are no longer formed, the zone fails to be replenished anteriorly but continues to be incorporated in C1 beta and ultimately C2, posteriorly. It is thus gradually eroded, and disappears until new lens fibres start to grow and elongate into C1 alpha once again.

If the capsule is ruptured by blunt trauma, it usually occurs posteriorly, with dehiscence of lens fibres into the vitreous. Water entry leads to the rapid development of a mature cataract.

Penetrating injury

Following penetration by a small object, the lens capsule may heal, with a resultant localized capsular and lens opacity (Figure 10.7). Any capsule rupture of significant size which fails to heal, leads to a rapidly progressive cataract. It appears that the lens is overwhelmed by the water influx, which passes from fibre to fibre.

Surgical injury to the anterior capsule occurs occasionally in peripheral iridectomy (Figure 12.16) and to the posterior capsule in vitrectomy. Even without actual injury to the posterior capsule, transient posterior subcapsular lens opacities are seen to occur during a vitrectomy procedure. These are translucent and spoke-shaped features and large vacuoles may form (Figure 12.17). They may represent over-hydrated groups of lens fibres.

Electric cataract

Electric cataract occurs as a result of a lightning strike or an industrial accident. Cataract may result with voltages as low as 220 volts (Hanna and Fraunfelder 1972). When an electrical charge strikes the head, current follows along the path of least resistance, through the eye to the brain, to the nerves and finally to ground. The skin burn on the head may be minor, but there may be burns at several exit wounds on other parts of the body. The event may cause memory loss, deafness, cataracts and, rarely, optic atrophy (Hanna and Fraunfelder 1975). If the electric shock is delivered equidistant from the two eyes, both eyes develop cataract. If the shock is to one side, the cataract develops on that side. Occasionally, a cataract of late onset develops in the fellow eye (anterior subcapsular vacuoles), which in turn may subsequently disappear (Fraunfelder and Hanna 1972).

Electroshock in animals causes the immediate appearance of fine anterior and posterior subcapsular vacuoles which coalesce and enlarge with time (Thomas and Hanna 1974). In humans, lens vacuoles have been seen within 1 day after injury. Fine vacuoles form a ring in the mid-periphery of the lens and may be missed without pupil dilatation. These vacuoles coalesce and gradually disappear so that it may appear almost normal apart from the presence of white, dust-like opacities in the epithelial region. Later, many greyish-white streaks appear which radiate towards the mid-periphery, following the course of the lens fibres. The cataract thus has some similarities to traumatic cataract, but in electric cataract the vacuoles have been shown to be extra-cellular (Hanna and Fraunfelder 1972). The streaks enlarge to form fine,

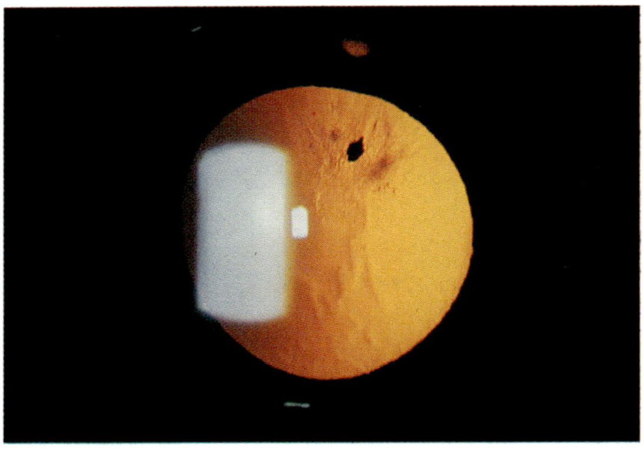

Figure 12.16 An anterior subcapsular cataract with groups of vacuolated fibres resulting from a surgical peripheral iridectomy. An iris pigment fleck is present on the capsule.

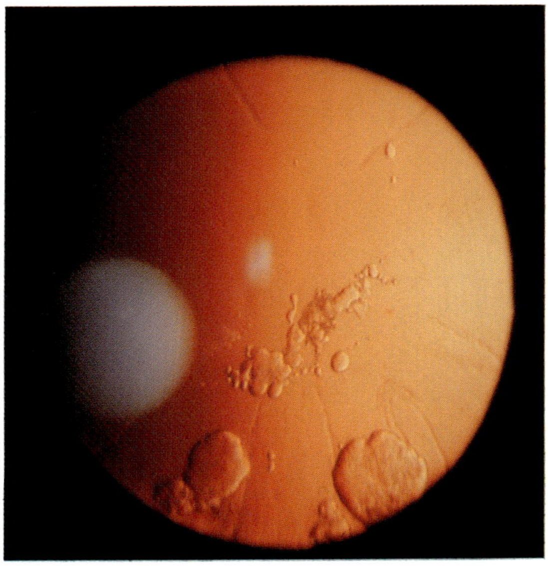

Figure 12.17 Posterior cortical vacuoles subsequent to vitrectomy with silicone oil injection. (Courtesy of J. Scott.)

elevated, lacy, curved, granular opacities which finally aggregate to form a white anterior subcapsular opacity. This is accompanied by a rapid fall in visual acuity.

The degree of cataract varies. It may regress completely giving a normal visual acuity or it may remain stationary for years and then develop into a mature cataract (Rhodes 1932; Long 1962, 1963; Kazdan 1969; Hanna and Fraunfelder 1975).

In experimental electric cataract the fine extracellular vacuoles almost disappear to leave dust-like particles made up of elongated epithelial cells surrounded by basal laminar material. The mid-peripheral opacities are islands of multilayered epithelial cells undergoing mitosis and giving rise to abortive lens fibres. In the final stage the opacities migrate to form a dense white anterior subcapsular opacity.

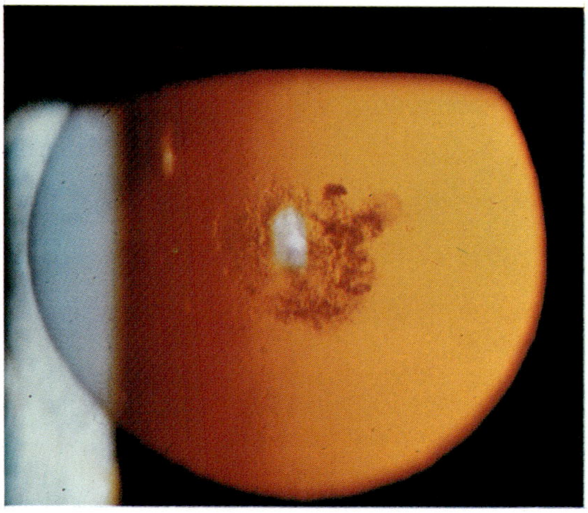

Figure 12.18 X-Ray cataract.

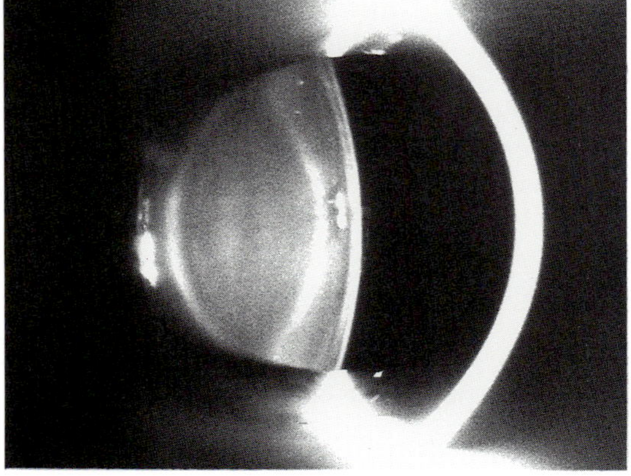

Figure 12.19 Radiation cataract.

Radiation cataract (Figures 12.18–12.20)

Ionizing radiation

Ionizing radiation is found in the electromagnetic band of wavelengths between 10 nm and 10^{-5} nm. It includes γ-rays (high energy photons) and X-rays (accelerated electrons), as well as heavy charged particles, and uncharged particles such as neutrons. They are all capable of causing a radiation cataract of typical appearance, differing only in the energy

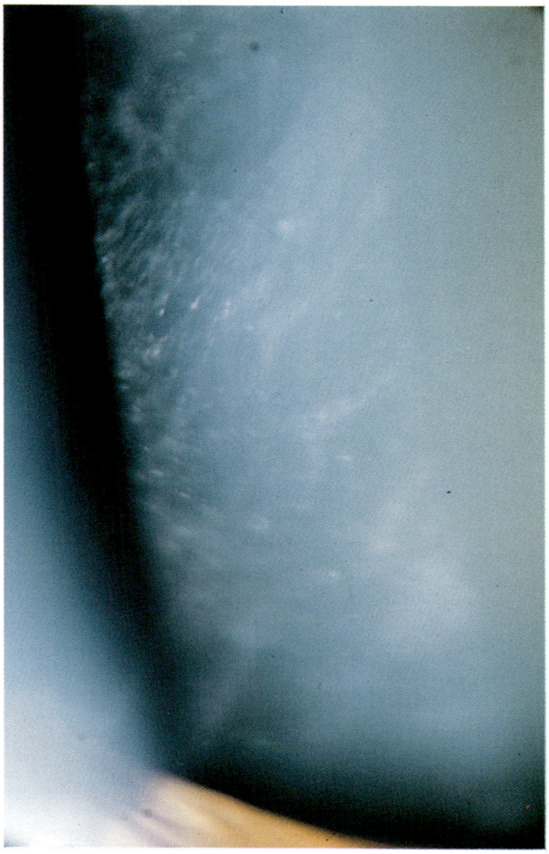

Figure 12.20 Neutron radiation cataract.

required to cause it and in the timing of its development.

The sources of ionizing radiation to which humans are exposed include natural ones such as cosmic rays, gamma rays, radon and thorium and artificial sources generated for diagnostic, therapeutic and industrial purposes. Soft X-rays (Grenz rays) are generated in an X-ray tube with a voltage of 8–25 kV, and hard X-rays with a voltage of 60–1000 kV. When electrons accelerated by a multimillion volt source hit a suitable target, gamma rays are emitted as photons.

When ionizing radiations such as X- or γ-rays pass through tissue they release electrons and positively charged ions which set up a process of ionization. Absorption, and hence the potential for causing the damage, is dependent on the atomic number of the elements concerned, with a higher atomic number leading to greater absorption for X- and γ-rays. The transfer of energy to a medium is expressed as the linear energy transfer (LET), a measure of absorption, which for neutrons is greater for elements with a lower atomic weight (e.g. the hydrogen of water). The LET of heavy charged particles and of neutrons is higher than that of X- and γ-rays and therefore determines the higher relative biological effectiveness of the former compared with the latter form of radiation (see Lerman, 1980).

Radiolysis of water Most of the effects of X-radiation on biological tissues come about from the ionization of water and the generation of free radicals (Lerman 1980). Ionization of water produces three reactive species which result directly or indirectly in tissue damage. These are: the hydroxyl radical, the hydrogen radical, and the hydrated electron.

Damage may also occur by the transfer of energy directly to the water of hydration of the functional groups of biopolymers.

1. $H_2O \rightarrow H_2O^+ + e^-$ [X- or γ-rays]
2. $H_2O + e^- \rightarrow H_2O^-$
3. $H_2O^+ \rightarrow H^+ + \bullet OH$ (hydroxyl radical)
4. $H_2O^- \rightarrow OH^- + \bullet H$ (hydrogen radical)

The hydrated electron is a powerful reducing agent which is highly reactive with compounds exhibiting unsaturated groups or halides. It therefore reacts strongly for instance, with thymidine and oxidized nucleotide (NAD^+).

Hydroxyl radicals cause the addition to double bonds and behave as electrophiles with aromatic compounds, from which they abstract hydrogen with the formation of carbon-centred free radicals. They are highly reactive with cysteine and tryptophan. The hydrogen radical has similar properties, but is less reactive.

The biological reactions of these radicals may be summarized as follows:

1. Radical : radical reactions
   $\bullet H + \bullet H \rightarrow H_2$
   $\bullet OH + \bullet OH \rightarrow H_2O_2$
   $\bullet OH + \bullet H \rightarrow H_2O$
2. Radical reactions with water and hydrogen peroxide
   $\bullet H + H_2O \rightarrow H_2 + \bullet OH$
   $\bullet OH + H_2O_2 \rightarrow H_2O + HO_2\bullet$
3. Radical reactions with biomolecules (R-H)
   $R\text{-}H + \bullet OH \rightarrow R\bullet + H_2O$
   $R\text{-}H + \bullet H \rightarrow R\bullet + H_2$
4. Reactions with molecular oxygen
   $\bullet H + O_2 \rightarrow HO_2\bullet$
   $R\bullet + O_2 \rightarrow RO_2\bullet$

Radiation damage to the cell DNA is vulnerable to damage by radiolysis either directly or by the action of radiolysis on its water of hydration. Radiolysis of bases acts by deamidation, demethylation, adduct formation at the 3,4, double bond of pyrimidine, or by oxidation and breakage of aromatic rings. Adenine and thymidine nucleotide are most vulnerable to these effects. This leads to depolymerization and dissociation of DNA and histones, and to single and double strand breaks in DNA. The former can be repaired by appropriate enzymes, while the latter leads to cell death. Damage to DNA leads to transcriptional errors and faulty RNA, and consequently to translational abnormalities and altered protein synthesis. The most sensitive phase of the cell cycle is the prophase, when DNA synthesis has been completed.

Radiolysis of DNA inhibits mitosis and may cause mutagenesis or cell death. Tissues with a high mitotic rate are in general most sensitive to damage.

Experimental radiation cataract is described on p. 113.

The first descriptions of radiation cataract in man related to the use of X-rays, with a delay of 5 years after exposure (Rohrschneider 1928) and radium, with a delay of 9 years (Meesman 1928). Since that time the occurrence of radiation cataract has been demonstrated with local ocular radiation therapy, head and whole body radiation therapy, in nuclear physicists and radiologists, before the risks were recognized in other industrial situations giving rise to ionizing radiation and in those who were exposed to nuclear explosions. Cataract has been recorded in uranium miners (Lerman 1962; Haye *et al.* 1965). Patients who were in the past exposed to Grenz and β-ray therapy applied locally to limbal lesions such as pterygium to inhibit corneal neovascularization, developed cataract despite the relatively poor penetration of these forms of radiation through tissue. This is because of the proximity of the limbus to the periphery of the lens and the germinative zone.

Studies of patients who developed cataract following the nuclear explosions at Nagasaki and Hiroshima demonstrated the dependence on dose as determined by distance from the hypocentre of the explosion (Cogan *et al.* 1950; Fillumore 1952; Ham 1953; Sinskey 1955; Tokunaga 1959; Miller *et al.* 1967; Merriam *et al.* 1972; Dodo 1975). The delay time depends on the dose and may be as short as 12 months.

Non-ionizing radiation

Infra-red radiation was well known to cause cataract in furnace workers and in glass-blowers prior to the availability of protective lenses. The mechanism is believed to involve energy absorption in the iris pigment epithelium causing a localized temperature rise. (Goldman 1935; Langley *et al.* 1960). In the rabbit, an additional, non-thermal mechanism appear to exist, in which posterior subcapsular cataract is induced by prolonged direct absorption of infra-red radiation by the lens in the range 1050–2000 nm (Wolbarsht *et al.* 1976, 1977). Prolonged industrial exposure to infra-red radiation over many decades increases the risk for all forms of cataract, including cortical spoke, nuclear and posterior subcapsular. Although posterior subcapsular cataract has been said to be characteristic of 'glass-blowers' cataract', it is ultimately no different in appearance to that which occurs in non-exposed subjects. The only pathognomonic feature of infra-red cataract is true exfoliation of the lens capsule. Here there is a linear splitting and detachment of the anterior capsule, which peels off from the periphery and coils up in the anterior chamber, while its central part remains attached to the lens. This exfoliated capsule remains clear, and the appearance is quite different to that of pseudoexfoliation (p. 136). Lydahl (1984), in a cross-sectional study of industrial exposure to infra-red radiation, showed that the level of exposure and risk for cataract was higher in glass-blowers than in workers in the iron and steel industry (Figure 12.21). The increased risk for cataract became evident in those over 60 years. Cataract and a higher exposure to radiation was found to be more frequent on the left side. This has been noted in the past, but has not been found in all studies. True exfoliation of the lens capsule was associated.

Ultraviolet radiation, and possibly also light in the visible blue region of the spectrum, has been implicated as a cause of cataract (Weale 1983). The cornea absorbs heavily in the UV but passes UV light in the region of 295–400 nm, which is absorbed by the lens. About 75% of UV light (300–400 nm) is transmitted by lenses under 10 years of age, but in those over 25 years, with the accumulation of chromophores, transmission drops down to 20% (Lerman 1980). The lens also absorbs some visible blue light, especially once senile nuclear yellowing has begun. The epidemiological evidence also implicates a high environmental temperature as a possible alternative, or additional, cause (see below). There is more recent epidemiological evidence from non-tropical regions to support a role for UV light, but the association is not strong (Taylor *et al.* 1988); it may have its effect by generating free radicals in the tissue. The type of cataract produced by UV has been reported as nuclear (Zigman 1979), which is the type that would be expected to result from the absorption by the yellowing aging lens. Posterior subcapsular cataract has also been reported (Sockow *et al.* 1989) and this could be due to lens epithelial damage. It is noted that spoke cataract occurs with most frequency in the lower nasal quadrant (Brown *et al.* 1993), which is the part of the lens most exposed to sunlight.

Microwave radiation has been demonstrated to cause cataract in the experimental animal, but exposure of man to such sources as radar is considered an unlikely cause (Joyner 1989). The effect is considered to be due to heating and possibly to specific properties of the radiation (p. 118).

Laser radiation in the visible and in the infra-red spectrum has been shown capable of causing localized opacities when used to perform iridotomies (Abraham and Miller 1975).

Environmental factors

The inter-relationship between the environment and the individual is necessarily complex. Cataracts occur at a younger age and with greater frequency in persons living in the equatorial regions of the world (Weale 1983). In these regions light levels are high (see non-ionizing radiation p. 205), but so are temperatures and this itself may be a factor. It has been shown in the experimental animal that the temperature within the lens rises when exposed to a hot environment and this may be damaging (Al-Ghadyan and Cotlier 1986). The relationship between temperature and presbyopia (p. 52) further suggests the damaging effect of temperature on the lens. Equatorial environments may also be associated with poor nutrition (see p. 200) and with diarrhoeal disease leading to dehydration (see p. 200). It is probable that all of these factors are co-cataractogenic.

Age-related (senile) cataract

It has been conventional to use the term 'senile cataract' to describe cataracts occurring without evident cause after the age of 50 years. It may be said that the vast majority of cataracts encountered are in this category, but this term is not really satisfactory, since environmental, toxic, nutritional and systemic factors are all contributory. Nowadays it is common to use the term 'age-related' instead. Age-related cataract takes the form of cortical, nuclear and subcapsular opacities, in that order of frequency. It is more prevalent in the female, even allowing for the excess of females in the ageing population.

The purpose of this section is to summarize some of the factors leading to age-related cataract. Almost all types of cataract increase with age, and age is the greatest risk factor. They result from the convergence of the effects of the multiple risk factors which affect an individual over their life span. Although heredity may play a small role in the occurrence of such cataracts, it is not excluded that genomic differences could influence susceptibility of an individual to different cataractogenic insults.

The major types of cataract commonly occur in some form of combination. However, although it is

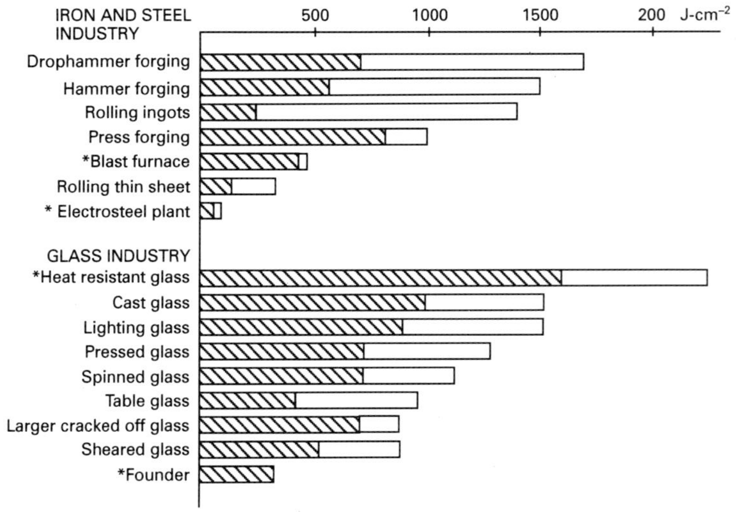

Figure 12.21 Industrial exposure to infrared radiation in a Scandinavian population. Maximal doses of exposure (3000–2600 nm) per eight hour day, registered for particular industrial processes (whole bars) and the mean doses for all jobs in each process (striped bars). *Dark protective glasses usually worn, but not considered here (Lydahl 1984).

likely that given patient populations are exposed to roughly the same form of cataractogenic insult, it is of interest that there are smaller numbers of patients who show subcapsular, spoke or nuclear cataract, in pure form. This clinical heterogeneity may imply differences in susceptibility within such populations, although it is also possible that degrees of exposure to insults also vary. One such difference in exposure within a population is diabetes mellitus. Diabetes greatly increases the risk of cataract (p. 176) but has little influence on cataract type (other than in the case of juvenile diabetic cataract).

An intriguing feature of human age-related cataract, found also in cataracts of known aetiology, and shared to a lesser extent by animal cataract, is the phenomenon of zonal constraint (i.e. the occurrence of specific cataract types within specific zones of the lens in a stereotyped and repeatable manner). Thus spoke-like senile lens opacities do not arise in the nucleus or perinucleus of the ageing lens, although the perinuclear cortex or peripheral nucleus may lay down lamellar cataracts which mimic these changes at an earlier period of life. Similarly, although nuclear scatter or brunescent nuclear cataract may spread to involve the perinuclear zone, it does not affect the superficial cortex. Retro-dot cataract, in the same way, is usually confined to the perinuclear cortex (p. 171). Other examples have been given in this book (p. 145).

The heterogeneity of cataract type and occurrence is a reminder that not all parts of the lens are equally exposed to a given cataractogenic influence. Thus the zones of exposure can roughly be thought of as four compartments (Figure 12.22).

1. *The pupillary compartment* is preferentially exposed to materials in the aqueous humour of the anterior chamber. The diffusion gradient for dissolved solutes in the aqueous will be from cornea to lens with respect to topically applied drugs. The pupillary zone of the lens, including the central epithelium and the superficial cortex, will be exposed to UV light within the cataractogenic waveband (300–400 nm). UV light will be progressively absorbed as it passes through the substance of the lens, so that little will reach the nucleus, with even less reaching the posterior cortex. It has been suggested that a greater amount of sunlight-derived UV light will reach the lower parts of the lens, and even more will reach the inferonasal quadrant (p. 205).
2. *The posterior chamber* is related to the peripheral epithelium and the lens equator, including the equatorial region of the lens fibres. This region of the lens will be exposed to the highest concentrations of blood-borne agents, including natural substances such as glucose, and drugs passing the blood–aqueous barrier. Some negatively charged substances are removed from the posterior chamber by the pigment epithelium of the iris.
3. *The vitreous compartment* is related to the posterior lens capsule and lens cortex, including the posterior suture system. This part of the lens will be exposed to lower concentrations of substances entering via the aqueous secretion and higher concentrations of substances arising from the retina (such as malondialdehyde resulting from lipid peroxidation in the degenerating

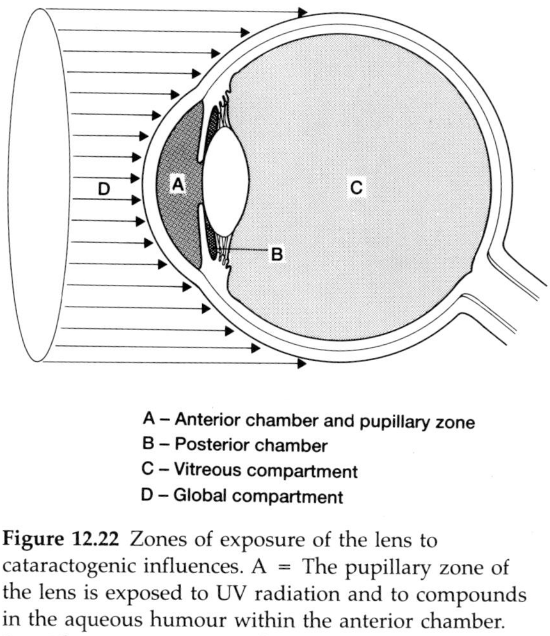

Figure 12.22 Zones of exposure of the lens to cataractogenic influences. A = The pupillary zone of the lens is exposed to UV radiation and to compounds in the aqueous humour within the anterior chamber. B = The zone exposed to the posterior chamber encounters agents which enter with the aqueous humour. The anterior lens is also influenced by changes in iris temperature. C = The vitreous body is in relation to the posterior lens surface. Agents within the vitreous humour may arise during inflammation or from the degenerating retina. D = The whole of the globe and lens will be exposed to certain forms of radiation, such as X radiation.

retina). It will be closest to toxic agents generated during vitreous surgery.

4. *The global compartment*: all parts of the lens are accessible to injury from some forms of insult, such as ionizing radiation or physical injuries from concussion or electric shock.

In the same way, the targets for damage within the lens will vary. Thus the lens epithelium and a proportion of the superficial cortex is nucleated and possesses organelles capable of aerobic in addition to anaerobic metabolism. There is little protein turnover in the nucleus of the lens although enzymes and some mRNA has been detected. The gamma crystallin content of the nucleus is enriched compared with the cortex, while the cytoskeletal content is depleted. The negligible turnover of the nuclear crystallins renders them vulnerable to post-translational modification. The epithelium and superficial cortical cells house the major Na^+/K^+, and Ca^{++}-activated ATPase pumps which provide most of the motive force for ion movement within the lens (p. 56). The pre-equatorial epithelium is the germinative zone of the lens, and site of most of the lens mitosis. Thus, the same insult, impinging on several sites of the lens, might have several different implications for cataract formation.

Predisposing factors to age-related (senile) cataract

A number of age-related changes in the lens are probably risk factors for cataract formation, although this relationship has yet to be demonstrated other than by inference.

Post-translational modification of proteins

There is a steady increase in post-translational modification of lens proteins by glycation, formation of mixed disulphides and other mechanisms (p. 98), which has been studied intensively in the crystallins. This affects the more stable crystallins of the nucleus more than those of the cortex. The process can be detected in the prenatal lens and continues relentlessly through the age span. It is expressed initially by the formation of water-soluble crystallin aggregates, chiefly of alpha crystallins, within which beta and gamma crystallins are incorporated. This is preceded by an unfolding of the crystallins due to surface charge changes, which, particularly in the case of the beta and gamma crystallins, exposes their previously buried thiol groups to oxidation. Disulphide bond formation leads to the formation of water-insoluble cross-linked aggregates whose large size is a basis for increased light-scattering. There is a steady increase in light-scattering by the lens with age (p. 23), affecting the nucleus more than the cortex. A number of authors have reported a progressive rise in the water-insoluble component of the crystallins of the lens with age in the absence of cataract, and although some of the reported insolubility may be an artefact due to preparative oxidation (Harding 1991), the inference remains that crystallin proteins, particularly of the nucleus, show an age-related unfolding which increases their risk of oxidative damage. It is likely that there is sufficient formation of water-insoluble disulphide cross-linked aggregates to account for an important part of the decreased transparency of the lens which occurs with age particularly after 45 years, although other factors also operate (see below).

Nuclear cataract is thought to be due to the presence of water-insoluble, disulphide and non-disulphide cross-linked aggregates (HM3 and HM4) within relatively intact fibres. Under transmission microscopy, the nuclear fibre membranes in nuclear cataract do not appear to be different from those of the normal nucleus, although these differ from those of the cortex (Kuszak *et al.* 1992). There are patchy membrane defects whose presence suggests that the fibres of the human nucleus retain their gross morphology by mechanisms which are independent of a need for a functional membrane. It is likely that the superficial cortical fibres and the ion pumps of the lens perform this function.

Nuclear cataract may be brunescent, or simply exhibit a scattering of light (white nuclear cataract) (p. 152). Pure light-scattering aggregates would be anticipated to occur following post-translational modification by carbamylation, mixed disulphides and the early stages of glycation. Brunescent cataract is associated with the presence of chromophores within the lens with specific light-absorbing and fluorescent properties. These chromophores, some of which arise as advanced glycation products, are discussed on p. 98. They account for some of the covalent, non-disulphide cross-links in the lens found in HM3.

As the degree of light scatter or brunescence associated with nuclear cataract increases in intensity there is a spread of these changes into the perinuclear cortex (C3 and C4) and in this respect there is no zonal constraint between the nucleus and deep cortex. However, retro-dots are almost entirely confined to the perinuclear cortex, although features resembling retro-dots are seen from time to time in the nucleus. Retro-dots are thought to be the precursor of 'spheroliths', the dense refractile opacities found in the 'nuclei' of Morgagnian cataracts. It is not clear, however, to what extent such 'nuclei' incorporate brunescent deep cortex. Retro-dot opacities are now known to be rich in calcium phosphate, and possibly also to contain calcium oxalate (Vrensen *et al.* 1994). Although a rise in calcium level is regarded as an important feature of cataract formation it is not known why these quasi-crystalline formations should localize in these regions of the lens.

In passing it may be noted that the deep cortex (C3) is a region which shows an age-related increase in the degree of light scatter from the fourth decade, with a spread to affect adjacent zones. The basis for this change is not known, but it is anticipated that membrane alterations will contribute to the altered light-scattering properties in addition to alterations in cytoplasmic proteins.

Channels, pumps and membrane permeability

There are age-related changes in lens membranes which are likely to be the result of various insults to the lens, which lower its resistance to further stresses. Takemoto *et al.* (1986) and Takemoto and Takehana (1986) have shown a conversion of MP26 to its degradation product MP22 in aged lenses. These studies originally suggested that the N-terminal proteolysis converts gap junctional protein to a non-functional protein which cannot be gated (i.e. closed) by calcium-calmodulin. Inability to gate-gap junctions would prevent the disengagement of normal from damaged fibres and would encourage the propagation of fibre damage by transmitting ionic disequilibrium from cell to cell. This interpretation must be a cautious one at this time, since there is some suggestion that MP26 may in fact represent a volume regulatory channel (aquaporin). However, the implications of its modification might be similar. There is morphological evidence that the number of gap junctions decreases in the older lens. Although, from what has gone before, it might be presumed that such a change would protect against the propagation of damage from fibre to fibre, so it can also be construed that loss of gap junctions would interfere with the long-term ionic homeostasis of the lens.

Garner and Spector (1980) demonstrated an alteration of the kinetics of $Na^{+}K^{+}$ATPase in diabetics, suggesting that this enzyme undergoes post-translational modification in this condition. Duncan *et al.* (1989), in a multicentre study, showed important age-related increases in membrane permeability in normal lenses, with a marked decline in membrane potential and resistance with age, and a rise in internal free sodium and calcium. There was a concomitant stimulation of transmembrane fluxes of Na^{+} and K^{+}. Duncan *et al.* inferred that with age there is an increasing contribution to membrane ion fluxes by channels which accommodate the passage of Na^{+}, K^{+} and Ca^{2+} ions. These membrane permeability changes were found to coincide exactly in degree with the rise in optical density with age (increased scattering), which had been reported for the normal lens by Weale (1982a), and are thought to make an important contribution to it.

Spoke cataracts are found in the superficial cortex, or more specifically in C2. They are fibre-based cataracts owing their shape entirely to the arrangement of fibres in the shell within which they occur (Bron and Brown 1986 p. 145). Such cataracts remain confined to C2 for considerable periods of time which may amount to years. Ultimately the fibre breakdown which characterizes the spoke opacity may spread to involve more superficial and deeper layers of the cortex. This progression leads to lens swelling or an intumescent cataract. However, although a short term centripetal spread was noted in a small study by Shun-Shin *et al.* (1989), the natural history of spoke cataract is not yet known in topographic terms, although there is information on the rate of progression for all major forms of cataract (Leske *et al.* 1991). Determination of its natural history should shed some light on the mechanism of spoke cataract.

Two features seen in ageing lenses which could shed light on the aetiology of spoke cataract are 'fibre folds' and water clefts (p. 140). Brown *et al.* (1989) demonstrated that so-called lamellar separation of the lens fibres, a common feature of the ageing lens, represents sheets of lens fibres within a fibre shell which have been ruptured at their equators, releasing their central limbs to take up an undulating folded condition. These have been termed appropriately 'fibre folds'. Remarkably, fine structural studies have indicated that the damaged fibres are sealed at the equator, presumably by the annealing mechanism referred to elsewhere (p. 97), so that the anterior and posterior segments of the fibres exhibiting folds remain intact. In almost 100% of cases fibre folds are found to be associated with the peripheral crescentic lens opacities (or 'shades') described by Obazawa *et al.* (1983). It must be assumed that these opacities represent the products of fibre breakdown at the sites of peripheral fibre rupture. Although peripheral fibre breaks would seem to be obvious candidates to initiate spoke cataracts, a relationship is not yet established (Brown *et al.* 1993).

Primary water clefts are optically empty features seen in the line of the sutures in C2, and extending with time into neighbouring cortical zones. They may take on vesicular features, which, with the radial disposition conferred by the suture, may simulate a cortical spoke. However, although water clefts often accompany spokes, they appear to be distinct from them. They have been shown to be associated with breakdown of the fibre tips and it is not clear to what extent the extracellular space is expanded in the sense of forming an actual 'cleft'. Like the peripheral break of the fibre fold, this feature too would seem to afford the opportunity to break down the fibre system to form a spoke cataract, this time from the apical and/or basal tip of the fibre. Once again, it appears that the annealing mechanism protects the fibre from dissolution, but the strength of this defence mechanism is not known.

Various aetiologies have been proposed for spoke cataract. Fisher (1970) suggested that spokes might arise as a result of the cumulative stresses brought about by accommodation. He was able induce spoke opacities in normal lenses by centrifugation. It will be important in the future to know whether spoke opacities always appear in cortex which has been exposed to such forces. Thus, if spoke opacities are found in cortex laid down after the age of about 45 years, this mechanism cannot be operative. Fisher (1970) calculated that their depth implied formation at a time when ciliary forces were at their greatest (i.e. at about 40 years). It has been suggested that spokes might arise as the result of compressive forces generated during compaction. There is no reason to believe that compaction raises intra-fibre pressure, since it is assumed that this process is accompanied by protein degradation, but a packing down of fibres during compaction could be conceived as altering suture registration and offering shearing damage to the fibre system. Kuszak, on the basis of SEM studies of cortical and corticonuclear cataracts, has proposed that spoke cataracts arise as a result of an abnormal construction of third and later suture generations (Kuszak *et al.* 1993) (p. 42). It is suggested that the incorporation of abnormally short fibres into the suture system results in the creation of asymmetrical sub-branches which are comparable in shape and size to spoke or cuneiform cataracts. It is also suggested that the peripheral location of such short fibres is responsible for the frequency of suture abnormalities in the infernonasal quadrant, a hypothesis invoked to explain the greater frequency of spoke cataract in this region. If the suture hypothesis is correct, then it is of interest to speculate whether the location and timing of closure of the fetal fissure could influence the location and construction of late generation sutures. Another explanation which has been advanced for the prevalence of the inferonasal cuneate cataract is the greater degree of exposure of this part of the lens to the UV fraction of sunlight.

Subcapsular cataract

The nature of subcapsular cataract is quite distinct from that of spoke and nuclear cataract. Anterior subcapsular cataract is caused by a metaplastic change in the central lens epithelium, while posterior subcapsular cataract is due to an epithelial dysplasia (Kuszak *et al.* 1993).

In anterior subcapsular cataract, central epithelial cells transform into elongated, spindle shaped myofibroblast-like cells which contain smooth muscle α-actinin. Their presence implies a metaplastic change. They lie within a connective tissue plaque between the anterior capsule and the epithelium. The connective tissue contains types I and III collagen and, in advanced plaques, type IV collagen, within a thin basal lamina, for which fibroblasts would be an unlikely source. Although a minor degree of anterior subcapsular haze frequently accompanies posterior subcapsular cataract, it is not certain that this change corresponds histologically to the entity described here. It is tempting to attribute anterior subcapsular cataract to a direct insult to the central epithelium, such as UV radiation. Johnson *et al.* (1988) have described such a change.

Posterior subcapsular cataract is due to a dysplastic change in the germinal epithelium. There is disorganization of the meridional row cells, absent or imperfect rotation of differentiating cells, and a posterior migration of their dysplastic products, the bladder or 'Wedl' cells. These cells possess many features of normal fibres, showing for instance membrane interdigitations, and synthesizing crystallins and cytoskeletal proteins. Kuszak and Deutsch (1991) suggest that the dysplastic cells migrate preferentially along the posterior, possibly abnormal, suture system and draw attention to a possible role in repair of lysomal structures found within the posterior opacity (Dark and Streeten 1977, Eshagian *et al.* 1980; Creighton *et al.* 1978; Gorthy *et al.* 1978). It is of interest that acid hydrolases are found to have a sutural location in some species such as the rat (Gorthy *et al.* 1980). Although the posterior migration theory of posterior subcapsular cataract has general credence, room should be left for the possibility that some posterior subcapsular cataracts are due to direct damage to a discoid zone of posterior fibre tips. Also, not all posterior subcapsular cataracts are observed to be associated with sutural opacities at the slit-lamp.

Cataract maturation

Maturation of cataracts involves a consolidation of the various processes described above. Cortical fibre breakdown may proceed to a state of massive water uptake and the swelling and increased capsular tension characterizing intumescent cataract. The lens is swollen and the anterior chamber shallows. The same process, proceeding at a slower pace, may lead to a state of hypermaturity, in which a shrunken lens, whose cortex is partially absorbed, exhibits a wrinkled capsule associated with organized connective tissue and calcium-containing deposits. Cortical fibre breakdown and digestion may proceed to any stage of liquefaction and absorption, and result in the full picture of Morgagnian cataract (p. 216). The liquefaction process, releasing crystallin fragments into the anterior chamber, may stimulate macrophage engulfment and induce phacolytic glaucoma. The fibre breakdown characteristic of cortical cataract is associated with a rise in lens calcium. Lens crystallin breakdown involves the participation of a number of calcium activated proteases (p. 104).

13

Cataract progress and prognosis

Change in lens dimensions

Lenses developing cataract are commonly smaller than healthy lenses of the same age (Weekers *et al.* 1973a,b; Perkins 1988). This change is seen most markedly in connection with subcapsular cataract (Figure 13.1) (Brown and Tripathi 1974). It is understandable that lens growth is interrupted with the formation of cataract and, in the case of subcapsular cataract, defective new fibre formation appears causative. It is probable that in subcapsular cataract the process actually involves lens shrinkage, which is evidenced by the change in shape sometimes seen in this condition, in which the cortex is very thin and the lens curvature becomes conoid, having taken on the shape of the nucleus (Figure 10.67a). This implies actual loss of the cortical substance; such cases followed sequentially have been seen to become smaller during the period of observation. To some extent the phenomenon may be explained by a failure of new growth in the presence of compaction, which is a normal phenomenon in the younger lens.

With the development of a mature cataract, the lens swells and the anterior chamber becomes shallowed, which may lead to angle closure glaucoma (Figure 13.2). The process of swelling can be very rapid in cataract occurring in young adults, or following capsule rupture.

As the cataract progresses to hypermaturity (Figures 13.3, 13.4) the lens again shrinks with loss of protein through the capsule.

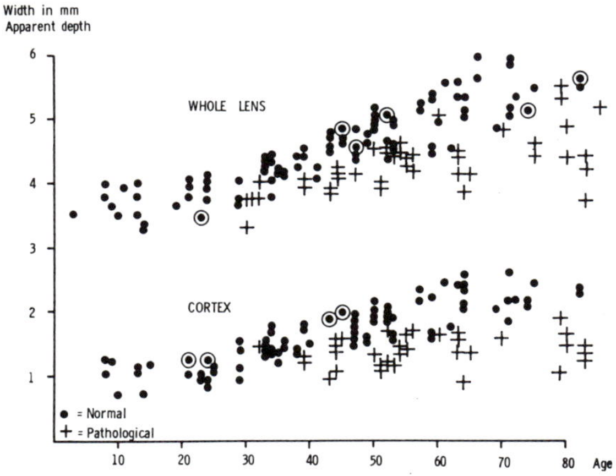

Figure 13.1 Reduced lens width and cortex width in presence of posterior subcapsular cataract (crosses) compared with normals (dots). (From Brown and Tripathi 1974 with permission.)

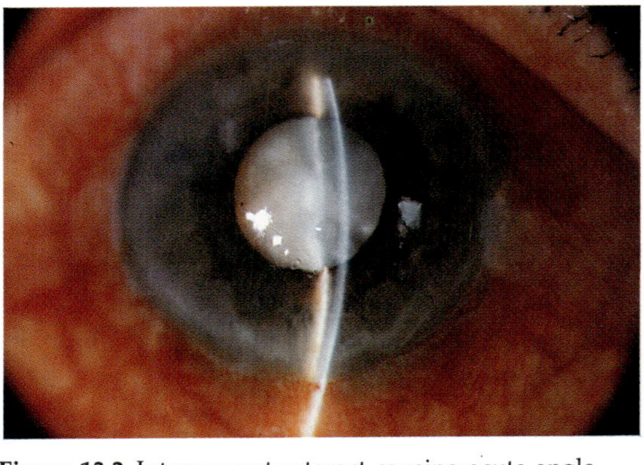

Figure 13.2 Intumescent cataract causing acute angle closure glaucoma.

Change in cataract

Once present, a cataract commonly increases both in terms of the area occupied and in the density of the opacity. The behaviour is very variable and relates to the cataract morphology.

Opacities that are the result of a temporary and not very severe insult to the lens cease to grow. As the lens grows, the affected fibres become compacted towards the lens centre, which results in a reduction in the diameter of lamellar opacities (Brown *et al.* 1988).

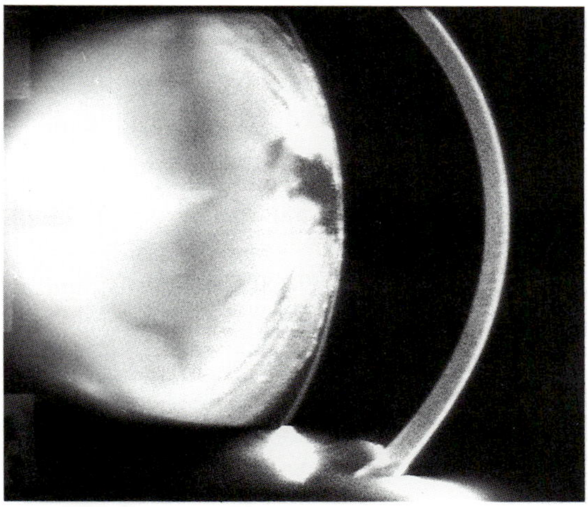

Figure 13.3 A hypermature lens in a young patient with anorexia nervosa showing shallowing of the anterior chamber. The lens anterior cortex contains a large water cleft.

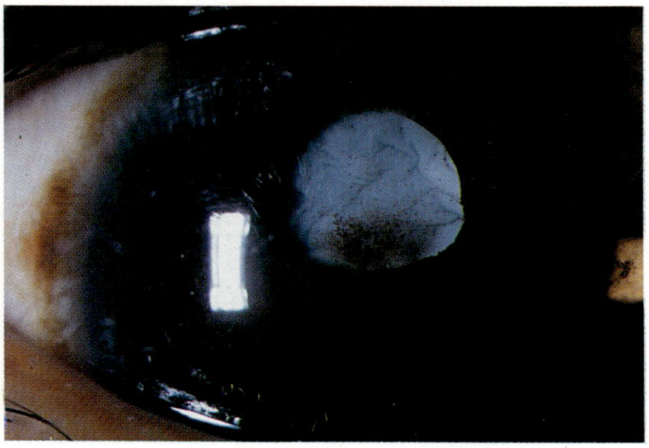

Figure 13.4 A hypermature cataract showing wrinkling of the anterior capsule indicating lens shrinkage.

The depth within the lens at which an opacity is found can be used to determine its time of origin in a lens which is showing continuing growth (Brown 1976). Many opacities, traumatic, glaucoma flecks and metabolic cataracts are subcapsular at their

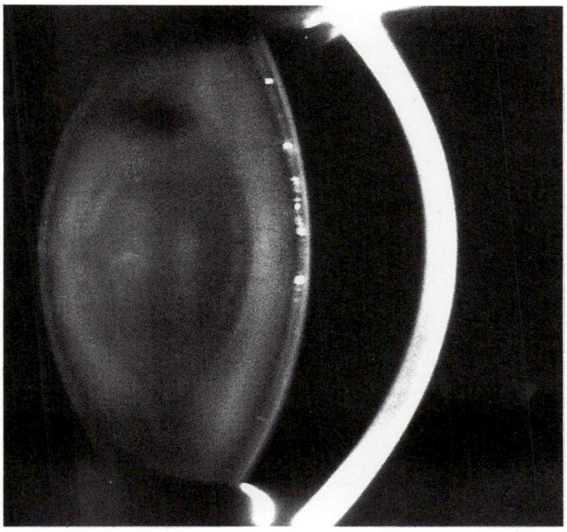

(a)

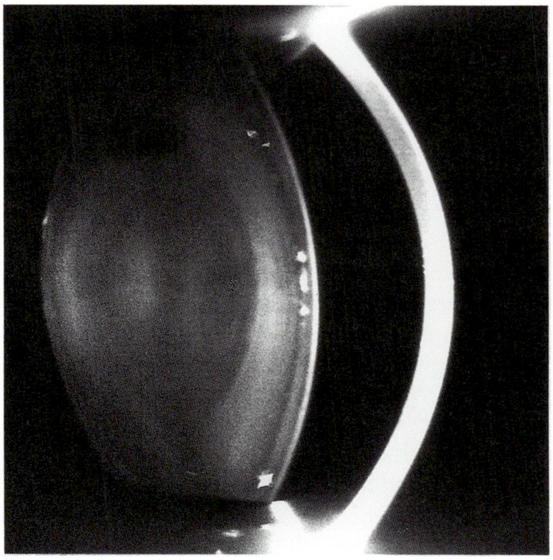

(b)

Figure 13.5(a) Glaucoma flecks at the time of their formation are immediately subcapsular **(b)** at 30 months, they already appear to have sunk into the lens, with the re-formation of C1α anterior to them.

inception and then appear to sink into the lens with time (Figures 10.39, 13.5). Extraneous material such as gold also shows the sinking-in effect. The lens grows at about 25 μm per year (p. 24) and the opacities appear to sink into the lens at twice this rate, which is made possible by the central compaction of the fibres.

The rate of growth may itself be influenced by the disease process. If growth rate is affected, it is more usually retarded, but examples also exist of accelerated lens growth, as if to 'catch up', following the development of posterior subcapsular cataract (Shun-Shin *et al.* 1991a).

Capsular opacity

The opacity in the capsule tends to remain static, but the lens may deteriorate with the laying down of subjacent cortical opacity in the form of discs, which may increase in number and diameter (see reduplication cataract – Figure 10.5).

Congenital and developmental cataract

The diameter of a congenital cataract is limited to that of the diameter of the lens at birth. If the cataract-forming process ceases at birth, which is common, then the diameter of the opacity becomes gradually reduced as the nucleus of the lens undergoes compaction, which is a normal feature of lens growth (Brown *et al.* 1988).

In cases in which the process of cataract formation does not cease at birth, which is seen in some familial cataracts, then developmental opacities are added. Developmental opacities (Figure 13.6) are those which are laid down in a lens which is otherwise developing normally. The tendency is probably genetically determined in all cases. The opacities formed consist of focal dot and coronary types (Figures 10.57, 10.58, 10.59, 10.60). Vision is good in youth and deteriorates gradually as more opacities are added over the years.

Age-related spoke cataract (Figures 9.5, 10.50, 10.51)

The opacity increases by spreading axially along the affected fibre and by spread to adjacent fibres. The axial spread occurs at an uneven rate. Some spokes increase rapidly over a period of a few months, while others in the same lens have periods of stagnation.

Age-related nuclear cataract (Figures 9.14, 9.15)

The light scattering and brown coloration increase gradually, but not necessarily at the same rate, so that one or other effect may be the more pronounced. The cataract is generally confined to the nucleus and to C4, but spread of brunescence into C3 does occur as nuclear brunescence deepens. Nuclear cataract may appear to occupy most of the lens when the cortex is thinned (Figure 10.67a).

Subcapsular cataract (Figures 9.10, 10.54, 10.55)

Subcapsular cataracts are first apparent at the posterior pole of the lens and gradually increase in area. The individual components within them have been shown to be in a state of flux (Shun-Shin *et al.* 1989).

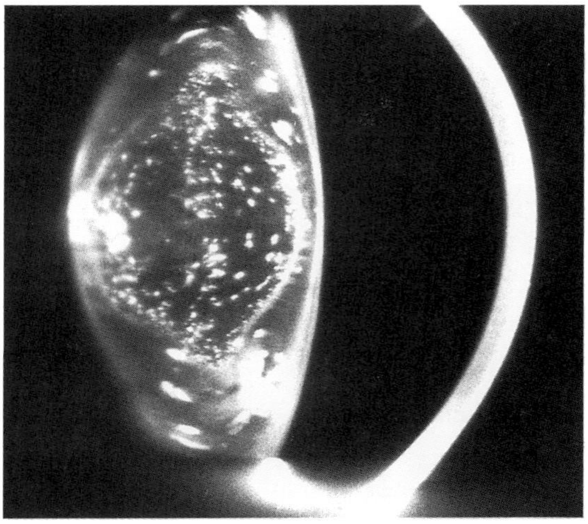

Figure 13.6 An example of a developmental cataract in a young adult, beginning with a congenital lamellar cataract to which coronary and cortical focal dot opacities are being added as the lens grows.

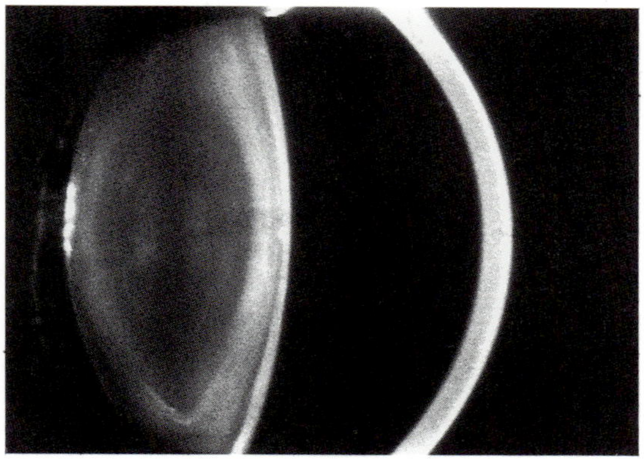

(a)

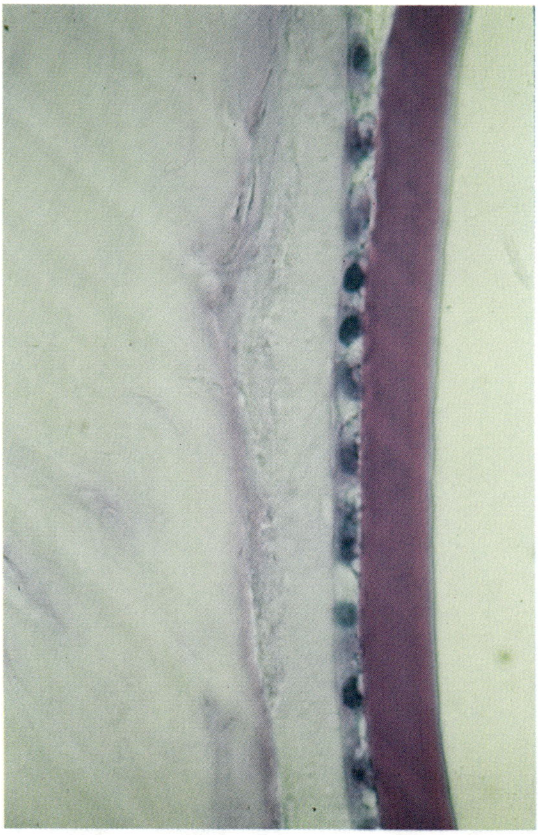

(b)

Figure 13.7(a) A small posterior subcapsular cataract, but with the loss of the anterior subcapsular clear zone (C1α). This cataract is likely to deteriorate rapidly. **(b)** Loss of anterior subcapsular clear zone. Histologically the superficial fibres show cataractous change. (Courtesy R. Tripathi.)

Anterior subcapsular changes are commonly associated with posterior subcapsular cataract and the first visible change is loss of the anterior subcapsular clear zone (Figure 13.7a), which histologically (Figure 13.7b) is shown to be due to actual cataract (Brown and Tripathi 1974). The state of the clear zone is useful in judging prognosis. An absent clear zone usually indicates a progressive cataract (Figure 10.67) and when the clear zone is present the condition is static or only slowly progressive. It will be recalled that the clear zone (C1α) maintains a near constant width during the life of the lens due to a maturation of the deeper fibres which increase their light-scattering properties as they are incorporated into C1α. It is likely that, in some cases at least, thinning of the clear zone results from a continuation of this process at a time when addition of fresh fibres to C1α has stopped. The clear zone may be seen to re-form once the stimulus causing the cataract has been removed; the cataract then progresses no further and is seen to sink into the lens with time. This is the finding in renal transplant patients (Shun-Shin *et al.* 1990) in whom a posterior opacity is first observed separated from the posterior pole at 1 year or later from the time of transplantation.

Loss of the subcapsular clear zone occurs as a temporary feature, without the development of cataract, following trauma and in acute iritis. Cataract does follow if the degree of trauma is severe, or if the response to treatment is poor.

Cataract maturation

A cataract is said to have become mature (Figure 13.8) once opacification appears to have become total. Formerly this name had clinical significance since this stage was awaited before operating.

Hypermature cataract (Figure 13.3)

Following or sometimes preceding maturation, the lens may absorb water and swell, becoming an intumescent cataract with a liability to angle closure glaucoma. This process may be very rapid in young lenses, especially following capsule perforation.

The cortex may undergo lysis and absorption, leading to lens shrinkage and capsule wrinkling (Figure 13.4). Calcareous deposits and opacities caused by epithelial hypertrophy may be seen in the capsule, and crystals may be seen in the cortex.

In the older eye this eventually leaves the harder nucleus free within the capsule as a Morgagnian cataract (Figure 13.9). The downward displacement of the nucleus may be mistaken for lens dislocation, which is also liable to affect the hypermature cataract (Figure 13.10). Occasionally the lens may release a snow-storm of flakes and crystals into the aqueous humour where they may circulate in a dramatic fashion (Berliner 1949).

Phacolytic glaucoma

This complication (Figure 13.1) follows cataract maturation and is the result of the leakage of lens proteins through the intact, but permeable, capsule. This incites a non-allergenic cellular response and the proteins are taken up by macrophages, which congregate on the surface of the lens and also become trapped in the trabecular meshwork, where they obstruct drainage.

The glaucoma is relatively acute and the appearance at the slit-lamp shows a very heavy anterior chamber flare and cellular reaction with relatively minor ciliary injection. A hypopyon may form due to macrophages.

Phacoallergic uveitis (phacoanaphylaxis)

This uncommon granulomatous uveitis occurs when the release of lens protein excites an allergic response. The release is usually the result of capsule rupture, but this is only rarely followed by phacoallergic uveitis. It is postulated that the secluded site of the lens fibres within the capsule from the time of first development of the lens in the embryo prevents the immune system from recognizing the lens proteins as 'self' and thus they are recognized as antigens. The condition may develop rapidly when lens protein is released in the contralateral eye following the previous release of

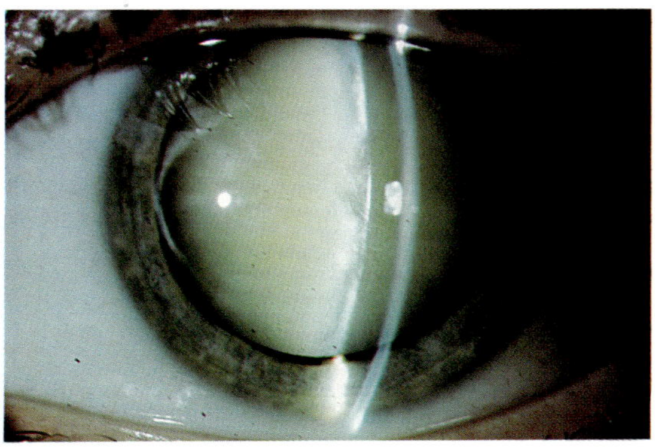

Figure 13.8 A mature cataract showing total opacification of the lens.

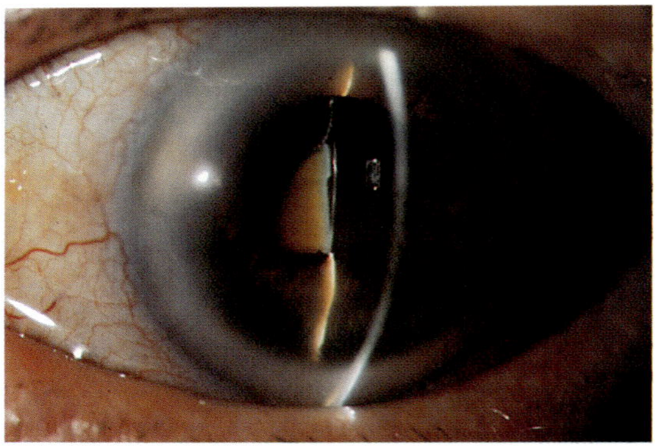

(a)

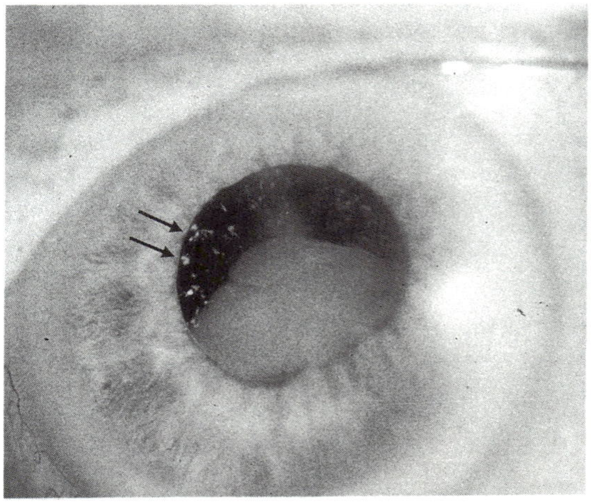

(b)

Figure 13.9(a) A Morgagnian hypermature cataract with the nucleus sunken within an otherwise empty capsular bag. **(b)** Morgagnian cataract, same patient as (a). The flecks of calcium salt on the lens capsule (arrows) identify the location of the capsule and clearly distinguish the sunken nucleus from a dislocated lens.

protein in the first eye, as in a planned extracapsular extraction.

The eye is acutely inflamed and painful. Soft lens matter seen in the anterior chamber helps to distinguish the condition from sympathetic ophthalmia. Secondary glaucoma is common.

After-cataract

Following extracapsular cataract surgery, with or without lens implant, there is a liability to reduction in vision due to capsule fibrosis or to epithelial cell proliferation to form Elschnig's pearls (Figure 13.12). These defects are more likely to occur in younger subjects, and contact between a posterior chamber implant and the capsule has an inhibitory effect. Opacification the posterior lens capsule after extracapsular lens extraction occurs in about 18.5–50% of cases (Apple *et al.* 1989; Solomon *et al.* 1991, 1994; Assia *et al.* 1991; Ohadi *et al.* 1991). The study by McDonnel *et al.* (1983) showed a 50% incidence in a 5 year follow-up. The incidence is nearly 100% in the paediatric age group within 2 years of follow-up (Nishi 1986; Maltzman *et al.* 1989).

It is caused by the metaplasia of residual lens epithelial cells and their migration over the posterior capsule as fibroblast-like cells with myoepithelial characteristics (Apple *et al.* 1989). Visual loss is due to contraction of 'fibroblastic' tissue and the formation of light-scattering opacity in and around the visual axis. Contraction of the capsule produces wrinkles which also degrade the retinal image.

The process of capsular opacification is due to the retention of epithelial cells at the time of surgery and their subsequent mitosis and migration. Manoeuvres which help to remove cells at the time of surgery or discourage migration in the post-operative period are thought to reduce the frequency of opacification. Riebsamen *et al.* (1988) described the aspiration of cells from the capsule using a limbal approach. Also, capsulorhexis combined with hydrodissection is thought to wash away more epithelial and nucleated cortical cells; a

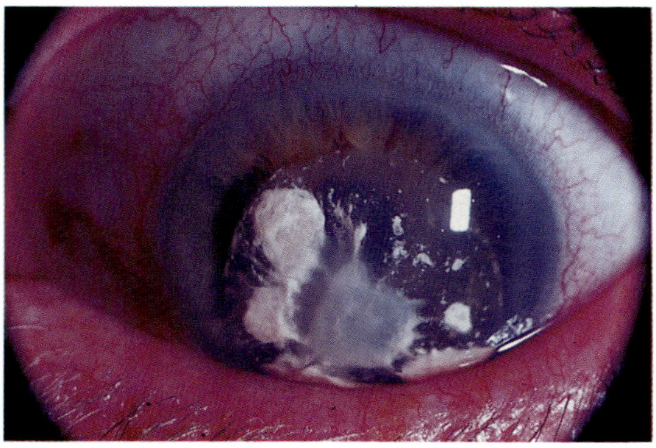

Figure 13.10 A calcified hypermature cataract dislocated into the anterior chamber.

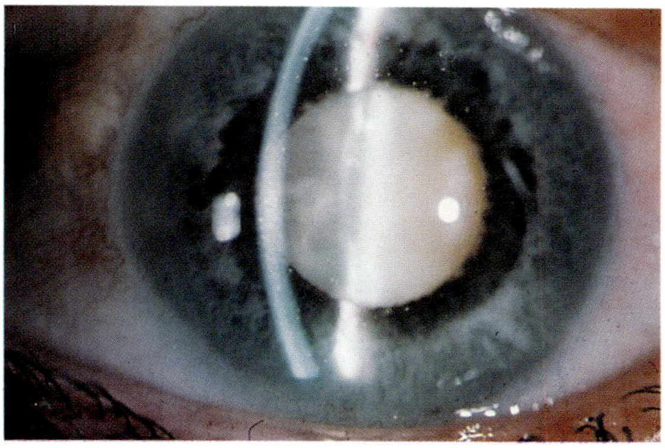

(a)

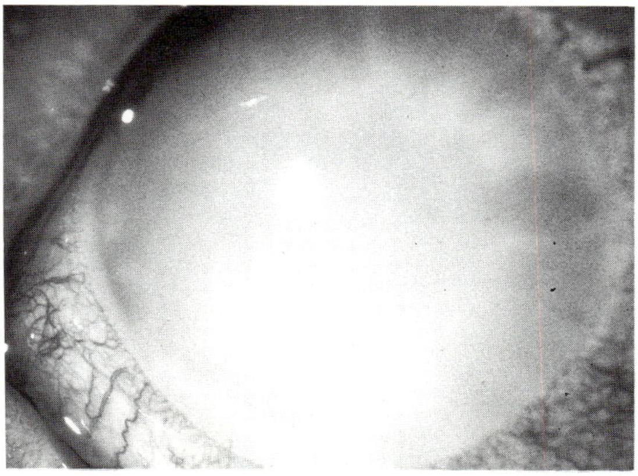

(b)

Figure 13.11 Phacolytic glaucoma. **(a)** A mature cataract with keratic precipitates on the corneal endothelium, but without inflammation. **(b)** In another patient the details of the iris are obscured by the presence of a cloud of lens protein and macrophages in the anterior chamber.

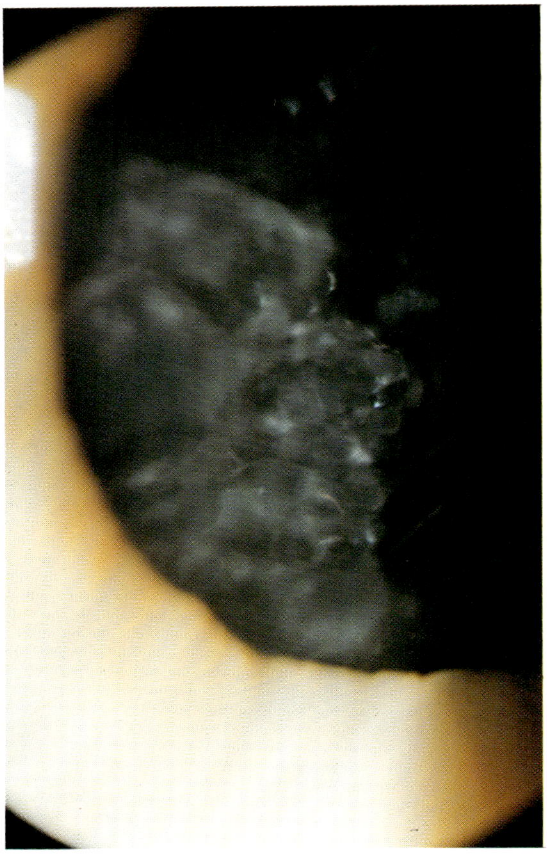

Figure 13.12 Elschnig's pearls.

large capsulotomy has been proposed in order to ensure a smaller residual number of cells (McDonnell *et al.* 1983) and a posterior convex implant optic (Lindstrom and Harris 1980; Harris and Aron-Rosa 1980; Sterling and Wood 1986; Santos *et al.* 1987; Selman and Lindstrom 1988; Born and Ryan 1990; Frezzotti and Caporossi 1990; Lowes 1990) or, experimentally, a biconvex optic (Hansen *et al.* 1988; Tetz *et al.* 1988), is believed to inhibit the migration of cells across the lens capsule and retard opacification. Since the likelihood of contact between the capsule and the lens implant is greater when there is a higher capsular tension, attempts to increase capsular tension have been made, including the use of a large, 'disc lens' or attention to haptic/loop design in order to maintain tension (Riebsamen 1988).

Various experimental studies have attempted to destroy epithelial cells *in situ*, using water (Hunold *et al.* 1989), fluorouracil (Solomon *et al.* 1990; Pearson *et al.* 1991) and colchicine (Legler *et al.* 1991). Colchicine inhibits mitosis and microtubular formation and could also retard epithelial migration. Daunorubicin has been used clinically, with some apparent success (Hartmann *et al.* 1989).

Soemmering's ring follows extracapsular extraction in the absence of an implant, when an adhesion is able to form between the cut edges of the anterior capsule, and the posterior capsule. Epithelial proliferation is then limited to forming a doughnut ring in the periphery.

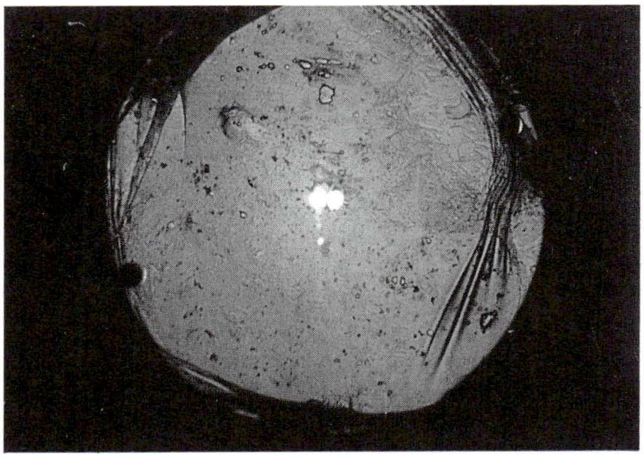

Figure 13.13(a) Posterior capsular opacification in a patient, 2 years after extracapsular cataract extraction. Note capsular folds and scattered Elschnig pearls.

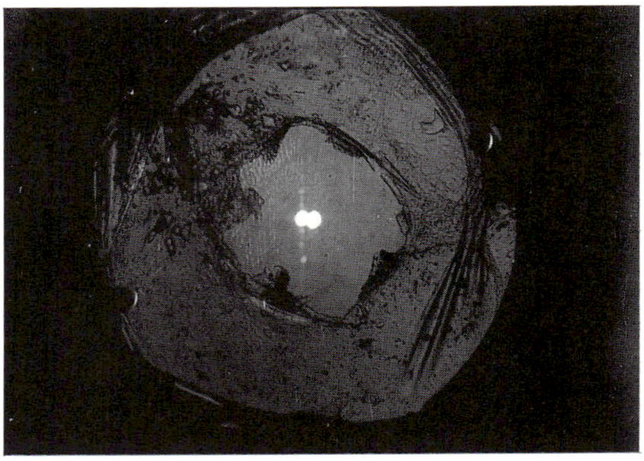

Figure 13.13(b) The same patient, at a later date, 3 days after YAG capsulotomy. Note the clear central gap of the capsulotomy and the presence of fresh pearls in the 4 o'clock position.

14

Vision in cataract

The most significant basic effect of cataract on vision, common to all types of cataract, is that of light scattering, so that the image received by the retina is desaturated by the contrast reducing effect of the scattered light. The degree of this effect depends on the proportion of the pupillary area that is occupied by the cataract. Once the pupil is fully occupied by dense opacity, the retina receives only scattered light and no formed image. Forward light scattering accounts for reduced contrast sensitivity, for glare and for reduced visual acuity. Objective methods of cataract assessment (see Chapter 7) can measure only backward scatter (light scattered away from the eye), rather than the forward scatter that affects the retina. It is reasonable to suppose that there is a relationship between forward scatter and backward scatter, but this has not been fully quantified (Elliott *et al.* 1991).

Light scattering in the lens is not unique to cataract and occurs in the normal ageing lens leading to increasing glare after the age of 50 (Carter 1982). This is likely to be the compounded result of the increase in lens thickness causing the light to traverse more fibre protoplasm plus a greater number of fibre membranes together with the increase in lens protein molecular size with age (Spector 1982).

There are a several demonstrable subjective ways in which vision is affected by cataract (Brown 1993) (Figures 14.1–14.3). Visual acuity is considered last because it has a relatively low level of importance to the patient, in spite of being the most commonly used assessment.

1. Myopic shift
2. Astigmatism

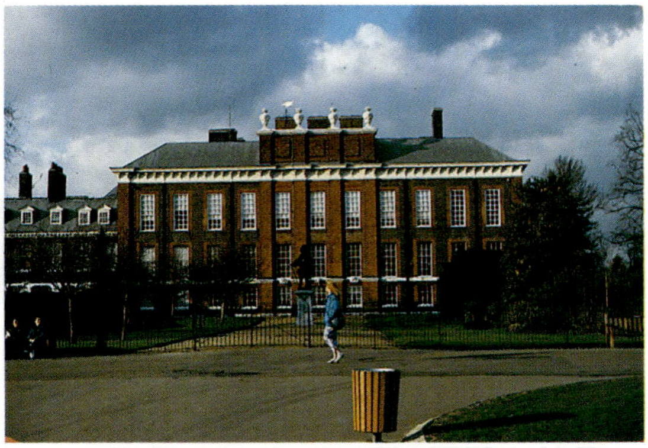

Figure 14.1 Normal view of the world in the absence of cataract.

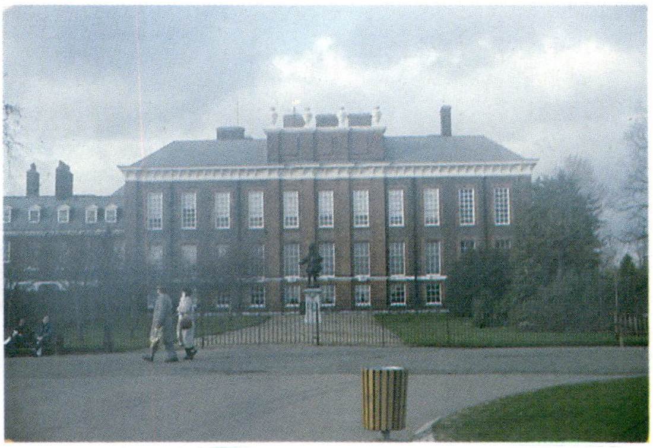

Figure 14.2 A simulated view through grade 3 spoke cataract. Note the reduction in contrast.

3. Monocular diplopia
4. Contrast sensitivity reduction
5. Glare
6. Colour shift
7. Reduced light transmission
8. Field loss
9. Visual acuity reduction

Myopic shift

The normal ageing human lens produces a gradual hypermetropic shift (Slataper 1950), which is offset by the development of nuclear cataract if this occurs. The patient may initially hail the change in vision as an improvement when they are enabled to give up their hypermetropic correction distance glasses, but as the condition progresses the vision deteriorates due to the other effects of the cataract.

Ageing patients not developing cataract, and those developing cortical or subcapsular cataract without nuclear cataract, show the continued hypermetropic shift, as does the healthy ageing eye. It is possible to predict that an ageing person is developing nuclear cataract if they show 0.5 or more myopic shift between refractions 2 years apart (Brown and Hill 1987).

Previously hypermetropic patients are usually happy to receive reduced strength glasses for best distance acuity, but the previously emmetropic patient is often uncomfortable with new minus lenses and a partial correction may be the best that is achievable.

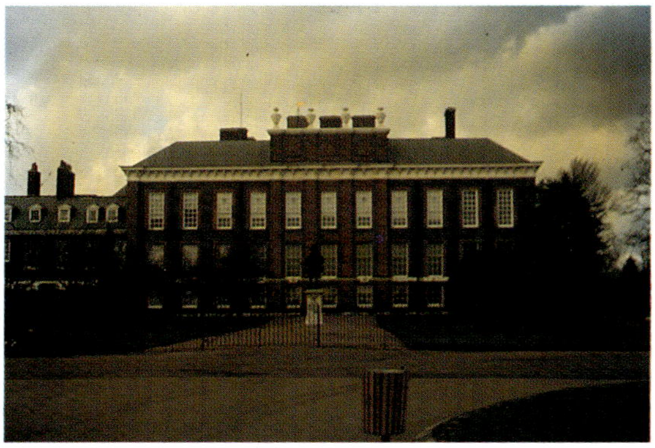

Figure 14.3 View through grade 3 brunescent cataract.

Astigmatism

This aspect of cataract vision appears not to have been researched. There is clinical experience that astigmatic shifts occur. Astigmatism is understandable in terms of an uneven change in refractive index in the lens and is seen in conjunction with cortical spoke cataract. Patients may be helped by the addition of, or change in, the astigmatic correction in their glasses.

Monocular diplopia

Monocular diplopia (Figure 14.4) is common in cataract, particularly with cortical spoke cataract and with water clefts in which conditions the

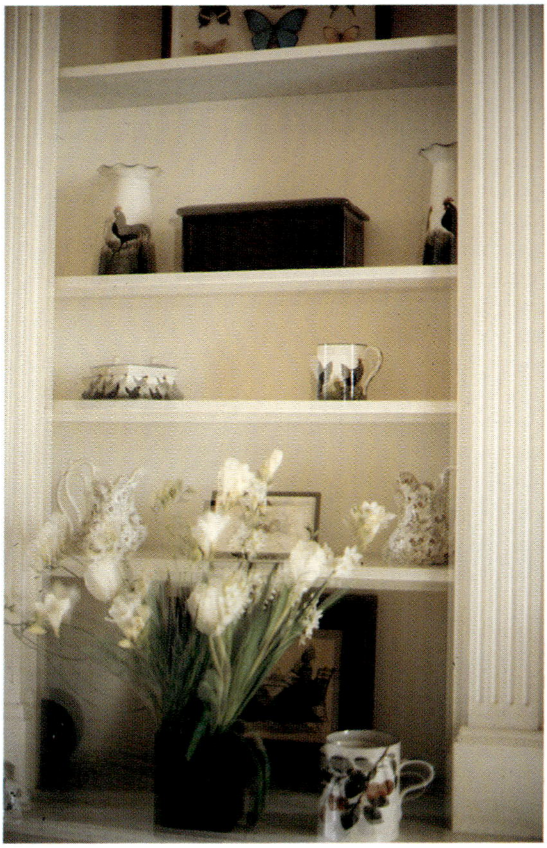

Figure 14.4 Monocular diplopia.

patient may experience multiple images (polyopia). Diplopia may also occur in nuclear cataract, in which the nucleus and cortex can produce separate images. The pin-hole test is useful as it will eliminate the monocular diplopia when it has a lenticular refractive cause.

It takes only a small prismatic effect due to refractive index changes to produce the double image. The picture illustrating monocular diplopia (Figure 14.4) was made with a prism of only 1 D covering part of the lens.

It is not usually possible to eliminate cataract monocular diplopia with glasses. However, the patient is made less aware of the doubled image when using the best possible correction, which is likely to include a cylinder.

Contrast sensitivity reduction

Contrast sensitivity (CS) testing is a research field in which the findings relate directly to the real world of the cataract patient (Elliott *et al.* 1990). All cataracts lower contrast sensitivity and it is the posterior subcapsular cataract which is most destructive of contrast sensitivity (Figure 14.5). The performance of the eye with cataract is reduced throughout the spatial frequency range. High spatial frequency CS losses in cataract correlate with Snellen VA losses and so, in cataract clinical trials, it is the low spatial frequency CS (1–2 cycles/degree) measurements that are the most informative. The patient has difficulty in distinguishing relatively large objects (low spatial frequency) of low contrast difference from their surroundings, although high spatial frequency objects of high contrast may be quite well seen (Elliott *et al.* 1989a). The effect is seen in Figure 14.2. Thus driving vision is impaired, while the ability to read may be retained. When a cataract is uniocular, the binocular contrast sensitivity test is affected at high spatial frequencies by binocular inhibition (Pardhan and Gilchrist 1991). Thus the vision of these patients is more affected than measurements on the good eye alone would indicate.

Glare

Even very minor degrees of cataract cause glare by the forward scattering of light. All forms of cataract cause glare, especially cortical (Figure 14.6) and posterior subcapsular. Glare affects the patient most severely when the light source is close to the object being looked at. This happens particularly in the context of night driving. Glare has a relatively weak effect at high contrast, such as with a Snellen chart, and is most accurately measured with a standardized glare source surrounding a contrast sensitivity test display (Elliott 1989b).

The subjective measurement of forward light scatter (Elliott *et al.* 1991) provides separately a

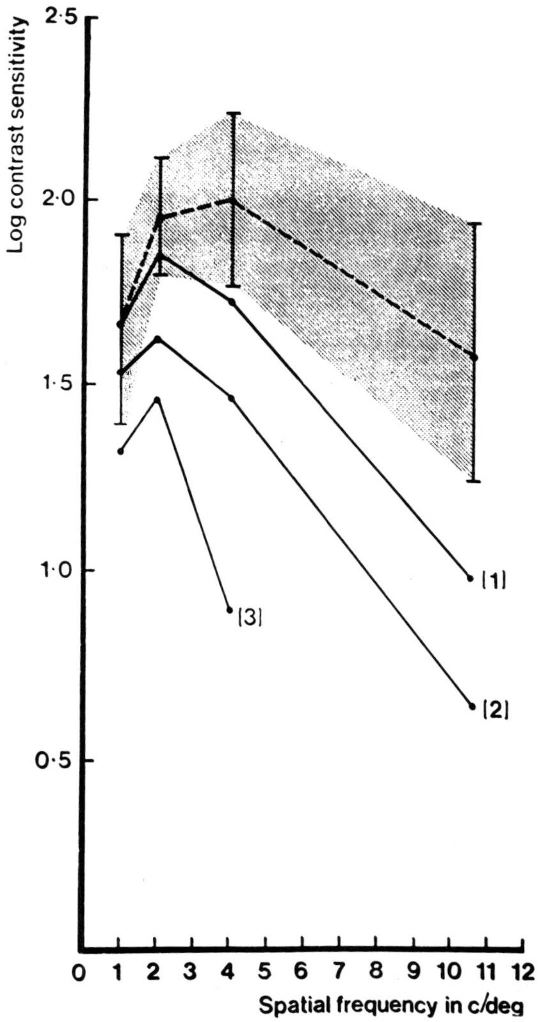

Figure 14.5 Contrast sensitivity in posterior subcapsular cataract compared with normals (broad band). (From Elliott 1989 with permission.)

measure of this effect of cataract which is the basic cause of contrast sensitivity reduction, of glare, and of visual acuity reduction. This is performed by the method of van den Berg (Ijspeert *et al.* 1990). The patient views a target of 1° surrounded by a ring of light emitting diodes (LEDs), which flicker. The flicker can be seen by the patient as superimposed on the target because of forward light scatter. The target is made to flicker in counterphase to the LEDs until it is indistinguishable. The amplitude of the luminance to produce zero perceived flicker corresponds directly to the amount of forward light scatter.

Glare is greater at short wave lengths and is reduced by a 550 nm cut off yellow filter (Tupper *et al.* 1985). This is an anticipated finding since short wave lengths are the more readily scattered and this effect is seen also in backward scattering in slit-image photography (Figure 3.13) in which the anterior portion of the lens appears blue.

Unlike contrast sensitivity reduction, some glare may be produced by opacities which do not lie within the pupil diameter, since these opacities will scatter light when receiving oblique rays and thus cause glare from light sources that are in the peripheral field.

Patients will benefit from the advice to use an adjustable reading light that is directed onto the page from an angle at which it cannot shine into their eyes. A hat or cap with a good brim can help to reduce glare from the sun. Tinted glasses can be useful in daylight, but the patient should avoid the temptation to drive with them at night. For patients who require glasses for driving, an anti-reflection coated glass helps by reducing reflections from the glass, but it will not remove glare from sources close to the point of fixation.

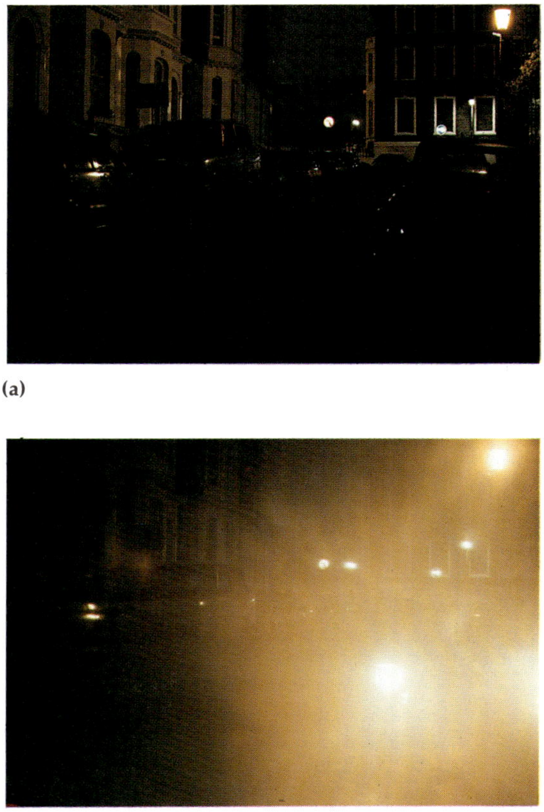

(a)

(b)

Figure 14.6(a) Normal night view. **(b)** Headlight glare in grade 3 cortical spoke cataract.

Colour shift

Patients with cataract are often unaware that their colour vision is defective (Figure 14.7) until it is restored to them by cataract surgery. The novel brightness of the colours seen through the lens implant is often far more amazing to the patient than the improvement in acuity.

The healthy ageing lens becomes progressively more absorbent at the blue end of the spectrum and this effect is exaggerated in cataract, particularly in nuclear brunescent cataract. Thus the patient with nuclear cataract is affected by reduced colour sense as well as by reduced contrast sensitivity and the myopic shift.

Reduced light transmission

The normal ageing lens passes progressively less light through to the retina (Boettner and Walter 1962; Weale 1987). This is accounted for in part simply by the increase in thickness of the lens with age. At the same time, the transparency of the ageing lens is becoming less, due to increased scattering and to increased absorption (Mellerio 1987). The inability of the ageing pupil to dilate in poor light is an additional factor in reducing retinal illumination. In poor light the absorption by the cataract becomes critical and vision is reduced.

The other effects of cataract also contribute to reduced vision in poor light. The contrast of objects is always lower than it is in direct sunlight, so that the patient's poor contrast sensitivity has a greater effect. Glare sources, such as headlights, are likely to be present in conditions of otherwise poor illumination.

Occasionally patients with cataract report improved vision in poor light. This occurs when there is a small diameter cataract placed centrally on the optic axis, so that vision improves with pupil dilatation.

There is no help to be gained from glasses in combating the reduced light transmission and patients are best advised to avoid wearing tinted glasses in poor light.

Field loss

Cataract can affect the visual field in one of two ways. With a pronounced spoke cataract a wedge-shaped shadow is thrown onto the retina (Figure 14.8) and this can cause an identifiable defect in the peripheral visual field (Lyne and Phillips 1969).

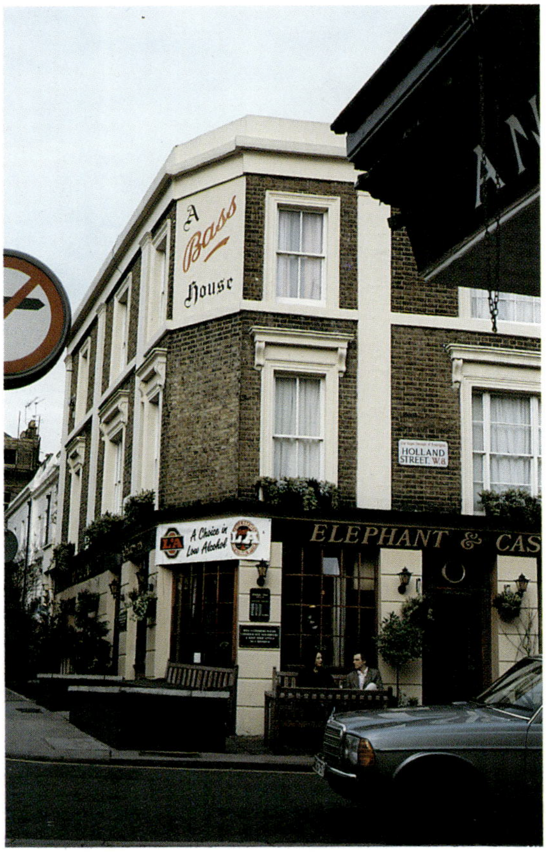

(a)

Figure 14.7(a) Normal view.

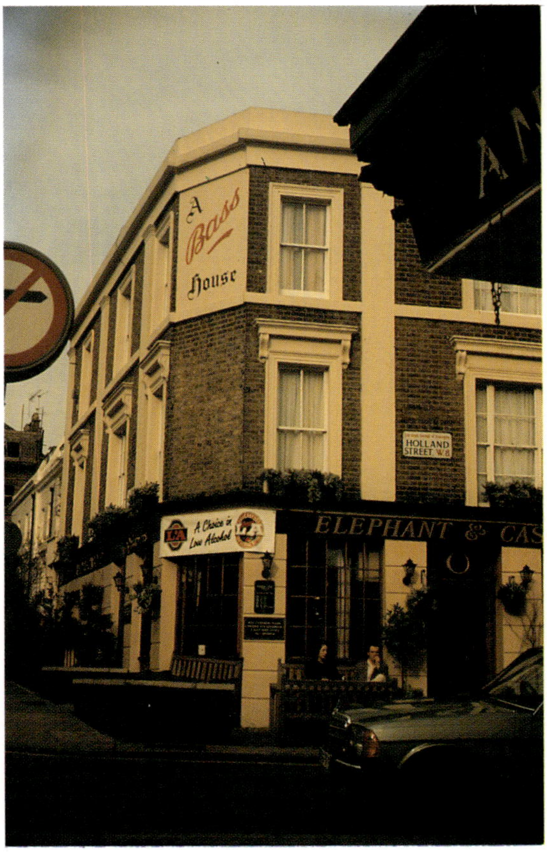

(b)

Figure 14.7(b) Shift of colour values in grade 3 brunescence.

The reduction in light transmission can cause an established glaucomatous field defect to appear to be increasing when tested with quantitative perimetry (Guthauser and Flammer 1988). An increase in the illumination of the test stimulus will reverse this effect, but the clinician is left with uncertainty about what is really happening at the retinal level.

Visual acuity reduction

Visual acuity testing is conducted under ideal circumstances, which are not normally met in the real world. The room is softly lit and all sources of glare are removed.

The test letters are of very high contrast, with nearly 100% difference between the letters and the background, which is not the same for most common objects in the environment. Even the print that the patient will commonly read at home, such as that in newspapers, does not begin to approach 100% contrast. There is a considerable lack of correlation between the visual acuity and the amount of cataract as measured photographically (Holden *et al.* 1993).

It is common to regard a VA of 6/12 as adequate to comply with the driving standard, but in poor light, or with glare from the headlights of other cars, the patient with cataract would be unlikely to meet this standard.

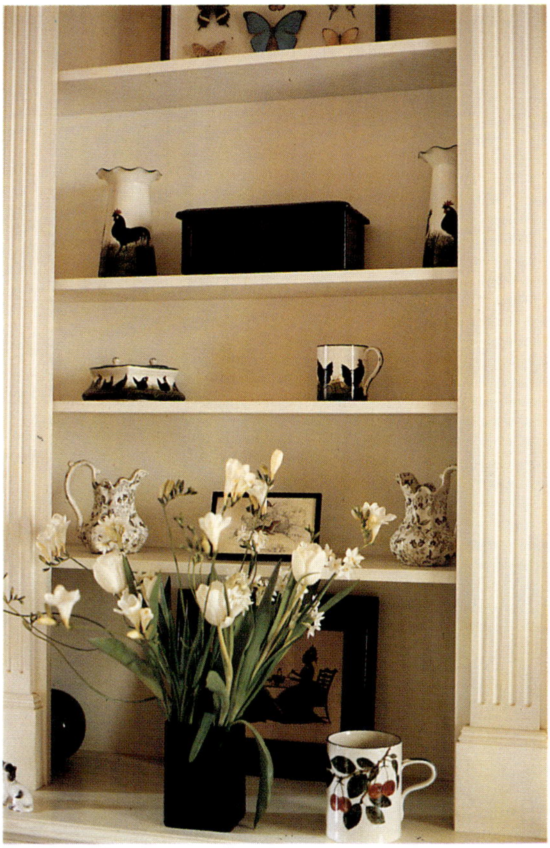

(a)

Figure 14.8(a) Normal view.

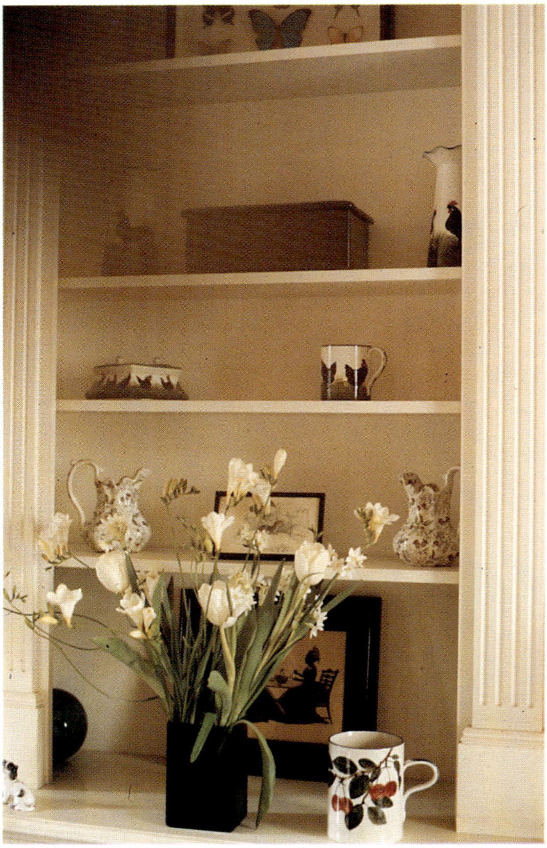

(b)

Figure 14.8(b) Field loss in the presence of a single prominent spoke cataract.

Conclusion

Cataract affects vision in many more ways than visual acuity testing alone would indicate. The nature of the effect varies with the degree of the cataract, with the cataract morphology, and with the amount of associated features, such as water clefts, vacuoles, retro-dots, and fibre folds. The assessment of a patient's visual disability is therefore not a simple task and cannot be based solely on visual acuity testing nor on the objective measurement of the amount of cataract.

Both contrast sensitivity and glare have been shown to correlate with the degree of the cataract as measured by cataract grading (Elliott *et al.* 1989) using the Oxford Grading System (p. 79), but the correlation is poor when measured photographically in early cataract, particularly for visual acuity (Holden *et al.* 1993).

The systems of classification and measurement are essential to ordered research work, but are necessarily an over simplification and tend to ignore the additional features associated with cataract including water clefts. These associated features are taken into account in the Oxford Clinical Cataract Classification and Grading System, but presently lack systems for measurement. Clinical experience suggests that these features affect vision, but the extent of the effect cannot be estimated until these features can be measured.

Patients developing cataract can best be helped by a careful refraction including a thorough search for astigmatic errors. Advice to use a magnifier for very small print is usually more helpful than giving strong reading glasses that necessitate a close reading distance. Advise the use of a good reading lamp that is directed only onto the page and does not shine into the eyes.

For many patients the need to drive is the crucial factor in determining the timing of cataract surgery. When it is becoming difficult to comply with the driving standard in the worst eye the patient should be considered for operation. Other occupational requirements should not be overlooked.

References

AASVED, H. (1969) The geographical distribution of fibrillopathia epitheliocapsularis. *Acta. Ophthalmol.*, **47**, 792–810

AASVED, H. (1971) Mass screening for fibrillopathia epitheliocapsularis, so-called senile exfoliation of pseudoexfoliation of the anterior lens capsule. *Acta. Ophthalmol.*, **49**, 334–343

ABBASSI, V., LOWE, C.U. and CALCAGNO, P.L. (1968) Oculocerebro-renal syndrome: a review. *Am. J. Dis. Child.*, **115**, 145–168

ABRAHAM, R.K. and MILLER, G.L. (1975) Outpatient argon laser iridectomies for angle closure glaucoma. *Trans. Am. Acad. Ophthalmol. Otolaryngol.*, **79**, 529

ADAMS, E. (1915) Congenital aphakia with microcornea. *Ophthal. Rec.*, **XXIV**, 581–

ADAMS, P.H. (1942) Doyne's discoid cataract (Coppock). *Br. J. Ophthalmol.*, **26**, 152

AL-GHADYAN, A.A. and COTLIER, E. (1986) Rise in lens temperature on exposure to sunlight or to high ambient temperature. *Br. J. Ophthalmol.*, **70**, 421–426

ALBERT, D.M., LAHAV, M., CARMICHAEL, L.E., *et al.* (1976) Canine herpes-induced retinal dysplasia and associated ocular anomalies. *Invest. Ophthalmol.*, **15**, 267–278

ALBERT, D.M., LAHAV, M., COLBY, E.D., *et al.* (1977) Retinal neoplasia and dysplasia. I: Induction of feline leukemia virus. *Invest. Ophthalmol. Vis. Sci.*, **16**, 325–337

ALCALA, J., KATAR, M. and MAISEL, H. (1982) Lipid composition of chick lens fiber cell gap junctions. *Curr. Eye Res.*, **2**, 569–578

ALCALA, J. and MAISEL, H. (1985) Biochemistry of lens plasma membranes and cytoskeleton. In *The Ocular Lens: Structure, Function and Pathology* (ed. H. Maisel), Marcel Dekker, New York, 169–222 [1799]

ALDEN, E.R., KALINA, R.E. and HODGSON, W.B. (1973) Transient cataracts in low birthweight infants. *J. Pediatr.*, **82**, 314–318

ALLANSMITH, M. and SENZ, E.H. (1960) Chondrodystrophia congenita punctata (Conradi's disease). *Am. J. Dis. Child.*, **100**, 109–116

ALT, A. (1906) A case of transitory lenticular opacity in both eyes in a diabetic patient. *Am. J. Ophthalmol.* **23**, 294–298

ALTER, M., TALBERT, O.R. and CROFFEAD, G. (1962) Cerebellar ataxia, congenital cataracts and retarded somatic and mental maturation: report of cases of Marinesco–Sjogren syndrome. *Neurology*, **12**, 836–847

ANDERSEN, A.C. and SCHULTZ, F.T. (1958) Inherited (congenital) cataract in the dog. *Am. J. Pathol.* **34**, 965–975

ANDERSEN, P.F. (1943) Craniofacial dysostosis (Crouzon's disease) as dominant hereditary disease. *Nord. Med.* **18**, 993–996

ANDERSEN, S.R.Y. and WARBURG, M. (1961) Norrie's disease: congenital bilateral pseudotumor of the retina with recessive X-chromosomal inheritance. Preliminary report. *Arch. Ophthalmol.*, **66**, 614–618

ANDERSON, R.S., TRUNE, D.R. and SHEARER, T.R. (1988) Histologic changes in selenite cortical cataract. *Invest. Ophthalmol. Vis. Sci.*, **29**, 1418–1427

ANDREWS, J.S. and LEONARD-MARTIN, T. (1981) Total lipid and membrane lipid analysis of normal animal and human lenses. *Invest. Ophthalmol.*, **21**, 39–45

APPLE, D.J., MAMALIS, N., LOFTFIELD, K., GOOGE, J.M., NOVAK, L.C., KAVKA-VAN NORMAN, D., BRADY, S.E. and OLSON, R.J. (1984) Complications of intraocular lenses: a historical and histopathological review. *Surv. Ophthalmol.*, **29**, 1–54

APPLE, D.J., KINCAID, M.C., OLSON, R.J. and MAMALIS, N. (1989) Intraocular Lenses: Evolution, Design, Complications and Pathology. Williams and Wilkins, Baltimore

ARNOTT, E.J., CRAWFORD, M.D.A. and TOGHILL, P.J. (1966) Anterior lenticonus and Alport's syndrome. *Br. J. Ophthalmol.*, **50**, 390–403

ASHTON, N., BARNETT, K.C., CLAY, C.E. *et al.* (1977) Congenital nuclear cataracts in cattle. *Vet. Rec.*, **100**, 505–508

ASTER, J.C., BREWER, G.J., HANASH, S.M. *et al.* (1984) Band 4.1-like proteins of the bovine lens. *Biochem. J.*, **224**, 609–616

ASTER, J.C., BRINN, K. MAISEL, H. *et al.* (1985) Phosphorylation of the band 4.1-like proteins of the bovine lens. *Biochem. Biophys. Res. Commun.*, **126**, 1166–1173

AXELSSON, U. (1969a) Glaucoma, miotic therapy and cataract. IV. Chronic simple glaucoma and cataract. *Acta Ophthalmol.* Suppl 47, 55–79

AXELSSON, U. (1969b) Glaucoma, miotic therapy and cataract. V. Studies on the lens in glaucoma eyes after discontinuance of echothiophate (Phospholine Iodide) therapy. *Acta Ophthalmol.* **47**, 1049–1056

AXELSSON, U. and HOLMBERG, Å. (1966) The frequency of cataract after miotic therapy. *Acta Ophthalmol.*, **44**, 421–429

BAGCHI, M. (1959) The effects of methionine-sulphoximine induced methionine deficiency on the crystalline lens of albino rats. *Indian J. Med. Res.*, **47**, 437–447

BAGCHI, M., ALCALA, J.R. and MAISEL, H. (1981) Delta-crystallin synthesis by the adult chicken lens. *Exp. Eye Res.*, **32**, 251–254

BAILLIE, H.D., HEALE, A.G. and PAL, D.K. (1970) Effects of metallic inclusions in a microwave field. *Non-ionizing Radiat.*, **3**, 159–163

BAKER, W.H. (1887) Congenital aphakia. *N.Y. Med. J.*, **46**, 595

BANE, W.M. (1944) Congenital cataracts. *Am. J. Ophthalmol.*, **27**, 651

BARAITSER, M. (1982) Marshall/Stickler syndrome. *J. Med. Genet.*, **19**, 139–140

BARANSKY, S. and CZERSKI, P. (1976) *Biological Effects of Microwaves.* Dowden Hutchinson & Ross, ??, PA.

BARDELLI, A.M., LASORELLA, G. and VANNI, M. (1989) Congenital and developmental cataracts and multi malformation syndromes. *Ophthalmic Pediatr. Genet.*, **10**, 293–298

BARNETT, K.C. (1978) Hereditary cataract in the dog. *J. Small Anim. Pract.*, **19**, 109–120

BARRIE, K.P., PEIFFER, R.L., GELATT, K.N. *et al.* (1979) Posterior lenticonus, microphthalmia, congenital cataracts, and retinal folds in an Old English Sheepdog. **15**, 715–717

BARTHOLOMEW, R.S. (1971) Pseudo-capsular exfoliation in the Bantu of South Africa. I. Early or pregranular stage. *Br. J. Ophthalmol.*, **55**, 693–699

BASSNETT, S. and DUNCAN, G. (1985) Direct measurement of pH in the rat lens by ion-sensitive microelectrodes. *Exp. Eye Res.*, **40**, 585–590

BASSNETT, S., STEWART, S., DUNCAN, G. *et al.* (1988) Efflux of chloride from the rat lens: influence of membrane potential and intracellular acidification. *Q.J. Exp. Physiol.*, **73**, 941–949

BECKER, B. (1964) Cataracts and topical corticosteroids. *Am. J. Ophthalmol.*, **58**, 872–873

BEEBE, D.C. and HYATT, G.A. (1992) A new embryo-specific growth factor in the anterior chamber: its role in establishing lens polarity. Proceedings of Xth ISER Meeting, Stresa, Italy [Abstract]. *Exp. Eye Res.*, **55**, 1

BEEBE, D.C., SILVER, M.H., BELCHER, K.S., *et al.* (1987) Lentropin, a protein that controls lens fibre formation, is related functionally and immunologically to the insulin-like growth factors. *Proc. Natl. Acad. Sci. USA*, **84**, 2327–2331

BEETHAM, W.P. (1940) Atopic cataracts. *Arch Ophthalmol.*, **24**, 21–37

BELLOWS, J.G. (1944a) *Cataract and Anomalies of the Lens.* Mosby, St Louis

BELLOWS, J.G. (1944b) The crystalline lens in diabetes mellitus. *Arch. Ophthalmol.*, **32**, 498–507

BELLOWS, J.G. and NELSON, D. (1944) Cataract produced by anoxia. *Arch. Ophthalmol.*, **31**, 250

BELOVA, S.F. and GORDON, Z.V. (1956) Deistve santimetrovykh volu na glaza. (Effect of 1 cm waves on the eye.) *Bull. Exp. Biol. Med.*, **41**, 327–330

BEN-SIRA, I., WEINBERGER, D., BODENHEIMER, J. *et al.* (1980) Clinical method for measurement of light back scattering from the *in vivo* human lens. *Invest. Ophthalmol. Vis. Sci.*, **19**, 435–437

BENEDEK, G.B. (1971) Theory of transparency of the eye. *Appl. Optics*, **10**, 459–473

BENEDEK, G.B., CHYLACK, L.T., LIBONDI, T. *et al.* (1987) Quantitative detection of the molecular changes associated with early cataractogenesis in the living human lens using quasielastic light scattering. *Curr. Eye Res.*, **6**, 1421–1432

BENSCH, K.S., FLEMING, J.E. and LOHMANN, W. (1985) The role of ascorbic acid in senile cataract. *Proc. Natl. Acad. Sci.*, USA, **82**, 7193–7196

BENSON, P.F., BROWN, S.P., CREE, J., *et al.* (1976) Phenotypic expression of galactokinase deficiency in heterozygous and homozygous subjects: *In vivo* and *in vitro* studies. *Birth Defects*, **12**, 1

BERGINER, V.M., SALEN, G. and SHEFER, S. (1984) Long-term treatment of cerebrotendinous xanthomatosis with chenodeoxycholic acid. *N. Engl. J. Med.*, **311**, 1649–1652

BERLINER, M.L. (1949) *Biomicroscopy of the Eye*, Paul Hoeber, New York, **2**, I.

BERLYNE, G.M., DANOVITCH, G.M., BEN ARI, J. *et al.* (1972) Cataracts of chronic renal failure. *Lancet*, **i**, 509–511

BERMAN, E.R. (1991) *Biochemistry of the Eye*, Plenum Press, New York

BERNSTEIN, H.N. (1983) Ophthalmologic considerations and testing in patients receiving long-term antimalarial therapy. *Am. J. Med.*, **1**, 25–34

BERNSTEIN, H.N., CURTIS, J., EARL, F.L. *et al.* (1970) Phototoxic corneal and lens opacities in dogs receiving a fungicide 2,6,dichloro-4-nitroaniline. *Arch. Ophthalmol.* **83**, 336–348

BERSON, E.L., SCHMIDT, S.Y. and SHIH, V.E. (1978) Ocular and biochemical abnormalities in gyrate atrophy of the choroid and retina. *Ophthalmology*, **85**, 1018–1027

BERTELSEN, T.I. and SELAND, J.H. (1972) Flat whole mount preparations of the lens capsule in fibrillopathia epitheliocapsularis, the so called senile exfoliation or pseudoexfoliation. *Acta Ophthalmol.*, **49**, 938–955

BESSEMS, G.J.H., BOURS, J., HOFMANN, D. *et al.* (1990) Molecular mass distribution of water-soluble crystallins from the human foetal lens during development. *J. Chromatogr.*, **529**, 277–286

BETTELHEIM, F.A. (1985) Physical basis of transparency. In *The Ocular Lens: Structure, Function and Pathology*, (ed. H. Maisel), Marcel Dekker, New York, 265–300

BETTELHEIM, F.A., ALI, S., WHITE, O. *et al.* (1986) Freezable and non-freezable water content of cataractous human lenses. *Invest. Ophthalmol. Vis. Sci.*, **27**, 122–125

BEUTLER, E., MATSAMOTO, F., KUHL, W. *et al.* Galactokinase deficiency as a cause of cataracts. *N. Engl. J. Med.*, **288**, 1203

BEYER, P., LAUSECKER, C., LEVY, J.M. *et al.* (1956) Une nouvelle observation d'arthrogryposis multiplex et de pterygium. *Arch. Fr. Pediatr.*, **13**, 286–293

BHUYAN, K.C. and BHUYAN, D.K. (1977) Regulation of hydrogen peroxide in eye humors. Effect of 3-amino-1H-1,2,4-triazole on catalase and glutathione peroxidase of rabbit eye. *Biochim. Biophys. Acta*, **497**, 641–651

BHUYAN, K.C., BHUYAN, D.K. and KATZIN, H.M. (1973) Amizol-induced cataract and inhibition of lens catalase in rabbit. Ophthalmic Res **5**, 236–247

BINDELS, J.G., SIEZEN, R.J. and HOENDERS, H.J. (1979) A model for the architecture of a-crystallin. *Ophthalmic Res.*, **11**, 441–452

BINKHORST, C.D. and GOBIN, M.H. (1970) Treatment of congenital and juvenile cataract with intraocular lens implants (pseudophakoi). *Br. J. Ophthalmol.*, **54**, 759–765

BISTNER, S.I., RUBIN, L.F. and SAUNDERS, L.Z. (1970) The ocular lesions of bovine viral diarrhea-mucosal disease. *Vet. Pathol.*, **7**, 275–286

BITO, L.Z. and MIRANDA, O.C. (1989) Accommodation and Presbyopia; in *Ophthalmology Annual*, (ed. R.D. Reinecke), Raven Press, New York, 103–128

BITO, L.Z., DE ROUSSEAU, C.J., KAUFMAN, P.L. *et al.* (1982) Age-dependent loss of accommodative amplitude in rhesus monkeys: an animal model for presbyopia. *Invest Ophthalmol. Vis. Sci.*, **23**, 23–31

BITO, L.Z., KAUFMAN, P.L., DE ROUSSEAU, C.J. *et al.* (1987a) Presbyopia: An animal model and experimental approaches for the study of the mechanism of acommodation and ocular ageing. *Eye*, **1**, 222–230

BITO, L.Z., KAUFMAN, P.L., NEIDER, M. *et al.* (1987b) The dynamics of accommodation (ciliary muscle contraction, zonular relaxation, and lenticular deformation) as a function of stimulus strength and age in iridectomized rhesus eyes. ARVO Suppl: *Invest. Ophthalmol. Vis. Sci.*, **28**, 318

BIXLER, D., HIGGINS, M. and HARTSFIELD, J.JR. (1984) The Nance-Horan syndrome: a rare X-linked ocular-dental trait with expression in heterozygous females. *Clin. Genet.*, **26**, 30–35

BJORKHEM, I. and SKREDE, S. (1989) Familial diseases with storage of sterols other than cholesterol. In *The Inherited Basis of Metabolic Disease* (eds C.R. Scriver, A.L. Beaudet, W.S. Sly *et al.*), 6th edn, McGraw-Hill, New York, 1283–1302

BLACK, R.L., OGLESBY, R.B., VON SALLMANN, L. *et al.* (1960) Posterior subcapsular cataracts induced by corticosteroids in patients with rheumatoid arthritis. *J. Am. Med. Assoc.*, **174**, 166–171

BLOEMENDAL, H. (1977) The vertebrate eye lens. *Science*, **197**, 127–138

BLOEMENDAL, H. (ed.) (1981) In *Molecular and Cellular Biology of the Eye Lens*, John Wiley, New York

BLOEMENDAL, H. (1985) Lens research: from protein to gene. *Exp. Eye Res.*, **41**, 429–448

BLONDIN, J., BARAGI, V., SCHWARTZ, E.R. *et al.* (1986) Dietary vitamin C prevents eye lens protein damage. ARVO Suppl: *Invest. Ophthalmol. Vis. Sci.*, **27**, 9

BOETTNER, E.A. and WALTER, J.R. (1962) Transmission of the ocular media. *Invest. Ophthalmol.*, **1**, 776–783

BONNEY, C.H., HUNTER, D.M., CONLEY, G.E. *et al.* (1977) Heavy-ion-induced cataractogenesis. *Aviat. Space Environ. Med.*, **48**, 731–733

BORCHMAN, D., PATERSON, C.A. and DELAMERE, N.A. (1989a) Ca^{2+}-ATPase activity in the human lens. *Curr. Eye Res.*, **8**, 1049–1054

BORCHMAN, D., PATERSON, C.A. and DELAMERE, N.A. (1989b) Oxidative inhibition of Ca^{2+}-ATPase in the rabbit lens. *Invest. Ophthalmol. Vis. Sci.*, **30**, 1633–1637

BORON, W.F., RUSSELL, J.M., BRODWICK, S.M., *et al.* (1978) Influence of cyclic AMP on intracellular pH regulation and chloride fluxes in barnacle muscle fibres. *Nature*, **276**, 511–513

BORN, C.P. and RYAN, D.K. (1990) Effect of intraocular lens optic design on posterior capsular opacification. *J. Cataract Refract. Surg.*, **16**, 188–192

BOURNE, M.C., CAMPBELL, D.A. and PYKE, M. (1938) Cataract associated with an hereditary retinal lesion in rats. *Br. J. Ophthalmol.*, **22**, 608–613

BOURS, J. (1987) A re-evaluation of lens wet weight, water content and water-soluble and -insoluble crystallins of the ageing human lens, compared with other species. In *Modern Trends in Aging Research* (eds Courtois and Fauchaux), INSERM **1**, 373–379

BOURS, J. and FODISCH, H.J. (1986) Human fetal lens: wet and dry weight with increasing gestational age. *Ophthalmic Res.*, **18**, 363–368

BOURS, J., FODISCH, H.J. and HOCKWIN, O. (1987) Age-related changes in water and crystallin content of the fetal and adult human lens, demonstrated by a microsectioning technique. *Ophthalmic Res.* **19**, 235–239

BOURS, J., HOFMANN, D., FÖDISCH, H.J. *et al.* (1989) The crystallin composition of human fetal and adult lens microsections, analyzed by agarose isoelectric focusing. In *Risk Factors for Cataract Development* (eds O. Hockwin, K. Sasaki, M.C. Leske), Dev. Ophthalmol. Karger, Basel, 188–191

BOURS, J., WEGENER, A., HOFMANN, D. *et al.* (1990) Protein profiles of microsections of the fetal and adult human lens during development and ageing. *Mechanisms of Ageing and Development*, **54**, 13–27

BOYD, M.W.J. and GRANT, A.P. (1959) Werner's syndrome (progeria of the adult): further pathological and biochemical observations. *Br. Med. J.*, **2**, 920–925

BRAKENHOFF, R.H., AARTS, H.J.M., REEK, F.H., LUBSEN, N.H. and SCHOENMAKERS, J.G.G. (1990) Human τ-crystallin genes. A gene family on its way to extinction. *J. Mol. Biol.*, **216**, 519–532

BRIDGES, C.H. and FLOWERS, A.I. (1958) Iridocyclitis and cataracts associated with an encephalomyelitis in chickens. *J. Am. Vet. Med. Assoc.*, **132**, 79–84

BRINI, A. and FLAMENT, J. (1973) Cataracta glaucomatosa acuta. *Exp. Eye Res.*, **16**, 19–28

BRITTEN, M.J.A., HALNAN, K.E. and MEREDITH, W.J. (1967) Radiation cataract. New evidence on radiation dosage to the lens. *Br. J. Radiol.*, **39**, 612

BROEKHUYSE, R.M. and KUHLMAN, E.D. (1974) Lens membranes. I: Composition of urea treated plasma membrane from calf lens. *Exp. Eye Res.*, **19**, 297–302

BROEKHUYSE, R. and KUHLMANN, E.D. (1980) Lens membranes. XI: Some properties of human lens main intrinsic protein (MIP) and its enzymatic conversion into a 22 000 dalton polypeptide. *Exp. Eye Res.*, **30**, 305–310

BRON, A.J. and BROWN, N.A.P. (1986) Lens structure and forms of cataract. In *The Lens: Transparency and Cartaract* (ed. G. Duncan), Eurage, 3–11

BRON, A.J. and BROWN, N.A.P. (1987) Perinuclear lens retrodots: a role for ascorbate in cataractogenesis. *Br. J. Ophthalmol.*, **71**, 86–95

BRON, A.J. and BROWN, N.A.P. (1994) Growth of the human lens: The lens as a clock. In *Congenital Cataracts* (eds E. Cotlier, S. Lambert and D Taylor), R.G. Landes Co., 203–235

BRON, A.J. and HABGOOD, J.O. (1976) Morgagnian cataract. *Trans. Ophthalmol. Soc.*, UK, **96**, 265–277

BRON, A.J., BROWN, N.A.P., SPARROW, J.M. *et al.* (1987) Medical treatment of cataract. *Eye*, **1**, 542–550

BRON, A.J. and LAMBERT, S.R. (1984) Specular microscopy of the lens. *Ophthalmic Res.*, **16**, 209

BROOKS, A.M.V. and GILLIES, W.E. (1987) The depevelopment of microneovascular changes in the iris in pseudoexfoliation of the lens capsule. *Ophthalmology*, **94**, 1090–1097

BROOKS, H.V., JOLLY, R.D. and PATERSON, C.A. (1983) The pathology of an inherited cataract of sheep. *Curr. Eye Res.*, **2**, 625–632

BROOKS, H.V., JOLLY, R.D., WEST, D.M. *et al.* (1982) An inherited cataract in New Zealand Romney sheep. *New Zealand Vet. J.*, **30**, 113–114

BROOKS, M.H. (1975) Lenticular abnormalities in endocrine dysfunction. In *Cataract and Abnormalities of the Lens* (ed. J.G. Bellows), Grune & Stratton, New York, 285–301

BROWN, A,L., (1924) Hereditary cataract. *Am. J. Ophthalmol.*, **7**, 36–38

BROWN, C.A. and BURMAN, D. (1973) Transient cataract in a diabetic child with hyperosmolar coma. *Br. J. Ophthalmol.*, **57**, 429–433

BROWN, H.G., IRELAND, M. and KUSZAK, J.R. (1990) Ultrastructural, biochemical and immunological evidence of receptor-mediated endocytosis in the crystalline lens. *Invest. Ophthalmol. Vis. Sci.*, **31**, 2579–2592

BROWN, J.D. (1988) Incontinentia pigmenti the development of pseudo glioma. *Br. J. Ophthalmol.*, **72**, 452–456

BROWN, N. (1970) Macrophotography of the anterior segment of the eye. *Br. J. Ophthalmol.*, **54**, 697–701

BROWN, N. (1971) The visibility of transparent objects in the eye by retro-illumination. *Br. J. Ophthalmol.*, **55**, 517–524

BROWN, N. (1972) Quantitative slit-image photography of the lens. *Trans. Ophthalmol. Soc. UK*, **92**, 303–317

BROWN, N. (1976) Dating the onset of cataract. *Trans. Ophthalmol. Soc. UK*, **96**, 18–23

BROWN, N.A.P. (1973) The change in shape and internal form of the lens of the eye on accommodation. *Exp. Eye Res.* **15**, 441–459

BROWN, N.A.P. (1974) The change in lens curvature with age. *Exp. Eye Res.* **19**, 175–183

BROWN, N.A.P. (1993) The morphology of cataract and visual performance. *Eye*, **7**, 63–67

BROWN, N.A.P. and BRON, A.J. (1987) An estimate of the human lens epithelial cell size *in vivo*. *Exp. Eye Res.*, **44**, 899–906

BROWN, N.A.P. and DAWSON, T. (1987) A new British ophthalmic camera. *Acta Ophthalmol. Suppl.*, **134**, 1253–1254

BROWN, N. and ELLIS, P. (1972) Anterior polar pyramidal cataract presenting as an anterior chamber foreign body. A case history. *Br. J. Ophthalmol.*, **56**, 57–59

BROWN, N.A.P. and HILL, A.R. (1987) Cataract: the relationship between myopia and cataract morphology. *Br. J. Ophthalmol.*, **71**, 405–414

BROWN, N. and HUNGERFORD, J. (1982) The influence of the size of the lens in ocular disease. *Trans. Ophthalmol. Soc. UK*, **102**, 359–363

BROWN, N.A.P., SPARROW, J.M., SHUN-SHIN, G.A. *et al.* (1991) The acuityscope: a resolution test target projection ophthalmoscope. *Int. Ophthalmol.*, **15**, 139–142

BROWN, N.A.P. and TRIPATHI, R. (1974) Loss of the anterior subcapsular clear zone of the lens. Prognostic significance in cataract formation. *Trans. Ophthalmol. Soc. UK*, **94**, 29–45

BROWN, N.A.P., BRON, A.J., AYLIFFE, W. *et al.* (1987a) The objective assessment of cataract. *Eye*, **1**, 234–246

BROWN, N.A.P., BRON, A.J. and SPARROW, J.M. (1987b) An estimate of the size and shape of the human lens fibre *in vivo*. *Br. J. Ophthalmol.*, **71**, 916–922

BROWN, N.A.P., BRON, A.J. and SPARROW, J.M. (1988) Central compaction in the process of lens growth as indicated by lamellar cataract. *Br. J. Ophthalmol.*, **72**, 538–544

BROWN, N.A.P., VRENSEN, G., SHUN-SHIN, G.A. *et al.* (1989) Lamellar separation in the lens: the case for fibre folds. *Eye*, **3**, 597–605

BROWN, N.P., HARRIS, M.L., SHUN-SHIN, G.A. *et al.* (1993) Is cortical spoke cataract due to lens fibre breaks? The relationship between fibre fold, fibre breaks, water clefts and spoke cataract. *Eye*, **7**, 672–679

BRUNSTING, REED and BLAIR (1955) No title. *Arch Dermatol.*, **72**, 237–

BURDE, R.M. and BECKER, B. (1970) Corticosteroid-induced glaucoma and cataracts in contact lens wearers. *J. Am. Med. Assoc.*, **213**, 2075–2077

BURNS, R.P., ANDERSON, R.S. and FEENEY-BURNS, L. (1980) Cataract-webbed trait in Peromyscus. II: Biomicroscopy and histology of eyes. *Invest. Ophthalmol. Vis. Sci.*, **19**, 31–42

BURNS, R.P. and FEENEY, L. (1975) Hereditary cataracts in deer mice (*Peromyscus maniculatus*). *Am. J. Ophthalmol.*, **80**, 370–378

BURTON, B.K., SUMNER, T., LANGER, L.O. JR. *et al.* (1986) A new skeletal dysplasia: clinical, radiologic, and pathologic findings. *J. Pediatr.*, **109**, 642–648

BUSCHKE, W. (1943) Classification of experimental cataracts in the rat. Recent observations on cataract associated with tryptophan deficiency and with some other experimental conditions. A.M.A. *Arch. Ophthalmol.*, **30**, 735–750

BUYSE, M. and BULL, M.J. (1978) A syndrome of osteogenesis imperfecta, microcephaly and cataracts. *Birth Defects*, **14**, 95–98

BYERS, P.H., SIEGEL, R.C., PETERSON, K.E. *et al.* (1981) Marfan syndrome: abnormal alpha-2 chain in type I collagen. *Proc. Natl. Acad. Sci. USA*, **78**, 7745–7749

CAIRD, F.I., PIRIE, A. and RAMSELL, T.G. (1969) *Diabetes and the Eye*, Blackwell Scientific, Oxford, 131

CAMERON, J.D. and MCCLAIN, C.J. (1986) Ocular histopathology of acrodermatitis enteropathica. *Br. J. Ophthalmol.*, **70**, 662–667

CAMMARATA, P.R., CANTUCROUCH, D., MORRILL, A. *et al.* (1986) Macromolecular organisation of the bovine lens capsule. *Tissue Cell*, **18**, 83–97

CAPELLA, J.A., KAUFMAN, H.E., LILL, F.J. *et al.* (1963) Hereditary cataracts and microphthalmia. *Am. J. Ophthalmol.*, **56**, 454–458

CARNEY, R.G. (1976) Incontinentia pigmenti. A world statistical analysis. *Arch. Dermatol.* **112**, 535

CARNEY, R.G. and CARNET, R.G.JR. (1970) Incontinentia pigmenti. *Arch. Dermatol.*, **102**, 157–162

CARPENTER, R.L. (1958) In *Proceedings of 2nd Triservice Conference on Biological Effects of Microwave Energy* USAF, New York, 146–168

CARPENTER, R.L. (1959) In *Proceedings of 3rd Triservice Conference on Biological Effects of Microwave Energy* RADC TR-597140, 279–290

CARPENTER, R.L., BIDDLE, D.K. and VAN UMMERSEN, C.A. (1960) In *Proceedings of the Third International Conference on Medical Electronics* (Part 3), London, 401–408

CARPENTER, R.L., HAGAN, G.J. and DONOVAN, G.L. (1977) In *Symposium on Biological Effects and Measurement of Radio Frequency/Microwaves* (ed. D.G. Hazzard), US Department of Health Education and Welfare, Rockville, 352–379

CARPER, D., RUSSELL, P. and SANYAL, S. (1985) Comparison of the lens crystallin proteins from normal, 'rd' and 'rds' mutant mice utilizing specific monoclonal antibodies. *Exp. Eye Res.*, **40**, 757–761

CARPER, D., SMITH-GILL, S.J. and KINOSHITA, J.H. (1986) Immunocytochemical localisation of the 27K β-crystallin polypeptide in the mouse lens during development using a specific monoclonal antibody: Implications for cataract formation in the Philly mouse. *Dev. Biol.*, **113**, 104–109

CARTER, A.H. (1960) An inherited blindness (cataract) in cattle. **20**, 108

CARTER, J.H. (1982) The effect of aging upon selected visual functions. In *Aging and Human Visual Function* (eds R. Sekuler, D. Kline and K. Dismukes), Liss, New York, 121–130

CARTIER, M., BREITMAN, M.L. and TSUI, L.-C. (1992) A frameshift mutation in the γE-crystallin gene of the *Elo* mouse. *Nature Genetics* **2**, 42–45

CARVER, J.A., AQUILINA, J.A. and TRUSCOTT, R.J.W. (1994) A possible chaperone-like quaternary structure for α-crystallin. *Exp. Eye Res.*, **59**, 231–234

CASHWELL, L.F.JR., HOLLEMAN, I.V., WEAVER, R.G. *et al.* (1989) Idiopathic true exfoliation of the lens capsule. *Ophthalmology*, **96**, 348–351

CASSADY, J.R. and LIGHT, A. (1957) Familial persistent pupillary membranes. *Arch. Ophthalmol.*, **58**, 438–448

CENEDELLA, R.J. (1983) Source of cholesterol for the ocular lens, studied with U 18666A: a cataract-producing inhibitor of lipid metabolism. *Exp. Eye Res.*, **37**, 33–43

CENEDELLA, R.J. (1987) Direct chemical measurement of DNA synthesis and net rates of rat lens epithelial cells *in vivo*: applied to the selenium cataract. *Exp. Eye Res.*, **44**, 677–690

CENEDELLA, R.J. (1989) Cell cycle specific effects of selenium on the lens epithelium studied *in vivo* by the direct chemical approach. *Curr. Eye Res.*, **8**, 429–433

CENEDELLA, R.J. and BIERKAMPER, G.G. (1979) Mechanism of cataract production by 3-β(2-diethylaminoethoxy) androst-5-en-17-one hydrochloride, U 18666A, an inhibitor of cholesterol biosynthesis. *Exp. Eye Res.*, **28**, 673–688

CERAMI, A. and CRABBE, M.J.C. (1986) Recent advances in ocular cataract research. *Trends Pharmaceutical Sci.*, 271–274

CERIMELE, D., COTTONI, F., SCAPPATICCI, S. *et al.* (1982) High prevalence of Werner's syndrome in Sardinia: description of six patients and estimate of the gene frequency. *Hum. Genet.*, **62**, 25–30

CHALUPECKY, H. (1897) Uber die Wirkung der Rontgenstrahlenzbl. *Prakt. Augenheilk.*, **21**, 386–401

CHAMBERLAIN, C.G. and MCAVOY, J.W. (1987) Evidence that fibroblast growth factor promotes lens fibre differentiation. *Curr. Eye Res.*, **6**, 1165–1169

CHAMBERS, C. and RUSSELL, P. (1991) Deletion mutation in an eye lens β-crystallin. *J. Biol. Chem.*, **266**, 6742–6746

CHARALAMPOUS, F.C. and HEGSTED, A. (1950) Effect of age and diet on development of cataracts in the diabetic rat. *Am. J. Physiol.*, **161**, 540–544

CHARLTON, J.M. and VAN HEYNINGEN, R. (1968) An investigation into the loss of proteins of low molecular size from the lens in senile cataract. *Exp. Eye Res.*, **7**, 47–55

CHASE, H.B. and CHASE, E.B. (1941) Studies on an anophthalmic strain of mice. I. Embryology of the eye region. *J. Morphol.*, **68**, 279–295

CHEN, C.J. and RICHARDSON, C.D. (1986) Bee sting-induced ocular changes. *Ann. Ophthalmol.*, **18**, 285–286

CHERRYHOLMES (1902) Congenital aphakia with microphthalmos. *Ophthal. Rec.*

CHIESA, R., GAWINOWICZ-KOLKS, M.A. and SPECTOR, A. (1987) The phosphorylation of the primary gene products of a-crystallin. *J. Biol. Chem.*, **262**, 1438–1441

CHIESA, R., MCDERMOTT, M.J. and SPECTOR, A. (1989) Differential synthesis and phosphorylation of the a-crystallin A and B chains during bovine lens fiber cell differentiation. *Curr. Eye Res.*, **8**, 151–158

CHRISTENBERRY, K.W., CONKLIN, J.W., UPTON, A.C. *et al.* (1963) Induction of cataracts in mice by 4-(*p*-dimethyl aminostyryl) quinoline. *Arch. Ophthalmol.*, **70**, 250–252

CHYLACK, L.T. (1975) Mechanism of hypoglycaemic cataract formation in the rat lens. I: The role of hexokinase instability. *Invest. Ophthalmol.*, **14**, 746

CHYLACK, L.T. and CHENG, H.M. (1978) Sugar metabolism in the crystalline lens. *Surv. Ophthalmol.*, **23**, 26–34

CHYLACK, L.T. JR. and FRIEND, J. (1990) Intermediary metabolism of the lens: A historical perspective 1928–1989. *Exp. Eye Res.*, **50**, 575–582

CHYLACK, L.T. and LESKE, M.C. (1986) Validity and reliability of photo-derived human cataract classification. ARVO Suppl: *Invest. Ophthalmol. Vis. Sci.*, **27**, 44

CHYLACK, L.T., CHENG, H.M., WHITE, O. *et al.* (1984) Variance associated with objective documentation *in vivo* of human cataractous change with Topcon S1-45 and Neitz lens photography. *Proc. Int. Eye Res.*, **111**, 143

CHYLACK, L.T. JR., LESKE, M.C., MCCARTHY, D. *et al.* (1989) Lens opacities classification system II (LOCS II). *Arch. Ophthalmol.*, **107**, 991–997

CHYLACK, L.T. JR., WOLFE, J.K., SINGER, D.M. *et al.*, (1993) The lens opacity classification system version III (LOCS III). *Arch. Ophthalmol.*, **111**, 831–836

CIBIS, P.A. and NOELL, W.K. (1955) Cataract induced by iodacetic acid. *Am. J. Ophthalmol.*, **40**, 379–382

CLARK, J.I. and BENEDEK, G.B. (1980a) The effects of glycols, aldehydes and acrylamide on phase separation and specification in the calf lens. *Invest. Ophthalmol.*, **19**, 771–776

CLARK, J.I. and BENEDEK, G.B. (1980b) Phase diagram for cell cytoplasm from the calf lens. *Biochem. Biophys. Res. Commun.*, **95**, 482–489

CLARK, J.I., OSGOOD, T.B. and TRASK, S.J. (1987) Inhibition of phase separation by reagents that prevent X-irradiation cataract *in vivo*. *Exp. Eye Res.*, **45**, 961–967

CLAYTON, R.M. (1979) In *Genetic Regulation in the Vertebrate Lens Cell* (eds J. Ebert, T. Okada), John Wiley & Sons, New York, 129

CLAYTON, R.M. (1985) Developmental genetics of the lens. In *The Ocular Lens: Structure, Function and Pathology* (ed. H. Maisel), Marcel Dekker, New York, 61–92

CLOUD, T.M., HAKIM, R. and GRIFFIN, A.C. (1960) Photosensitization of the eye with methoxsalen. *Arch. Ophthalmol.*, **64**, 346–351

CLOUD, T.M., HAKIM, R. and GRIFFIN, A.C. (1961) Photosensitization of the eye with methoxsalen. *Arch. Ophthalmol.*, **66**, 689–694

COGAN, D.G., MARTIN, S.F., KIMURA, S.J. *et al.* (1950) Ophthalmologic study of atomic bomb survivors in Japan. *Trans. Am. Ophthalmol. Soc.*, **40**, 62–87

COGAN, D.G., GOFF, J.L. and GRAVES, E. (1952a) Experimental radiation cataract. II: Cataract in rabbit following single exposure to fast neutrons. *Arch. Ophthalmol.*, **47**, 584–929

COGAN, D., DONALDSON, D. and REESE, A.B. (1952b) Clinical and pathological characteristics of radiation cataract. *Arch. Ophthalmol.*, **47**, 55–70

COHEN, S.M.Z., BROWN, F.R. and MARTYN, L. *et al.* (1983) Ocular histopathologic and biochemical studies of the cerebrohepatorenal syndrome (Zellweger's syndrome) and its relationship to neonatal adrenoleukodystrophy. *Am. J. Ophthalmol.*, **96**, 488–501

COLE, D.F. (1984) Ocular fluids. In *The Eye* (ed. H. Davson), 3rd edn, Academic Press, New York, 269–390

COLE, H.N., GIFFEN, H.K., SIMMONS, J.T. *et al.* (1945) Congenital cataracts in sisters with congenital ectodermal dysplasia. *JAMA*, **129**, 723–728

COLLINS, E.T. (1894) Lectures on the anatomy and pathology of the eye. *Lancet*, **2**, 1329–1337

COLLINS, W.J. (1905) Crystalline lens in health and in cataract. *Br. Med. J.*, **2**, 1440–1445

CONNEALLY, P.M., WILSON, A.F., MERRITT, A.D. *et al.* (1978) Confirmation of genetic heterogeneity in autosomal dominant forms of congenital cataracts from linkage studies. *Cytogenet. Cell Genet.*, **22**, 295–297

CONSUL, B.N. and NAGPAL, P.N. (1968) Quantitative study of the variations in the levels of glutathione and ascorbic acid in human lenses with senile cataract. *Ear Nose Throat J.*, **47**, 336–340

COOK, C.A., KORETZ, J.F., PFAHNL, A., HYUN, J. and KAUFMAN, P.L. (1994) Accommodation and presbyopia in the human eye. Aging of the human crystalline lens and anterior segment. *Vision Res.*, in press

COOPER, K.E., TANG, J.H., RAE, J.L. *et al.* (1986) A cation channel in frog lens epithelia responsive to pressure and calcium. *J. Membr. Biol.*, **93**, 259–269

COOPER, R.L., CONSTABLE, I.J. and DAVIDSON, L. (1984) Aqueous humor catecholamines. *Curr. Eye Res.*, **3**, 809–813

COPPIN, C.M., KAPLAN, E.D., THOMSON, J.A. *et al.* (1986) Specificity of initial hydrogen peroxide damage to crystallins in calf lenses [abstract]. *Invest. Ophthalmol. Vis. Sci.*, **27**, 278

CORDES, F.C. (1961) Cataract types. A manual. *Am. Acad. Ophthalmol.*, **1**, 1

COSTAGLIOLA, C., IULIANO, G., MENZIONE, M. *et al.* (1988)

Systemic human diseases. Oxidative risk factors in cataractogenesis. I: Diabetes. *Ophthalmic Res.*, **20**, 308–316

COSTELLO, M.J., MCINTOSH, T.J. and ROBERTSON, J.D. (1989) Distribution of gap junctions and square array junctions in the mammalian lens. *Invest. Ophthalmol. Vis. Sci.*, **30**, 975–989

COTLIER, E. (1981) Senile cataracts: Evidence for acceleration by diabetes and deceleration by salicylate. *Can. J. Ophthalmol.*, **16**, 113–118

COTLIER, E. and APPLE, D. (1973) Cataracts induced by the polypeptide antibiotic polymyxin B sulfate. *Exp. Eye Res.*, **16**, 69

COTLIER, E. and RICE, P. (1971) Cataracts in the Smith–Lemli–Opitz syndrome. *Am. J. Ophthalmol.*, **72**, 955–959

COTLIER, E., FOX, J., BOHIGIAN, G., *et al.* (1968) Pathogenic effects of rubella virus on embryos and newborn rats. *Nature*, **217**, 38–40

COWAN, T.H. (1961) Pigmentation and colouration of the lens. *Surv. Ophthalmol.*, **6**, 630–647

CREIGHTON, M.O., TREVITHICK, J.R., MOUSA, G.Y. *et al.* (1978) Globular bodies: A primary cause of the opacity in senile and diabetic posterior cortical subcapsular cataracts. *Can. J. Ophthalmol.*, **13**, No. 3

CREWS, S.J. (1963) Posterior subcapsular lens opacities in patients on long term corticosteroid treatment. *Br. Med. J.*, **1**, 1644–1647

CREWS, S.J. and BUNDEY, S.E. (1982) Is there an X-linked form of congenital cataract? [letter] *Clin. Genet.*, **21**, 351–353

CRIDLAND, A.B. (1918) Three cases of hereditary cortical cataract, with a chart showing the pedigree of a family in which they occurred. *Trans. Ophthalmol. Soc. UK*, **38**, 375–376

CROFT, L.R. (1972) The amino acid sequence of y-crystallin (fraction II) from calf lens. *Biochem. J.*, **128**, 961–970

CROME, L., DUCKETT, S. and FRANKLIN, A.W. (1963) Congenital cataracts, renal tubular necrosis and encephalopathy in two sisters. *Arch. Dis. Child.*, **38**, 505–515

CROSS, H.E. (1976) Differential diagnosis and treatment of dislocated lenses. *Birth Defects*, **12**, 335–346

CRUYSBERG, J.R.M., SENGERS, R.C.A., PINCKERS, A. *et al.* (1986) Features of a syndrome with congenital cataract and hypertrophic cardiomyopathy. *Am. J. Ophthalmol.*, **102**, 740–749

CURTIN, V.T., JOYCE, E.F. and BALLIN, N. (1967) Ocular pathology in the oculo-cerebro-renal syndrome of Lowe. *Am. J. Ophthalmol.*, **64**, 533–543

CURTIS, P.B., HAUGE, S.M. and KRAYBILL, H.R. (1932) The nutritive value of certain animal protein concentrates. *J. Nutr.*, **5**, 503–517

DA SILVA, E.O., JANOVITZ, D. and DE ALBUQUERQUE, S.C. (1980) Ellis-van Creveld syndrome: report of 15 cases in an inbred kindred. *J. Med. Genet.*, **17**, 349–356

DAILY, L., WAKIM, K.G., HERRICK, J.F. *et al.* (1950) The effects of microwave diathermy on the eye. *Am. J. Ophthalmol.*, **33**, 1241–1254

DAILY, L., ZELLER, E.A., WAKIM, K.G. *et al.* (1951) Influence of microwaves on certain enzyme systems in lens of eyes. *Am. J. Ophthalmol.*, **34**, 1301–1306

DAISLEY, K.W. (1955) Synthesis of glutathione by normal and X-irradiated lenses. *Biochem. J.*, **60**, 1

DALGLEISH, R., WILLIAMS, G. and HAWKINS, J.R. (1986) Length polymorphism in the pro alpha-2(1) collagen gene: an alternative explanation in a case of Marfan syndrome. *Hum. Genet.*, **73**, 91–92

DARK, A.J. and STREETEN, B.W. (1977) Ultrastructural study of cataract in myotonia dystrophica. *Am. J. Ophthalmol.*, **84**, 666–674

DARK, A.J. and STREETEN, B.W. (1990) Precapsular film on the aging human lens: Precursor of pseudoexfoliation? *Br. J. Ophthalmol.*, **74**, 717–722

DARNELL, J., LODISCH, H. and BALTIMORE, D. (1990) *Molecular Cell Biology* Scientific American Books

DAS, B.N., THOMPSON, J.R., PATEL, R. *et al.* (1990) The prevalence of age related cataract in the Asian community of Leicester: A community based study. *Eye*, **4**, 723–726

DASLER, W. and WANG, H.L.S. (1972) Studies on cataracts induced in rats by N2-phenyl-B-hydrazinopropronitrile. *Invest. Ophthalmol.*, **11**, 236–240

DAVID, L.L. and SHEARER, T.R. (1986) Purification of calpain II from rat lens and determination of endogenous substrates. *Exp. Eye Res.*, **42**, 227–238

DAVIS, M.D., HILLER, R., MAGLI, Y.L. *et al.* (1979) Prognosis for life in patients with diabetes: relation to severity of retinopathy. *Trans. Am. Ophthalmol. Soc.*, **77**, 144–170

DAVSON, H. (1980) *Physiology of the Eye*. 4th edn, Churchill Livingstone, London & Edinburgh

DAVSON, H. (1990) *Physiology of the Eye*. 5th edn, MacMillan Press, London, 1–830

DAY, P.L. (1934) Vitamin G deficiency. *Am. J. Public Health*, **24**, 603–608

DAY, P.L. and DARBY, W.J. (1936) The inverse relation between growth and incidence of cataract in rats given graded amounts of vitamin G-containing foods. *J. Nutr.*, **12**, 387–394

DAY, P.L., LANGSTON, W.C. and O'BRIEN, C.S. (1931) Cataract and other ocular changes in vitamin G deficiency: experimental study on albino rats. *Am. J. Ophthalmol.*, **14**, 1005–1009

DE BERNADINIS, E. (1950) *Ann. Ottalm.*, **76**, 91

DE BUSK, F.L. (1972) The Hutchinson–Gilford progeria syndrome. *J. Pediatr.*, **80**, 697–724

DE BUSTRO, S., THOMPSON, J.J. (1988) Nuclear sclerosis after vitrectomy for idiopathic epiretinal membranes. *Am. J. Ophthalmol.*, **105**, 160–164

DE JONG, P.T.V.M., BLEEKER-WAGENMAKERS, E.M., VRENSEN, G.F.J.M. *et al.* (1990) Crystalline cataract and uncombable hair. *Ophthalmology*, **97**, 1181–1187

DE PABLO, F., CALDES, T., PEREZ-VILLAMIL, B. *et al.* (1992) The paracrine role of insulin-like growth factor 1 in embryonic differentiation. none [1], 1

DE ROETTH, A. (1966) Lens opacities in glaucoma patients

on phospholine iodide therapy. *Am. J. Ophthalmol.*, **62**, 619–628

DELAYE, M. and TARDIEU, A. (1983) Short range order of crystallin proteins accounts for eye lens transparency. *Nature*, **302**, 415–417

DELAYE, M., CLARK, J.J. and BENEDEK, G.B. (1982) Identification of the scattering elements responsible for lens opacification in cold cataracts. *Biophys. J.*, **37**, 647–656

DELLAMERE, N.A. and PATERSON, C.A. (1978) The influence of calcium-free EGTA solution upon membrane permeability in the crystalline lens of the frog. *J. Gen. Physiol.*, **71**, 581–593

DELLAMERE, N.A. and PATERSON, C.A. (1981) Hypocalcaemic cataract. In *Mechanisms of Cataract Formation in the Human Lens* (ed. G. Duncan), Academic Press, New York, 219–236

DELLEMAN, J.W., BEEKERS-WAGEMAKERS, E.M. and VAN VEELEN A.W.C. (1977) Opacities of the lens indicating carrier status of the oculo-cerebro-renal (Lowe) syndrome. *J. Pediatr. Ophthalmol.*, **14**, 205

DELMARCELLE, Y., FRANCOIS, J., COLLIGNON-BRACH, J. *et al.* (1976) Biometrie oculaire clinique. *Bull. Soc. Belge. Ophtalmol.*, **172**, 1

DEN DUNNEN, J.T., JONGBLOED, R.J.E., GEURTS VAN KESSEL, A.H.M. *et al.* (1985) Human lens y-crystallin sequences are located in the p12-qter region of chromosome 2. *J. Genet. Hum.*, **70**, 217–221

DETLEFSON, J.A. and YAPP, W.W. (1920) The inheritance of congenital cataract in cattle. *Am. Nat.*, **54**, 277–280

DI PAOLA, M., BIANCHI, M. and BAARLI, J. (1978) Lens opacification in mice exposed to 14-MeV neutrons *Radiat. Res.*, **73**, 340–350

DIEGAARDE, P.J., WIERINGA, B., BLEEKER-WAGEMAKERS, E. *et al.* (1989) Physical fine mapping of a deletion spanning the Norrie gene. *Hum. Genet.*, **84**, 22–26

DIETHELM, W. (1947) Ueber Ectopia lentis ohne Arachnodaktylie und ihre Beziehungen zur Ectopia lentis et pupillae. *Ophthalmologica*, **114**, 16–32

DIETZ, H.C. *et al.* (1991) The Marfan syndrome locus: confirmation of assignment to chromosome 15 and identification of tightly linked markers at 15q15-q21.3. *Genomics*, **9**, 355–361

DIKSHIT, S.K. and AVASTHI, P.N. (1965) Posterior lenticular opacities in children on corticosteroid therapy. *Indian J. Pediatr.*, **32**, 93–96

DODO, T. (1975) Review of thirty years study of Hiroshima and Nagasaki atomic bomb survivors. II. Biological effects H. cataracts. *J. Rad. Res. (Tokyo)*, **16** (Suppl.), 132–137

DOGGART, J.H. (1957) Congenital cataract. *Trans. Ophthalmol. Soc. UK*, **77**, 31–37

DRANCE, S.M. (1969) *Symposium on Ocular Therapy*, 4

DUB, B. (1891) Beitrage zur Kenntnis der Cataracta zonularis. *A. von Graefes Arch. Ophthalmol.*, **37**, 26–38

DUFOUR, R. (1968) Experience with intraocular silicone injection. In *New and Controversial Aspects of Retinal Detachment* (ed. A. McPherson), Harper & Row, New York, 377–382

DUKE-ELDER, S. (1925) Changes in refraction in diabetes mellitus. *Br. J. Ophthalmol.*, **9**, 167–187

DUKE-ELDER, S. (1961) The blood vessels of the orbit. In *System of Ophthalmology: Anatomy of the Visual System* (eds S. Duke-Elder, K. Wybar), Vol. 2, Henry Kimpton, London, 467–479

DUKE-ELDER, S. (1969) In *System of Ophthalmology*, Vol. 9 Henry Kimpton, London, p. 19

DUNCAN, G. (1969a) Relative permeabilities of the lens membranes to sodium and potassium. *Exp. Eye Res.*, **8**, 315–325

DUNCAN, G. (1969b) The site of the ion restricting membranes in the toad lens. *Exp. Eye Res.*, **8**, 406–412

DUNCAN, G. (1974) Comparative physiology of the lens membranes. In *The Eye* (ed. H. Davson), Academic Press, New York, 357–398

DUNCAN, G. (ed.) (1981) *Mechanisms of Cataract Formation in the Human Lens*. Academic Press, London

DUNCAN, G. and HIGHTOWER, K.R. (1986) Age-related changes in human lens membrane physiology. Colloq INSERM, **147**, 341–348

DUNCAN, G. and JACOB, T.J.C. (1984) Calcium and the physiology of cataract. In *Human Cataract Formation, Ciba. Found. Symp.*, **106**, 132–152

DUNCAN, G., EMPTAGE, N.J. and HIGHTOWER, K.R. (1988a) *p*-chloro-mercuriphenyl sulphonate activates a quinine-sensitive potassium conductance in frog lens. *J. Physiol.*, **404**, 637–648

DUNCAN, G., STEWART, S., PRESCOTT, A.R. *et al.* (1988b) Membrane and junctional properties of the isolated frog lens epithelium. *J. Membr. Biol.*, **102**, 195–204

DUNCAN, G., HIGHTOWER, K.R., GANDOLFI, S.A. *et al.* (1989) Human lens membrane cation permeability increases with age. *Invest. Ophthalmol. Vis. Sci.*, **30**, 1855–1859

DUNCAN, G., DART, C., CROGHAN, P.C. *et al.* (1992) Evidence for a Na^{+}–$Cl^{-}H^{+}$–$HCO3^{-}$ exchange system in the mammalian lens. *Exp. Eye Res.*, **54**, 941–946

DUNCAN, G., MARCANTONIO, J.M. and TOMLINSON, J. (1991) Lens calcium and cataract. In *Presbyopia Research* (eds G. Obrecht and L.W. Stark), Plenum Press, New York, 33–40

DUNIA, I., MANENTI, S., ROUSSELET, A. *et al.* (1987) Electron microscopic observations of the reconstituted proteoliposomes with the purified major intrinsic membrane protein of the eye lens fibres. *J. Cell Biol.*, **105**, 1679–1689

DYER, D.G., BLACKLEDGE, J.A., KATZ, B.M., HULL, C.J., ADKISSON, H.D., THORPE, S.R., LYONS, T.J. and BAYNES, J.W. (1991) The Maillard reaction in vivo. *Z. Ernahrungswiss*, **30**, 29–45

EBBERS, R.W. and SEARS, D. (1975) Ocular effects of a 325 mm ultraviolet laser. *Am. J. Optom. Physiol. Opt.*, **52**, 216–223

ECKERSKORN, U., KOKKAS, K., HOCKWIN, O., *et al.* (1989a) Physiologic changes of lens transparency during ageing: a Scheimpflug photography study. *Dev. Ophthalmol.*, **17**, 72–74

ECKERSKORN, U., MEINKE, K., MEINKE, C. *et al.* (1989b) Disease profile in an ophthalmologist's private practice: analysis of patients seen in 1987. *Dev. Ophthalmol.*, **17**, 17–20

EDERER, F., HILLER, R. and TAYLOR, H.R. (1981) Senile lens changes and diabetes in two population studies. *Am. J. Ophthalmol.*, **91**, 381–395

EDWARDS, G.A., BERNARDINO, V.B., BABCOCK, V.I. *et al.* (1975) Cataracts in bleomycin-treated rats. *Am. J. Ophthalmol.*, **80**, 538–542

EDWARDS, A., GUPTA, J.D. and HARLEY, J.D. (1973) Photomicrographic evaluation of drug-induced cataracts on cultured embryonic chick lens. *Exp. Eye Res.*, **15**, 495–498

EHLING, U.H., FAVOR, J., KRATOCHVILOVA, J. *et al.* (1982) Dominant cataract mutations and specific-locus mutations in mice induced by radiation or ethylnitrosourea. *Mutation Res.*, **92**, 181–192

EISSLER, R. and LONGENECKER, L.P. (1962) The common eye findings in mongolism. *Am. J. Ophthalmol.*, **54**, 398–406

ELBERGER, A.J. (1979) The role of the corpus callosum in the development of interocular eye alignment and the alignment and the organization of the visual field in the cat. *Exp. Brain Res.*, **36**, 71–85

ELENA, P.P., KOSINA-BOIX, M., MOULIN, G. *et al.* (1987) Autoradiographic localization of beta-adrenergic receptors in rabbit eye. *Invest. Ophthalmol. Vis. Sci.*, **28**, 1436–1441

ELLIOTT, D.B., GILCHRIST, J., PICKWELL, L.D. *et al.* (1989a) The subjective assessment of cataract. *Ophthal. Physiol. Opt.*, **9**, 16–19

ELLIOTT, D.B., GILCHRIST, J. and WHITAKER, D. (1989b) Contrast sensitivity and glare sensitivity changes with three types of cataract morphology: are these techniques necessary in clinical evaluation of cataract? *Ophthal. Physiol. Opt.*, **9**, 25–30

ELLIOTT, D.B., HURST, M.A. and WEATHERILL, J. (1990) Comparing clinical tests of visual function in cataract with the patient's perceived visual disability. *Eye*, **4**, 712–717

ELLIOTT, D.B., HURST, M.A. and WEATHERILL, J. (1991) Comparing clinical tests of visual loss in cataract patients using a quantification of forward light scatter. *Eye*, **5**, 601–606

ELSAS, F.J., MAUMENEE, I.H., KENYON, K.R. *et al.* (1977) Familial aniridia with preserved ocular function. *Am. J. Ophthalmol.*, **83**, 718–724

EMPTAGE, N.J., DUNCAN, G. and CROGHAN, P.C. (1992) Internal acidification modulates membrane and junctional resistance in the isolated lens of the frog (*Rana pipiens*). *Exp. Eye Res.*, **54**, 33–39

ENOCH, I.M. (1976) Retinal stretch and accommodation. In *Current Concepts in Ophthalmology* (eds H.E. Kaufman and T.J. Zimmerman), Mosby, Saint Louis, 59–78

ESHAGIAN, J. and STREETEN, B.W. (1980) Human posterior subcapsular cataract. An ultrastructural study of the posterior migrating cells. *Arch. Ophthalmol.*, **98**, 134–143

ESHAGIAN, J., MARCH, W.F., GOOSENS, W. *et al.* (1978) Ultrastructure of cataract in myotonic dystrophy. *Invest. Ophthalmol. Vis. Sci.*, **17**, 289–293

ESHAGIAN, J., RAFFERTY, N.S. and GOOSSENS, W. (1980) Ultrastructure of human cataract in retinitis pigmentosa. *Arch. Ophthalmol.*, **98**, 2227–2230

EVA, P.R., PASCOE, P.T. and VAUGHAN, D.G. (1982) Refractive change in hyperglycaemia: hyperopia, not myopia. *Br. J. Ophthalmol.*, **66**, 500–505

EVANS, T.C. (1948) Effects of small daily doses of fast neutrons on mice. *Radiology*, **30**, 811–832

EVANS, T.C., RICHARDS, R.D. and RILEY, E.F. (1960) Histologic studies .of neutron and X-irradiated mouse lenses. *Radiat. Res.*, **13**, 737–750

EVERETT, C.A., GLENISTER, P.H., TAYLOR, D.M. *et al.* (1994) Mapping of six dominant cataract genes in the mouse. *Genomics* (in press), 1–21

FAGERHOLM, P.P. and PHILLIPSON, B.T. (1985) Cataract in retinitis pigmentosa. An analysis of cataract surgery results and pathological lens changes. *Acta Ophthalmol.*, **63**, 50–58

FAGERHOLM, P.P., PHILIPSON, B.O. and CARLSTRÖM, D. (1981/82) Calcification in the human lens. *Curr. Eye Res.*, **1**, 629–633

FAGERHOLM, P.P., PHILLIPSON, B.T. and LINDSTROM, A. (1981) Normal human lens – the distribution of protein. *Exp. Eye Res.*, **33**, 615–620

FAGERHOLM, P., PHILLIPSON, B.T. and LYDAHL, E. (1990) Subcapsular zones of discontinuity in the human lens. *Ophthal. Res. Suppl.*, **22**, 51–55

FALLS, H.F. and COTTERMAN, C.W. (1943) Genetic studies on ectopia lentis: a pedigree of simple ectopia of the lens. *Arch. Ophthalmol.*, **30**, 610–620

FARBER, D.N. (1949) Cataract in dystrophia myotonica. *Arch. Ophthalmol.*, **41**, 450–459

FARELL, J.W., MORGEN, K.S. and BLACK, S. (1988) Lensectomy in an infant with Cri du Chat syndrome and cataracts. *J. Pediatr. Ophthalmol Strabismus*, **25**, 131–135

FARNSWORTH, P.N. and BURKE, P.A. (1977) Three-dimensional architecture of the suspensory apparatus of the lens of the Rhesus monkey. *Exp. Eye Res.*, **25**, 563–576

FARNSWORTH, P.N. and SHYNE, S.E. (1979) Anterior zonular shifts with age. *Exp. Eye Res.*, **28**, 291–297

FARNSWORTH, P.N., BURKE, P.A. and KESTIN, W.T. (1978) Suspensory apparatus of the human lens. ARVO Suppl: *Invest. Ophthalmol. Vis. Sci.*, **17**, 233

FAULKNER, H.W. (1971) Pseudo-exfoliation of the lens among Navajo Indians. *Am. J. Ophthalmol.*, **72**, 206–207

FAVOR, J. and PRETSCH, W. (1990) Genetic localization and phenotypic expression of X-linked cataract (*Xcat*) in *Mus musculus*. *Genet. Res.*, **56**, 157–162

FEENEY-BURNS, L., BURNS, R.P. and ANDERSON, R.S. (1980) Ultrastructure and acid phosphatase activity in hereditary cataracts of Deer mice. *Invest. Ophthalmol. Vis. Sci.*, **19**, 777–788

FEINGOLD, J., BOIS, E., CHOMPRET, A. *et al.* (1985) Genetic heterogeneity of Alport syndrome. *Kidney Int.*, **27**, 672–677

FILLUMORE, P.G. (1952) The medical examination of Hiroshima patients with radiation cataracts. *Science*, **116**, 322–323

FINE, B.S. and YANOFF, M. (1972) *Ocular Histology. A Text and Atlas*, Harper & Row, New York

FISHER, R.F. (1969a) The elastic constants of the human lens capsule. *J. Physiol.*, **201**, 1–19

FISHER, R.F. (1969b) The significance and shape of the lens and capsular energy changes in accommodation. *J. Physiol.*, **201**, 21–47

FISHER, R.F. (1970) Senile cataract: a comparative study between lens fibre stress and cuneiform formation. *Trans. Ophthalmol. Soc. UK*, **90**, 93–109

FISHER, R.F. (1971) The elastic constant of the human lens. *J. Physiol.*, **212**, 147–180

FISHER, R.F. (1973) The Human Lens in Relation to Cataract [Discussion]. *Ciba Found. Symp.*, **19**, 114

FISHER, R.F. (1977) The force of contraction of the human ciliary muscle during accommodation. *J. Physiol.*, **270**, 51–74

FITZSIMMONS, T.D., FAGERHOLM, P., HÄRFSTRAND, A. and SCHENHOLM, M. (1992) Hyaluronic acid in exfoliation syndrome. *Opthalmology (Suppl)*, **99**, 134

FLACH, A.J., DOLAN, B.J., SUDDUTH, B. *et al.* (1983) Amiodarone-induced lens opacities. *Arch. Ophthalmol.*, **101**, 1554–1556

FLAYE, D.E., SULLIVAN, K.N., CULLINAN, T.R. *et al.* (1989) Cataracts and cigarette smoking: The City Eye Study. *Eye*, **3**, 379–384

FLECKENSTEIN, A. (1983) In *Calcium Antagonism in Heart and Smooth Muscle. Experimental Facts and Therapeutic Prospects*, John Wiley, New York, 201–286

FLESCHNER, C.R. and CENEDELLA, R.J. (1988), Specific restriction of cholesterol from cortical lens gap junctional membrane U18 666A cataracts. *Curr. Eye Res.*, **7**, 1029–1034

FONSECA (1938) *Arch. Clin. Ophthalmol.*, **5**, 23

FORBES, J.E., HOLDEN, R., HARRIS, M. *et al.* (1992) Growth of the human crystalline lens in childhood. Proceedings of Xth ISER Meeting, Stresa, Italy [Abstract]. *Exp. Eye Res.*, **55**, 172

FORSIUS, H. (1988) Exfoliation syndrome in various ethnic populations. (Suppl. 184). *Acta. Ophthalmol.*, **66**, 71–85

FOULDS, W.S. (1987) Is your vitreous really necessary? The role of the vitreous in the eye with particular reference to retinal attachment, detachment and the mode of action of vitreous substitutes. *Eye*, **1**, 641–664

FRACCARO, M., MORONE, G., MANFREDINI, U. *et al.* (1967) X-linked cataract. *Ann. Hum. Genet.*, **31**, 45–50

FRANCESCHETTI, A.T. (1976) Fabry disease: Ocular manifestations. *Birth Defects*, **12**, 195–208

FRANCHESCHETTI, A. (1927) Ectopia lentis et pupillae congenita als rezessives Erbleiden und ihre Manifestierung durch Konsanguintaet. *Klin. Monatsbl. Augenheilk.*, **78**, 351–362

FRANCOIS, J. (1963) *Congenital Cataracts*. Van Gorcum, Assen, Netherlands

FRANCOIS, J. (1982) Genetics of cataract. *Ophthalmologica*, **184**, 61

FRANCOIS, J. (1983) Francois dyscephalic syndrome. *Dev. Ophthalmol.*, **7**, 13

FRANCOIS, J. and RABAEY, M. (1958) Permeability of the capsule for the lens proteins. *Acta. Ophthalmol.*, **36**, 837–844

FRANKS, W.A., MILLER, M.H., HITCHINGS, R.A. and JEFFREY, M.N. (1990) Secondary angle closure in association with pseudoexfoliation of the lens capsule. *Acta Ophthalmol.* **68**, 350–352

FRASER, G.R. and FRIEDMANN, A.I. (1967) *The Causes of Blindness in Childhood. A Study of 776 Children with Severe Visual Handicaps*, Johns Hopkins University Press, Baltimore, 59

FRASER, F.C. and SCHABTACH, G. (1963) 'Shrivelled': A hereditary degeneration of the lens in the house mouse. *Genet. Res.*, **3**, 383–387

FRASER, P.J., DUNCAN, G. and TOMLINSON, J. (1990) Nuvan and cataracts in atlantic salmon (Salmo salar) [letter] *Exp. Eye Res.*, **50**, 443–447

FRAUNFELDER, F. and BURNS, R. (1962) Production of unilateral reversible cataracts in the hamster. *Proc. Soc. Exp. Biol. Med.*, **110**, 72–74

FRAUNFELDER, F.T. and BURNS, R.P. (1966) Effect of lid closure in drug-induced experimental cataracts. *Arch. Ophthalmol.*, **76**, 599–601

FRAUNFELDER, F.T. and HANNA, C. (1972) Electric cataracts. I: Sequential changes, unusual and prognostic findings. *Arch. Ophthalmol.*, **87**, 179–183

FREZZOTTI, R. and CAPOROSSI, A. (1990) Pathogenesis of posterior capsular opacification: Part I: Epidemiological and clinico-statistical data. *J. Cataract Refract. Surg.*, **16**, 347–352

FRIEDBURG, D. (1973) Enzyme activity patterns in clear human lenses and in different types of human senile cataract. *Ciba Found. Symp.*, **19**, 117–133

FRIEDENWALD, J.S. (1930) Permeability of the lens capsule with special reference to the etiology of senile cataract. *Arch. Ophthalmol.*, **3**, 182–193

FRIEDENWALD, J.S. and RYTEL, D. (1955) Contribution to the histolpathology of cataracts. *Arch. Ophthalmol.*, **53**, 825–831

FUJINAGA, Y. (1969) On the histological study of cataract in atomic bomb survivors. *Acta. Soc. Ophthalmol. Jpn.*, **73**, 1094–1097

FUKUI, H.N., OBAZAWA, H. and KINOSHITA, H.J. (1976) Lens growth in the Nakano mouse. *Invest. Ophthalmol.*, **15**, 422–425

FUKUI, H.N., IWATA, S., EPSTEIN, D.L. *et al.* (1977) Cataractogenic effects of boron hydride disulphide compound. *Exp. Eye Res.*, **16**, 654–657

FUKUI, H.N., MEROLA, L.M. and KINOSHITA, J.H. (1978) A possible cataractogenic factor in the Nakano mouse lens. *Exp. Eye Res.*, **26**, 477–485

FUKUI, H.N., MEROLA, L.M., FUKUSHI, S. *et al.* (1980) Nakano mouse cataract. In *Red Blood Cell and Lens Metabolism* (ed. S.K. Srivastava), Elsevier, North Holland, 389–404

GAJEWSKI, A.K., MAJEWSKA, J., SLOWIKOWSKA, M.G. *et al.* (1977) Types and rate of cataract development in mice irradiated at different ages. *Radiat. Res.*, **71**, 471–480

GANDOLFI, S.A., DUNCAN, G., TOMLINSON, J. *et al.* (1990) Mammalian lens inter-fiber resistance is modulated by calcium and calmodulin. *Curr. Eye Res.*, **9**, 533–541

GARADI, R., LOU, M. and WHITNEY, A. (1986) Ascorbic acid protection against oxidative damage to lens Na^+K^+ AT-Pase and transport systems. ARVO Suppl.: *Invest. Ophthalmol. Vis. Sci.*, **27**, 277

GARBER, A.T., STIRK, L. and GOLD, R. (1983) Abnormalities of crystallins in the lens of the cat^{Fraser} mouse. *Exp. Eye Res.*, **36**, 165–169

GARBER, A.T., WINKLER, G., SHINOHARA, T., *et al.* (1985) Selective loss of a family of gene transcripts in a hereditary murine cataract. *Science*, **227**, 74–77

GARDENER, R.J.M. and BROWN, N. (1976) Lowe's syndrome. Identification of the carriers by lens examination. *J. Med. Genet.*, **13**, 449–454

GARLAND, D., ZIGLER, J.S., JR. and KINOSHITA, J. (1986) Structural changes in bovine lens crystallins induced by ascorbate, metal and oxygen. *Arch. Biochem. Biophys.*, **251**, 771–776

GARNER, A., FIELDER, A.R., PRIMAVESI, R. *et al.* (1982) Tapetoretinal degeneration in the cerebro-hepato-renal (Zellweger) syndrome. *Br. J. Ophthalmol.*, **66**, 422–431

GARNER, M.H., GARNER, W.H., JENKINS, G. *et al.* (1986a) Effect of H_2O_2 on Na/K ATPase kinetics. *Invest. Ophthalmol. Vis. Sci.*, **24**, 74

GARNER, M.H., GARNER, W.H. and SPECTOR, A. (1986b) H_2O_2 modification of Na, K-ATPase. *Invest. Ophthalmol. Vis. Sci.*, **27**, 103–107

GARNER, M.H. and SPECTOR, A. (1980) Comparison of the 10,000 and 43,000 dalton polypeptide populations isolated from the water soluble and insoluble fractions of human cataractous lenses. *Proc. Natl Acad. Sci. USA*, **77**, 1274–1277

GARNER, M.H. and SPECTOR, A. (1986) ATP hydrolysis kinetics by Na,K-ATPase in cataract. *Exp. Eye Res.*, **42**, 339–348

GARNER, W.H., GARNER, M.H. and SPECTOR, A. (1983), H_2O_2-induced uncoupling of bovine lens Na^+K^+-ATPase. *Proc. Natl. Acad. Sci. USA*, **80**, 2044–2048

GEERAETS, W.J., HAM, W.T., MUELLER, H.A. *et al.* (1971) Effects of acute and protracted ionizing radiation on the rabbit lens. *Acta Ophthalmol.*, **49**, 817–855

GEERAETS, W.J., HARREL, W., GUERRY, D. *et al.* (1965) Aging, anomalies and radiation effect of the rabbit lens. *Acta Ophthalmol.*, **43**, 3–21

GEHRING, P.J. and BUERGE, J.F. (1969) The distribution of 2,4 dinitrophenol relative to its cataractogenic activity in ducklings and rabbits. *Toxic. Appl. Pharmacol.*, **15**, 574

GELATT, K.N. (1971) Cataracts in cattle. *J. Am. Vet. Med. Assoc.*, **159**, 195–200

GELATT, K.N. (1972) Cataracts in the golden retriever dog. *Vet. Med. Small Anim. Clin.*, **67**, 1113–1115

GELATT, K.N. (1975) Congenital cataracts in a litter of rabbits. *J. Am. Vet. Med. Assoc.*, **167**, 598–599

GELATT, K.N. (1991) The metabolic basis of ophthalmic diseases in animals. *Anim. Eye Res.*, **10**, 1–16

GELATT, K.N. and DAS, N.D. (1984) Animal models for inherited cataracts: a review. *Curr. Eye Res.*, **3**, 765–778

GELATT, K.N., SAMUELSON, D.A., BARRIE, K.P. *et al.* (1983a) Biometry and clinical characteristics of congenital cataracts and microphthalmia in the Miniature Schnauzer. *J. Am. Vet. Med. Assoc.*, **183**, 99–102

GELATT, K.N., SAMUELSON, D.A., BAUER, J.E. *et al.* (1983b) The inheritance of congenital cataracts and microphthalmia in the Miniature Schnauzer. *Am. J. Vet. Res.*, **44**, 1130–1132

GELATT, K.N., WHITLEY, R.D., LAVACH, J.D. *et al.* (1979) Cataracts in Chesapeake Bay retrievers. *J. Am. Vet. Med. Assoc.*, **175**, 1176–1178

GELATT, K.N., BRUSS, M., DECOSTANZA, S.M. *et al.* (1982) Reduced oxidized, and protein-bound glutathione concentrations in normal and cataractous lenses in the dog. *J. Am. Vet. Med. Assoc.*, **43**, 1215–1217

GENTRY, R.F., BRAUNE, M.O. and ROTHENBACHER, H. (1968) Recovery of virus from cataracts following field exposure to avian encephalomyelitis. *105th Proceedings of the American Veterinary Medical Association*, 145

GERNET, H. (1964a) Achsenlänge und Refraktion lebender Augen von Neugeborenen. *A von Graefes Arch. Ophthalmol.*, **166**, 530–536

GERSON, R.J., MACDONALD, J.S., ALBERTS, A.W. *et al.* (1990) On the etiology of subcapsular lenticular opacities produced in dogs receiving HMG-CoA reductase inhibitors. *Exp. Eye Res.*, **50**, 65–78

GIBLIN, F.J. and REDDY, V.N. (1978) Oxidation of protein sulfydryl groups and formation of high molecular weight protein in X-ray induced cataract. Third International Congress, Osaka. *Exp. Eye Res. Suppl.*, **1**, 170

GIBLIN, F.J., MCCREADY, J.P., KODAMA, T. *et al.* (1984) A direct correlation between the levels of ascorbic acid and H_2O_2 in aqueous humour. *Exp. Eye Res.*, **38**, 87–93

GIBLIN, F.J., MCCREADY, J.P., SCHRIMSCHER, L. *et al.* (1987) Peroxide-induced effects on lens cation transport following inhibition of glutathione reductase activity in vitro. *Exp. Eye Res.*, **45**, 77–91

GIESER, S.J., CAREY, J.C. and APPLE, D.J. (1986) Human chromosomal disorders and the eye. In *Goldberg's Genetic and Metabolic Eye Disease* (ed. W.A. Renie), 2nd edn, Little Brown, Boston,

GIFFORD, D.H.A. (1957) A clinical and pathological study of exfoliation of the lens capsule. *Trans. Am. Ophthalmol. Soc.*, **55**, 189–216

GIFFORD, S.R. (1924) Congenital anomalies of the lens as seen with the slit-lamp. *Am. J. Opthalmol.*, **7**, 678

GIFFORD, S.R. (1927) Zum kongenitalen Star des Embryonalkerns. *Klin. Monsatsbl. Augenheilk.*, **78**, 191

GIFFORD, S.R., BENNETT, A.E. and FAIRCHILD, N.M. (1929)

Cataract in myotonic dystrophy. *Arch. Ophthalmol.*, **1**, 335–345

GIFFORD, S.R. and PUNTENNEY, I. (1937) Coralliform cataract and a new form of congenital cataract with crystals in the lens. *Arch. Ophthalmol.*, **17**, 885–892

GILES, C.L., MASON, G.L., DUFF, I.F. *et al.* (1962) The association of cataract formation and systemic corticosteroid therapy. *J. Am. Med. Assoc.*, **182**, 719–722

GINSBERG, J. *et al.* (1980) Further observations of ocular pathology in Down's syndrome. *J. Pediatr. Ophthalmol. Strabismus*, **17**, 166

GINSBERG, J., BOFINGER, M.K. and ROUSH, J.R. (1977) Pathologic features of the eye in Down's syndrome with relationship to other chromosomal anomalies. *Am. J. Ophthalmol.*, **83**, 874–880

GIRSCH, S. and PERACCHIA, C. (1985) Lens cell-to-cell channel protein. I: Self assembly into liposomes and permeability regulation by calmodulin. *J. Membr. Biol.*, **83**, 217–225

GITZELMAN, R. (1967) Hereditary galactokinase deficiency, a newly recognized cause of juvenile cataracts. *Pediatr. Res.*, **1**, 14

GITZELMANN, R. (1972) Deficiency of uridine diphosphate galactose 4-epimerase in blood cells of an apparently healthy infant. *Helv. Paediat. Acta*, **27**, 125–130

GJESSING, H.G.A. (1920) Untersuchung in maximaler mydriasis von 4768 Augen im Alter von 3 Monaten bis zu 87 1/2 Jahren mit punktuell abbildenen Licht, und Zurar in besonderem Hinblick auf die Vogtsche sog. Coronarkatarakt. *Klin. Monatsbl. Augenheilk.*, **65**, 233–265

GOBLIN, F.J., MCREADY, J.P., SCHRIMSCHER, L. *et al.* (1987) Peroxide induced effects on lens cation transport following inhibition of glutathione reductase activity *in vitro*. *Exp. Eye. Res.*, **45**, 77–91

GOLDBERG, M.F. and CUSTIS, P.H. (1992) Retinal and other manifestations in nine cases of incontinentia pigmenti [abstract]. *Invest. Ophthalmol. Vis. Sci.*, **33**, 1084

GOLDBERG, M.F. and HARDY, J.M.B. (1971) X-linked cataract. In *Clinical Delineation of Birth Defects. VIII: The Eye*, (ed. D. Bergsma), Williams & Wilkins, Baltimore

GOLDMANN, H. (1935) La genêse de la cataracte des verriers. *Ann. Oculist. (Paris)*, **172**, 13–41

GOLDMANN, H. and RABINOWITZ, A. (1928) No title. Klin. Monatsbl. Augenheilk., **81**, 771

GOLTZ, R.W., HENDERSON, R.R., HITCH, J.M. *et al.* (1970) Focal dermal hypoplasia syndrome. A review of the literature and report of two cases. *Arch. Dermatol.*, **101**, 1–11

GOOD, W.V., BRODSKY, M.C., EDWARDS, M.S. and HOYT, W.F. (1991) Bilateral retinal hamartomas in neurofibromatosis. *Br. J. Ophthalmol.*, **75**, 109

GOODENOUGH, D.A., DICK, J.S.B. II. and LYONS, J.E. (1980) Lens metabolic cooperation: a study of mouse lens transport and permeability visualized with freeze substitution autoradiography and electron microscopy. *J. Cell. Biol.*, **86**, 576–589

GORIN, M.B., YANCEY, S.B., CLINE, J. *et al.* (1984) The major intrinsic protein (MIP) of the bovine lens fibre membrane: characterization and structure based on cDNA cloning. *Cell Tissue Res.*, **39**, 49–59

GORTHY, W.C. (1977) Cataracts in the aging rat lens. Morphological characterization and evaluation as a model for human senile cataracts. *Ophthalmic Res.*, **9**, 329–342

GORTHY, W.C. (1978) Cataracts in the aging rat lens. Morphology and acid phosphatase histochemistry of incipient forms. *Exp. Eye Res.*, **27**, 301–322

GORTHY, W.C. (1979) Developmental ocular abnormalities in rats with X-ray induced cataract mutation. *Invest. Ophthalmol. Vis. Sci.*, **18**, 939–946

GORTHY, W.C. and ABDELBAKI, Y.Z. (1974) Morphology of a hereditary cataract in the rat. *Exp. Eye Res.*, **19**, 147–156

GORTHY, W.C. and ANDERSON, J.W. (1980) Special characteristics of the polar regions of the rat lens: morphology and phosphatase histochemistry. *Invest. Ophthalmol. Vis. Sci.*, **19**, 1038–1052

GORTHY, W.C., MORRILL, D.J., and ANDERSON, J.W. (1980) Anterior polar cataract development in mutant wistar rats. An ultrastructural study. In *Aging of the Lens* (eds F. Regnault, D. Hockwin and Y. Courtois), Elsevier, North Holland, 207–222

GRAINGER, R.M., HENRY, J.J., SAHA, M.S. *et al.* (1992) Recent progress on the mechanisms of embryonic lens formation. *Eye*, **6**, 117–122

GRANSTROM, K.O. (1933) Refraktionsveranderungen bei diabetes mellitus. *Acta Ophthalmol.*, **11**, 1–161

GRAW, J., KRATOCHVILOVA, J. and SUMMER, K.-H. (1984) Genetical and biochemical studies of a dominant cataract mutant in mice. *Exp. Eye Res.*, **39**, 37–45

GRAW, J., FAVOR, J., NEUHÄUSER-KLAUS. A. *et al.* (1986) Dominant cataract and recessive specific locus mutations in offspring of X-irradiated male mice. *Mutation Res.* **159**, 47–54

GRAW, J., SUMMER, K., MICHEL, C. *et al.* (1985) Catalase and superoxide dismutase activities in lenses of cataractous NOP-mice *Exp. Eye. Res.*, **41**, 577–579

GRAW, J., KRATOCHVILOVA, J., LOBKE, A. *et al.* (1989) Characterization of Scat (suture cataract), a dominant cataract mutation in mice. *Exp. Eye Res.*, **49**, 469–477

GREEN, E.L. (1981) Catalog of mutant genes and polymorphic loci. In *Genetic Variants and Strains of the Laboratory Mouse* (ed. M.C. Green), Fisher, Stuttgart & New York, 8–28

GREEN, H., BOCHER, C.A. and LEOPOLD, I.H. (1959) Anaerobic carbohydrate metabolism of crystalline lens. *Am. J. Ophthalmol.*, **39**, 106–113

GREEN, M.C. (1981) In *Genetic Variants and Strains of the Laboratory Mouse* (ed. M.C. Green), Gustav Fischer Verlag, Stuttgart, 8

GREEN, M.C. (1989) Catalog of mutant genes and polymorphic loci. In *Genetic Variants and Strains of the Laboratory Mouse*, (eds M.F. Lyon, A.G. Searle), 2nd ed., Oxford University Press, 12–403

GREGORY, P.W., MEAD, S.W. and REGAN, W.M. (1943) A congenital hereditary eye defect of cattle. *J. Heredity*, **34**, 125–128

GROM, E. (1975) An inquiry in the history of the crystalline lens. In *Cataract and Abnormalities of the Lens* (ed. J.G. Bellows), Grune and Stratton, New York

GRUBER, M. (1945) Ueber primaere familiaere Linsendyplasie. *Ophthalmologica*, **110**, 60–73

GRUIJTERS, W.T.M., KISTLER, J., BULLIVANT, S. *et al.* (1987) Immunolocalization of MP70 in lens fibers 16–17 nm intercellular junctions. *J. Cell Biol.*, **104**, 565–572

GRZEDZIELSKI, J. (1935) Zur Histologie der Rontgenkatarakt. **95**, 360–369

GUBLER, M., LEVY, M., BROYER, M. *et al.* (1981) Alport's syndrome: a report of 58 cases and a review of the literature. *Am. J. Med.*, **70**, 493–505

GUGGENMOOS-HOLZMANN, I., ENGEL, B., HENKE, V. *et al.* (1989) Cell density of human lens epithelium in women higher than in men. *Invest. Ophthalmol. Vis. Sci.*, **30**, 330–332

GUNN, R.M. (1895) Peculiar coralliform cataract with crystals (? of cholesterine) in the lens. *Trans. Ophthalmol. Soc. UK*, **15**, 119

GUTHAUSER, U. and FLAMMER, J. (1988) Quantifying visual field damage caused by cataract. *Am. J. Ophthalmol.*, **106**, 480–484

GUZEK, J.P., HOLM, M., COTTER, J.B., CAMERON, J.A., RADEMAKER, W.J., WISSINGER, D.H., TONJUM, A.M. and SLEEPER, L.A. (1987) Risk factors for intraoperative complications in 1000 extracapsular cataract cases. *Ophthalmology*, **94**, 461–466

HAFT, A.S. (1953) Idiopathic hypoparathyroidism and cataract. Report of four cases. *Arch. Ophthalmol.*, **50**, 455

HALBERTSMA, K.T.A. (1934) Familiare aangeboren cataract. *Ned. Tijdschr. Geneeskd.*, **78**, 1705–1709

HALL, E.J. (1963) Radiation cataractogenesis. In *Radiology for the Radiobiologist* (ed. E.J. Hall), Harper & Row, New York, 343–349

HALL, W.K., BOWLES, L.L., SYDENSTRICKER, V.P. *et al.* (1948) Cataracts due to deficiencies of phenylalanine and of histidine in the rat. A comparison with other types of cataracts. *J. Nutr.*, **36**, 277–295

HAM, W.T. (1953) Radiation cataract. *Arch. Ophthalmol.*, **50**, 618–643

HAMAI, Y. and KUWABARA, T. (1975) Early cytologic changes of Fraser cataract: An electron microscopic study. *Invest. Ophthalmol. Vis. Sci.*, **14**, 517–527

HAMAI, Y., FUKUI, H.N. and KUWABARA, T. (1974) Morphology of hereditary mouse cataract. *Exp. Eye Res.*, **18**, 537–546

HAMMERSTEIN, W. and SCHOLT, W. (1974) Familiaere Form einer 'Cataracta centralis': klinisch-genetische Studie mit Koppelungsdaten. *A von Graefes Arch. Klin. Exp. Ophthalmol.*, **189**, 9–19

HAMMING, N.A., APPLE, D.J. and GOLDBERG, M.F. (1976) Histopathology and ultrastructure of busulphan induced cataract. *A von Graefes Arch. Klin. Exp. Ophthalmol.*, **200**, 139–147

HANNA, C. (1975) Chalcosis of the lens. In *Cataract and Abnormalities of the Lens*, (ed. J.G. Bellows), Grune & Stratton, New York, 279

HANNA, C. and FRAUNFELDER, F.T. (1972) Electric cataracts. II: Ultrastructural lens changes. *Arch. Ophthalmol.*, **87**, 184–191

HANNA, C. and FRAUNFELDER, F.T. (1975) Electrical cataract. In *Cataract and Abnormalities of the Lens*, (ed. J.G. Bellows), Grune & Stratton, New York, 224–230

HANNA, C., JARMAN, R.V., KEATTS, J.G. *et al.* (1968) Virus-induced cataracts. *Arch. Ophthalmol.*, **79**, 59–63

HANSEN, E. and SELLEVOLD, O.J. (1969) Pseudoexfoliation of the lens capsule. II. Development of the exfoliation syndrome. *Acta Ophthalmol.*, **47**, 161–173

HANSEN, S.O., SOLOMON, K.D., MCKNIGHT, G.T., WILBRANDT, T.H., GWIN, T.D., O'MORCHOE, D.J.C., TETZ, M.R. and APPLE, D.J. (1988) Posterior capsular opacification and intraocular lens decentration: part I: Comparison of various posterior chamber lens designs implanted in the rabbit model. *J. Cataract Refract. Surg.*, **14**, 605–613

HAPPLE, R. (1979) X-linked dominant ichthyosis. *Clin. Genet.*, **15**, 239–240

HAPPLE, R. (1981) Cataracts as a marker of genetic heterogeneity in chondrodysplasia punctata. *Clin. Genet.*, **19**, 64–66

HAPPLE, R. and KUCHLE, H.J. (1983) Sectorial-cataract: a possible example of lyonisation [letter]. *Lancet*, **ii**, 909–920

HAPPLE, R., MATTHASS, H.-H. and MACHER, E. (1977) Sex-linked chondrodysplasia punctata? *Clin. Genet.*, **11**, 73–76

HARCH, C., CHASE, H.B. and GONSALVES, N.I. (1978) Studies on anophthalmic strain of mice. VI. Lens and cup interaction. *Dev. Biol.*, **63**, 352–357

HARDING, J.J. (1988) Case-control studies and risk factors for cataract: discussion paper. *J. R. Soc. Med.*, **81**, 585–587

HARDING, J.J. (1991) *Cataract: Biochemistry, Epidemiology and Pharmacology*. Chapman & Hall, London, 1–333

HARDING, J.J. (1993) Pathophysiology of cataract. *Curr. Opin. Ophthalmol.*, **4**, 14–21

HARDING, J.J. and CRABBE, M.J.C. (1984) The lens: development, proteins, metabolism and cataract. In *The Eye* (ed. H. Davson), 3rd edn, Academic Press, London, 207–492

HARDING, J.J. and DILLEY, K.J. (1976) Structural proteins of the mammalian lens: a review with emphasis on changes in development, aging and cataract. *Exp. Eye Res.*, 22, 1–73

HARDING, J.J. and VAN HEYNINGEN, R. (1988) Drugs, including alcohol, that act as risk factors for cataract, and possible protection against cataract by aspirin-like analgesics and cyclopenthiazide. *Br. J. Ophthalmol.*, **72**, 809–814

HARDING, J.J. and VAN HEYNINGEN, R. (1989a) Risk factors for cataract. *Br. J. Ophthalmol.*, **73**, 579–580

HARDING, J.J. and VAN HEYNINGEN, R. (1989b) Beer, cigarettes and military work as risk factors for cataract. *Dev. Ophthalmol.*, **17**, 13–16

HARDING, C.V., CHYLACK, J.T.JR., SUSAN, S.R. *et al.* (1983) Calcium-containing opacities in the human lens. *Invest. Ophthalmol. Vis. Sci.*, **24**, 1194–1202

HARDING, J.J., RIXON, K.C. and MARRIOTT, F.H.C. (1977) Men have heavier lenses than women of the same age. *Exp. Eye Res.*, **25**, 651

HARDING, J.J., HARDING, R.S. and EGERTON, M. (1989) Risk factors for cataract in Oxfordshire: Diabetes, peripheral neuropathy, myopia, glaucoma and diarrhoea. *Acta. Ophthalmol.*, **67**, 510–517

HARLEY, J.D. *et al.* (1974) Maternal enzymes of galactose metabolism and the inexplicable infantile cataract. *Lancet*, **ii**, 259

HARMAN, N.B. (1909) Congenital cataract, a pedigree of five generations. *Trans. Ophthalmol. Soc. UK*, **29**, 101–108

HARMAN, N.B. (1910a) Congenital cataract. In *Treasury of Human Inheritance*, part 4, Cambridge University Press, Cambridge, 126–169

HARMAN, N. (1910b) Ten pedigrees of congenital and infantile cataract, lamellar, coralliform, discoid, posterior polar with microphthalmia. *Trans. Ophthalmol. Soc. UK*, **30**, 251

HARNISCH, J.P., BARRACH, H.J., HASSELL, J.R. and SINHA, P.K. (1981) Identification of a basement membrane proteoglycan in exfoliation material. *Graefes. Arch. Klin. Exp. Ophthalmol.*, **215**, 273–278

HARRIS, J.E. and GEHRSITZ, L.O. (1951) Significance of changes in potassium and sodium content of the lens. *Am. J. Ophthalmol.*, **34**, 131

HARRIS, J.E. and GRUBER, L. (1969) The reversal of Triparanol-induced cataracts in the rat. *Doc. Ophthalmol.*, **26**, 324–333

HARRIS, M.L., BROWN, N.A.P. and BRON, A.J. (1994) Application of charge couple device Scheimpflug and retroillumination cameras to lens toxicity monitoring in man. *Ophthalmic Res.*, Suppl. **26**, 44–47

HARRIS, M.L., SMITH, G.T.H. and BROWN, N.A.P. (1991) Inter and intra observer reproducibility of the new Oxford CCD Scheimpflug camera. *Eye.*, **5**, 487–490

HARRIS, M.L., BROWN, N.A.P., SHUN-SHIN, G.A. and SMITH, G.T.H. (1992) Capsular 'pits' in the human lens. *Br. J. Ophthalmol.*, **76**, 248–249

HARRIS, M.L., HANNA, K.J., SHUN-SHIN, G.A., HOLDEN, R. and BROWN, N.A.P. (1993) Verification of a new method for the analysis of retro-illumination photographs for use in longitudinal studies of cataract. *Eye*, **7**, 572–577

HARRIS, W.S., AARON-ROSA, D.S., BYRON, H.M. *et al.* (1985) Management of posterior capsule after cataract extraction. *CLAO J.* **11**, 273–288

HARRISON, R. (1960) Bilateral lens opacities. Associated with use of di-isopropyl fluorophosphate eyedrops. *Am. J. Ophthalmol*, **50**, 153–154

HARSHMAN, J.P. (1948) Glaucoma associated with subluxation of the lens in several members of family. *Am. J. Ophthalmol.*, **31**, 833–836

HARTMANN, C., WIEDEMANN, P., WELLER, M., PHARMAKAKIS, N. and HEIMANN, K. (1981) Identification of a basement membrane proteoglycan in exfoliation material. *Graefes. Arch. Klin. Exp. Ophthalmol.*, **215**, 273–278

HARTMANN, C., WIEDEMANN, P., WELLER, M., PHARMAKAKIS, N. and HEIMANN, K. (1989) In vitro changes in the lens epithelium and corneal endothelium caused by the cytostatic drug daunomycin *Fortschr Ophthalmol*, **86**, 167–171

HAYE, C., JAMMET, H. and DOLFUS, M.A. (1965) *L'Oeil et les radiations ionisantes.* Masson, New York, 422–426

HAYES, B.P. and FISHER, R.F. (1984) Ultrastructural appearances of a lens with marked polychromatic lustre: evidence of diffraction as a cause. *Br. J. Ophthalmol.*, **68**, 850–858

HECKENLIVELY, J.R. (1982) The frequency of posterior subcapsular cataract in the hereditary retinal degenerations. *Am. J. Ophthalmol.*, **93**, 733–738

HECKENLIVELY, J.R. (1988) *Retinitis Pigmentosa.* J.B. Lippincott, Philadelphia

HEINE, L. (1898) Beitrage zur Physiologie und Pathologie der Linse. *A von Graefes Arch. Ophthalmol.*, **46**, 525–552

HELVE, J. and NIEMINEN, H. (1976) Autofluorescence of the human diabetic lens in vivo. *Am. J. Ophthalmol.*, **81**, 491–494

HENDERSON, M.J., HOLTON, J.B. and MACFAUL, R.. (1983) Further observations in a case of uridine diphosphate galactose-4-epimerase deficiency with a severe clinical presentation. *J. Inherit. Metab. Dis.*, **6**, 17–20

HENDIND, P. and PROSE, P. (1967) Anterior polar cataract. Electron-microscopic evidence of collagen. *Am. J. Ophthalmol.*, **63**, 768–771

HENKE, E., LEADER, M., TAJIMA, S. *et al.* (1985) A 38 base pair insertion in the pro alpha-2(1) collagen gene of a patient with Marfan syndrome. *J. Cell. Biochem.*, **27**, 161–174

HENRY, J.C., KRUPIN, T., SCHMITT, M. *et al.* (1987) Long term follow up of pseudoexfoliation and the development of elevated intraocular pressure. *Ophthalmology*, **94**, 545–552

HERBST, C. (1901) *Formative Reize in der Tierischen Ontogenese. Ein Beitrag zum Verstandnis der tierischen Embryonalentwicklung*, Arthur Georgi, Leipzig

HERVA, R., VON WENDT, L., VON WENDT, G. *et al.* (1987) A syndrome with juvenile cataract, cerebellar atrophy, mental retardation and myopathy. *Neuropediatrics*, **18**, 164–169

HESS, C. (1911) Pathologie und Therapie des Linsensystems. In *Graefe-Saemisch Handbuch* 3rd edn, Graefe-Saemisch Handbuch Gesamten Augenheilk. **1**, 35

HESS, H.H., NEWSOME, D.A., KNAPKA, J.J. *et al.* (1981) Effects of sunflower seed supplements on reproduction and growth of RCS rats with hereditary retinal dystrophy. *Lab. Anim. Sci.*, **31**, 482–488

HESS, H.H., NEWSOME, D.A., KNAPKA, J.J. *et al.* (1983a) Slit-lamp assessment of age of onset and incidence of cataracts in pink-eyed, tan-hooded retinal dystrophic rats. *Curr. Eye Res.*, **2**, 265–269

HESS, H.H., NEWSOME, D.A., KNAPKA, J.J. *et al.* (1983b) Slit-lamp assessment of onset of cataracts in black-eyed, black-hooded retinal dystropic rats. *Invest. Ophthalmol. Vis. Sci.*, **24**, 654–657

HETHERINGTON, J., JR. (1988) Capsular glaucoma management philosophy. (Suppl. 184). *Acta. Ophthalmol.*, **66**, 138–140

HEYWOOD, R. (1971) Juvenile cataracts in the beagle dog. *J. Small Anim. Pract.*, **12**, 171–177

HIETANEN, J. and TARKKANEN, A. (1989) Glycoconjugates in exfoliation syndrome: A lectin histochemical study of the ciliary body and lens. *Acta. Ophthalmol.*, **67**, 288–294

HIGHTOWER, K.R. (1986) Membrane -SH groups and permeability. ARVO Suppl: *Invest. Ophthalmol. Vis. Sci.*, **27**, 8

HIGHTOWER, K.R. and HARRISON, S.E. (1987) The influence of calcium on glucose metabolism in the rabbit lens. *Invest. Ophthalmol. Vis. Sci.*, **28**, 1433–1436

HIGHTOWER, K.R., MCCREADY, J.P. and GOUDSMIT, E.M. (1987) Calcium-induced opacification is dependent upon lens pH. *Curr. Eye Res.*, **6**, 1415–1420

HIGHTOWER, K.R., RILEY, M.V. and MCCREADY, J. (1989) Regional distribution of calcium in alloxan diabetic rabbit lens. *Curr. Eye Res.*, **8**, 517–522

HILBERT, R. (1912) Schichtstarbildung durch vier Generationen einer Familie. *Munch. Med. Wochenschr.*, **59**, 1272–1273

HILLER, R. and KAHN, H.A. (1976) Senile cataract extraction and diabetes. *Br. J. Ophthalmol.*, **60**, 283–286

HILLER, R., SPERDUTO, R.D. and EDERER, F. (1983) Epidermiologic associations with cataract in the 1971–1972 National Health and Nutrition Examination Survey. *Am. J. Ophthalmol.*, **118**, 239–248

HILLER, R., SPERDUTO, R.D. and KRUEGGER, D.E. (1982) Pseudoexfoliation, intraocular pressure and senile lens changes in a population-based study. *Arch. Ophthalmol.*, **100**, 1080–1082

HIRSCH, S.E., APPLETON, B., FINE, B.S. *et al.* (1977) Effects of repeated microwave irradiations to the albino rabbit eye. *Invest. Ophthalmol.*, **16**, 315–319

HIRTH, R.S., GREENSTEIN, E.T. and PEER, R.L. (1974) Anterior capsular opacities (spurious cataracts) in beagle dogs. *Vet. Pathol.*, **11**, 181–194

HITTNER, H.M., KRETZER, F.L. and MEHTA, R.S. (1977) Zellweger syndrome: lenticular opacities indicating carrier status and lens abnormalities characteristic of homozygotes. *Arch. Ophthalmol.*, **99**, 1

HITTNER, H.M., KRETZER, F.L. and MEHTA, R.S. (1981) Zellweger syndrome: lenticular opacities indicating carrier status and lens abnormalities characteristic of homozygotes. *Arch. Ophthalmol.*, **99**, 1977–1982

HOCKWIN, O. (1962) Early changes of lens metabolism after X-irradiation. *Exp. Eye Res.*, **1**, 422–426

HOCKWIN, O. and DRAGOMIRESCU, V. (1981) Die Scheimpflug-photographie des Vorden Augenabschnittes. *Acta Ophthalmol.*, Suppl., **2**, 129–136

HOCKWIN, O. and WEGENER, A. (1987) Syn and co-cataractogenesis. *Concepts Toxicol.*, **4**, 241–249

HOCKWIN, O., POONAWALLA, N., NOLL, E. *et al.* (1973) Durchlässigkeit der isolierten Rinderlinsenkapsel für Aminosäuren und wasserlösliche Eiweiße. *A von Graefes Arch. Ophthalmol.*, **188**, 75–181

HOCKWIN, O., DRAGOMIRESCU, V. and LASER, H. (1982) Measurement of lens transparency and of its disturbance by densitometric image analysis of Scheimpflug photographs. *A von Graefes Arch. Klin. Exp. Ophthalmol.*, **219**, 255–262

HOCKWIN, O., WEGENER, A., BESSEMS, G. *et al.* (1992) Models and methods for testing toxicity: lens. In *Manual of Oculotoxicity Testing of Drugs* (eds O. Hockwin, K. Green, L.F. Rubin), Gustav Fischer Verlag, Stuttgart, 255–317

HOGAN, M.J., ALVARADO, J.A. and WEDDELL, J.E. (1971) *Histology of the Human Eye.* W.B. Saunders, Philadelphia

HOGG, D., GORIN, M.B., HEINZMANN, C., *et al.* (1987) Nucleotide sequence for the cDNA of the bovine βB2 crystallin and assignment of the orthologous human locus to chromosome 22. *Curr. Eye Res.*, **6**, 1335–1342

HOLDEN, R., HESLER, J., FORBES, J. and BROWN, N.A.P. (1993) Visual performance and objectively measured grades of cataract. *Optom. Vis. Sci.*, **70**, 982–985

HOLLINS, M. (1974) Does the central human retina stretch during accommodation? *Nature*, **251**, 729

HOOK, E.B. (1982) Epidemiology in Down Syndrome. In *Down Syndrome: Advances in Biomedicine and the Behavioral Sciences* (eds S.M. Pueschel, J.E. Rynders), The Ware Press

HOOK, E.B. *et al.* (1965) Trisomy 18 in a 15-year-old female. *Lancet*, **ii**, 910

HORAN, M.B. and BILLSON, F.A. (1974) X-linked cataract and Hutchinsonian teeth. *Aust. Paediatr. J.* **10**, 98–102

HORVEN, E. (1937) Exfoliation of the superficial layer of the lens capsule (Vogt) and its relation to glaucoma simplex. *Br. J. Ophthalmol.*, **21**, 625–637

HORVEN, I. and HUTCHINSON, B.T. (1967) Exfoliation syndrome (case reports of 31 and 35 year old patients). *Acta. Ophthalmol.*, **45**, 294–298

HORWITZ, J. (1993) The function of alpha crystallin. *Invest. Ophthalmol. Vis. Sci.*, **34**, 10–22

HOSOKAWA, Y. (1967) Experimental study on radiation cataract. 1: relative biological effectiveness of fast neutrons and X-rays for lenticular damage in rabbits. *Acta Soc. Ophthalmol. Jpn.*, **71**, 126–134

HOSOKAWA, M., ASHIDA, Y. TSUBOYAMA, T. *et al.* (1988) Cataract in Senescence Accelerated Mouse (SAM). 2: Development of a new strain of mouse with late-appearing cataract. *Exp. Eye Res.*, **47**, 629–640

HOULE, R.E. and GRANT, W.M. (1973) Zinc chloride keratopathy and cataracts. *Am. J. Ophthalmol.*, **75**, 992–996

HOYT, C. and LAMBERT, S. (1990) Childhood glaucoma. In *Pediatric Ophthalmology* (ed. D. Taylor) Blackwell Scientific, 319–332

HUGGERT, A. (1946a) The thickness of the cortex of the crystalline lens in different ages. *Acta Ophthalmol.*, **24**, 43–62

HUGGERT, A. (1946b) Are the discontinuity zones of the crystalline lens iso-indiccal surfaces? *Acta Ophthalmol.*, **24**, 417–421

HUGGERT, A. (1953) The appearance of the band of dysjunction of the lens in diabetes mellitus. *Am. J. Ophthalmol.*, **31**, 227–234

HUNOLD, W., WIRTZ, M., KREINER, C., GREITE, J.H. and KADEN, P. (1989) Linsen-Epithel-Nekrose-Faktor (LENF) zur Nachstarverhutung. *Fortschr. Ophthalmol.*, **88**, 386–389

IIMURO, A., TAKENHANA, M. and IWATA, S. (1987) Influence of calmodulin antagonists on Ca^{2+} transport in the lens. *Ophthalmic Res.*, **19**, 95–101

IJSPEERT, J.K., DEWARD, P.W.T., VAN DEN BERG, T.J.T.P. *et al.* (1990) The intraocular straylight function in 129 healthy volunteers; dependence on angle, age and pigmentation. *Vision Res.*, **30**, 699–707

IKEDA, A., SEKI, Y., YOSHI, I. *et al.* (1981) An immunohistochemical study of lens development in a mutant small eye and cataractous mouse. *Arch. Histol. Jap.*, **44**, 237–249

INANA, G., HOTTA, Y. and ZINTZ, C. *et al.* (1988) Expression defect of ornithene aminotransferase gene in gyrate atrophy. *Invest. Ophthalmol. Vis. Sci.*, **29**, 1001–1005

INGOLIA, T.D. and CRAIG, E.A. (1982) Four small Drosophila heat shock proteins are related to each other and to mammalian a-crystallin. *Proc. Natl. Acad. Sci. USA*, **79**, 2360–2364

IRELAND, A.W., HORNEBROOK, J.W., NEALE, F.C. *et al.* (1968) The crystalline lens in chronic surgical hypoparathyroidism. none**122**, 408

IRELAND, M.E. and JACKS, L.A. (1989) Initial characterization of lens beta-adrenergic receptors. *Invest. Ophthalmol. Vis. Sci.*, **30**, 2190–2194

IRELAND, M. and MAISEL, H. (1984a) Phosphorylation of chick lens proteins. *Curr. Eye Res.*, **3**, 961–968

IRELAND, M. and MAISEL, H. (1984b) A cytoskeletal protein unique to lens fibre cell differentiation. *Exp. Eye Res.*, **38**, 637–645

IRELAND, M.E. and MAISEL, H. (1987) Adrenergic stimulation of lens cytoskeletal phosphorylation. *Curr. Eye Res.*, **6**, 489–496

IRELAND, M.E. and MAISEL, H. (1988) Isoproterenol treatment causes cytoskeletal reorganization in chicken lens fiber cells. *Invest. Ophthalmol. Vis. Sci.*, **29**, 1356–1360

IWATA, S. (1979) Experimental implantation of crystalline lens. *Doc. Ophthalmol. Proc. Series*, **21**, 201–207

IWATA, S. (1985) Calcium-pump and its modulator in the lens: A review. *Curr. Eye Res.*, **4**, 299–304

IWATA, S. and KINOSHITA, J.H. (1971) Mechanism of development of hereditary cataract in mice. *Invest. Ophthalmol.*, **10**, 504–512

JACKSON, R.C. (1955) Temporary cataracts in diabetes mellitus. *Br. J. Ophthalmol.*, **39**, 629–631

JACOB, T.J.C. and DUNCAN, G. (1982) Glucose-induced membrane permeability changes in the lens *Exp Eye Res*, **34**, 445–453

JACQUES, P.F., CHYLACK, L.T., MCGANDY, R.B. *et al.* (1988) Antioxidant status in persons with and without senile cataract. *Arch. Ophthalmol.*, **106**, 337–340

JAEGER, E.A. (1980) Ocular findings in Down's syndrome. *Trans Am. Ophthalmol. Soc.*, **78**, 808

JAEGER, W. (1983) Green ring of the anterior lens capsule. *Acta XXIV International Congress of Ophthalmology* **1**, 63–65

JAFFE, N.S. and HORWITZ, J. (1992) Lens and cataract. In *Textbook of Ophthalmology* (eds S.M. Podos, M. Yanoff), vol. 3, Gower Medical Publishing, New York & London

JAHNS, H. (1938) Angeborener Star in drei Generationen. *Klin. Monatsbl. Augenheilk.*, **100**, 481–482

JANKIEWICZ, H. and FREEBERG, D.D. (1956) A six-generation pedigree of congenital zonular cataract. *Am. J. Optom.*, **33**, 555–557

JAUREGUY, B.M. and HALL, J.G. (1979) Isolated congenital ectopia lentis with autosomal dominant inheritance. *Clin. Genet.*, **15**, 97–109

JAY, B., BLACH, R.K. and WELLS, R.S. (1968) Ocular manifestations of ichthyosis. *Br. J. Ophthalmol.*, **52**, 217–226

JEDZINIAK, J.A., CHYLACK, L.T.JR., CHENG, H.M. *et al.* (1981) The sorbitol pathway in the human lens: Aldose reductase and polyol dehydrogenase. *Invest. Ophthalmol. Vis. Sci.*, **20**, 314–326

JENSEN, A.D., CROSS, H.E. and PATON, D. (1974) Ocular complications in the Weill-Marchesani syndrome. *Am. J. Ophthalmol.*, **77**, 261–269

JERNIGAN, H.M.JR., KADOR, P.F. and KINOSHITA, J.H. (1981) Carrier mediated transport of choline in rat lens. *Exp. Eye Res.*, **32**, 709–718

JOHANSEN, E.V. (1947) *Undesogelser over det indbyrdes Storrelsesforhold mellum Cornea og Lens crystallina hos Mennesket*, Enjar Munksgaard, Copenhagen

JOHNSON, G., MINASSIAN, D. and FRANKEN, S. (1989) Alterations of the anterior lens capsule associated with climatic keratopathy. *Br. J. Ophthalmol.*, **73**, 229–234

JOHNSON, G.J. and OVERALL, M. (1978) Histology of sphenoidal degeneration of the cornea in Labrador. *Br. J. Ophthalmol.*, **62**, 53–61

JOHNSON, S.S. and NEVIN, N.C. (1976) Ocular manifestations in patients and female relatives of families with the oculocerebrorenal syndrome of Lowe. In *The Eye and Inborn Errors of Metabolism*, (eds D. Bergsma, A.J. Bron, and E. Cotlier), Liss, New York, 569–577

JORDAN, M. (1955) Stammbaumuntersuchungen bei Cataracta stellata coralliformis. *Klin. Monatsbl. Augenheilk.*, **126**, 475

JOSEPH, R. (1957) Congenital total cataract – possibly recessive. *Br. J. Ophthalmol.*, **41**, 444–445

JOYNER, K.H. (1989) Microwave cataract and litigation: A case study. *Acta Ophthalmol. Suppl.*, **57**, 545–549

KADOR, P., FUKUI, H.N., FUKUSHI, S. *et al.* (1980a) Philly

mouse: A new model of hereditary cataract. *Exp. Eye. Res.*, **30**, 59–68

KADOR, P.F., JERNIGAN, H.M.JR. and KINOSHITA, J.H. (1980b) Accumulation and incorporation of radiolabeled choline into cultured rabbit lens: evidence for a choline transport system. *Exp. Eye Res.*, **30**, 1–11

KADOR, P., UGA, S. and PIATIGORSKY, J. (1980c) The Philly mouse hereditary cataract. In *Aging of the Lens* (eds F. Regnault, O. Hockwin and Y. Courtois), Elsevier, North Holland, 157–170

KAISER-KUPFER, M., KUWABARA, T., and ASKANAS, A. *et al.* (1981) Systemic manifestations of gyrate atrophy of the choroid and retina. *Ophthalmology*, **88**, 302–306

KAISER-KUPFER, M., LUDWIG, I.H. and DE MONASTERIO, F.M. *et al.* (1985) Gyrate atrophy of the choroid and retina. Early findings. *Ophthalmology*, **92**, 394–401

KAISER-KUPFER, M.I., FREIDLIN, V., DATILES, M.B. *et al.* (1989) The association of posterior capsular lens opacities with bilateral acoustic neuromas in patients with neurofibromatosis type 2. Arch. Ophthalmol., **107**, 54

KALANT, H. (1959) Physiological hazards of microwave radiation: a survey of published literature. *Can. Med. Assoc. J.*, **81**, 575–582

KANSKI, J.J. and MCALLISTER, J.A. (1989) *Glaucoma. A Colour Manual of Diagnosis and Treatment*. Butterworth, Washington, 1–152

KAREL, I. (1969) Clinical picture of congenital diffuse tapetoretinal degeneration in 42 cases. *Acta Univ. Carol. Med. Monogr. Praha*, **15**, 259–335

KARR, D.J. and SCOTT, W.E. (1986) Visual acuity results following the treatment of persistent primary hyperplastic vitreous. *Arch. Ophthalmol.*, **104**, 662–667

KAYE, L.D., ROTHNER, A.D., BEAUCHAMP, G.R., MEYERS, S.M. and ESTES, M.L. (1992) Ocular findings associated with neurofibromatosis type II. *Ophthalmology*, **99**, 1424–1429

KAZDAN, M.S. (1969) Electric cataract: A report of two cases. *Can. J. Ophthalmol.*, **4**, 104–105

KAZUHIKO, U., KUMIKO, N. and NORIO, O. (1986). Haemorrhage in the lens: Spontaneous occurrence in congenital cataract. *Br. J. Ophthalmol.*, **70**, 593–595

KEIZER, D.P.R. (1952) Congenitale cataract. *Ned. Tijdschr. Geneeskd.*, **96**, 763–765

KERN, H.L. and HO, C.K. (1974) No title *Ophthalmic Res.*, **6**, 166–174

KERN, H.L. and ZOLOT, S.L. (1987) Transport of vitamin C in the lens. *Curr. Eye Res.*, **6**, 885–896

KERN, H.L., BELLHORN, R.W. and PETERSON, C.M. (1977) Sodium cyanate-induced ocular lesions in the beagle. *J. Pharmacol. Exp. Ther.*, **200**, 10–16

KHATAMI, M., ROEL, L.E., LI, W. and ROCKEY, J.H. (1986) Ascorbate regeneration in bovine ocular tissues by NADPH-dependent semidehydroascorbate reductase. *Exp. Eye Res.*, **43**, 167–175

KHAN, H.A., LEIBOWITZ, H.M., GANLEY, J.P. *et al.* (1977) The Framingham Eye Study. 1: Outline and major prevalence findings. *Am. J. Ophthalmol.*, **106**, 17–32

KHU, P.M. and KASHIWAGI, T. (1993) Quantifying nuclear opacification in color Scheimpflug photographs. *Invest. Ophthalmol. Vis. Sci.* **34**, 130–136

KIMURA, S. and IKUI, H. (1951) Atom-bomb radiation cataract. *Am. J. Ophthalmol.*, **34**, 811–816

KINOSHITA, J.H. (1964) Selected topics in ophthalmic biochemistry. *Arch. Ophthalmol.*, **72**, 554

KINOSHITA, J.H. (1965a) Pathways of glucose metabolism in the lens. *Invest. Ophthalmol.*, **4**, 619–628

KINOSHITA, J.H. (1965b) Cataracts in galactosemia. The Jonas S. Friedenwald Memorial Lecture. *Invest. Ophthalmol.*, **5**, 786–799

KINOSHITA, J.H. (1974) Mechanisms initiating cataract formation. *Invest. Ophthalmol.*, **13**, 713

KINOSHITA, J.H. and MEROLA, L.O. (1973) Cyanate effects on the lens. *in vitro*. *Invest. Ophthalmol.*, **12**, 544–547

KINOSHITA, J.H., MEROLA, L.O., SATOH, K. *et al.* (1962) Osmotic changes caused by the accumulation of dulcitol in the lenses of rats fed with galactose. *Nature*, **194**, 1085–1087

KINOSHITA, J.H., FUTTERMAN, S., SATOH, K. *et al.* (1963) Factors affecting the formation of sugar alcohols in ocular lenses. *Biochim. Biophys. Acta*, **74**, 340

KINSEY, V.E. (1973) Studies on the crystalline lens. XIX: Quantitative aspects of active and passive transport of sodium. *Exp. Eye. Res.*, **15**, 699–710

KINSEY, V.E. and MERRIAM, F.C. (1950) Studies on the crystalline lens. II: Synthesis of glutathione in the normal and cataractous rabbit lens. A.M.A. *Arch. Ophthalmol.*, **44**, 370–380

KIRBY, T.J. (1967) Cataracts produced by triparanol (MER-29). *Trans. Am. Ophthalmol. Soc.*, **65**, 493–543

KIRBY, T.J., ACHOR, R.W.P., PERRY, H.O. *et al.* (1962) Cataract formation after triparanol therapy. *Arch. Ophthalmol.*, **68**, 486

KISTLER, J. and BULLIVANT, S. (1987) Protein processing in lens intercellular junctions: Cleavage of MP70 to MP38. *Invest. Ophthalmol. Vis. Sci.*, **28**, 1687–1692

KISTLER, J., KIRKLAND, B. and GOODENOUGH, D.A. (1985) Identification of a 70 000 daltons protein in lens membranes junctional domains. *J. Cell Biol.*, **101**, 28–35

KIVLIN, J.D., FINEMAN, R.M., CRANDALL, A.S. *et al.* (1986) Peter's anomaly as a consequence of genetic and non genetic syndromes. *Arch. Ophthalmol.*, **104**, 61–64

KLASS, A.M. and BERNS, R.P. (1964) Modifications of hypothermic lens opacity in hamsters by closure of eyelids. *Exp. Eye Res.*, **3**, 213–217

KLEIFELD, O. and HOCKWIN, O. (1960) The importance of oxygen for the metabolism of the lens. *A von Graefes Arch. Ophthalmol.*, **162**, 346–349

KLEIN, D. (1956) Cataracte congenitale familiale: consanguinite des parents. *J. Génét. Hum.* **5**, 283–284

KLEMETTI, A. (1988) Intraocular pressure in exfoliation syndrome. *Acta. Ophthalmol.*, Suppl. **66**, 54–58

KNAPP, F.N. (1926) Familial cataract: a study through five generations. *Am. J. Ophthalmol.*, **9**, 683–684

KNORR, H.L., JUNEMANN, A., HANDEL, A. and NAUMANN, G.O. (1991) Morphometric and qualitative changes in corneal endothelium in pseudoexfoliative syndrome. *Fortschr Ophthalmol.*, **88**, 786–789

KNOX, P. (1976) Carcinogenic nitrosomides and cell cultures. *Nature*, **259**, 671–673

KOCH, H.R., KREMER, F., LINNER, E. *et al.* (1974) On the influence of the monolateral carotid ligation upon the formation of radiation cataract in rats. *Ophthalmic Res.*, **6**, 175–182

KOLIOPOULOS, J. and PALIMERIS, G. (1975) A typical Hallermann-Streiff Francois syndrome in three successive generations. *J. Pediatr. Ophthalmol.*, **12**, 235–239

KONSTAS, A.G., MARSHALL, G.E. and LEE, W.R. (1990) Immunogold localisation of laminin in normal and exfoliative iris. *Br. J. Ophthalmol.*, **74**, 450–457

KONYUKHOV, B.V. and VAKHRUSHEVA, M.P. (1969) Abnormal development of eyes in mice homozygous for the fidget gene. *Teratology*, **2**, 147–157

KORETZ, J. and HANDELMAN, G.H. (1986) The 'lens paradox' and image formation in accommodating human eyes; in 'The Lens: Transparency and Cataract', (ed. Duncan, G.) *Eurage*, 57–64

KORETZ, J.F., HANDLEMAN, G.H. and BROWN, N.A.P. (1984) Analysis of human crystalline lens curve as a function of accommodative state and age. *Vision Res.*, **24**, 1141–1151

KORETZ, J.F., KAUFMAN, P.L., NEIDER, M.W. *et al.* (1989) Accommodation and presbyopia in the human eye – aging of the anterior segment. *Vision Res.*, **29**, 1685–1692

KRAMER, P.O., EMERY, A.F., GUY, A.W. *et al.* (1975) The ocular effects of microwaves on hypothermic rabbits: a study of microwave cataractogenic mechanisms. *Ann. NY Acad. Sci.*, **247**, 155–165

KRAMER, P.O., HARRIS, C., GUY, A.W. *et al.* (1976) Proceedings: Study of the effects of chronic low level microwave radiation on rabbits. In *Biological Effects of Electromagnetic Waves* (eds C.C. Johnson and M.L. Shore), US DHEW Publication (FDA) 77–8010, 49–60

KRATOCHVILOVA, J. (1981) Dominant cataract mutations detected in offspring of gamma-irradiated male mice. *J. Hered.*, **72**, 302–307

KRATOCHVILOVA, J. and FAVOR, J. (1988) Phenotype characterization and genetic analysis of twenty dominant cataract mutations detected in offspring of irradiated male mice. *Genet. Res.*, **52**, 125–134

KRATOCHVILOVA, J. and FAVOR, J. (1992) Allelism test of 15 dominant cataract mutations in mice. *Genet Res.*, **59**, 199–203

KREHBIEL, J.D. (1972) Cataracts in bobwhite quail. *J. Am. Vet. Med. Assoc.*, **161**, 634–637

KREIBIG, W. (1954) Zur operativen Behandlung des akuten Glaukomanfelles. *Klin. Monatsbl. Augenheilk.*, **125**, 39–44

KRETZER, F.L., HITTNER, H.M. and MEHTA, R.S. (1981) Ocular manifestations of the Smith–Lemli–Opitz syndrome. *Arch. Ophthalmol.*, **99**, 2000

KRILL, A.E., WOODBURY, G. and BOWMAN, J.E. (1969) X-chromosomal-linked sutural cataracts. *Am. J. Ophthalmol.*, **68**, 867–872

KRONEVI, T., HOLMBERG, B. and BORG, K. (1977) Lens lesions in the elk. *Acta Vet. Scand.*, **18**, 159–167

KRUCKMANN, J. (1940) Ueber den histoligischen Befund einer Röntgen-katarakt. *Klin. Monatsbl. Augenheilk.*, **104**, 621–628

KUBESOVA (1949) Cited by Duke-Elder in *System of Ophthalmology* vol. XI, Henry Kimpton, London, 1969 *Cesk. Oftalmol.*, **5**, 149

KUCK, J.F.R. and KUCK, K.D. (1983) The Emory mouse cataract: loss of soluble protein, glutathione, protein sulfhydryl and other changes. *Exp. Eye Res.*, **36**, 351–362

KUCK, J.F.R., KUWABARA, T. and KUCK, K.D. (1981) The Emory mouse cataract: An animal model for human senile cataract. *Curr. Eye Res.*, **1**, 643–649

KUSZAK, J.R. and BROWN, H.G. (1991) Embryology and anatomy of the lens. In *Principles and Practice of Ophthalmology in The Harvard System* (eds D. Albert and F. Jacobiec), Saunders, Philadelphia

KUSZAK, J.R. and DEUTSCH, T.A. (1991) Anatomy of aged and senile cataractous lenses. In *Principles and Practice of Ophthalmology* (eds D. Albert, F. Jacobiec), W B Saunders, Philadelphia

KUSZAK, J.R., BERTRAM, B.A., MASCAI, M.S. and RAE, J.L. (1984) Sutures of the crystalline lens: A review. *Scanning Electron Microsc.*, **III**, 1369–1378

KUSZAK, J.R., BERTRAM, B.A. and RAE, J.L. (1986) The ordered structure of the crystalline lens. In *Cell and Developmental Biology of the Eye. Development of Order in the Visual System* (eds S.R. Hilfer and J.B. Sheffield), Springer-Verlag, New York, 35–60

KUSZAK, J.R., KHAN, A.R. and CENEDELLA, R.J. (1988) An ultrastructural analysis of plasma membrane in the U18666A cataract. *Invest. Ophthalmol. Vis. Sci.*, **29**, 261–267

KUSZAK, J.R., ENNESSER, C.A., BERTRAM, S. *et al.* (1989) The contribution of cell to cell fusion to the ordered structure of the crystalline lens. *Lens Eye Toxic Res.*, **6**, 639–673

KUSZAK, J.R., MAISEL, H. and HARDING, C.V. (1978) Gap junctions of chick lens fibre cells. *Exp. Eye Res.*, **27**, 495–498

KUSZAK, J.R., MASCAI, M.S., BLOOM, K.J., RAE, J.L. and WEINSTEIN, R.S. (1985) Cell-to-cell fusion of lens fibre cells *in situ*: correlative light, scanning electron microscopic and freeze-fracture studies. *J. Ultrastruct. Res.*, **93**, 144–160

KUSZAK, J.R., PETERSON, K.L. and BROWN, H.G. (1992) Electron microscopic observations of the crystalline lens. In *Electron Microscopy of the Visual System: The Anterior Segment of the Eye* (special issue), *J. Electron. Microsc.*, **1**, 619

KUSZAK, J.R., PETERSON, K.L., SIVAK, J.G. and HERBERT, K.L.

(1994) The interrelationship of lens anatomy and optical quality. II. Primate lenses. *Exp. Eye Res.*, **59**, 521–535

KUSZAK, J.R., DEUTSCH, T.A. and BROWN, H.G. (1993) Anatomy of aged and senile cataractous lenses, (chapter 39). In *Principles and Practice of Ophthalmology* (eds F.A. Jakobiec and D. Albert), W B Saunders, Philadelphia

KUWABARA, T. (1975) Maturation of the lens cell: A morphological study. *Exp. Eye Res.*, **20**, 427–443

KUWABARA, T., KINOSHITA, J.N. and COGAN, D.G. (1969) Electron microscopic study of galactose-induced cataract. *Invest. Ophthalmol.*, **8**, 133–149

KWAN, M., NUNIKOSKI, J. and HUNT, T.K. (1972) In vivo measurements of oxygen tension in the cornea, aqueous humor and anterior lens of the open eye. *Invest. Ophthalmol.*, **11**, 108–114

LA VAIL, M.M., SIDMAN, R.L. and GERHARDT, C. (1975) Congenic strains of RCS rats with inherited retinal degeneration and their congenic controls. *J. Hered.*, **66**, 242–244

LAHIRI, L.M. (1938) Night blindness and cataract in bullocks. (A deficiency disease?) *Indian Vet. J.*, **15**, 58

LAING, R.A. and BURSELL, S.E. (1981) *In vivo* photomicrography of the crystalline lens. *Arch. Ophthalmol.*, **99**, 688–690

LAMB, H.D. (1937) Anterior capsular cataract. An example of true metaplasia. *Arch. Ophthalmol.*, **17**, 877–879

LAMBERT, B.W. and KINOSHITA, J.H. (1967) The effects of ionizing irradiation on lens cation permeability, transport, and hydration. *Invest. Ophthalmol.*, **6**, 624–634

LAMPE, P.D. and JOHNSON, R.G. (1989) Phosphorylation of MP26, a lens junction protein, is enhanced by activators of protein kinase. *Immunol. Rev.*, **107**, 145–155

LANGLEY, R.K., MORTIMER, C.B. and MCCULLOCH, C. (1960) The experimental production of cataracts by exposure to heat and light. *Arch. Ophthalmol.*, **63**, 473–488

LARSEN, J.S. (1971) The saggittal growth of the eye. *Acta Ophthalmol.*, **49**, 427–440

LATIES, A.M. (1969) Localization in cornea and lens of topically-applied irreversible cholinesterase inhibitors. *Am. J. Ophthalmol.*, **68**, 848–857

LAYDEN, W.E. and SHAFFER, R.N. (1974) Exfoliation syndrome. *Am. J. Ophthalmol.*, **78**, 835–841

LAYDEN, W.E., RITCH, R., KING, D.G. and TEEKHASAENEE, C. (1990) Combined exfoliation and pigment dispersion syndrome. *Am. J. Ophthalmol.*, **109**, 530–534

LEAVER, P.K., GREY, R.H.B. and GARNER, A. (1979) Silicone oil injection in the treatment of massive preretinal retraction. II: Late complications in 93 eyes. *Br. J. Ophthalmol.*, **63**, 361–367

LEE, J.B. and BENEDICT, W.L. (1950) Hereditary nuclear cataract. *Arch. Ophthalmol.*, **44**, 643–650

LEE, B., GODFREY, M., VITALE, E., *et al.* (1991) Linkage of Marfan syndrome and a phenotypically related disorder to two different fibrillin genes. *Nature.*, **352**, 330–334

LEGLER, U.F.C., ASSIA, E.I., APPLE, D.J. and POWERS, T. (1991) The effect of colchicine in a sustained drug delivery system on posterior capsular opacification. *Ophthalmol. Times*, **9**, 17

LEHMANN, A.R., FRANCIS, A.J. and GIANELLI, F. (1985) Prenatal diagnosis of Cockayne's syndrome. *Lancet*, **I**, 486–488

LEIBOWITZ, H.M., KRUEGER, D.E., MAUNDER, L.R. *et al.* (1980) The Framingham Eye Study Monograph: An ophthalmological and epidemiological study of cataract, glaucoma, diabetic retinopathy, macular degeneration and visual acuity in a general population of 2631 adults. *Surv. Ophthalmol. Suppl.*, **24**, 335–610

LEONARD, A. and MAISIN, J.R. (1965) Hereditary cataract induced X-irradiation of young rats. *Nature*, **205**, 615–616

LERMAN, S. (1962) Radiation cataractogenesis. *NY J. Med.*, **52**, 3075–3085

LERMAN, S. (1967) The structural proteins of the ocular lens. *Surv. Ophthalmol.*, **12**, 112–129

LERMAN, S. (1972) Lens proteins in aging and cataract formation. In *Contemporary Ophthalmology* (ed. J. Bellow), Williams & Wilkins, Baltimore

LERMAN, S. (1980) *Radiant Energy and the Eye*, MacMillan, New York, 251–301

LERMAN, S. and BORKMAN, R.F. (1976) *Ophthalmic Res.*, **8**, 335–353

LERMAN, S., ASHLEY, D.L., LONG, R.C. *et al.* (1982) Nuclear magnetic resonance analyses of the cold cataract: whole lens studies. *Invest. Ophthalmol. Vis. Sci.*, **23**, 218–226

LERMAN, S., MORAN, M. and MATHEWS, N. (1989) Photographic and spectroscopic correlations of human cataracts. *Ophthalmic Res.*, **21**, 18–26

LESKE, M.C., CHYLACK, L.T., KHU, P. *et al.* (1987) Evaluation of a simple classification system based on standard photographs. ARVO Suppl: *Invest. Ophthalmol. Vis. Sci.*, **28**, 323

LESKE, M.C., CHYLACK, L.T.JR., WU, S.-Y. *et al.* (1991) The LSC Group. Longitudinal changes in lens photographs with the LOCS II method. (Abstract) *ARVO Suppl.: Invest. Ophthalmol. Vis. Sci.*, **32**, 1244

LETSON, R.D. and DESNICK, R.J. (1978) Punctate lenticular opacities in type II mannosidosis. *Am. J. Ophthalmol.*, **85**, 218–224

LEWIS, B.S., HARDING, J.J., QUINLAN, M. and BRON, A.J. (1994) Lenses with retrodots do not have a high oxalate content. *Dev. Ophthalmol.*, **26**, 1–3

LEWIS, W.H. (1904) Experimental studies on the development of the eye in Amphibia. I: On the origin of the lens: *Rana palustris*. *Am. J. Anat.*, **3**, 505–536

LI, Y., BULLER, B., FUHRMANN, C., *et al.* (1992) The autosomal dominant familial exudative vitreretinopathy locus maps on 11q and is closely linked to D11S533. *Am. J. Hum. Genet.*, **51**, 749–754

LI, Z.-Y., STREETEN, B.W. and WALLACE, R.N. (1988) Association of elastin with pseudoexfoliative material. An immunoelectron microscopic study. *Curr. Eye Res.*, **7**, 1163–1172

LI, Z.Y., STREETEN, B.W. and WALLACE, R.N. (1991) Vitronectin localizes to pseudoexfoliative fibers in ocular conjunctival sites by immunoelectron microscopy. *ARVO Suppl.: Invest. Ophthalmol. Vis. Sci.*, **32**, 777

LINDSTROM, R.L. and HARRIS, W.S. (1980) Management of the posterior capsule following posterior chamber lens implantation. *J. Am. Intraocul. Implant Soc.*, **6**, 255–258

LITTLE, J., IKEDA, A., ZWAAN, J. *et al.* (1965) The immunologic specificity of human lens proteins. *Exp. Eye Res.*, **4**, 187–195

LIU, C.S.C., BROWN, N.A.P., LEONARD, T.J.K. *et al.* (1988) The prevalence and morphology of cataract in patients on allopurinol treatment. *Eye*, **2**, 600–606

LO, W.K. (1987) *In vivo* and *in vitro* observations on permeability and diffusion pathways of tracers in rat and frog lenses. *Exp. Eye Res.*, **45**, 393–406

LO, W.K. and HARDING, C.V. (1983) Tight junctions in the lens epithelia of human and frog: freeze fracture and protein tracer studies. *Invest. Ophthalmol. Vis. Sci.*, **24**, 396

LO, W.K. and HARDING, C.V. (1986) Structure and distribution of gap junctions in lens epithelium and fibre cells. *Cell Tissue Res.*, **244**, 253–263

LONG, J.C. (1962) A clinical and experimental study of electric cataract. *Trans. Am. Ophthalmol. Soc.*, **60**, 471–516

LONG, J.C. (1963) Electric cataract. *Am. J. Ophthalmol.*, **56**, 108–133

LOREDO, A., RODRIGUEZ, R.S. and MURILLO, M.L. (1972) Cataracts after short-term corticosteroid treatment. *N. Eng. J. Med.*, **286**, 160–

LOUIS, C.F., MICKELSON, J.R., TURNQUIST, J. *et al.* (1987) Regulation of lens cyclic nucleotide metabolism by calcium plus calmodulin. *Invest. Ophthalmol. Vis. Sci.*, **28**, 806–814

LOWE, R.F. (1949a) Some thoughts on cataract development. *Trans. Ophthalmol. Soc. Aust.*, **9**, 215–225

LOWE, R. (1949b) The eyes in mongolism. *Br. J. Ophthalmol.*, **33**, 131

LOWE, R.F. and CLARK, B.A.J. (1973a) Posterior corneal curvature. Correlations in normal eyes and in eyes involved with primary angle-closure glaucoma. *Br. J. Ophthalmol.*, **57**, 464–470

LOWE, R.F. and CLARK, B.A.J. (1973b) Radius of curvature of the anterior lens surface. Correlations in normal eyes and in eyes involved with primary angle-closure glaucoma. *Br. J. Ophthalmol.*, **57**, 471–474

LOWES, M. (1990) The effect of posterior vaulting of intraocular lens implants on capsular opacification. *Eur. J. Implant Refract. Surg.*, **2**, 47–52

LOWRY, R.B. (1982) Early onset of Cockayne syndrome. (Editorial). *Am. J. Med. Genet.*, **13**, 209–210

LOWRY, R.B., MACLEAN, R., MCLEAN, D.M. *et al.*, (1971) Cataracts, microcephaly, kyphosis and limited movement in two siblings: a new syndrome. *J. Pediatr.*, **79**, 282–284

LUBSEN, N.H., RENWICK, J.H., TSUI, L.C. *et al.* (1987) A locus for a human hereditary cataract is closely linked to the gamma-crystallin gene family. *Proc. Natl. Acad. Sci. USA*, **84**, 489–492

LUBSEN, N.H., AARTS, H.J.M. and SCHOENMALZERS, J.J.G. (1988) The evolution of lenticular proteins: the b(beta) and g(gamma) crystallin super gene family. *Prog. Biophys. Mol. Biol.*, **51**, 47–76

LUBSEN, N.H., PEEK, R., MCAVOY, J.W. *et al.* (1992) Gene pulses and targeted mRNA breakdown control crystallin RNA levels during BFGF directed rat lens fibre cell differentiation. Proceedings of Xth ISER Meeting, Stresa, Italy [Abstract]. *Exp. Eye Res.*, **55**, 2

LUCAS, V.A. and ZIGLER, J.S. (1987) Transmembrane glucose carriers in the monkey lens. *Invest. Ophthalmol. Vis. Sci.*, **28**, 1404–1412

LUCAS, V.A. and ZIGLER, J.S. (1988) Identification of the monkey lens glucose transporter by photoaffinity labelling with cytochalasin B. *Invest. Ophthalmol. Vis. Sci.*, **29**, 630–635

LÜLLMANN, H., LÜLLMANN-RAUCH, R. and WASSERMAN, O. (1975) *Crit. Rev. Toxicol.*, **4**, 185–

LUTJEN-DRECOLL, E., TAMM, E. and KAUFMANN, P.L. (1988a) Age changes in rhesus monkey ciliary muscle: light and electron microscopy. *Exp. Eye Res.*, **47**, 885–889

LUTJEN-DRECOLL, E., TAMM, E. and KAUFMANN, P.L. (1988b) Age related loss of morphologic response to pilocarpine in rhesus monkey ciliary muscle. *Arch. Ophthalmol.*, **106**, 1591–1598

LUTJEN-DRECOLL, E., TAMM, E. and ROHEN, J.W. (1992) Morphology of aging processes in the ciliary body. Proceedings of Xth ISER Meeting, Stresa, Italy [Abstract]. *Exp. Eye Res.*, **55**, 173

LUYCKX, J. (1966) Measure des composantes optiques de l'oeil du nouveau-né par échographie ultrasonique. *Arch. Ophthalmol. (Paris)*, **26**, 159–170

LYDAHL, E. (1984) Infrared radiation and cataract. *Acta Ophthalmol.* **Suppl. 166**

LYFORD, J.H. and ROY, F.H. (1974) Arrhinencephaly unilateralis, uveal coloboma and lens reduplication. *Am. J. Ophthalmol.*, **77**, 315–318

LYNE, A.J. and PHILLIPS, C.I. (1969) Visual field defect due to opacities in the optical media. *Br. J. Ophthalmol.*, **53**, 119–122

LYON, M.F., JARVIS, S.E., SAYERS, I. *et al.* (1981) Lens opacity: a new gene for congenital cataract on chromosome *10* of the mouse. *Genet. Res.*, **38**, 337–341

LYONS, T.J., SILVESTRI, G., DUNN, J.A. *et al.* (1991) Role of glycation in modification of lens crystallins in diabetic and non-diabetic senile cataracts. *Diabetes*, **40**, 1010–1015

MCAVOY, J.W. and VAN HEYNINGEN, R. (1976) Changes in the cells of the lens bow and epithelium of tryptophan-deficient rats. Colloq INSERM, **60**, 245–250

MCAVOY, J.W., PALFREY, L.J. and VAN HEYNINGEN, R. (1979) A light microscope study of the lens of the tryptophan deficient rat. *Exp. Eye Res.*, **28**, 533–538

MCAVOY, J.W., CHAMBERLAIN, C.G., DE IONGH, R.U. *et al.* (1992) The role of fibroblast growth factor in eye lens development. *Ann. NY Acad. Sci.*, 1

MCDONNELL, P.J., ZARBIN, M.A. and GREEN, W.R. (1983)

Posterior capsule opacification in pseudophakic eyes. *Ophthalmology.*, **90**, 1548–1553

MACDONALD, E.B., DOUGLAS, R. and HARDEN, P.A. (1983) A Caucasian family with the i phenotype and congenital cataracts. *Vox Sang.*, **44**, 322–325

MACDONALD, W.B., FITCH, K.D. and LEWIS, I.C. (1960) Cockayne's syndrome: a heredo-familial disorder of growth and development. *Pediatrics*, **25**, 997–1007

MCFALL-NGAI, M.J., DING, L.L., TAKEMOTO, L.J. *et al.* (1985) Spatial and temporal mapping of the age-related changes in human lens crystallins. *Exp. Eye Res.*, **41**, 745–758

MACKAY, G., STEWART, C.P. and ROBERTSON, J.D. (1932) A note on the inorganic constituents of normal and cataractous human crystalline lenses. *Br. J. Ophthalmol.*, **16**, 193–201

MACKEEN, D., FINE, S. and FINE, B.S. (1973) Production of cataracts in rabbits with the ultraviolet laser. A preliminary report. *Ophthalmic Res.*, **5**, 317–324

MCKUSICK, V.A. (1972) *Heritable Disorders of Connective Tissue*, 4th edn, Mosby, St Louis

MCKUSICK, V.A. (1988) *Mendelian Inheritance in Man*, 8th edn, Johns Hopkins University Press, Baltimore,

MCKUSICK, V.A. (1992) Mendehan Inheritance and Man, 10th edn. John Hopkins University Press, Baltimore

MCLAREN, D.S. (1959) The eye and related glands of the rat and pig in protein deficiency. *Br. J. Ophthalmol.*, **43**, 78–87

MCLAREN, D.S. (1980) *Nutritional Ophthalmology*, 2nd edn, Academic Press, London,

MAHTO, R.S. (1972) Ocular features of hypothyroidism. *Br. J. Ophthalmol.*, **56**, 546–549

MAISEL, H. (1963) The immunologic specificity of lens antigens. *Am. J. Ophthalmol.*, **55**, 1208–1216

MAISEL, H. (ed.) (1985) *The Ocular Lens: Structure, Function and Pathology*, Marcel Dekker, New York

MAISEL, H. and PERRY, M. (1972) Electron microscopic observations on some structural proteins of the chick lens. *Exp. Eye Res.*, **14**, 7–12

MALTZMANN, B.A., HAUPT, E. and NOTIS, C. (1989) Relationship between age at time of cataract extraction and time interval before capsulotomy for opacification. *Ophthalmic Surg.*, **20**, 321–324

MANDELL, R.B. (1967) Corneal contour of the human infant. *Arch. Ophthalmol.*, **77**, 345–348

MANN, I. (1921) Congenital absence of the lens, with special reference to an aphakic human embryo. *Br. J. Ophthalmol.*, **5**, 301–307

MANN, I. (1956) *Developmental Abnormalities of the Eye*, 2nd edn, British Medical Association, London

MANN, I. (1957) *Developmental Abnormalities of the Eye*, 2nd edn, Lippincott, Philadelphia

MANN, I. (1964) The Development of the Eye. 3rd edn. *Br. Med. Assoc., Lond.*

MANSCHOT, W.A. (1963) Primary congenital aphakia. *Arch. Ophthalmol.*, **69**, 571–577

MANSKI, W. and SPECTOR, A. (1972) I. Immunochemical studies on alpha crystallin subunits. *Exp. Eye Res.*, **13**, 194–204

MANZITTI, E., DARNEL, A., GAMIO, S. and BENOZZI, J. (1994) Eye length in congenital cataracts; in *Congenital Cataracts*, (eds E. Cotlier, S. Lambert and D. Taylor) R. G. Landes Co., 251–259

MARAINI, G. and MANGILI, R. (1973) Differences in proteins and in the water balance of the lens in nuclear and cortical types of senile cataract; in *The Human Lens in Relation to Cataract. (Ciba Foundation Symposium 19)*, (eds K.M. Elliott and D.W. Fitzsimmons) Elsevier Excerpta Medica, Amsterdam, London, New York, 79–97

MARAINI, G and PESCATORI, A. (1972) Changes in weight and in protein-water ratio of the lens in human senile cataracts. *Ophthalmic Res.*, **3**, 108–113

MARCANTONIO, J.M., DUNCAN, G. and RINK, H. (1986) Calcium-induced opacification and loss of protein in the organ-cultured bovine lens. *Exp. Eye Res.*, **42**, 617–630

MARINESCO, G., DRAGANESCO, S. and VASILIU, D. (1931) Nouvelle maladie familiale caracterisee par une cataracte congenitale et un arret du development somato-neuro-psychique. *Encephale*, **26**, 97–109

MARNER, E. (1949) A family with eight generations of hereditary cataract. *Acta Ophthalmol.*, **27**, 537–551

MARSHALL, J. and GRINDLE, C.F.J. (1978) Fine structure of the cornea and its developments. *Trans Ophthalmol. Soc. UK*, **98**, 320–328

MARTSOLF, J.T., HUNTER, A.G.W. and HAWORTH, J.C. (1978) Severe mental retardation, cataracts, short stature and primary hypogonadism in two brothers. *Am. J. Med. Genet.*, **1**, 291–299

MASAKI, S. and WATANABE, T. (1988) Suppression of mouse lens γ-crystallin encoded by *Len-1* in the mutant mouse with eye lens obsolescence (*Elo*). *Exp. Eye Res.*, **47**, 727–735

MASAKI, S. and WATANABE, T. (1989) Linkage analysis of the mutation locus in the eye lens obsolescence (Elo) mouse. *Genomics*, **5**, 259–263

MATHIAS, R.T., RAE, J.L. and EISENBERG, R.S. (1981) The lens as a non uniform spherical syncytium. *Biophys. J.*, **34**, 61–83

MATHOLONE, M.B.R. (1967) Eye and skin changes in psychiatric patients treated with chlorpromazine. *Br. J. Ophthalmol.*, **51**, 86–93

MATSUZAWA, A. and WADA, E. (1988) Retarded and distinct progress of lens opacification in congenic hereditary cataract mice, Balb/c-nct/nct. *Exp. Eye Res.*, **47**, 705–711

MAUMENEE, I. (1979) Hereditary cataracts. **86**, 1554–1558

MAUMENEE, I. (1988) Cited by McKusick (1992) concerning Nance-Horan syndrome [McKusick number 302350]

MAYER, H. and IRION, K.M. (1985) New approach to area image analysis of scheimpflug photos of the anterior eye segment. *Ophthalmic Res.*, **17**, 106–110

MEESMANN, A. (1928) Beitrag zur Rontgen-Radiumstrahlenschadigung der menschlichen Linse. *Klin. Monatsbl. Augenheilk.*, **8**, 1259–1269

MEHTA, P.D. and LERMAN, S. (1972) Alpha crystallin subunits in the bovine lens. *Can. J. Ophthalmol.*, **7**, 218–222

MEISSNER, M. (1933) Augenaertzliches aus dem Blindeninstitut. *Z. Augenheilk.*, **80**, 48–58

MELLERIO, J. (1987) Yellowing of the human lens: Nuclear and cortical contributions. *Vision Res.*, **27**, 1581–1587

MENKES, J.H., SCHIMSCHOCK, J.R. and SWANSON, P.D. (1968) Cerebrotendinous xanthomatosis: the storage of cholestanol within the nervous system. *Arch. Neurol.*, **19**, 47–53

MERIN, S. (1986) Congenital cataracts. In *Goldberg's Genetic and Metabolic Eye Disease* (ed. W.A. Renie), 2nd edn, Little Brown, Boston

MERIN, S. and CRAWFORD, J.S. (1971a) The etiology of congenital cataracts: A survey of 386 cases. *Can. J. Ophthalmol.*, **6**, 178–182

MERIN, S. and CRAWFORD, J.S. (1971b) Hypoglycaemia and infantile cataract. *Arch. Ophthalmol.*, **86**, 495–498

MERIN, S., CRAWFORD, J.S. and CARDARELLI, J. (1971) Hyperplastic persistent pupillary membrane. *Am. J. Ophthalmol.*, **72**, 717–719

MERIN, S., LAPITHIS, A.G., HOROWITZ, D. *et al.* (1972) Childhood blindness in Cyprus. *Am. J. Ophthalmol.*, **74**, 538–542

MERKEL, F. and ORR, A.W. (1891–1892) Das Auge des Neugeborenen an einem schematischen Durchschnitt erläutert. *Arb. Anat. Inst. Wiesbaden*, **1**, 271–299

MERRIAM, G.R., SZECHTER, A. and FOCHT, E.F. (1972) The effects of ionizing radiation on the eye. *Front. Radiation Ther. Onc.*, **6**, 346–385

MERRIAM, G.R. and SZECHTER, A. (1973) The effect of age on the radomisation of rat lenses. *Trans. Am. Ophthalmol. Soc.*, **71**, 88–110

MEYER, E.T. (1954) Familial ectopia lentis and its complications. *Br. J. Ophthalmol.*, **38**, 163–172

MICHON, J. and KINOSHITA, J.H. (1968) Experimental miotic cataract. II: Permeability, cation transport and intermediary metabolism. *Arch. Ophthalmol.*, **79**, 611

MILLER, D. (1958) A case of anorexia nervosa in a young woman with development of subcapsular cataract. *Trans. Ophthalmol. Soc. UK*, **78**, 217–222

MILLER, J.E. (1975) Aging changes in extraocular muscle; in *Basic Mechanisms of Ocular Motility and their Clinical Implications*, (eds G. Lennerstrand and P. Bach-y-Rita) Pergamon Press, Oxford, 47–61

MILLER, P.J., JOHNSTON, R.L., HOEFER, J.A. *et al.* (1954) The riboflavin requirement of the baby pig. *J. Nutr.*, **52**, 405–413

MILLER, R.J., FUJINO, T. and NEFZGER, M.D. (1967) Lens findings in atomic bomb survivors. A review of major ophthalmic surveys at the Atomic Bomb Casualty Commission 1949 to 1962. *Arch. Ophthalmol.*, **78**, 697–704

MINASSIAN, D.C., MEHRA, V. and JONES, B.R. (1984) Dehydrational crises from severe diarrhoea or heatstroke and risk of cataract. *Lancet* **i**, 751–753

MITCHELL, W.J., and MARTIN, J.R. (1992) Herpes simplex virus type I replicates in the lens and induces cataracts in mice. *Lab. Invest.*, **66**, 32–38

MIZUNO, K. and MUROI, S. (1979) Cycloscopy of pseudoexfoliation. *Am. J. Ophthalmol.*, **87**, 513–518

MODAK, S.H. (1972) A model for transcriptional control in terminally differentiating lens fibre cells. In *Cell Differentiation* (eds R. Harris, P. Allin, D. Viza), Munksgaard, Copenhagen, 339–342

MODAK, S.P. (1972) Programmed life-cycle of lens cells. *Ophthalmic Res.*, **3**, 23

MOLNÁR, L. (1970) Refraktionsänderung des Auges im Laufe des Lebens. *Klin. Monatsbl. Augenheilk.*, **156**, 326–339

MONACO, M.A., SAMUELSON, D.A. and GELATT, K.N. (1984–1985) Morphology and postnatal development of the normal lens in the dog and congenital cataract in the miniature Schnaazer. *Lens Res.*, **2**, 393–433

MONJAN, A.A., SILVERSTEIN, A.M. and COLE, G.A. (1972) Lymphocytic choriomeningitis virus-induced retinopathy in newborn rats. *Invest. Ophthalmol.*, **11**, 850–856

MOORE, L.A. (1939) Relationship between carotene, blindness due to constriction of the optic nerve, papillary oedema and nyctalopia in calves. *J. Nutr.*, **17**, 443–459

MOROSS, T., VAITHILINGAM, S.S., STYLES, S. *et al.* (1984) Autosomal dominant anterior polar cataracts associated with a familial 2 : 14 translocation. *J. Med. Genet.*, **21**, 52–53

MORTON, W.R., DRANCE, S.M. and FAIRCLOUGH. M. (1969) Effect of echothiophate iodide on the lens. *Am. J. Ophthalmol.*, **68**, 1003–1010

MOSIER, M.A., OCCHIPINTI, J.R. and BURSTEIN, N.L. (1986) Autofluorescence of the crystalline lens in diabetes. *Arch. Ophthalmol.*, **104**, 1340–1343

MUGGLETON-HARRIS, A.L. and HIGBEE, N. (1987) An *in vivo* and *in vitro* study of the embryonic and adult Lop mutant congenital cataractous lens. *Exp. Eye Res.*, **44**, 805–815

MUGGLETON-HARRIS, A.L., FESTING, M.F.W. and HALL, M. (1987) A gene location for the inheritance of the Cataract Fraser (Cat^{Fr}) mouse congenital cataract. *Genet. Res.*, **49**, 235–238

MURPHREE, A.L., BEAUDET, A.L., PALMER, E.A., *et al.* (1976a) Cataract in mannosidosis. *Birth Defects*, **12**, 319

MURPHREE, A.L., BEAUDET, A.L., PALMER, E.A. and NICHOLS, B.L., JR. (1976b) Cataract in mannosidosis; in *The Eye and Inborn Errors of Metabolism*, (eds D. Bergsma, A.J. Bron, and E. Cotlier) Alan R. Liss, New York, 319–325

NAGARAJ, R.H., SELL, D.R., PRABHAKARAM, M. *et al.* (1991) High correlation between pentosidine protein crosslinks and pigmentation implicates ascorbate in human lens senescence and cataractogenesis. *Proc. Natl. Acad. Sci. USA*, **88**, 10257–10261

NAGATA, M., MATSUURA, H. and FUJINAGA, Y. (1986) Ultrastructure of posterior subcapsular cataract in human lens. *Ophthalmic Res.*, **18**, 180–184

NAKAJIMA, A. (1964) Population genetic study of blinding diseases in Japan. Proceedings of the 2nd International

Congress, Rome, *Hum. Genet.*, **3**, 1961

NAKANO, T., YAMAMOTO, S., KUTSUKAKE, G. *et al.* (1960) Hereditary cataract in mice. *Jpn. J. Clin. Ophthalmol.*, **14**, 196–200

NANCE, W.E., WARBURG, M., BIXLER, D. *et al.* (1974) Congenital X-linked cataract, dental anomalies and brachymetacarpalia. *Birth Defects*, **10**, 285–291

NATIONAL INSTITUTES OF HEALTH CONSENSUS DEVELOPMENT CONFERENCE (1988) Statement of neurofibromatosis. *Arch. Neurol.*, **45**, 575–580

NAUMANN, G.O. (1988) Exfoliation syndrome as a risk factor for vitreous loss in extracapsular cataract surgery. (Suppl. 184). *Acta. Ophthalmol.*, **66**, 129–131

NEIDER, M.W., CRAWFORD, K., TRUE, B., KAUFMAN, P.L. and BITO, L.Z. (1986) Functional studies of accommodation and presbyopia in rhesus monkeys. ARVO Suppl. *Invest. Ophthalmol. Vis. Sci.*, **27**, 81

NELSON, L.B. and MAUMENEE, I.H. (1971) Ectopia lentis. *Surv. Ophthalmol.*, **162**, 151

NENE, V., DUNNE, D.W., JOHNSON, K.S. *et al.* (1986) Sequence and expression of a major egg antigen from *Schistosoma mansoni*. Homologies to heat shock proteins and alpha-crystallins. *Immunol. Rev.*, **21**, 179–188

NETTLESHIP, E. (1909) Seven new pedigrees of hereditary cataract. *Trans. Ophthalmol. Soc. UK*, **29**, 188–211

NETTLESHIP, E. (1912) A pedigree of presenile or juvenile cataract. *Trans. Ophthalmol. Soc. UK*, **32**, 337–352

NETTLESHIP, E. and OGILVIE, F.M. (1906) A peculiar form of hereditary cataract. *Trans. Ophthalmol. Soc. UK*, **26**, 191–206

NICHOLL and QUINLAN (1994) Chaperone activity of α-crystallins modulates interediate filament assembly. *EMBO J.*, **13**, 945–953

NICHOLSON, D.H., HARKNESS, D.R., BENSON, W.E. *et al.* (1976) Cyanate-induced cataracts in patients with sickle-cell hemoglobinopathies. *Arch. Ophthalmol.*, **94**, 927–930

NIEDEN, A. (1887) *Z. Prak. Augenheilk.*, **11**, 353

NIESEL, P. (1982) Visible changes of the lens with age. *Trans. Ophthalmol. Soc. UK*, **102**, 327–330

NISHI, O. (1986) Incidence of posterior capsule opacification in eyes with and without posterior chamber intraocular lenses. *J. Cataract Refract. Surg.*, **12**, 519–522

NOBLE, L.B. and MAUMENEE, I.H. (1986) Ectopia Lentis. In *Goldberg's Genetic and Metabolic Eye Disease* (ed. W.A. Renie), 2nd edn, Little Brown, Boston

NOGA, E.J., WOLF, E.D. and CARDEILHAC, P.T. (1981) Cataracts in cichlid fish. *J. Am. Vet. Med. Assoc.*, **179**, 1181–1182

NORDMANN, J. (1954) *Biologie du Cristallin*, Masson et Cie, Paris

NORDMANN, J. (1966) Early postnatal cataracts. *Am. J. Ophthalmol*, **61**, 1256–1263

NORDMANN, J., FINK, H. and HOCKWIN, O. (1974) Die Wachstumskurve der menschlichen Linse. *Graefes Arch. Klin. Exp. Ophthalmol.*, **191**, 165–175

NORRIE, G. (1927) Causes of blindness in children; twenty five years experience of Danish institutes for the blind. *Acta Ophthalmol.*, **5**, 357–386

OBAZAWA, H., FUJIWARA, T. and KAWARA, T. (1983) The maturing process of the senile cataractous lens. XXIV International Congress of Ophthalmology. *Am. Acad. Ophthalmol.*, [1], 1

OCCHIPINTI, J.R., MOSIER, M.A. and BURSTEIN, N.L. (1986) Autofluorescence and light transmission in the aging crystalline lens. *Ophthalmologica*, **192**, 203–209

ODA, S., WATANABE, K., FUJISAWA, H. *et al.* (1980) Impaired development of lens fibers in genetic microphthalmia, eye lens obsolescence Elo, of the mouse. *Exp. Eye Res.*, **31**, 673–681

ODA, S., WATANABE, T. and KONDO, K. (1980) A new mutation, eye lens obsolescence, *Elo* on chromosome 1 in the mouse. *Jpn. J. Genet.*, **55**, 71–75

OGATA, H., OKUBO, Y. and AKABANE, T. (1949) Phenotype *i* associated with congenital cataracts. *Br. J. Ophthalmol.*, **33**, 601–629

OGATA, H., OKUBO, Y. and AKABANE, T. (1979) Phenotype i associated with congenital cataract in Japanese. *Transfusion*, **19**, 166–168

OHADI, C., MOREIRA, H. and MCDONNELL, P.J. (1991) Posterior capsule opacification. *Curr. Opin. Ophthalmol.*, **2**, 46–52

OHRLOFF, C. and HOCKWIN, O. (1983) Lens metabolism and aging: enzyme activities and enzyme alterations in lenses of different species during the process of aging. *J. Gerontol.*, **38**, 271–277

OKUN, E. (1967) *Ber. Dtsch. Ophthal. Ges.*, **68**, 150

OLESEN, H.P., JENSEN, D.A. and NORM, M.S. (1974) Congenital hereditary cataract in cocker spaniels. *J. Small Anim. Pract.*, **15**, 741–750

OLMSTED, E., PRASAD, S., SHEFFER, J. *et al.* (1966) Ocular lesions induced in C57 mice by the suckling mouse cataract agent (SMCA). *Invest. Ophthalmol.*, **5**, 413–420

OPITZ, J.M. (1972) Ocular anomalies in malformation syndromes. *Trans. Am. Acad. Ophthalmol. Otolaryngol.*, **76**, 1193–1202

ORTWERTH, B.J. and OLESEN, P.R. (1988) Glutathione inhibits the glycation and crosslinking of lens proteins. *Exp. Eye Res.*, **47**, 737–750

ORZALESI, N., SORCINELI, R. and GUISO, G. (1981) Increased incidence of cataract in male subjects deficient in glucose 6-phosphate dehydrogenase. *Arch. Ophthalmol.*, **99**, 69–70

OSBORNE, N.N. (1991) Agonist-induced stimulation of cAMP in the lens: presence of functional beta-receptors. *Exp. Eye Res.*, **52**, 105–106

ØSTERBERG, G. (1935) Topography of the layer of rods and cones in the human retina. *Acta Ophthalmol.*, **Suppl. 6**, 1–102

PAGENSTECHER, A. (1925) Irismissbildung in drei Generationen (Teilweise Verdoppelung des mesodermalen Teiles der Iris). *Klin. Monatsbl. Augenheilk.*, **74**, 128

PAGET, O.E. (1953) Cataracta hereditaria subcapsularis: Ein neues, dominates Allel bei der Hausmaus. *Zeitschrift für induktive Abstammungs- und Vererbungslehre*, **85**,

238–244

PAGET, O. and BAUMGARTNER-GAMAUF, M. (1953) *Osten Zool. S.*, **85**, 238

PALMQUIST, B.M., FAGERHOLM, P.P. and PHILIPSON, B.T. (1986) Nuclear vacuoles in nuclear cataract. *Acta Ophthalmol.*, **64**, 63–66

PALMQUIST, B.M., PHILIPSON, B. and BARR, P.O. (1984) Nuclear cataract and myopia during hyperbaric oxygen therapy. *Br. J. Ophthalmol.*, **68**, 113–117

PARDHAN, S. and GILCHRIST, J. (1991) The importance of measuring binocular contrast sensitivity in unilateral cataract. *Eye*, **5**, 31–35

PARMALEE, J.T., ROBINSON K.R. and PATTERSON, J.W. (1985) Effects of calcium on the steady outward currents at the equator of the rat lens. *Invest. Ophthalmol.*, **26**, 1343–1348

PARMALEE, J.T. (1986) Measurement of steady currents around the frog lens. *Exp. Eye Res.*, **42**, 433–441

PARMIGIANI, C.M. and MCAVOY, J.W. (1991) The roles of laminin and fibronectin in the development of the lens capsule. *Curr. Eye Res.*, **10**, 501–511

PARROW, R.D. (1955) Hereditary cataract in two families. *Acta Paediatr.*, **44**, 460–464

PARVING, A. and WARBURG, M. (1977) Audiological findings in Norrie's disease. *Audiology*, **16**, 124–131

PATTERSON, C.A. (1971) International Ophthalmology; in *Side Effects of Drugs in Ophthalmology.* vol. 11, No. 2, Little Brown & Co, Boston

PATTERSON, C.A. (1971) International Ophthalmology; in *Side Effects of Drugs in Ophthalmology.* Little Brown & Co., Boston, **11**, 1

PAU, H. (1951) Linsenquellung im physiologischen Milieu. *A von Graefes Arch. Ophthalmol.*, **15**, 352

PAU, H. and KRANTZ, J. (1992) The increasing sclerosis of the human lens with age and its relevance to accommodation and presbyopia. *A von Graefes Arch. Klin. Exp. Ophthalmol.*, **229**, 294–296

PAU, H., GRAF, P. and SIES, H. (1990) Glutathione levels in human lens: regional distribution in different forms of cataract. *Exp. Eye Res.*, **50**, 17–20

PAVONE, L., LA ROSA, M., SORGE, G. *et al.* (1981) Ocular manifestations in a family with probably X-linked cataracts. *Clin. Genet.*, **20**, 243–246

PEARCE, W.G. (1972) Ocular and genetic features of Cockayne's syndrome. *Can. J. Ophthalmol.*, **7**, 435–444

PEARSON, P.A., SOLOMON, K.D., VAN METER, W.S. and ASHTON, P. (1991) Pharmacologic inhibition of posterior capsule opacification. ARVO Suppl: *Invest. Ophthalmol. Vis. Sci.*, **32**, 1235

PEIFFER, R.L. and GELATT, K.N. (1974) Cataracts in the cat. *Feline Pract.*, **4**, 34–38

PEIFFER, R.L. and GELATT, K.N. (1976) Cataracts in a woolly monkey. *Mod. Vet. Pract.*, **57**, 609–610

PEIFFER, R.L., DEKKER, C.D. and SIEGEL, F.L. (1983) Ocular lesions in mice following intracerebral injection of herpes simplex virus type I. *Invest. Ophthalmol. Vis. Sci.*, **24**, 1070–1078

PEPIN, B., MIKOL, J., GOLDSTEIN, B., *et al.* (1980) Familial mitochondrial myopathy with cataract. *J. Neurol. Sci.*, **45**, 191–203

PERACCHIA, C., GIRSCH, S.J., BERNARDINI, G. *et al.* (1985) Lens junctions are communicating junctions. *Curr. Eye Res.*, **4**, 1155–1169

PERCY, D.H., OLANDER, H.J. and CARMICHAEL, L.E. (1968) Encephalitis in the newborn pup due to a canine herpes virus. *Vet. Pathol.*, **5**, 135–145

PERCY, D.H., CARMICHAEL, L.E., ALBERT, D.M. *et al.* (1971) Lesions in puppies surviving infection with canine herpes virus. *Vet. Pathol.*, **8**, 37–53

PEREIRA, L. *et al.* (1993) Genomic organization of the sequence coding for fibrillin, the defective gene product in Marfan syndrome. *Mol. Genet.*, (in press)

PERKINS, E.S. (1984) Cataract: refractive error, diabetes and morphology. *Br. J. Ophthalmol.*, **68**, 293–297

PERKINS, E.S. (1988) Lens thickness in early cataract. *Br. J. Ophthalmol.*, **72**, 348–353

PETERSEN, H.P. (1954) Teleangiectasis and cataract. *Acta Ophthalmol.*, **32**, 565–571

PFLUGK, A. VON (1909) Die Fixierung der Wirbeltierlinsen insbesondere der Linse des neugeborenen Menschen. *Klin. Monatsbl. Augenheilk.*, **47**, 1–14

PHILIPSON, B.T. (1973) Changes in the lens related to reduction in transparency. *Exp. Eye Res.*, **16**, 29–39

PHILIPSON, B.T. and FAGERHOLM, P.P. (1973) Lens changes responsible for increased light scattering in some types of senile cataract. *Ciba Found. Symp.*, **19**, 45–58

PIATIOGORSKY, J., KADOR, P.F. and KINOSHITA, H.J. (1980) Differential synthesis and degradation of protein in the hereditary Philly mouse cataract. *Exp. Eye Res.*, **30**, 69–78

PICNALOSA, B., TONI, F. and LIGUORI, G. (1989) Considerations on posterior chamber intraocular lens implantation in patients with pseudoexfoliation syndrome. *Doc. Ophthalmol.*, **71**, 49–53

PIERSCIONEK, B.K. (1990) Presbyopia: effect of refractive index. *Clin. Exp. Optom.*, **73**, 23–30

PIERSCIONEK, B.K. and AUGUSTEYN, R.C. (1991) Structure/function relationship between optics and biochemistry of the lens. **8**, 229–243

PIERSCIONEK, B.K. and CHAN, D.Y.C. (1989) Refractive index gradient of human lenses. *Optom. Vis. Sci.*, **66**, 822–829

PIERSCIONEK, B.K., CHAN, D.Y.C., ENNIS, J.P. *et al.* (1988) Nondestructive method of constructing three-dimensional gradient index models for crystalline lenses. 1: Theory and experiment. *Am. J. Optom. Physiol. Opt.*, **65**, 481–491

PIRIE, A. (1957) The biochemistry of the eye. *Bibl. Ophthalmol.*, **49**, 287

PIRIE, A. (1965) Glutathione peroxidase in lens and a source of hydrogen peroxide in aqueous humour. *Biochem. J.*, **96**, 244–253

PIRIE, A. (1968) Color and solubility of the proteins of human cataract. *Invest. Ophthalmol.*, **7**, 634–650

PIRIE, A. and OVERALL, M. (1972) Effect of vitamin A deficiency on the lens epithelium of the rat. *Exp. Eye Res.*, **13**, 105–109

PIRIE, A. and REES, J.R. (1970) Diquat cataract in the rat. *Exp. Eye Res.*, **9**, 198–203

PIRIE, A., VAN HEYINGEN, R. and BOAG, J.W. (1953) Changes in lens during the formation of x-ray cataracts in rabbits. *Biochem. J.*, **54**, 682–688

PIRIE, A., REES, J.R. and HOLMBERG, N.J. (1970) Diquat cataract: formation of the free radical and its reaction with constituents of the eye. *Exp. Eye Res.*, **9**, 204–214

PITTS, D.C., CULLEN, A.P. and HACKER, P.D. (1977) Ocular effects of ultraviolet radiation from 295–365 nm. *Invest. Ophthalmol.*, **16**, 932–939

PLATSCH, K.D. and WIEDERHOLT, M. (1981) Effect of ion substitution and ouabain on short circuit current in the isolated human and rabbit lens. *Exp. Eye Res.*, **32**, 615–625

POHJOLA, S. (1966) The glucose content of the aqueous humor in man. *Acta Ophthalmol. Suppl.*, **28**, 11–80

POLYAK, S.L. (1957) The Vertebrate Visual System. University of Chicago Press, Chicago

PRCHAL, J.T., CONRAD, M.E. and SKALKA, H.W. (1978) Association of presenile cataracts with heterozygosity for galactosaemic states and with riboflavin deficiency. *Lancet*, **I**, 12–13

PRCHAL, J., SKALKA, H., CLEMENTS, R.S. *et al.* (1980) Diabetes and risk of cataract development. *Metab. Pediatr. Syst. Ophthalmol.*, **4**, 185–189

PRESCOTT, A.R., DUNCAN, G., RAWLINS, D. *et al.* (1991) Dye communication properties in three regions of the intact frog lens. In *Eye Lens Membranes and Aging* (eds G.F.J.M. Vrensen and J. Clauwaert), Eurage, 59

PRINCE, A.M. and RITCH, R. (1986) Clinical signs of the pseudoexfoliation syndrome. *Ophthalmology.*, **93**, 803–807

PRINCE, J. (1956) Comparative Anatomy of the Eye. Charles C. Thomas, Springfield, Illinois

PRUETT, R.C. (1983) Retinitis pigmentosa: Clinical and observations and correlations. *Trans. Am. Ophthalmol. Soc.*, **76**, 693–735

QUINLAN, P., ODA, S., BREITMAN, M.L. *et al.* (1987) The mouse eye lens obsolescence (*Elo*) mutant: studies on crystallin gene expression and linkage analysis between the mutant locus and the γ-crystallin genes. *Genes and Development*, **1**, 637–644

QUINLAN, R.A., CARTER, J.M., HUTCHESON, A.M. *et al.* (1992) The 53kDa polypeptide component of the bovine fibre cell cytoskeleton is derived from the 115kDa beaded filament protein: evidence for a fibre cell specific intermediate filament protein. *Curr. Eye Res.*, **11**, 909–921

RABL, C. (1900) Concerning the structure and development of the lens. *Z. Wiss. Zool.*, **67**, 1–138

RABL, C. (1903) *Über den Bau und Entwicklung der Linse*, Leipzig

RADOS, A. (1947) Central pulverulent (discoid) cataract and its hereditary transmission. *Arch. Ophthalmol.*, **38**, 57–77

RAE, J.L. and KUSZAK, J.R. (1983) The electrical coupling of epithelium and fibers in the frog lens. *Exp. Eye Res.*, **36**, 317–326

RAE, J.L. (1974) The movement of procion dye in the crystalline lens. *Invest. Ophthalmol.*, **13**, 147–150

RAE, J.L. (1985) The application of patch clamp methods to ocular epithelia. *Curr. Eye Res.*, **4**, 409–420

RAE, J.L. and MATHIAS, R.T. (1985) The physiology of the lens. In *The Ocular Lens: Structure, Function and Pathology* (ed. H. Maisel). Marcel Dekker, New York, 93–121

RAE, J.L. and STACEY, T.R. (1979) Lanthanum and procion yellow as extracellular markers in the crystalline lens of the rat. *Exp. Eye Res.*, **28**, 1–21

RAFFERTY, N.S. (1965) Propagation and prolongation of mitotic activity in the formation of injury-induced lentomas in Rana pipiens. *Anat. Rec.*, **153**, 111–127

RAFFERTY, N.S. and SCHOLZ, D.L. (1984) Polygonal arrays of microfilaments in epithelial cells of the intact lens. *Curr. Eye Res.*, **3**, 1141–1149

RAFFERTY, N.S. and SCHOLZ, D.L. (1989) Comparative study of actin filament patterns in lens epithelial cells. Are these determined by the mechanism of lens accommodation? *Curr. Eye Res.*, **8**, 569–579

RAITTA, C. and SETALA, K. (1986) Intraocular lens implantation in exfoliation syndrome and glaucoma. *Acta. Ophthalmol.*, **64**, 130–133

RAMSAY, M.S., YANOFF, M. and FINE, B.S. (1972) The ocular histopathology of homocystinuria. A light and electron microscopic study. *Am. J. Ophthalmol.*, **74**, 377–385

RAO *et al.* (1994) Chaperone-like activity of α-crystallin. *J. Biol. Chem.*, **269**, 13266–13272

RATHBUN, W.B. (1984) Lenticular glutathione synthesis: Rate-limiting factors in its regulation and decline. *Curr. Eye Res.*, **3**, 101–108

RATHBUN, W.B. and BOVIS, M.G. (1986) Activity of glutathione peroxidase and glutathione reductase in the human lens related to age. *Curr. Eye Res.*, **5**, 381–385

RATHBUN, W.B., BOVIS, M.G. and HOLLESCHAU, A.M. (1986) Glutathione peroxidase, glutathione reductase and glutathione-S-transferase activities in the rhesus monkey lens as a function of age. *Curr. Eye Res.*, **5**, 195–199

RAZOOLI and BENJAMIN (in press) *Eye*

REDDY, D.V.N. and KINSEY, V.E. (1962) Studies on the crystalline lens. Quantitative analysis of free amino acids and related compounds. *Invest. Ophthalmol.*, **1**, 635–641

REDDY, V.N., TAURA, T., GARADI, R. *et al.* (1986) Effects of glutathione depletion on lens membrane permeability and on membrane protein disulfide formation. ARVO Suppl: *Invest. Ophthalmol. Vis. Sci.*, **27**, 8

REES, J.R. and PIRIE, A. (1967) Possible reactions of 1,2-naphthaquinone in the eye. *Biochem. J.*, **102**, 853–863

REESE, A.B. (1955) Persistent hyperplastic primary vitreous. *Am. J. Ophthalmol.*, **40**, 317–331

REESE, P.D., TUCK-MULLER, C.M. and MAUMENEE, I.H. (1987)

Autosomal dominant congenital cataract associated with chromosomal translocation [t (3;4) (p2 6 2–5)]. *Arch. Ophthalmol.*, **105**, 1382–1384

RENWICK, J.H. (1970) Eyes on chromosomes. *J. Med. Genet.*, **7**, 239–243

RENWICK, J.H. and LAWLER, S.D. (1963) Probable linkage between a congenital cataract locus and the Duffy blood group locus. *Ann. Hum. Genet.*, **27**, 67–84

REPO, L.P., TERASVIRTA, M.E. and TUOVINEN, E.J. (1990) Generalised peripheral iris transluminance in the pseudoexfoliation syndrome. *Ophthalmology.*, **97**, 1027–1029

REVEL, J.P., NICHOLSON, B. and YANCEY, S.B. (1985) Chemistry of gap junctions. *Immunol. Rev.*, **47**, 263–279

REVEL, J.P., YANCEY, S.B., NICHOLSON, B. *et al.* (1987) Sequence diversity of gap junction proteins. In *Junctional Complexes of Epithelial Cells* (eds G. Bok and S. Clark), *Ciba Found. Symp.*, **125**, 108–127

RHODES, D.H. (1932) Electric cataract. *Am. J. Ophthalmol.*, **15**, 1059

RIAD, M. (1938) Congenital familial cataract with cholesterin deposits. *Br. J. Ophthalmol.*, **22**, 745–749

RICHARDS, J., MAUMENEE, I.H., ROWE, S. *et al.* (1984) Congenital cataract possibly linked to haptoglobin. (Abstract) *Cytogenet. Cell Genet.*, **37**, 570

RICHARDSON, A.W., LOMAX, D.H., NICHOLS, J. *et al.* (1952) The role of energy, pupillary diameter, and alloxan diabetes in the production of ocular damage by microwave irradiations. *Am. J. Ophthalmol.*, **35**, 993–1000

RIEBSAMEN, D., TRINKMANN, R., KOHL, M. and LEGLER, U. (1988) Ergebnisse der Nachstarpeeling Methode mit dem Saug-Spulsystem. *Fortschr. Ophthalmol.*, **85**, 497–498

RIECK, P., DAVID, T., TASSIN, J. *et al.* (1992) Role of the mitotoxin FGF-Saporin on lens epithelial growth and corneal endothelial healing. Proceedings of Xth ISER Meeting, Stresa, Italy [abstract]. *Exp. Eye Res.*, **55**, 110

RIGDON, R.H., FERGUSON, T.M. and COUCH, J.R. (1959) Spontaneous cataracts in turkeys. *Am. J. Vet. Res.*, **20**, 961–964

RIISE, R. (1967) Hereditary 'ant-egg-cataract'. *Acta Ophthalmol. Suppl.*, **45**, 341

RILEY, E.F. (1970) Comparison of the cytological effects produced by ionizing radiation of different let. Nine-year summary of activities. Iowa State University Radiation Research Laboratory, *USAEC Report*, 1, 1024–1040

RILEY, V.M. (1983) The chemistry of the aqueous humor. In *Biochemistry of the Eye*, (ed. R.E. Anderson), Plenum, New York, 79–95

RILEY, V.M., MEYER, R.F. and YATES, E.M. (1980) Glutathione in the aqueous humor of human and other species. *Invest. Ophthalmol. Vis. Sci.*, **19**, 94–96

RINALDI, E., ALBINI, L., COSTAGLIOLA, C., DE ROSSA, G. *et al.* (1984) High frequency of lactose absorbers among adults with idiopathic senile and presenile cataract in a population with a high prevalence of primary adult lactose malabsorption. *Lancet.*, **I**, 355–357

RINTOUL, D.A., CUNDY, K.V. and CENEDELLA, R.J. (1987) Physical properties of membranes and membrane lipids from the fibre cell of the U18666A-cataractous rat. *Curr. Eye Res.*, **6**, 1343–1348

ROBERTS, S.R. and HELPER, L.C. (1972) Cataracts in Afghan hounds. *J. Am. Vet. Med. Assoc.*, **160**, 427–432

ROBINSON, K.R. and PATTERSON, J.W. (1983) Localization of steady current in the lens. *Curr. Eye Res.*, **12**, 843–847

ROHEN, J.W. (1952) Der Ziliarkorper als funktionelles System. *Morph. Jahrbuch.*, **92**, 415

ROHEN, J. (1961) Comparative and experimental studies on the iris of primates. *Am. J. Ophthalmol.*, **52**, 384–396

ROHEN, J.W. (1979) Scanning electron microscopic studies of the zonular apparatus in human and monkey eyes. *Invest. Ophthalmol. Vis. Sci.*, **18**, 133–144

ROHRSCHNEIDER, W. (1928) Klinischer Beitrag zur Entstehung und Morphologie der Rontgenkataract. *Klin. Monatsbl. Augenheilk.*, **81**, 254–259

ROMER, A. (1926) Untersuchung ueber die Erblichkeit der Spiesskatarakt (Vogt). *Arch. Klaus-Stift. Vererb-Forsch.*, **2**, 207–220

ROSE, R.C. and BODE, A.M. (1992) Tissue-mediated regeneration of ascorbic acid: is the process enzymatic? *Enzyme.*, **46**, 196–203

ROSS, W.M., CREIGHTON, M.O. and TREVITHNICK, J.R. (1982) Modelling cortical cataractogenesis. 3: *In vivo* effects of vitamin E on cataractogenesis in diabetic rats. *Can. J. Ophthalmol.*, **17**, 61–66

ROSSIER, B.C., GEERING, K. and THRAEHENBUHL, J.P. (1987) Regulation of the sodium pump: how and why? *Trends Biochem. Sci.*, **12**, 484–487

ROTH, A. and EPSTEIN, D. (1980) Exfoliation syndrome. *Am. J. Ophthalmol.*, **89**, 477–481

ROTH, J., BROWN, N., CATERALL, M. *et al.* (1976) The effect of fast neutron radiation on the human eye. *Br. J. Ophthalmol.*, **60**, 236–244

ROTHMUND, A. (1868) Ueber Cataracte in Verbindung mit einer eigenthuemlichen Hautdegeneration. *A von Graefes Arch. Klin. Exp. Ophthalmol.*, **14**, 159–182

ROULEAU, G.A., WERTELECKI, W., HAINES, J.L., HOBBS, W.J., TROFATTER, J.A., SEIZINGER, B.R., MARTUZA, R.L., SUPERNEAU, D.W., CONEALLY, P.M. and GUSELLA, J.F. (1987) Genetic linkage of bilateral acoustic neurofibromatosis to a DNA marker on chromosome 22. *Nature.*, **329**, 246–248

ROY, D., SPECTOR, A. and FARNSWORTH, P.N. (1979) Human lens membrane: comparison of major intrinsic polypeptides from young and old lenses isolated by a new methodology. *Exp. Eye Res.*, **28**, 353–358

ROY, F.H. *et al.* (1968) Ocular manifestations of the Rubinstein-Taybi syndrome: case report and review of the literature. *Arch. Ophthalmol.*, **79**, 272–278

RUBENSTEIN, R.A. and EGGLESTON, T.F. (1965) Congenital cataracts associated with congenital ichthyosiform erythroderma. *J. Pediatr. Ophthalmol.*, **2**, 53

RUBIN, L.F. and MATTIS, P.A. (1966) Dimethyl sulphoxide:

lens changes in dogs during oral administration. *Science*, **153**, 83–84

RUBIN, L.F. and FLOWERS, R.D. (1972) Inherited cataract in a family of standard poodles. *J. Am. Vet. Med. Assoc.*, **161**, 207–208

RUBIN, L.F., KOCH, S.A. and HUBER, R.J. (1969) Hereditary cataracts in miniature schnauzers. *J. Am. Vet. Med. Assoc.*, **154**, 1456–1458

RUSSELL, P., FUKUI, H.N., TSUNEMATSU, Y. *et al.* (1977) Tissue culture of lens epithelial cells from normal and Nakano mice. *Invest. Ophthalmol.*, **16**, 243–246

RUSSELL, P., ZELENKA, P., MARTENSEN, T. *et al.* (1987) Identification of the EDTA-extractable protein in lens as calpactin I. *Curr. Eye Res.*, **6**, 533–538

RYAN, H. (1970) Cataracts of dysplasia epiphysealis punctata. *Br. J. Ophthalmol.*, **54**, 197–199

SAEBO, J. (1949) An investigation into the mode of heredity of congenital and juvenile cataracts. *Br. J. Ophthalmol.*, **33**, 601–629

SAKAI, L.Y., KEENE, O.R. and ENGVALL, E. (1986) Fibrillin, a new 350-KD glycoprotein, is a component of extracellular microfibrils. *J. Cell. Biol.*, **103**, 2499–2509

SAKAI, L.Y. *et al.* (1991) Purification and partial characterisation of fibrillin, a cysteine-rich structural component of connective tissue microfibrils. *J. Biol. Chem.*, **266**, 14763–14770

SAKURAGAWA, M., KUWABARA, T., KINOSHITA, J.H. *et al.* (1975) Swelling of the lens fibers. *Exp. Eye Res.*, **21**, 381–394

SALZANO, F.M. (1961) Osteopetrosis: review of dominant cases and frequency in a Brazilian state. *Acta Genet. Med. Gemellol.*, **10**, 353–358

SAMPAOLESI, R., ZARATE, J. and CROXATO, O. (1988) The chamber angle in exfoliation syndrome: Clinical and pathological findings. (Suppl. 184). *Acta Ophthalmol.*, **66**, 48–53

SANCHEZ, J.M., BARREIRO, C. and FREILIJ, H. (1985) Two brothers with Martsolf's syndrome. *J. Med. Genet.*, **22**, 308–310

SANDBERG, H.O. (1976) The alpha-crystallin content of aqueous humour in cortical, nuclear, and complicated cataracts. *Exp. Eye Res.*, **22**, 75–84

SANFORD, S.E. and DUKES, T.W. (1978) Acquired bilateral cortical cataracts in mature sows. *J. Am. Vet. Med. Assoc.*, **173**, 852–853

SANTOS, B.A., DELMONTE, M.A., PASTORA, R. and O'DONNELL, F.E. (1987) Comparative study of the effects of optic design on lens epithelium in vitro. *J. Cataract Refract. Surg.*, **13**, 127–130

SANYAL, S. and HAWKINS, R.K. (1979) Dysgenetic lens (dyl) – a new gene in the mouse. *Invest. Ophthalmol. Vis. Sci.*, **18**, 642–645

SAS, D.F., SAS, M.J., JOHNSON, K.R. *et al.* (1985) Junctions between lens fiber cells are labelled with a monoclonal antibody shown to be specific for MP26. *J. Cell. Biol.*, **100**, 216–225

SCAMMON, R.E. and ARMSTRONG, E.L. (1925) On the growth of the human eyeball and optic nerve. *J. Comp. Neurol.*, **38**, 165–219

SCAMMON, R.E. and HESDORFFER, M.B. (1937) Growth in mass and volume of the human lens in postnatal life. *Arch. Ophthalmol.*, **17**, 104–112

SCAMMON, R.E. and WILMER, H.A. (1950) Growth of the components of the human eyeball. II. Comparison of the calculated volumes of the eyes of the newborn and of adults, and their components. *Arch. Ophthalmol.*, **43**, 620–637

SCHACHAT, A.P. and MAUMENEE, I.H. (1982) The Bardet-Biedl syndrome and related disorders. *Arch. Ophthalmol.*, **100**, 285–288

SCHÄFFER (1925) *Arch. Derm. Syph.*, (Berlin), **148**, 425

SCHEIE, H.G. and ALBERT, D.M. (1969) *Adler's Textbook of Ophthalmology*, 8th edn, W B Saunders, Philadelphia

SCHEPENS, C.L. (1974) Discussion of rationale of surgical procedures. In *Retina Congress* (eds R.C. Pryett and C.D.J. Regan), Appleton-Century-Crofts, New York, 316

SCHIAVO, D.M. and FIELD, W.E. (1974) The incidence of ocular defects in a closed colony of beagle dogs. *Lab. Anim. Sci.*, **24**, 51–56

SCHLÖTZER-SCHREHARDT, U., DÖRFLER, S. and NAUMANN, G.O.H. (1992a) Immunohistochemical localization of basement membrane components in pseudoexfoliative material of the lens capsule. *Curr. Eye Res.*, **11**, 343–355

SCHLÖTZER-SCHREHARDT, U.M., KOCA, M.R., NAUMANN, G.O.H. and VOLKHÖLZ, H. (1992b) Pseudoexfoliation syndrome: Ocular manifestation of a systemic disorder? *Arch. Ophthalmol.*, **110**, 1752–1756

SCHUTGENS, R.B.H., HEYMANS, H.S.A. and WANDERS, R.J.A. *et al.* (1986) Peroxisomal disorders; a newly recognized group of genetic diseases. *Eur. J. Pediatr.*, **144**, 430–440

SCOTT, J.D. (1979) Lens changes in retinal detachment. *Trans. Ophthalmol. Soc. UK*, **99**, 241–243

SCOTT, J.D. (1982) Lens epithelial proliferation in retinal detachment. *Trans. Ophthalmol. Soc. UK*, **102**, 385–389

SCOTT-EMUAKPOR, A.B., HEFFELFINGER, J. and HIGGINS, J.V. (1977) A syndrome of microcephaly and cataracts in four siblings: a new genetic syndrome? *Am. J. Dis. Child.*, **131**, 167–169

SEIZINGER, B.R., ROULEAU, G., OZELIUS, L.J., LANE, A.H., ST. GEORGE-HYSLOP, P., HUSON, S., GUSELLA, J.F. and MARTUZA, R.L. (1987) Common pathogenetic mechanism for three tumor types in bilateral acoustic neurofibromatosis. *Science*, **236**, 317–319

SELAND, J.S. (1974) Ultrastructural changes in the normal human lens capsule from birth to old age. *Acta Ophthalmol.*, **52**, 688–706

SELL, D.R., NAGARAJ, R.H., GRANDHEE, S.K. *et al.* (1991) Pentosidine: a molecular marker for the cumulative damage to proteins in diabetes, aging and uremia. *Diabetes Metab. Rev.*, **7**, 239–251

SELLARS, S.L. and BEIGHTON, P.H. (1978) Deafness in osteodysplasty of Melnick and Needles. *Arch. Otolaryngol.*, **104**, 225–227

SELLMAN, T.R. and LINDSTROM, R.L. (1988) Effect of a plano-convex posterior chamber lens on capsule opacification from Elschnig pearl formation. *J. Cataract Refract. Surg.*, **14**, 68–72

SENGERS, R.C.A., TERHAAR, B.G.A., TRIJBELS, J.M.F. *et al.* (1975) Congenital cataract and mitochondrial myopathy of skeletal and heart muscle associated with lactic acidosis after exercise. *J. Pediatr.*, **86**, 873–880

SHAFFER, R.N. and HETHERINGTON, J., JR. (1966) Anticholinesterase drugs and cataracts. *Am. J. Ophthalmol.*, **62**, 613–618

SHEARER, T.R., DAVID, L.L. and ANDERSON, R.S. (1987) Selenite cataract: a review. *Curr. Eye. Res.*, **6**, 289–300

SHEARER, T.R., DAVID, L.L., ANDERSON, R.S. *et al.* (1992) Review of selenite cataract. *Curr. Eye Res.*, **11**, 357–369

SHOKEIR, M.H.K. and LOWRY, R.B. (1985) Juvenile cataract in Hutterites. *Am. J. Med. Genet.*, **22**, 495–500

SHUN-SHIN, G.A., BROWN, N.A.P., BRON, A.J. *et al.* (1989) The dynamic nature of posterior subcapsular cataract. *Br. J. Ophthalmol.*, **73**, 522–527

SHUN-SHIN, G.A., RATCLIFFE, P., BRON, A.J. *et al.* (1990) The lens after renal transplantation. *Br. J. Ophthalmol.*, **74**, 267–271

SHUN-SHIN, G.A., BRON, A.J. and BROWN, N.A.P. (1991a) Growth spurt in a lens with posterior subcapsular cataract. *Int. Ophthalmol.*, **15**, 87–91

SHUN-SHIN, G.A., VRENSEN, F.J.M., BROWN, N.P. *et al.* (1991b) Does the pathogenesis of waterclefts reside in the lens fibre membrane? In *Lens Membranes and Aging* (eds G.F.J.M. Vrensen, and J.C. Clauwert), Eurage, 261–267

SHUN-SHIN, G.A., BRON, A.J., BROWN, N.P. *et al.* (1992a) The relationship between central nuclear scatter and perinuclear retrodots in the human crystalline lens. *Eye*, **6**, 407–410

SHUN-SHIN, G.A., VRENSEN, G., BROWN, N.P. *et al.* (1992b) The morphology of christmas tree cataracts. Association of Eye Research 33rd Meeting (June), Aachen [Abstract].

SHUN-SHIN, G.A., VRENSEN, J.M., BROWN, N.A.P., WILLEKENS, B., SMEETS, H. and BRON, A.J. (1993) Morphological characteristics and chemical composition of Christmas tree cataract. *Invest. Ophthalmol. Vis. Sci.*, **34**, 3489–3496

SIDDALL, J.R. (1965) The ocular toxic findings with prolonged and high dosage chlorpromazine intake. *Arch. Ophthalmol.*, **74**, 460–464

SIEBINGA, I., VRENSEN, G.F.J.M., DE MUL, F.F.M. and GREVE, J. (1991) Age-related changes in local water and protein content of human eye lenses measured by Raman microspectroscopy. *Exp. Eye Res.*, **53**, 233–239

SIEZEN, R.J., THOMSON, J.A., KAPLAN, E.D. *et al.* (1987) Human lens gamma-crystallins: isolation, identification, and characterization of the expressed gene products. *Proc. Natl. Acad. Sci. USA*, **84**, 6088–6092

SIEZEN, R.J., WU, E., KAPLAN, E.D., THOMSON, J.A. and BENEDEK, G.B. (1986) *Invest. Ophthalmol. Vis. Sci.*, **27**, 214

SILVER, J. and HUGHES, A.F.W. (1974) The relationship between morphogenetic cell death and the development of congenital anophthalmia. *J. Comp. Neurol.*, **157**, 281–301

SIMON, K.A. (1962) Diabetes and lens changes in myotonic dystrophy. *Arch. Ophthalmol.*, **67**, 312–315

SIMON (1994) Human dander. An important cause of infantile eczema. *J. Am. Med. Assoc.*, **125**, 350–335

SIMS, K.B., LEBO, R.V., BENSON, G., SHALISH, C., SHUBACK, D., CHEN, Z.Y., BRUNS, G., *et al.* (1992) The Norrie disease gene maps to a 150 Kb region on chromosome Xp11.3. *Hum. Mol. Genet.*, **1**, 83–89

SINSKEY, R.M. (1955) The status of lenticular opacities caused by atomic radiation. *Am. J. Ophthalmol.*, **39**, 285–293

SIPPEL, T.O. (1962) Respiration and glutathione in the growing rat lens. *Invest. Ophthalmol.*, **1**, 629–634

SIPPEL, T.O. (1966) Energy metabolism in the lens during development of galactose cataract in rats. *Invest. Ophthalmol.*, **5**, 576

SIVAK, J.G., HERBERT, K.L., PETERSON, K.L. and KUSZAK, J.R. (1994) The interrelationship of lens anatomy and optical quality. I. Non-primate lenses. *Exp. Eye Res.*, **59**, 505–520

SJÖGREN, T. (1947) Hereditary congenital spinocerebellar ataxia combined with congenital cataract and oligophrenia. *Acta Psychiatr. Neurol. Scand. Suppl.*, **46**, 286–289

SJÖGREN, T. (1950) Hereditary congenital spinocerebellar ataxia accompanied by congenital cataract and oligophrenia: a genetic and clinical investigation. *Confin. Neurol.*, **10**, 293–308

SJÖGREN, T. (1970) Klinische und vererbungmedizinische Untersuchungen über Oligophrenie mit kongenitaler Katarakt. *Z. Ges. Neurol. Psychiatr.*, **152**, 263

SKALKA, H.W. and PRCHAL, J.T. (1980) Presenile cataract formation and decreased activity of galactosemic enzyme. *Arch. Ophthalmol.*, **98**, 269–273

SKUTA, G.L., PARISH, R.K., HODAPP, E. *et al.* (1987) Zonular dialysis during extracapsular cataract extraction in pseudoexfoliation syndrome. *Arch. Ophthalmol.*, **105**, 632–634

SLACK, J.M.W. (1991) *From egg to embryo* 2nd edn, Cambridge University Press, Cambridge

SLATAPER, F.J. (1950) Age norms of refraction and vision. *Arch. Ophthalmol.*, **43**, 466–481

SLINEY, D.H. (1986) Physical factors in cataractogenesis: Ambient ultraviolet radiation and temperature. *Invest. Ophthalmol. Vis. Sci.*, **27**, 781–790

SLINGSBY, C. and MILLER, L.R. (1983) *Exp. Eye Res.*, **37**, 517–530

SMITH, G.T.H., SHUN-SHIN, G.A. and BRON, A.J.B. (1990a) Spontaneous reabsorption of a rubella cataract. *Br. J. Ophthalmol.*, **74**, 564–565

SMITH, G.T.H., SMITH, R., BROWN, N.A.P. *et al.* (1990b) Changes in light scatter and width measurements in the human lens cortex with age. *Br. J. Ophthalmol.*,

SMITH, G., PIERSCIONEK, B.K. and ATCHISON, D.A. (1991) Optical modelling of the human lens. *Ophthalmic Physiol. Opt.*, **11**, 359–369

SMITH, P. (1910) A pedigree of Doyne's discoid cataract. *Trans. Ophthalmol. Soc. UK*, **30**, 37–42

SMITH, R.S., HOFFMAN, H. and CISAR, C. (1969) Congenital cataracts in the rat. *Arch. Ophthalmol.*, **81**, 259–263

SMITH, T.W., ALBERT, D.M., ROBINSON, N. *et al.* (1974) Ocular manifestations of Marek's disease. *Invest. Ophthalmol.*, **13**, 586–592

SMITH PRIESTLEY, (1883) Disease of the crystalline lens and capsule. I. On the growth of the crystalling lens. *Trans. Ophthalmol. Soc. UK*, **3**, 79–99

SOLOMON, C., LIGHT, A.E. and DE BEER, E.J. (1955) Cataracts produced in rats by 1,4-dimethanesulfonoxybutane (Myleran). *Arch. Ophthalmol.*, **54**, 850–857

SOLOMON, K.D., VAN METER, W.S., PEARSON, P.A., BLANDFORD, D. and SMITH, T.J. (1990) Sustained drug delivery systems in cataract surgery. ARVO Suppl: *Invest. Ophthalmol. Vis. Sci.*, **31**, 351

SOLOMON, K.D., APPLE, D.J., MAMALIS, N., GWIN, T.D., WILBRANDT, T.H., HANSEN, S.O., TETZ, M.R., LETCHINGER, S.L., BROWN, S.F. and LEGLER, U.F.C. (1991) Complications of intraocular lenses with special references to an analysis of 2500 explanted intraocular lenses (IOLs). *Eur. J. Implant Refract. Surg.*, **3**, 195–200

SOLOMON, K.D., LEGLER, U.F.C. and KOSTICK, A.M.P. (1992) Capsular opacification after cataract surgery. *Curr. Opin. Ophthalmol.*, **3**, 46–51

SPAETH, G.L. and FROST, P. (1965) Fabry's disease: its ocular manifestations. *Arch. Ophthalmol.*, **74**, 760

SPAETH, G.L. and VON SALLMANN, L. (1966) Corticosteroids and cataracts *Int. Ophthalmol. Clin.*, **6**, 915

SPARKES, R.S. and GRAHAM, C.B. (1972) Camurati–Engelmann disease: genetics and clinical manifestations with a review of the literature. *J. Med. Genet.*, **9**, 73–85

SPARROW, J.M., BRON, A.J., BROWN, N.A.P. *et al.* (1986) The Oxford clinical cataract classification and grading system. *Int. Ophthalmol.*, **9**, 207–225

SPARROW, J.M., HILL, A.R., AYLIFFE, W. *et al.* (1988) Human lens nuclear colour matching and brunescence grading *in vivo*. *Int. Ophthalmol.*, **11**, 139–149

SPARROW, J.M., BROWN, N.A.P., SHUN-SHIN, G.A. *et al.* (1990) The Oxford modular cataract image analysis system. *Eye*, **4**, 638–648

SPARROW, J.M., BRON, A.J., BROWN, N.A.P. *et al.* (1992) Autofluorescence of the crystalline lens in early and late onset diabetes. *Br. J. Ophthalmol.*, **76**, 25–31

SPECTOR, A. (1982) Aging of the lens and cataract formation. In *Aging and Human Visual Function* (eds R. Sekuler, D. Kline and K. Dismukes), Liss, New York, 27–43

SPECTOR, A. (1984). The search for a solution to senile cataracts. Proctor Lecture. *Invest. Ophthalmol. Vis. Sci.*, **25**, 130–146.

SPECTOR, A. and GARNER, W.H. (1981) Hydrogen peroxide and human cataract. *Exp. Eye Res.*, **33**, 673–681

SPEMANN, H. (1901) Uber Correlationen in die Entwicklung des Auges. *Verh. Anat. Ges.*, **15**, 61–79

SPENCER, R.P. (1976) Change in weight of the human lens with age. *Ann. Ophthalmol.*, **8**, 440–441

SPRANGER, J.W., OPITZ, J.M. and BIDDER, U. (1971) Heterogeneity of chondrodysplasia punctata. *Humangenetik*, **11**, 190–212

SRINIVASAN, B.D. and HARDING, C.V. (1965) Cellular proliferation in the lens. *Invest. Ophthalmol.*, **4**, 452–470

STAMBOLIAN, D. (1988) Galactose and cataract. *Surv. Ophthalmol.*, **32**, 333–349

STAMBOLIAN, D., LEWIS, R.A., BUETOW, K., BOND, A. and NUSSBAUM, R. (1990) Nance-Horan syndrome: localization within the region Xp 21.Xp 22.3 by linkage analysis *Am. J. Hum. Genet.*, **47**, 13–19

STANESCU, B. and DRALOANDS, L. (1972) Cerebro-hepatorenal (Zellweger's) syndrome: ocular involvement. *Arch. Ophthalmol.*, **87**, 590–592

STERLING, S. and WOOD, T.O. (1986) Effect of intraocular lens convexity on posterior capsule opacification. *J. Cataract Refract. Surg.*, **12**, 655–657

STEVENS, R.E., DATILES, M.B., ANSARI, H.H. *et al.* (1989) Idiopathic presenile cataract formation and galactosaemia. *Br. J. Ophthalmol.*, **73**, 48–51

STEVENSON, R.E., SCHROER, R.J., TAYLOR, H.A. *et al.* (1982) Dislocated lens, dolichostenomelia, and joint stiffness. *Proceedings of the Greenwood Genetic Center*, 16–22

STIEREN, E. (1907) A study in atavistic descent of congenital cataract through four generations. *Ophthalmic Rev.*, **16**, 234–238

STIRLING, R.J. and GRIFFITHS, P.G. (1991) Scanning EM studies of normal human lens fibres and fibre from nuclear cataracts. *Eye*, **5**, 86–92

STREETEN, B.W. (1992) Anatomy of the zonular apparatus. (Chapter 14); in *The Biomedical Foundations of Ophthalmology*, (eds T.D. Duane and E.A. Jaeger) Harper & Row, Philadelphia; 1–23

STREETEN, B.W., GIBSON, S.A. and LI, Z.-Y. (1986) Lectin binding to pseudoexfoliative material and the ocular zonules. *Invest. Ophthalmol. Vis. Sci.*, **27**, 1516–1521

STREETEN, B.W., DARK, A.J., WALLACE, R.N., LI, Z.-Y. and HOEPNER, J.A. (1990) Pseudoexfoliative fibrillopathy in the skin of patients with ocular pseudoexfoliation. *Am. J. Ophthalmol.*, **110**, 490–499

STREETEN, B.W., LI, Z.-Y., WALLACE, R.H., EAGLE, R.C. and KESHGEGIAN, A.A. (1992) Pseudoexfoliative fibrillopathy in visceral organs of a patient with pseudoexfoliation syndrome. *Arch Ophthalmol.*, **110**, 1757–1762

STREIFF, E.B. (1952) Keratocone et retinite pigmentaire. *Bull. Soc. Ophthalmol. Fr.*, 323–326

STURROCK, G.D. and TRIPATHI, R.C. (1976) Pigmented lens striae. *Br. J. Ophthalmol.*, **60**, 287–293

SUGAR, H.S. (1976) The exfoliation syndrome: Source of fibrillar material on the capsule. *Surv. Ophthalmol.*, **21**, 59–64

SUMMANEN, P. and TONJUN, A.M. (1988) Exfoliation syndrome among Saudis. (suppl. 184). *Acta. Ophthalmol.*, **66**, 102–111

SUMMERS, I., WISTOW, G., NAREBOR, M. *et al.* (1984) X-ray studies of the lens specific proteins: the crystallins. *Pep.*

Protein Rev., **3**, 147–168

SUNDE, O.A. (1956) On the so called exfoliation of the anterior lens capsule. *Acta. Ophthalmol.*, Suppl. **45**, 1–85

TAKEMOTO, L. and TAKEHANA, M. (1986) Main intrinsic polypeptide (MIP 26K) from human lens membrane: characterization of low-molecular weight forms in the aging human lens. *Exp. Eye Res.*, **43**, 661–667

TAKEMOTO, L.J., AZARI. P. and GORTHY, W.C. (1975) Role of sulfhydryl groups in the formation of a hereditary cataract in the rat. *Exp. Eye Res.*, **20**, 1–13

TAKEMOTO, L., TAKEHANA, M. and HORWITZ, J. (1986) Covalent changes in MIP 26K during aging of the human lens membrane. *Invest. Ophthalmol. Vis. Sci.*, **27**, 443–446

TAKEMOTO, L., TAKEMOTO, D., BROWN, G. *et al.* (1987) Cleavage from the N-terminal region of βBp crystallin during aging of the human lens. *Exp. Eye Res.* **45**, 385–392

TAKEMOTO, L., KUCK, J. and KUCK, K. (1988) Changes in the main intrinsic polypeptide (MIP 26K) during opacification of the Emory mouse lens. *Exp. Eye Res.*, **47**, 329–336

TAKKI, K. and SIMELL, O. (1976) Gyrate atrophy of the choroid and retina with hyperornithenemia. *Birth Defects*, **12**, 373–384

TANAKA, M., RUSSELL, P., SMITH, S. *et al.* (1980) Membrane alterations during cataract development in the Nakano mouse lens. *Invest. Ophthalmol. Vis. Sci.*, **19**, 619–629

TARDIEU, A. and DELAYE, M. (1986) Eye lens transparency analysed by X-ray and light scattering, *The Lens: Transparency and Cataract* (ed. G. Duncan) Eurage, Rijswijk, 49–56

TARKKANEN, A. (1962) Pseudoexfoliation of the lens capsule: A clinical study of 418 patients with special reference to glaucoma, cataract, and changes of the vitrous. *Acta. Ophthalmol.*, Suppl. **71**, 1–98

TARKKANEN, A. (1986) Exfoliation syndrome. *Trans. Ophthalmol. Soc. UK*, **105**, 233–236

TARKKANEN, A. and KARJALAINEN, K. (1966) Cataract formation during miotic treatment for chronic open-angle glaucoma. *Acta Ophthalmol.*, **44**, 932–939

TARR, K.H. and CONSTABLE, I.J. (1980) Late complications of pterygium treatment. *Br. J. Ophthalmol.*, **64**, 496–505

TASKER, W.G., MASTRI, A.R. and GOLD, A.P. (1970) Chondrodystrophica calcificans congenita (dysplasia epiphisealis punctata). *Am. J. Dis. Child.*, **119**, 122

TAURA, T., GOBLIN, F.J. and REDDY, V.N. (1985) Further observations on the effect of galactose on the development of X-ray induced cataract in mice. *Exp. Eye Res.*, **41**, 527–543

TAYLOR, A., HAAS, A.L., JAHNGEN, J. *et al.* (1986) Age related changes of *in vivo* eye lens ubiquitin and ubiquitin conjugates and plausible role in cataract formation. ARVO Suppl., *Invest. Ophthalmol. Vis. Sci.*, **27**, 277

TAYLOR, H.R., HOLLOWS, F.C. and MORAN, D. (1977) Pseudoexfoliation of the lens in Australian aborigines. *Br. J. Ophthalmol.*, **61**, 473–475

TAYLOR, H.R., WEST, S.K., ROSENTHAL, F.S. *et al.* (1988) Effect of ultraviolet radiation on cataract formation. *N. Engl. J. Med.*, **319**, 1429–1433

TEICHER, L.S. and CASPARI., E.W. (1978) The genetics of blind – a lethal factor in mice. *J. Hered.*, **69**, 86–90

TEIR, H. and GRENQUIST-NORDEN, B. (1990) Peripheral cataracts and trinitrotoluene exposure. A follow-up study. *Acta Ophthalmol.*, **68**, 49–51

TEMTAMY, S.A. and SHALASH, B.A. (1974) Genetic heterogeneity of the syndrome: microphthalmos with congenital cataract. *Birth Defects*, **10**, 292–293

TERRIEN, F. and PRELAT (1959) *Bull. Soc. Pediatr.* (Paris), **11**, 370

TETSUMOTO, K., SCHLÖTZER-SCHREHARDT, U., KUCHLE, M., DORFLER, S. and NAUMANN, G.O. (1992) Precapsular layer of the anterior lens capsule in early pseudoexfoliation syndrome. *Graefes Arch. Klin. Exp. Ophthalmol.*, **230**, 252–257

TETZ, M.R., O'MORCHOE, D.J.C., GWIN, T.D., WILBRANDT, T.H., SOLOMON, K.D., HANSEN, S.O. and APPLE, D.J. (1988) Posterior capsular opacification and intraocular lens decentration: part II. Experimental findings on a prototype circular IOL design. *J. Cataract Refrac. Surg.*, **14**, 614–623

THEILER, K., VARNUM, D.S. and STEVENS, L.C. (1978) Development of Dickie's small eye, a mutation in the house mouse. *Anat. Embryol.*, **155**, 81–86

THOMAS, A.H. and HANNA, C. (1974) Electric cataracts. III: Animal model. *Arch. Ophthalmol.*, **91**, 469–473

THOMAS, D.M. and SCHEPLER, K.L. (1980) Raman spectra of normal and ultraviolet-induced cataractous rabbit lens. *Invest. Ophthalmol.*, **19**, 904–912

THOMAS, R.C. (1989) Bicarbonate and pHi response. *Nature*, **337**, 601

THOMPSON, J.S. and THOMPSON, M.W. (1980) *Genetics in Medicine*, 3rd edn, Saunders, Philadelphia,

THOMSON, J.A. and AUGUSTEYN, R.C. (1985) Ontogeny of lens crystallins. *Exp. Eye Res.*, **40**, 393–410

THOMSON, M.S. (1936) Poikiloderma congenitale. *Br. J. Dermatol.*, **48**, 221–234

TITARELLI, R., CATALINO, P. and BUCCI, M.G. (1961) Contributo allo studio della cataratta sperimentale da leucinol. *Bull. Ocul.*, **40**, 619–634

TOKUNAGA, T. (1959) Atomic bomb radiation cataract in Nagasaki. *Acta Soc. Ophthalmol. Jpn.*, **63**, 1211–1230

TOMLINSON, J., BANNISTER, S.C., CROGHAN, P.C. *et al.* (1992) Analysis of rat lens $45Ca^{2+}$ fluxes: evidence for NA^+–Ca^{2+} exchange. *Exp. Eye Res.*, **52**, 1

TOMLINSON, J. and DUNCAN, G. (1991) Membrane models for cortical cataract: pCMPS-induced changes in lens Na^+, Ca^{2+} and transparency can be modified by channel antagonists. In *Eye Lens Membranes and Aging*, (eds G.F.J.M. Vrensen and J. Clauwaert), Eurage, 1, 73–86

TORRIGLIA, A. and ZIGMAN, S. (1988) The effect of near-UV light on NaK-ATPase of the rat lens. *Curr. Eye Res.*, **7**, 539–548

TORRIGLIA, A., PAXHIA, T., ZIGMAN, S. *et al.* (1986) A study of the mechanism of lens Na^+–K^+–ATPase inhibition by near UV light. ARVO Suppl., *Invest. Ophthalmol. Vis. Sci.*, **27**, 49

TOSCH, C. (1958) Beitrag zur Stammbaumforschung der Cataracta floriformis. *Klin. Monatsbl. Augenheilk.*, **133**, 60–66

TOTTER, J.R. and DAY, P.L. (1942) Cataract and other ocular changes resulting from tryptophan deficiency. *J. Nutr.*, **24**, 159–166

TOWNES, P.L. (1976) Ectopia lentis et pupillae. *Arch. Ophthalmol.*, **94**, 1126–1128

TRAVERS, M. (1990) Structural correlates of shape change in the primate crystalline lens. *D. Phil. Thesis.*

TRAYHURN, P. and VAN HEYNINGEN, R. (1972) The role of respiration in the energy metabolism of the bovine lens. *Biochem. J..*, **129**, 507–509

TRAYHURN, P. and VAN HEYNINGEN, R. (1973a) The metabolism of amino acids in the bovine lens: their oxidation as a source of energy. *Biochem. J.*, **136**, 67–75

TRAYHURN, P. and VAN HEYNINGEN, R. (1973b) The metabolism of glutamine in the bovine lens: glutamine as a source of glutamate. *Exp. Eye Res.*, **17**, 149–154

TREVITHICK, J.R., CREIGHTON, M.O., ROSS, W.M. *et al.* (1980) Modelling cortical cataractogenesis. II: *In vitro* effects on the lens of agents preventing glucose and sorbitol cataracts. *Can. J. Ophthalmol.*, **16**, 32–38

TRIPATHI, R.C., CIBIS, G.W. and TRIPATHI, B.J. (1986) Pathogenesis of cataracts in patients with Lowe's syndrome. *Ophthalmology*, **93**, 1046–1051

TRIPATHI, R.C., MILLARD, C.B. and TRIPATHI, B.J. (1989) Protein composition of human aqueous humor: SDS-PAGE analysis of surgical and post-mortem samples. *Exp. Eye Res.*, **48**, 117–130

TROKEL, S. (1962) The physical basis for transparency of the crystalline lens. *Invest. Ophthalmol.*, **1**, 493–501

TROPE, G.E. and RUMLEY, A.G. (1985) Catecholamines in human aqueous humor. *Invest. Ophthalmol. Vis. Sci.*, **26**, 399–401

TRUE-GABELT, B., POLANSKY, J.R. and KAUFMAN, P.L. (1987) Ciliary muscle muscarinic receptors, ChAt and AChE in young and old rhesus monkeys. ARVO Suppl: *Invest. Ophthalmol. Vis. Sci.*, **28**, 65

TRUSLOVE, G.M. (1956) The anatomy and development of the fidget mouse. *J. Genet.*, **54**, 64–86

TRUSLOVE, G.M. (1962) A gene causing ocular retardation in the mouse. *J. Embryol. Exp. Morphol.*, **10**, 652–660

TSO, M.O.M., FINE, B.S. and THORPE, H.E. (1975) Kayser–Fleischer ring and associated cataract in Wilson's disease. *Am. J. Ophthalmol.*, **79**, 479–488

TSUNEMATSU, Y., FUKUI, H.N. and KINOSHITA, H.N. (1978) Studies on primary cultures of adult lens cells from normal and hereditary cataractous mice. *Exp. Eye Res.*, **26**, 671–685

TULLOH, C.G. (1955) Heredity of posterior polar cataract with report of a pedigree. *Br. J. Ophthalmol.*, **39**, 374–379

TUPPER, B., MILLER, D. and MILLER, R. (1985) The effect of 55 nm cut off filter on the vision of cataract patients. *Ann. Ophthalmol.*, **17**, 67–72

UGA, S., KADOR, P.F. and KUWABARA, T. (1980) Cytological study of Philly mouse cataract. *Exp. Eye Res.*, **30**, 79–92

UNAKAR, N.J., TSUI, J.Y., KUCK, J.F. *et al.* (1986) Sodium-potassium-dependent-ATPase activity in Emory mouse lens. *Curr. Eye Res.*, **5**, 263–271

USHER, C.H. (1924) A pedigree of congenital dislocation of lenses. *Biometrika*, **16**, 273–282

VAIL, D. (1966) Travaux d'ophtalmologie modern (dedicated to J. Mauras). Paris, 343–

VALERIO, M. (1963) Les dangers de la cortisonothérapie locale prolongée. *Buli Mem. Soc. Fr. Ophthalmol.*, **76**, 572–580

VALK, L.E.M. and BINKHORST, P.G. (1956) A case of familial dwarfism, with choroideremia, myopia, posterior polar cataract and zonular cataract. *Ophthalmologica*, **132**, 299

VAN CREVELD, S., KOZLOWSKI, K., PIETRON, K. *et al.* (1971) Metaphyseal chondrodysplasia calcificans: a report of two cases. *Br. J. Radiol.*, **44**, 773–779

VAN DEN EIJNDEN-VAN RAAIJ, A.J.M., DE LEEUW, A.L.M. and BROEKHUYSE, R.M. (1985) Bovine lens calmodulin: Isolation, partial characterization and calcium-independent binding to lens membrane proteins. *Curr. Eye Res.*, **4**, 905–912

VAN DEN EIJNDEN-VAN RAAIJ, A.J.M., FREIJEN, A. and SNOEK, G.T. (1987) EDTA-extractable proteins from calf lens fibre membranes are phosphorylated by Ca^{2+}-phospholipid-dependent protein kinase. *Exp. Eye Res.*, **45**, 215–225

VAN DEN EIJNDEN-VAN RAAIJ, A.J.M., DE LEEUW, A.L.M. and BROEKHUYSE, R.M. (1985) Bovine lens calmodulin. Isolation, partial characterization and calcium-independent binding to lens membrane proteins. *Curr. Eye Res.*, **4**, 905–912

VAN DEN EIJNDEN-VAN RAAIJ, A.J.M., FREIJEN, A. and SNOEK, G.T. (1987) EDTA-extractable proteins from calf lens fibre membranes are phosphorylated by Ca2+-phospholipid-dependent protein kinase. *Exp. Eye Res.*, **45**, 215–225

VAN DORP, D.B. and DELLEMAN, J.W. (1979) A family with X-chromosomal recessive congenital cataract, microphthalmia, a peculiar form of the ear and dental anomalies. *J. Pediatr. Ophthalmol. Strabismus*, **16**, 166–171

VAN HEYNINGEN, R. (1959a) Formation of polyols by the lens of the rat with 'sugar' cataract. *Nature*, **184**, 194–195

VAN HEYNINGEN, R. (1959b) Metabolism of xylose by the lens. 2: Rat lens *in vivo* and *in vitro*. *Biochem. J.*, **73**, 197–207

VAN HEYNINGEN, R. (1962a) The sorbitol pathway in the lens. *Exp. Eye Res.*, **1**, 396

VAN HEYNINGEN, R. (1962b) The lens. In *The Eye* (ed. H.

Davson), Academic Press, New York, 213–287

VAN HEYNINGEN, R. (1963) Changes in weight and adenosine triphosphate content in the lens of the xyolse-fed rat. *Exp. Eye Res.*, **2**, 362

VAN HEYNINGEN, R. (1969a) The lens: metabolism and cataract. In *The Eye* (ed. H. Davson), 2nd edn, Academic Press, New York, 381–488

VAN HEYNINGEN, R. (1969b) The metabolism of D-glyceraldehyde by the lens. *Biochem. J.*, **112**, 211–220

VAN HEYNINGEN, R. (1972) The human lens. II: Some observations on cataracts removed in Oxford, England. *Exp. Eye Res.*, **13**, 148–154

VAN HEYNINGEN, R. (1976) Experimental studies on cataract: Proctor lecture. *Exp. Eye Res.*, **15**, 685

VAN HEYNINGEN, R. (1977) The biochemistry of the lens – selected topics. In *Scientific Foundations of Ophthalmology*, (eds E.S. Perkins and D.W. Hill), Heinemann, London, 44

VAN HEYNINGEN, R. and HARDING, J.J. (1972) Some changes in the lens of the dimethyl sulphoxide fed rabbit. *Exp. Eye Res.*, **14**, 91–98

VAN HEYNINGEN, R. and HARDING, J.J. (1986) Risk factors for cataract: diabetes, myopia and sex. In *Modern Trends in Aging Research*, (eds Y. Courtois, D. Forette and D. Knook)

VAN HEYNINGEN, R. and HARDING, J.J. (1988) A case-control study of cataract in Oxfordshire: some risk factors. *Br. J. Ophthalmol.*, **72**, 804–808

VAN HEYNINGEN, R. and LINKLATER, J. (1975) The metabolism of the bovine lens in air and nitrogen. *Exp. Eye Res.*, **20**, 393–396

VAN HEYNINGEN, R. and LINKLATER, J. (1976) Metabolism of ^{14}C palmitic acid by lens. *Invest. Ophthalmol.*, **15**, 427–443

VAN LEEN, R.W., VAN ROOZENDAAL, K.E.P., LUBSEN, N.H. and SCHOENMAKERS, J.G.G. (1987) Differential expression of crystallin genes during development of the rat eye lens. *Dev. Biol.*, **120**, 457–464

VANNAS, A. (1969) Fluorescein angiography of the vessels of the iris in pseudoexfoliation of the lens capsule, capsular glaucoma and some other forms of glaucoma. *Acta. Ophthalmol.*, Suppl. **105**, 9–75

VARMA, S.D., KUMAR, S. and RICHARDS, R.D. (1979) Light-induced damage to ocular lens cation pump: prevention by vitamin C. *Proc. Natl. Acad. Sci. USA*, **76**, 3504–3506

VARNUM, D.S. and STEVENS, L.C. (1968) Aphaki a new mutation in the mouse. *J. Hered.*, **59**, 147–150

VERREY, F. (1957) Uber Cataracta congenita. *Ophthalmologica*, **133**, 302

VINDING, T. and NEILSON, N.V. (1984) Two cases of acutely developed cataract in diabetes mellitus. *Acta Ophthalmol.*, **62**, 373–377

VOGT, A. (1921) *Atlas of Slit-Lamp Microscopy of the Living Eye*, Springer-Verlag, Berlin

VOGT, A. (1922) Atlas der Spaltlampenmikroskopie des lebenden Auges mit Anleitung zur Technik und Methodik der Untersuchung. (Julius Springer, 1921). *Graefes Arch. Ophthalmol.*, **107**, 196

VOGT, A. (1930) Neve von Linskap selglaukom. *Klin. Monatsbl. Augenheilk.*, **84**, 1–2

VOGT, A. (1931) Lehrbuch und Atlas der Spaltlampenmikroskopie des lebenden Auges (Linse und Zonula); 2nd ed. Springer-Verlag, Berlin

VOGT, A. and LÜSSI, U. (1919) Weitere Untersuchungen über das Relief der menschlichen Linsen kernoberflache. *A von Graefes Arch. Ophthalmol.*, **100**, 157–167

VON PFLUGK, A. (1909) Die Fixierung der Wirbeltierlinsen insbesondere der Linse des neugeborenen Menschen. *Klin. Monatsbl. Augenheilk.*, **47**, 1–14

VON SALLMANN, L. (1950a) Report on studies on the effect of X-ray irradiation on the rabbits lens. NYO-1508, *USAEC Report*,

VON SALLMANN, L. (1950b) Experimental studies on early lens changes after roentgen irradiation. *Trans. Am. Ophthalmol. Soc.*, **48**, 228–242

VON SALLMANN, L. (1957) The lens epithelium in the pathogenesis of cataract. *Am. J. Ophthalmol.*, **44**, 1598–1670

VON SALLMANN, L. (1959) Early lenticular lesions resulting from ionizing radiation. *Trans. Am. Acad. Ophthalmol. Otolaryngol.*, **63**, 439–448

VON SALLMANN, L. (1965) Cytologic studies on lens epithelium: A comparison of effects of X-rays, Myleran and TEM. *Invest. Ophthalmol.*, **4**, 471–479

VON SALLMANN, L., CARAVAGGIO, L., MUNOZ, C.M. *et al.* (1957) Species differences in the radiosensitivity of the lens. *Am. J. Ophthalmol.*, **43**, 693–704

VON SALLMANN, L. and GRIMES, P. (1966) The effect of triethylene melamine on DNA synthesis and mitosis in the lens epithelium. *Doc. Ophthalmol.*, **20**, 1–12

VON SALLMANN, L., GRIMES, P. and COLLINS, E. (1959) Mimosine cataract. *Am. J. Ophthalmol.*, **47**, 107–117

VON SALLMANN, L., GRIMES, P. and COLLINS, E. (1963) Triparanol-induced cataract in rats. *Arch. Ophthalmol.*, **70**, 522

VON SALLMANN, L. and MUNOZ, C.M. (1951) Experimental studies on early lens changes after roentgen irradiation. I: Morphological and cytochemical changes. *Arch. Ophthalmol.*, **45**, 149–164

VON SALLMANN, L., MUNOZ, C.M. and DRUNGIS, A. (1953) Effects of beta irradiation on the rabbit lens. *Arch. Ophthalmol.*, **50**, 727–736

VOORTER, C.E.M., MULDERS, J.W.M., BLOEMENDAL, H. *et al.* (1986) Some aspects of the phosphorylation of a-crystallin A. *Immunol. Rev.*, **160**, 203–210

VRENSEN, G. and WILLEKENS, B. (1988) Conservation mechanisms in cataractous human lenses: Ultrastructural aspects. *Ophthalmic Res.*, **20**, 84–84

VRENSEN, G. and WILLEKENS, B. (1990) Biomicroscopy and scanning electron microscopy of early opacities in the ageing human lens. *Invest. Ophthalmol. Vis. Sci.*, **31**, 1582–1591

VRENSEN, G., KAPPELHOF, J. and WILLEKENS, B. (1990a)

Morphology of the aging human lens II ultrastructure of clear lens. *Lens Eye Toxic. Res.*, **7**, 1–30

VRENSEN, G., VAN MARLE, J., WILLEKENS, B. and VAN VEEN, H. (1990b) Square arrays in early cortical lens opacities. *Invest. Ophthalmol. Vis. Sci.*, **31**, 2476–2481

VRENSEN, G.F.J.M., WILLEKENS, B., DE JONG, P.T.V.M., SHUN-SHIN, G.A., BROWN, N.A.P. and BRON, A.J. (1994) Heterogeneity in ultrastructure and elemental composition of perinuclear lens retrodots. *Invest. Ophthalmol. Vis. Sci.*, **35**, 199–206

WAARDENBURG, P.J. (1924) Ueber das Erblichkeitsmoment bei der angeborenen Ekotpie der Pupille und der Linse. *Genetica*, **6**, 337–382

WAARDENBURG, P.J. (1949) Gross remants of the pupillary membrane, anterior polar cataract and microcornea in a mother and her children. *Ophthalmologica*, **118**, 828

WAARDENBURG, P.J., FRANCESCHETTI, A. and KLEIN, D. (1961) *Genetics and Ophthalmology*, Charles C Thomas, Springfield ILL, 851–888

WAGNER, B.J., MARGOLIS, J.W., GARLAND, D.L. *et al.* (1986) Bovine lens neutral proteinase preferentially cleaves an oxidatively modified form of glutamine synthetase. ARVO Suppl., *Invest. Ophthalmol. Vis. Sci.*, **27**, 273

WAGNER, H. (1938) Ein bisher unbekanntes erbleiden des auges (Degeneratio hyaloideo retinalis herediteria), beobachtet im Karifon Zurich. Klin. Monatsbl. Augenheilk., **100**, 840–856

WAGNER, F. (1952) Beiderseitiges Linsenkolobom bei Arachnodaktylie (Status dysraphicus). *Klin. Monatsbl. Augenheilk.*, **120**, 640–643

WAGNER, H. (1940) Recessive vererbter angeborener Star. *Klin. Monatsbl. Augenheilk.*, **104**, 337–338

WALLS, G.L. and HEATH, G.G. (1959) Dominant ectopia lentis et pupillae. *Am. J. Hum. Genet.*, **11**, 166–168

WALSH, F.B. and WEGMAN, M.E. (1937) Pedigree of hereditary cataract, illustrating sex-limited type. *Bull. Johns Hopkins Hosp.*, **61**, 125–135

WALSHE, J.M. (1976) The eye in Wilsons disease. *Birth Defects*, **3**, 187

WANG and SPECTOR (1994) The chaperone activity of bovine α-crystallin. *J. Biol. Chem.*, **269**, 13601–13608

WARBURG, M. (1961) Norrie's disease, a new hereditary bilateral pseudotumour of the retina. *Acta Ophthalmol.*, **39**, 757–772

WARBURG, M. (1963) Norrie's disease (atrofia bulborum hereditaria). *Acta Ophthalmol.*, **41**, 134–146

WARBURG, M. (1966) Norrie's disease, a congenital progressive oculo-acoustico-cerebral degeneration. *Acta Ophthalmol. Suppl.*, **89**, 1–147

WARBURG, M. (1970) Focal dermal hypoplasia. Ocular and general manifestations with a survey of the literature. *Acta Ophthalmol.*, **48**, 525–536

WARKANY, J. (1971) *Congenital Malformations: Notes and Comments*, Year Book, Chicago

WATANABE, H. and SHEARER, T.R. (1989) Lens crystallins in aqueous and vitreous humour in selenite overdose cataract. *Curr. Eye Res.*, **8**, 479–486

WATSON, P.G., JAKEMEN, C., OZTURK, M. *et al.* (1990) The complications of trabeculoplasty (a 20-year follow-up). *Eye*, **4**, 425–438

WATZKE, R.C. (1967) Silicone retinopiesis for retinal detachment. A long-term clinical evaluation. *Arch. Ophthalmol.*, **77**, 185–196

WATZKE, R.C., STEVENS, T.S. and CARNEY, R.G. (1976) Retinal vascular changes of incontinentia pigmenti. *Arch. Ophthalmol.*, **94**, 743–746

WEALE, R.A. (1963) *The Aging Eye*. H.K. Lewis, London

WEALE, R.A. (1980) A note on a possible relation between refraction and a disposition for senile cataract. *Br. J. Ophthalmol.*, **64**, 311–314

WEALE, R.A. (1981) Human ocular aging and ambient temperature. *Br. J. Ophthalmol.*, **65**, 869–870

WEALE, R.A. (1982a) On the anatomy of ocular optics. *2nd International Symposium on Visual Optics, Tucson, Arizona*. In press

WEALE, R.A. (1982b) *A Biography of the Eye: Development, Growth, Age*, H. K. Lewis, London

WEALE, R.A. (1983) Senile cataract: The case against light. *Ophthalmology*, **90**, 420–423

WEALE, R.A. (1986) Real light scatter in the human crystalline lens. *A von Graefes Arch. Klin. Exp. Ophthalmol.*, **224**, 463–466

WEALE, R.A. (1987) Senescent vision: Is it all the fault of the lens? *Eye*, **1**, 217–221

WEBER, E. (1940) Weitere Untersuchungen ueber den kongenitalen, vererbten Kernstar (Cataracta nuclearis diffusa congenita hereditaria Vogt). *Schweiz. Med. Wochenschr.*, **70**, 295–297

WEEKERS, R., DELMARCELLE, Y., LUYCKX-BACUS, J. *et al.* (1973) Morphological changes of the lens with age and cataract. In *The Human Lens in Relation to Cataract*, Ciba Found. Symp., **19**, 25–39

WEIDLE, E.G. (1987) Lenticular chrysiasis in oral chrysiotherapy. *Am. J. Ophthalmol.*, **103**, 240–241

WEILL, J.C., LECA, G., VINCENT, A. *et al.* (1980) Messenger RNA for cataractous lens proteins are also present on normal lens polyribosomes. *Eur. J. Biochem.*, **111**, 593–601

WEINGEIST, T.A., HERMSEN, V., HANSON, J.W. *et al.* (1982) Ocular and systemic manifestations of Stickler's syndrome: A preliminary report. *Birth Defects*, **18**, 539–560

WEINSTOCK, M. and STEWART, H.C. (1961) Occurrence in rodents of reversible drug-induced opacities of the lens. *Br. J. Ophthalmol.*, **45**, 408–414

WELEBER, R.G. and KENNAWAY, N.G. (1988) Gyrate atrophy of the choroid and retina. In *Retinitis Pigmentosa* (ed. J.R. Heckenlively), Lippincott, Philadelphia, 198–220

WENDA, L. (1949) La syndrome des sclérotiques bleues. *Arch. Ophthalmol.*, **9**, 44–47

WERNER, O. (1904) Ueber Katarakt in Verbindung mit Sclerodermie. Kiel Diss **1**, 1

WEST, S., MUNOZ, B., EMMETT, E.A. and TAYLOR, H.R. (1989) Cigarette smoking and risk of nuclear cataract. *Arch.*

Ophthalmol., **107**, 1166–1169

WEST, S., ROSENTHAL, F., NEWLAND, H.S. *et al.* (1985) A comparison of methods for typing and grading lens opacities for field surveys. *ARVO Suppl: Invest. Ophthalmol. Vis. Sci.*, **26**, 119

WETTKE-SCHAFER, R. and KANTNER, G. (1983) X-linked dominant inherited diseases with lethality in hemizygous males. *Hum. Genet.*, **64**, 1–23

WHITNALL, S.E. and NORMAN, R.M. (1940) Microphthalmia and the visual pathways. A case associated with blindness and imbecility, and sex-linked *Br. J. Ophthalmol.*, **24**, 229–244

WILLEKENS, B. and VRENSEN, G. (1982) The three dimensional organization of the lens fibers in the rhesus monkey. *Graefes Arch. Klin. Exp. Ophthalmol.*, **219**, 112–120

WILLIAMS, M.R., DUNCAN, G., CROGHAN, P.C. *et al.* (1992) pH regulation in tissue-cultured bovine lens epithelial cells. *J. Membr. Biol.*, **129**, 179–187

WILLIAMS, R.J., MCKEE, A. and FINCH, E.D. (1975) Ultrastructural changes in the rabbit lens induced by microwave radiation. *Ann. NY Acad. Sci.*, **247**, 166–174

WILLIAMSON, A.P., BLATTNER, R.J. and SIMONSEN, L. (1957) Cataracts following mumps virus in early chick embryos. *Proc. Soc. Exp. Biol. Med.*, **96**, 224–228

WILSON, J.G. and FRASER, F.C. (1977) *Handbook of Teratology*, Plenum Press, New York

WILSON, D.K., BOHREN, K.M., GABBAY, K.H. and QUIOCHO, F.A. (1992) An unlikely sugar substrate site in the 1.65 A structure of the human aldose reductase holoenzyme implicated in diabetic complications. *Science*, **257**, 81–84

WINDER, A.F., FELLS, P., JONES, R.B., KISSUN, R.D., MENZIES, I.S. and MOUNT, J.N. (1982) Galactose intolerance and the risk of cataract. *Br. J. Ophthalmol.*, **66**, 438–441

WINDER, A.F., FIELDER, A.R., MOUNT, J.N. and MENZIES, I.S. (1985) Direct and maternal aspects of the risk of cataract with partial disorders of galactose metabolism. *Clin. Genet.*, **28**, 199–206

WINKLER, B.S. (1987) In vitro oxidation of ascorbic acid and its prevention by GSH. *Biochim. Biophys. Acta.*, **925**, 258–264

WINSTANLEY, J. (1961) Iris atrophy in primary glaucoma. *Trans. Ophthalmol. Soc. UK*, **81**, 23–38

WINTROBE, M.M., BUSCHKE, W., FOLLIS, R.H. *et al.* (1944) Riboflavin deficiency in swine. *Johns Hopkins Hosp. Bull.*, **75**, 102–114

WISE, P.H., WEIR, B.J., HIME, J.M. *et al.* (1968) Implications of hyperglycaemia and cataract in a colony of Tuco-Tuco (*Ctenomys talarum*). *Nature*, **219**, 1374–1376

WISTOW, G. and PIATIGORSKY, J. (1987) Recruitment of enzymes as lens structural proteins. *Science*, **236**, 1554–1556

WISTOW, G.J. and PIATIGORSKY, J. (1988) Lens crystallins: the evolution and expression of proteins for a highly specialized tissue. *Immunol. Rev.*, **57**, 479–504

WITKOP-OOSTENRIJK, G.A. (1956) Microphthalmus, Microcornea en aageboren Cataract. *Ned. Tijdschr. Geneeskd.*, **100**, 2910–2913

WOINOW, M. (1974) Ueber die Brechungscoefficienten der verschiedenen Linsenschichten. *Klin. Monatsbl. Augenheilk.*, **12**, 407–408

WOLFF, S.P., WANG, G.M. and SPECTOR, A. (1987) Pro-oxidant activation of ocular reductants. 1: Copper and riboflavin stimulate ascorbate oxidation causing lens epithelial cytotoxicity *in vitro*. *Exp. Eye Res.*, **45**, 777–789

WOLOSIN, J.M., ALVAREZ, L.J. and CANDIA, O.A. (1988) Cellular pH and Na^+–H^+ exchange activity in lens epithelium of *Bufo marinus* toad. *Am. J. Physiol.*, **255**, C595–C602

WOOD, D.C., SWEET, D., VAN DOLAH, J. *et al.* (1967) A study of DMSO and steroids in rabbit eyes. *Ann. NY Acad. Sci.*, **141**, 346–380

WORGUL, B.V. (1992) Lens. (Chapter 15); in *The Biomedical Foundations of Ophthalmology*, (eds T.D. Duane and E.A. Jaeger). Harper and Row, Philadelphia; 1–35

WORGUL, B.V. and ROTHSTEIN, H. (1975) Congenital cataracts associated with disorganized meridional rows in a new laboratory animal: The degu (*Octodon degus*). **23**, 1–4

WORGUL, B.V., BITO, L.Z. and MERRIMAN, G.R. (1977) Intraocular inflammation produced by X-irradiation of the rabbit eye. *Exp. Eye Res.*, **25**, 53–61

YAKELY, W.L. (1978) A study of heritability of cataracts in the American cocker spaniel. *J. Am. Vet. Med. Assoc.*, **172**, 814–817

YAKELY, W.L., HEGREBERG, G.A. and PADGETT, G.A. (1971) Familial cataracts in the American cocker spaniel. *Vet. Med. Small Anim. Clin.*, **7**, 127–135

YAMAGUCHI, H., OKUBO, Y. and TANAKA, M. (1972) A note on possible close linkage between the Ii blood locus and a congenital cataract locus. *Proc. Jpn. Acad.*, **48**, 625–628

YAMAMOTO, Y., HAYASAKA, S. and SETOGAWA, T. (1988) Family with amoidia microcornea, and spontaneously reabsorbed cataract. *Arch. Ophthalmol.*, **106**, 502–505

YANOFF, M. (1988) Intraocular pressure in exfoliation syndrome. *Acta. Ophthalmol.*, Suppl. **184**, 59–61

YANOFF, M. (1975) Pathology of cataract. In *Cataract and Abnormalities of the Lens* (ed. J.G. Bellows), Grune & Stratton, New York, 155–190

YANOFF, M. and FINE, S.B. (1989) *Ocular Pathology. A Text and Atlas*. 3rd edn, Lippincott, Philadelphia

YANOFF, M., FINE, B.S. and SCHAFFER, D.B. (1973) Histopathology of transient neonatal lens vacuoles: A light and electron microscopy study. *Am. J. Ophthalmol.*, **76**, 363–370

YEH, S., SCHOLZ, D.L., LIOU, W. *et al.* (1986) Polygonal arrays of actin filaments in human lens epithelial cells. *Invest. Ophthalmol. Vis. Sci.*, **27**, 1535–1540

YOON, S.-H., SKALKA, H. and PRCHAL, J.T. (1989) Presence of erythroid and non-erythroid spectrin transcripts in human lens and cerebellum. *Invest. Ophthalmol. Vis. Sci.*, **30**, 1860–1866

YORIO, T. and BENTLEY, P.J. (1976) The effects of hyperosmotic agents on the electrical properties of the amphibian lens in vitro. *Exp. Eye Res.*, **22**, 195–208

YOSHIOKA, H., TESHIMA, T. and ENDO, Y. (1965) *Acta Soc. Ophthalmol. Jpn.*, **69**, 545

YOUNG, R.W. (1991) *Age-Related Cataract*. Oxford University Press, Oxford

YOUNG, R.W. and OCUMPAUGH, D.E. (1966) Autoradiographic studies on the growth and development of the lens capsule in the rat. *Invest. Ophthalmol.*, **5**, 583–593

ZAMPIGHI, G.A., HALL, J.E., EHRING, G.R. *et al.* (1989) The structural organization and protein composition of lens fiber junctions. *J. Cell. Biol.*, **108**, 2255–2275

ZAMPIGHI, G.A., HALL, J.E. and KREMAN, M. (1985) Purified lens junctional protein forms channels in planar lipid films. *Proc. Natl. Acad. Sci. USA*, **82**, 8468–8472

ZEIMER, R.C. and NOTH, R.M. (1984) A new method of measuring in vivo the lens transmittance, and study of lens scatter, fluorescence and transmittance. *Ophthalmic Res.*, **16**, 246–255

ZEITER, H.J. (1963) Congenital microphthalmus. A pedigree of four affected siblings and an additional report of 44 sporadic cases. *Am. J. Ophthalmol.*, **55**, 910–922

ZELENKA, P.S. (1980) Changes in phosphatidylinositol metabolism during differentiation of lens epithelial cells into lens fiber cells in the embryonic chick. *J. Biol. Chem.*, **255**, 1296–1300

ZELENKA, P.S. (1984) Lens lipids. *Curr. Eye Res.*, **3**, 1337–1359

ZELLWEGER, H. (1987) The cerebro-hepato-renal syndrome and other peroxisomal disorders. *Dev. Med. Child. Neurol.*, **29**, 821–829

ZIGLER, J.S. and HESS, H.H. (1985) Cataracts in the Royal College of Surgeons rat: evidence for initiation by lipid peroxidation products. *Exp. Eye Res.*, **41**, 67–76

ZIGLER, J. and LUCAS, V.A. (1986) Oxidative stress and the cultured rhesus monkey lens [abstract]. ARVO Suppl: *Invest. Ophthalmol. Vis. Sci.*, **27**, 7

ZIGLER, J.S., CARPER, D.A. and KINOSHITA, J.H. (1981) Changes in lens crystallins during cataract development in the Philly mouse. *Ophthalmic Res.*, **13**, 237–251

ZIGMAN, S. and VAUGHAN, T. (1974) Near-ultraviolet light effects on the lenses and retinas of mice. *Invest. Ophthalmol.*, **13**, 462–465

ZIGMAN, S., YULO, T. and SCHULTZ, J. (1974) Cataract induction in mice exposed to near ultraviolet light. *Ophthalmic Res.*, **6**, 259–270

ZOUZIAS, D. and MANSKI, W. (1972) II: Immunochemical studies on alpha crystallin subunits. *Exp. Eye Res.*, **13**, 205–218

ZUCLICH, J.A. and CONNOLLY, J.S. (1976) Ocular damage induced by near-ultraviolet laser radiation. *Invest. Ophthalmol.*, **15**, 760–764

ZWAAN, J. and WILLIAMS, R.M. (1969) Cataracts and abnormal proliferation of the lens epithelium in mice carrying the cat Fr gene. *Exp. Eye Res.*, **8**, 161–167

Index